POTTER'S
HERBAL
CYCLOPAEDIA

Potter's New Cyclopaedia of Botanical Drugs & Preparations
was first published in 1907 and subsequently reprinted in revised editions in
1915, 1923, 1932, 1939, 1950, 1956, 1968, 1970, 1971, 1973, 1980, 1982 &
1985. It was then rewritten in 1989 and reprinted in 1989, 1994 & 1998.

This totally revised, enlarged and rewritten edition was first published in 2003
to coincide with the 190th birthday of Potter's Herbal Medicine
and their 50th year in Wigan.

Published in the United Kingdom by
The C.W. Daniel Company Limited
1 Church Path, Saffron Walden,
Essex CB10 1JP

ISBN 0 85207 361 5

Production in association with
Book Production Consultants plc,
25–27 High Street, Chesterton Cambridge CB4 1ND
Designed by Marion Hughston
Printed and bound in Britain by the
Cromwell Press, Trowbridge, Wiltshire.

POTTER'S HERBAL CYCLOPAEDIA

The Authoritative Reference work on Plants with a Known Medical Use

By Elizabeth M. Williamson BSc., PhD, MRPharmS., FLS

based on a work by R.C. Wren

Index compiled by Ann Griffiths

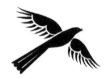

SAFFRON WALDEN

THE C.W. DANIEL COMPANY LIMITED

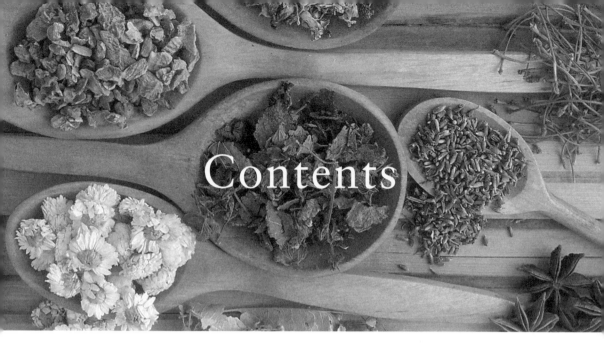

Contents

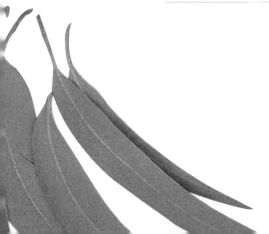

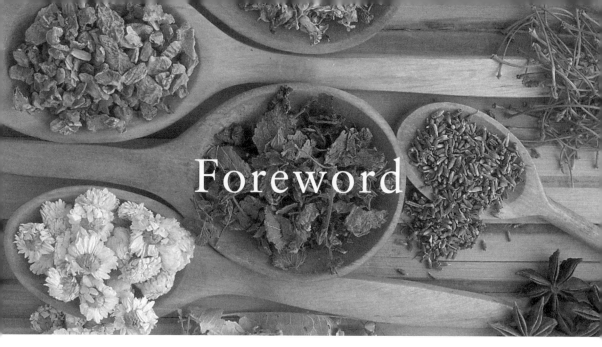

Foreword

H umans have always employed plants in a multitude of ways, in a tradition spanning all their evolution. The selection of medicinal plants is a conscious process by indigenous peoples, which has led to an enormous number of medicinal plants being used by all cultures of the world. At least 10–20 % of all species of higher plants (i.e. 25,000 to 50,000 species) are thought to have some sort of medicinal usage. The earliest documented record, which relates to medicinal plants, dated from around 60,000 BC, was found in the grave of a Neanderthal man in Shanidar IV, an archaeological site in Iraq. Pollen from six species of plants, which were presumably employed as medicines or in rituals, was discovered and identified:

- *Achillea* sp. (yarrow, Asteraceae),
- *Althea* sp. (mallow, Malvaceae),
- *Centaurea solstitialis* L. (knapweed, Asteraceae),
- *Ephedra altissima* (ephedra, Ephedraceae)
- *Muscari* sp. (grape hyacinth, Hyacinthaceae)
- *Senecio* sp. (ragwort/groundsel, Asteraceae)*.

*Leroi-Gourhan, A (1975) 'Flowers found with Shanidar IV, a Neanderthal burial in Iraq'. Science 190: 562–564, and Heinrich M, Pieroni A and Bremner P (2003). 'Medicinal Plants and Phytomedicines'. In: The Cultural History of Plants. Arcadia Publ. (Editorial Advisor: Sir Ghillean Prance).

These plants were presumably of major cultural importance to the people of Shanidar, although these reports have been criticised because pollen does not usually survive well in the Middle East, and there is good evidence that ants often hoard pollen in a similar context **. So although this may be a finding with no direct bearing on the Neanderthal culture of Shanidar, the species are still used in Iraq and elsewhere, and it may equally be the first record of their tradition in existence.

Of these six genera, *five* figure prominently in the latest edition of *Potter's Cyclopedia* (the only exception being grape hyacinth) and this testifies to the long tradition certain plants have as medicines. Summarizing the scientific information about the most important and widely used 630 botanical drugs is a tremendous task and Liz Williamson has done an excellent job not only in updating monographs included in earlier editions, but also by adding a further 70 plants. Data on the botany and general biology, pharmaceutical usage, pharmacology, regulatory status and, if available, clinical studies have been included.

The first edition of 'Potters' was published in 1907 thus the nine editions of this established handbook span over 95 years of development in the field of medicinal plant research and usage. Colleagues in the field of Pharmacognosy and Phytotherapy of the School of Pharmacy, University of London, have been closely associated with this publication for several decades. I am therefore even more delighted to see this tradition continued, and to see a new version after a gap of nearly 15 years since the publication of the previous edition. Who would spend so much time and effort on such a monumental undertaking? It takes a Yorkshire woman with an enormous dedication to the subject, as well as an interest in the applied side of pharmacy, to attempt such a task!

The discipline of pharmacognosy had been central both to research and teaching in pharmacy until the last century. However, in the 1970s and 80s, more and more schools of pharmacy gave up our oldest sub-discipline, only to find that, if pharmacists do not see themselves as

** Sommer J D (1999) 'The Shanidar IV flower burial': a re-evaluation of Neanderthal burial ritual. *Cambridge Archaeological Journal* 9(1):127.

specialists in medicinal plants, patients and the population in general will turn to other (and often much less reliable) sources. This popular demand for something 'natural' has led to increased medical and pharmaceutical attention to 'alternative' and 'complementary' therapies. Medicinal plants have always been a central part of our arsenal for curing diseases and many botanical drugs are available as high-quality phytomedicines. The scientific basis clearly distinguishes such medicines from 'alternative and complementary' forms of treatment. The emphasis on quality, efficacy and safety is at the core of the science-based study of medicinal plants. Recent developments in the field of pharmacognosy have seen a significant upsurge of scientific interest and engagement in this discipline. Many patients wish to use plant-based (natural) medicines, which have been well studied, and they expect and obtain health benefits from them. New plants (and new uses for well-known ones) are being discovered, as simultaneously there is an increased use of remedies from African, Ayurvedic and Traditional Chinese herbal medicine. This changing picture shows that the use of botanical medicines evolves, rather than remaining based only on historical use, a fact recognized by the inclusion in this book of a significant number of plants originating from other medical systems. This ninth edition will surely help practising community pharmacists to serve their patients in the best way possible.

All health professions require a concise, up-to-date and science-based overview of the most important medicinal plants used in Europe and North America. Dr Williamson has taken on this challenging task and has – surely with many hard spells in between – completed this excellent overview useful to herbalists, pharmacists, nurses, medical doctors and lay people interested in the scientific background of phytotherapy and medicinal plant use.

Prof. Dr Michael Heinrich
Centre for Pharmacognosy and Phytotherapy
The School of Pharmacy, Univ. London,
Email: phyto@ams1.ulsop.ac.uk

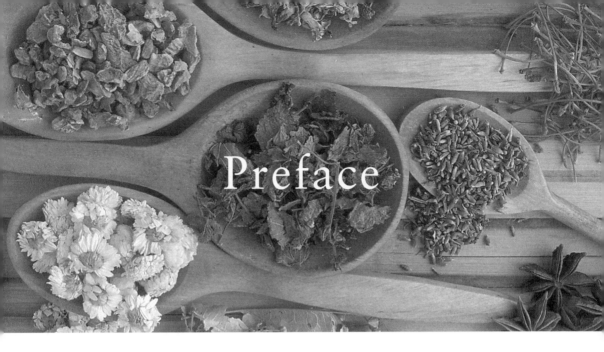

Preface

'If we built enough factories to produce enough aspirin to treat everyone in the world with a headache, the smoke from the chimneys would destroy the ozone layer completely'
O Akerele, World Health Organization, Geneva, Switzerland, 1994.

There is an increasing use of plant medicines, herbs and their extracts throughout Europe and America, but it must be remembered that, for the majority of people in the world, medicinal plants are the main source of medicines. They are used as phytomedicines, and also as isolated ingredients in conventional drugs, and new substances, for example taxol from Yew tree bark, *Taxus baccata*, and irinotecan from *Camptotheca acuminata*, continue to be introduced. As well as European medical herbalism, the popularity of ancient Asian holistic medical systems such as Traditional Chinese Medicine (TCM) and Ayurveda is also rising. It is therefore important that reliable information regarding all of these should be available for patients, healthcare professionals (herbalists, general physicians, pharmacists, nurses) and scientists. *Potter's Herbal Cyclopaedia* (formerly 'Potter's New Cyclopaedia of Botanical Drugs and Preparations') brings together as much information as is currently available from the scattered scientific literature and provides a concise account of the general characters of over 620 herbs, together with a summary of the actions and uses. Each is referenced so that the reader may refer to the original source. The monographs are not intended to be entirely consistent in length or detail, since many have been adequately covered elsewhere (see Review Reference list), and also the amount of information actually available for each varies widely. For some herbs this book provides the only readily available information. With its continuing popularity as a book of reference, 'Potter's' covers over 100 years of British herbal history, and in this edition I have retained many of the features of the early editions. These include the Biblical References, for which thanks are due to Timothy Whittaker, and quotes from the herbalists and philosophers of the past.

The very first edition of the Cyclopaedia was written by Richard Cranfield Wren, FLS. Wren was an acknowledged authority on the cultivation, identification and preparation of herbal drugs, and was deeply concerned with the botanical authentication of the various species used in medicine and as home remedies at the time. In the second edition, published in 1915, he collaborated with E M Holmes, FLS., who was curator of the Pharmaceutical Society Museum, to produce an updated version of the botanical aspects of the first edition. A third edition, in 1923, contained 200 line drawings reproduced from Bentham's *Handbook of the British Flora.* The fourth edition was published in 1932, written by R W Wren, FLS., MPS (the son of R C Wren), in conjunction with H A Potter, Ph.C. A further revision was undertaken in 1956, for the seventh edition, where Wren attempted to give a more philosophical background to herbal medicine. Reference was made not only to the herbalists of antiquity such as Paracelsus, Galen, Dioscorides, Pliny and Theophrastos, but also to English herbalists including John Gerard, Nicholas Culpeper and others, and biblical references to herbs were included. This historical aspect has been kept, and further added to by Timothy Whittaker, the chief chemist at Potter's Herbal Medicines.

Henry Potter trained as a pharmacist at the School of Pharmacy, University of London, where he was a contemporary of Jesse Boot. The

School was attached at that time to the Pharmaceutical Society of Great

Britain, providing the link with E M Holmes. Potters have always looked to scientific research to improve the quality control of their products and knowledge of their effects, and were instrumental in setting up the British Herbal Medicine Association (BHMA). They also took the decision to apply for product licences, so that herbal medicines could be prescribed on the NHS, and this is still the case. The BHMA had appointed a scientific committee, even before the advent of any regulatory control, to produce the British Herbal Pharmacopoeia, to help ensure quality of the raw materials. Dr Elizabeth Williamson and Professor Fred Evans, of the School of Pharmacy (who were members of this committee at the time), then produced a revised edition of the Cyclopaedia in 1988, continuing the collaboration between the School and Potter's.

This edition took the important step of including chemical constituents and pharmacological and clinical data, together with references to the medical and scientific literature. Scientific data is of variable quality and it is often necessary to see the original paper to validate (or repudiate) claims made. This approach continues and, although every effort has been made to select good experimental evidence, sometimes it is necessary to put in what is available rather than what is desirable! In some instances, the regulatory status of the herb (in the UK) has been included. For example, controlled drugs (CD; controlled by the Misuse of Drugs Act); prescription only medicine (POM); Pharmacy medicines (P), available only through a registered Pharmacy; and general sales list (GSL; comprising drugs available for sale to the general public). For many drugs there is no regulatory status, and they are not under legal control. A new piece of legislation, the Traditional Use Directive, will be introduced shortly and will help to put on a legitimate footing those herbs which have been in use for at least 30 years. These plants are referenced in the Cyclopaedia to the 1956 edition of Potter's [R1] as an indication of historical use. Some preparations and their dosages are given but often are not, since they may not be clear, or self-medication may not be appropriate. The book is not intended to be a handbook for treatment or to replace the expertise of the medical herbalist, physician or pharmacist, but it is hoped that it will be the initial reference point when wanting to know about a particular plant. Although expanded, it is unfortunately still not possible to include all of the medicinal plants used throughout the world. I hope readers will forgive any glaring omissions as well as any errors, which are unavoidable in a volume containing so many plants and despite the meticulous checking of Timothy Whittaker. I hope to increase the number of entries still further for the next edition; many of the additions are either newer introductions to the West, or are very important in TCM and Ayurveda. None of the original entries has been removed although some may be more of historical than current interest. Inclusion in this book is not an endorsement as modern safety concerns have meant that some herbs are no longer considered suitable for human use.

I am as always indebted to Potter's for allowing me complete academic freedom as before, and for all their help: to Tony Hampson for support in so many ways, and to Timothy Whittaker for advice on modern herbal use and careful checking of the manuscript. Mr Harry Hall (see Introduction) unfortunately passed away before the new revision was started, and I hope he would have approved the new expanded version. Due to the retirement of Professor Fred Evans I have continued the new revision alone, along the lines we set previously, although we have now changed the title to *Potter's Herbal Cyclopaedia* to reflect the content more accurately. This edition is dedicated particularly to Fred, as well as all those with a belief in the power of plants and their preparations to correct human disease conditions in a natural manner.

Elizabeth M Williamson
Centre for Pharmacognosy and Phytotherapy
The School of Pharmacy, University of London.

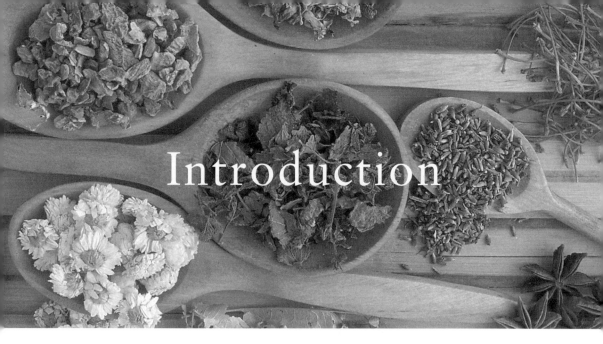

Introduction

O ne of the first things to strike the reader of this edition of the Cyclopaedia is the proliferation of scientific literature references available about herbs today.

After only a brief scan, it is apparent just how extensive the research work has been, and especially how many papers have been written since the last edition fourteen years ago. This explosion of investigative work opens up new lines of enquiry into how a herb is extracted to best advantage, and where the analytical laboratory needs to be looking in its quest for improved control methods, all of which in due course, lead to better quality herbal medicines that can be used with confidence.

For the help it gives in this area, I really welcome this new edition. More than ever, the consumer wants confidence in his purchases, and a reliability, that will bring him back to the use of a herbal medicine next time too. All over the world this volume will help those who develop new and improved formulations of herbs to do their best for the user, as it helps me.

It has been both a pleasure and a privilege to be involved in this work.

Timothy J. Whittaker B.Sc(Pharm), FIRCH
Chief Chemist: October 2002

INTRODUCTION TO THE 1988 EDITION BY (THE LATE) HARRY HALL, MPS

Former Technical Director, Potter's Herbal Medicines.

The plant kingdom has been mankind's main source of medicine since prehistoric times. So that in 1812 when Henry Potter first set up his business in Farringdon Street, London, as a Supplier of Herbs and Dealer in Leeches, there already existed a vast store of knowledge which had been passed down through the centuries. Much of this traditional information on the medicinal virtues of herbs has been documented in the ancient mediaeval Herbals, not only from Britain but also from the Americas, the Middle East, India and Asia.

Henry Potter first saw his herbal business expand in leaps and bounds. When in 1846 it passed to his nephew Henry Potter 2nd and his son, Henry Potter 3rd, the solid foundation for a business had been established. 'Potter's' was set to become Europe's leading manufacturer of herbal remedies. Henry Potter 3rd had one son, Henry Arthur, who had qualified as a pharmacist and, in 1896, had become a partner in the firm. In the same year his future colleague, R C Wren, FLS, who was then general manager, also became a partner. The special talents which the two brought to the business, which had now become known as Potter & Clarke Limited, led to the rapid development of the company as manufacturing chemists and druggists, specializing in the extraction of crude drugs for the herbal and pharmaceutical industry, and for the well-known range of Potter's proprietary herbal remedies.

R C Wren was particularly interested in the study of medicinal plants and, as the herbal business increased, he saw that there was an urgent need for a reference work, which would serve as a complete guide for all those who used or handled botanical drugs. This was to include common and botanical titles, synonyms and therapeutic actions, with preparations and dosage. Under the title 'Potter's Cyclopaedia of Botanical Drugs and Preparations as compiled by R C Wren', the first edition of the modern Herbal appeared in 1907.

After reorganisation in 1952, Potter's became known as Potter's (Herbal Supplies) Limited. They had then moved to their new location in Wigan, Lancashire, where the production of modern licensed herbal remedies has continued with renewed vigour. As with all other medicines, the latest and most sophisticated scientific techniques have been and continue to be used to control the manufacture and quality of a very comprehensive range of these traditional remedies. To this day, Potter's Herbal Medicines continues its heritage by continuing to make available a full range of safe natural herbal medicines, which comply fully with all modern regulatory and legal requirements. Potter's is a government regulated licensed manufacturer of herbal medicines.

I first came to know Potter's Cyclopaedia in the third edition, published in 1923, when it really became my first textbook. Coming from a herbal background I had decided to consolidate my interest in herbal medicine within a qualification in pharmacy. This was to lead to my joining Potter's as a pharmacist in 1935 where close involvement in the herbal industry often required reference to the Cyclopaedia, then in its later editions. Now, in this edition, there is to be found a very concise and unique combination of the old with the new. The principal constituents of each herb are now given as they have been discovered in research into plant chemistry. Much of this new information on constituents is supportive of the known traditional therapeutic properties of many herbs, so it is particularly gratifying to me to have been associated in some way with Dr F J Evans and Dr Elizabeth Williamson of London University in their re-writing of the Cyclopaedia into this modern state-of-the-art form. This new Potter's Cyclopaedia will prove invaluable to all those concerned with herbal medicine and with the scientific background to traditional herbal usage.

H HALL, M.R.Pharm.S. (1987).

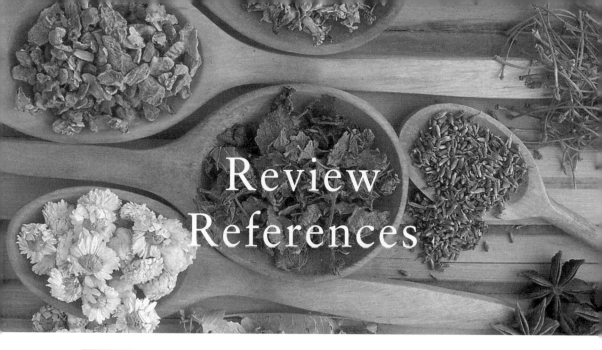

Review References

These are standard works, which are accepted as authoritative references. With the exception of 'R1', all are referenced to primary sources. 'R1' however is significant in that any plant with this annotation has been in use for over 30 years, which has implications for the Traditional Use Directive. This legislation will require evidence of traditional use for regulatory purposes, although at the time of printing it is not yet in force.

R1. Potter's New Cyclopaedia of Botanical Drugs and Preparations. R C Wren. C W Daniels, Saffron Walden 1956.
NB: Inclusion indicates historical usage of > 30 yrs.

R2. Herbal Remedies CD4. Eds Brendler, Gruenwald, Jaenicke. Phytopharm Consulting GmbH, Berlin. Medpharm Scientific Publishers Stuttgart, Germany, 2001

R3. Trease and Evans Textbook of Pharmacognosy. 15th Ed. W C Evans. W B Saunders, UK, 2002

R4. Tachenbuch der Drogenkunde 8th Ed. H Hoppe. De Gruyter, Berlin, Germany,1981

R5. Chinese Drugs of Plant Origin. W Tang and G Eisenberg. Springer-Verlag, Berlin, Germany, 1992

R6. Selected Medicinal Plants of India. Bharatiya Vidya Bhavan's Ayurveda Research Centre. Chemexcil, Bombay, India, 1992

R7. Herbal Medicines. J Barnes, L A Anderson and J D Phillipson (2nd Ed.) Pharmaceutical Press UK, 2002

R8. Rational Phytotherapy. V Schultz, R Hansel and V Tyler. Springer-Verlag, Berlin, Germany,1998

R9. Teedrogen. M Witchl. Medpharm Scientific Publishers Stuttgart, Germany, 1997

R10. The Merck Index, 11th Edn. Ed. S. Budavari. Merck and Co, Inc. USA, 1989

R11. Botanical Influences on Illness. M Werbach and M Murray. Third Line Press, USA, 1994

R12. Medicinal Plants of the World Vol 1. I Ross. Humana Press, Totowa, USA, 1999

R13. Medicinal Plants of the World Vol 2. I Ross. Humana Press, Totowa, USA, 2000

R14. Martindale, The Extra Pharmacopiea 31st Edn. Pharmaceutical Press, UK, 1997

R15. British Herbal Pharmacopoeia, HMSO, UK, 1990

R16. Major Herbs of Ayurveda. The Dabur Research Foundation. Ed. E M Williamson. Churchill Livingstone, Edinburgh, UK, 2002/3.

R17. Principles and Practice of Phytotherapy. S Mills and K Bone. Churchill Livingstone, Edinburgh, UK, 2000

R18. Essential Oil Safety. R Tisserand and T Balacs. Churchill Livingstone, Edinburgh, UK, 1995

R19. Encyclopedia of Common Natural Ingredients used in Food, Drugs and Cosmetics. A Y Leung. Wiley, New York, USA, 1980

R20. Pharmacology and Applications of Chinese Materia Medica Vol. 1. Eds H Chan and P But. World Scientific, Singapore, 1986

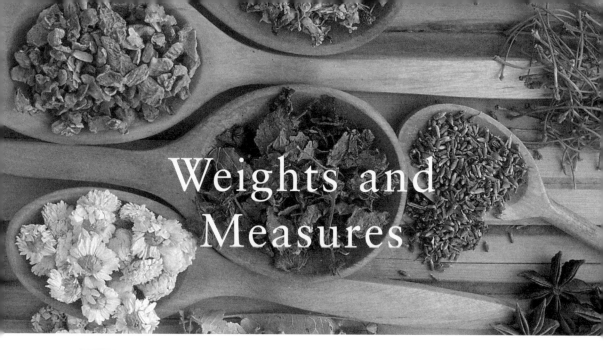

Weights and Measures

Weights and Measures: Conversation Table for Metric and Imperial Weights and Measures with Approximate Domestic Equivalents and Abbreviations.

Imperial:	Metric:	Approximate Domestic Equivalent
1 drachm (60 grains)	3.888 grammes (g)	4 g
1 ounce (oz)	28.3495 g	30 g
1 pound (lb)	453.59 g	500 g, 0.5 kilogrammes (kg)
1 fluid drachm (60 minims)	3.552 millilitres (ml)	4 ml
1 fluid ounce (fl oz)	28.4123 ml	30 ml
1 pint (pt) (20 oz)	0.5682 litres (l)	500 ml, 0.5 l
1 gallon (gal) (8 pt)	4.5459 l	4 l
1 inch (in)	2.54 centimetres (cm)	2.5 cm, 25 millimetres (mm)
1 foot (ft)	30.48 cm	30 cm
1 yard (yd)	0.9144 metres (m)	1 m
	5 ml	1 teaspoonful (tsp)
	10 ml	1 dessertspoonful (dsp)
1/2 fl oz	15 ml	1 tablespoon (tblsp)
1 1/2 fl oz (3–4 tblsp)		1 wineglassful
4–5 fl oz (5–10 tblsp)		1 teacupful

N.B. 10 millimetres = 1 centimetre; 100 centimetres = 1 metre;
1000 millilitres = 1 litre

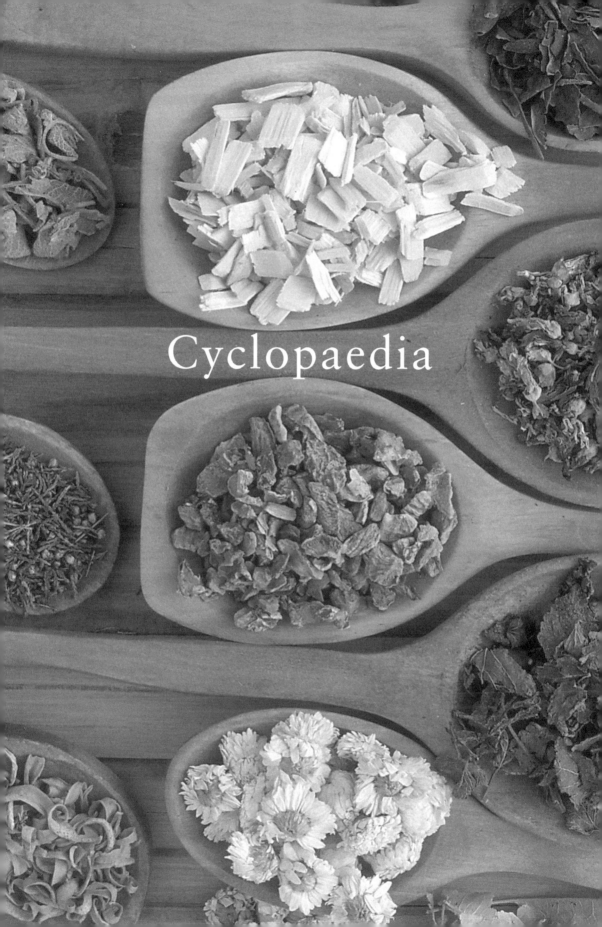

Cyclopaedia

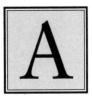

ABELMOSCHUS
ABELMOSCHUS MOSCHATUS MEDIK
Fam. Malvaceae

SYNONYMS: Ambrette Seed, Muskseed, *Hibiscus abelmoschus* L. *Bamia abelmoschus* R. Br.

HABITAT: The plant is indigenous to Africa, India, Java and South America and is widely cultivated in tropical regions.

DESCRIPTION: An annual or biennial herb with large, bright yellow flowers with crimson centres and bristly hairs. The seeds are kidney-shaped, compressed, about 3 mm in diameter, with numerous striations concentric about the hilum, contained in a pyramid-shaped capsule. They are greyish-brown with a musky odour and oily taste.

PART USED: Seeds.

CONSTITUENTS: (i) Volatile oil, containing farnesyl acetate, ambrettolide (a macrocyclic lactone, hexadec-7-en-16-olide), ambrettolic acid and related compounds (ii) Sterols including beta-sitosterol and its glucoside (iii) Fixed oil composed of esters of palmitic, linoleic and stearic acids (iv) Mucilage [R2,R19;1,2,3].

MEDICINAL USE: Traditionally used in Africa for snakebite, as an antispasmodic in digestive complaints and in Chinese medicine for headache. It is more often used as a flavouring or fragrance ingredient.

SPECIFIC REFERENCES: 1. Maurer B *et al* (1977) *Helv. Chim. Acta* 60:1155. 2. Srivastava K *et al* (1969) *Planta Med.* 17:189. 3. Opdyke D (1975) *Food Cosmet. Toxicol.* 13:705 and 707.

ABRUS PRECATORIUS
ABRUS PRECATORIUS L.
Fam. Fabaceae

SYNONYMS: Indian Liquorice, Wild Liquorice, Jequirity, Prayer Beads, Crab's Eyes.

HABITAT: India, South America, West Africa.

DESCRIPTION: Seeds oval, rounded at the ends, about 3 mm diameter, hard and polished, vermilion red with the upper third black; very hard and tough.

PART USED: Seeds, leaves, roots.

CONSTITUENTS: Seeds: (i) Proteins; toxalbumins known as abrins I, II and III, and agglutinins APA I and II [1] (ii) Alkaloids and amines; precatorine, trigonelline, abrine, *N*-methyltryptamine, *N*-methyltryptophan and hypaphorine [2] (iii) Triterpenes including the Abrus saponins I and II, abrisapogenol, abricin, abrusgenic acid, campesterol and others [3,4] (iv) Flavonoids and anthocyanins; abrectorin, precatorins I, II and III, xyloglucosyldelphinidin and others [4,5,6]. Roots and aerial parts: (i) Quinones known as abruquinones A-G, in the root [R12,R16] (ii) Isoflavonoids including abrusalactone (iii) Triterpenes including abrusosides A-E, abrusgenic acid in the aerial parts, and the sweetening agent glycyrrhizin (see Liquorice) in both [R12,R16;7,8].

MEDICINAL USE: Irritant, abortifacient. It has also been used as a contraceptive but this cannot be recommended as it is so poisonous, and has caused fatalities. Usually seed preparations are treated to denature the toxins before internal use. The seeds are also teratogenic; the proteins are the toxins and cause agglutination of erythrocytes, haemolysis and enlargement of the lymph glands. A paste of the seeds is used in Ayurveda, applied topically, for skin complaints and eye infections. The root is used in tropical Africa as an anti-emetic and to treat infestations with *Bilharzia* and tapeworm, as well as for many other disorders. Pharmacological effects including anti-platelet, anti-allergic, anti-inflammatory, and other activities have been described for the aerial parts and roots, and anti-fertility effects in both male and female animals for the seeds. Anti-tumour and immunomodulating effects have been observed for the proteins, which have lethal effects on molluscs and insects. The abrusides and glycyrrhizin are sweetening agents [see R12, R16;12 and refs therein;19,10,11].

SPECIFIC REFERENCES: 1. Hegde R *et al* (1991) *Anal. Biochem.* 194(1):101. 2. Ghosal S *et al* (1971) *Phytochem.* 10:195. 3. Kinjo J *et al* (1991) *Chem. Pharm. Bull.* 39(1):116. 4. Ma C-M *et al* (1998) *Chem. Pharm. Bull.* 46(6):982. 5. Bharadwaj D *et al* (1980) *Phytochem.* 19:2040. 6. Karawya M *et al* (1981) *Fitoterapia* 52(4):175. 7. Chiang T *et al* (1983) *Planta Med.* 49(3):165. 8. Kennelly E *et al* (1996) *Phytochem.* 41(5):1381. 9. Anam E (2001) *Phytomedicine* 8(1):24. 10. Wang J-P *et al* (1995) *Eur. J. Pharmacol.* 273(1–2):73. 11. Singh S *et al* (1999) *Phytother. Res.* 13(3):210. 12. Aslam M (1998) *Pharm. J.* 261:822.

ABSCESS ROOT
POLEMONIUM REPTANS L.
Fam. Polemoniaceae

SYNONYMS: American Greek Valerian, False Jacob's Ladder, Sweatroot.

HABITAT: North America.

DESCRIPTION: Rhizome slender, 2–5 cm long, about 3 mm diameter, with the bases of numerous stems on the upper surface, and tufts of slender, smooth, wiry, pale roots below.

PART USED: Rhizome.

CONSTITUENTS: Triterpene saponins (unspecified) [R2].

Medicinal use: Diaphoretic, astringent and expectorant, it has been used in febrile and inflammatory conditions [R1]. An infusion produces copious sweating. No recent research is available.

ACACIA BARK
ACACIA ARABICA WILLD
A.DECURRENS WILLD
Fam. Mimosaceae

SYNONYMS: Babul Bark, Wattle Bark.

HABITAT: A. arabica: India, North Africa, *A. decurrens:* Australia.

DESCRIPTION: The bark appears in commerce as hard, rusty-brown pieces 3–10 mm thick, readily dividing into layers, fissured externally and striated and fibrous internally. *A. decurrens* is smoother than *A. arabica.*

PART USED: Bark.

CONSTITUENTS: Condensed tannins, catechins [R3], mucilage and flavonoids [R4].

MEDICINAL USE: Astringent [R1], but seldom used. The herbalist Joseph Miller in 1722 stated that, "It helps ulcers in the mouth and fastens loose teeth." Formerly used in the tanning industry.

BIBLICAL REFERENCES: Exodus 25–27, 30, 35–38; Deuteronomy 10:3; Isaiah 41:19. The references are to Shittim Wood, a variety of acacia (probably *A. arabica*) which was chosen for constructing the Holy Tabernacle and its furniture, due to its availability and hardness.

ACACIA GUM
ACACIA SENEGAL (L.) WILLD
AND OTHER SPECIES
Fam. Mimosaceae

SYNONYMS: Gum Acacia, Gum Arabic, Gum Senegal.

HABITAT: West and North Africa, particularly the Sudan.

DESCRIPTION: The gum exudes from the tree naturally, and can be tapped from incisions made in the bark. The commercial gum appears in rounded or angular, often cracked, transparent pieces, the finest is known as Kordofan gum. Acacia gum is soluble 1:2 in water; the mucilage is usually made with hot or boiling water.

CONSTITUENTS: High molecular weight polysaccharides 80–90%, composed of arabic acid, an acidic arabinogalactan, residues of neutral sugars including galactose, arabinose and rhamnose, and galacturonic and glucuronic acids; oxidizing enzymes and amylases [R2,R3;1].

MEDICINAL USE: Demulcent, used for making emulsions and as an ingredient in compounds for the treatment of diarrhoea, catarrh etc. [R1]. It is used widely in the food industry as a stabilizer and flavour fixative, and in chewing gum. *In vitro* tests demonstrated antibacterial and anti-protease activities [2], and a clinical trial showed it to be more effective in preventing plaque formation than sugar-free gum [3].

SPECIFIC REFERENCES: 1. Menzies A R *et al* (1996) *Food Add.*

Contam. 18(8):991. 2. Clark D *et al* (1993) *J. Clin. Periodont.* 20(4):238.
3. Gazi, M (1991) *J. Clin. Periodont.* 18(1):75.

ACONITE

ACONITUM NAPELLUS L.
A. carmichaeli Debx
A. kusznezoffii Reichb.
A. heterophyllum Wall.
A. uncinatum L. var *japonicum*
and other species
Fam. Ranunculaceae

SYNONYMS: Wolfsbane, Monkshood, Friar's Cap, Blue Rocket *(A. napellus)*.

HABITAT: *A. napellus* is indigenous to Central Europe, and according
to Pliny is named after the Black Sea Port, Aconis. It is cultivated and
naturalized extensively. The others are Oriental species and are
widespread throughout the Far East.

DESCRIPTION: The plant is robust, erect, with violet-blue flowers
occurring in racemes, followed by capsules of angular, wrinkled seeds.
The root is blackish, conical, with a 5–7 pointed star in the centre of
the fracture, which is white and starchy.

PART USED: Root, occasionally leaves.

CONSTITUENTS: (i) In all species, terpenoid alkaloids, including
aconitine, aconine, hypaconitine, neopelline, picraconitine, napelline,
benzoylaconine, *N*-desethylaconitine, oxo-aconitine, lappaconitine etc.,
traces of ephedrine and sparteine (ii) Aconitic, itaconic acids
(iii) sugars and starch [R2,R3,R5;1,2].

MEDICINAL USE: Sedative, anodyne, febrifuge [R1]. It is a powerful
poison affecting the heart and central nervous system and therefore
rarely used internally except homoeopathically and in Chinese and
Indian medicine. Topically it is used for bruises, sciatica, rheumatic
pain etc. It causes a tingling sensation followed by numbness. It must
be borne in mind when using, that absorption through the skin may
cause systemic poisoning. Aconitine has a short-lived cardiotonic action
followed by cardiac depression, weakening of contractility, and cardiac
arrest, and is sometimes used as a pharmacological tool to induce
arrhythmia. Aconine, the hydrolysed alkaloid, is very much less toxic.
Aconitine has a transient hypotensive activity whereas the herb, after
heat treatment, has a transient pressor activity. A decoction of the herb
or the total alkaloids increases coronary flow and causes vasodilation
of the blood vessels in the limbs in animals. Aconitine has analgesic
activity, anti-inflammatory activity and local anaesthetic activity.
In Chinese medicine Aconite is the principal constituent of many
prescriptions for shock; and preparations with the aconitine are
available for various forms of heart disease. *Aconitum* species have
been shown to have antihistaminic, anti-tumour, antiviral, antibacterial
and antipyretic activity in laboratory tests. [R2,R5,R6;3,4] There is
an old story that wolves, tearing up roots of plants for food in winter,

5

mistake this plant and die from its poison, hence the name
'Wolfsbane'.

PREPARATIONS: Aconite, Belladonna and Chloroform Liniment BPC
1968; Aconite Tincture and Strong Aconite Tincture BPC 1949;
Aconite Liniment BPC 1968.

SPECIFIC REFERENCES: 1. Konno C et al (1982) J. Nat. Prod. 45:128.
2. Hikino H et al (1983) J. Nat. Prod. 46:178. 3. Kimura I et al (1996)
Biol. Pharm. Bull. 19 (11):1440. 4. Kolev S et al (1996) Hum. Exp.
Toxicol. 15:839.

ACORNS
QUERCUS ROBUR L.
Fam. Fagaceae

DESCRIPTION: The fruit of the oak tree.

CONSTITUENTS: Tannins, flavonoids, sugar, starch, albumin and
fixed oil [R4].

MEDICINAL USE: Astringent; an old remedy for diarrhoea, where they
are powdered or grated and washed down with water [R1]. Roasted
acorns have been used as a substitute for coffee during wartime.

ADDER'S TONGUE, AMERICAN
ERYTHRONIUM AMERICANUM KER-GAWL
Fam. Liliaceae

SYNONYMS: Serpent's Tongue, Dog's Tooth Violet, Yellow Snowdrop.

HABITAT: North America.

DESCRIPTION: Flowers; yellow, star-shaped, about 2 cm across, with 6
stamens. Leaves; two only, about 6 cm long by 2–3 cm wide, minutely
wrinkled and with parallel veins. Corms spindle-shaped, up to about
2 cm long. Taste: sweetish.

PART USED: Fresh leaves, roots.

CONSTITUENTS: Little information available. (i) Alpha-methylenebuty-
rolactone (ii) Tuliposides [R2].

MEDICINAL USE: Emetic, emollient [R1]. The fresh leaves have use as
a poultice for ulcers, together with an infusion taken internally. The
aqueous extract has some activity against Gram positive and Gram
negative bacteria [1].

SPECIFIC REFERENCES: 1. Cavallito C et al (1946) J. Chem. Soc.
66:2332.

ADDER'S TONGUE, ENGLISH
OPHIOGLOSSUM VULGATUM L.
Fam. Ophioglossaceae

SYNONYMS: Serpent's Tongue

HABITAT: Moist meadows in Great Britain, it flowers in April or May.

DESCRIPTION: The plant has a solitary leaf, lanceolate with forked veins and bearing a stalked, linear spike of spore-cases, in double row which resembles an adder's tongue.

PART USED: Herb.

CONSTITUENTS: Flavonoids including quercetin glycosides [R2].

MEDICINAL USE: Similar to that of American Adder's Tongue (q.v.) [R1]. An ointment has been made by boiling the herb in oil or fat, for use on wounds. The water extract is reputed to be soothing to tired eyes.

ADRUE
CYPERUS ARTICULATUS L.
Fam. Cyperaceae

SYNONYMS: Guinea Rush.

HABITAT: Europe, Africa and Latin America.

DESCRIPTION: Blackish, top-shaped tubers, with bristly remains of former leaves, sometimes connected in twos or threes by narrow underground stems. Transverse section pale, showing a central column with darker vascular bundles. Taste: bitter; odour: aromatic, recalling that of lavender.

PART USED: Root.

CONSTITUENTS: Sesquiterpene ketones including cyperenone and cyperone (= articulone) [R2;1].

MEDICINAL USE: Anti-emetic, carminative, anti-epileptic and sedative in peptic disorders [R1]. In Chinese medicine it is used as an anti-haemorrhagic. A water extract has been found to reduce spontaneous epileptiform discharges *in vitro* by inhibition of NMDA neurotransmission [2]. The essential oil has insect repellant and anti-feedant activity [3].

SPECIFIC REFERENCES: 1. Pinder A (1976) *Tetrahedron* 23:2172. 2. Burn E *et al* (1996) *J. Ethnopharmacol.* 54(2–3):103. 3. Abubakar M *et al* (2000) *Phytother. Res.* 14(4):281.

AGAR
GELIDIUM AMANSII LAM., AND OTHER SPECIES OF *GELIDIUM AND GRACILARIA*
Fam. Rhodophyceae

SYNONYMS: Agar-Agar, Japanese Isinglass.

HABITAT: The main species from which agar is prepared are indigenous to Japan, but many other countries now produce it.

DESCRIPTION: Agar is the dried mucilaginous extract, obtained by boiling, filtering and drying. It occurs in translucent strips or as a powder; it is colourless and tasteless and capable of absorbing up to 200 times its volume of water to form a jelly.

7

PART USED: Extract.

CONSTITUENTS: The structure is complex. Most agars consist of two major polygalactoses, the neutral agarose and the sulphonated polysaccharide agaropectin, with traces of amino acids and free sugars [R2,R4].

MEDICINAL USE: Nutritive, bulk-laxative, occasionally made into an emulsion with liquid paraffin for the treatment of constipation [R1]. The extract has antioxidant activity [1], and an enzyme degraded polysaccharide fraction has been found to have immunopotentiating activity [2] and anti-tumour activity [3] in mice. It is widely used to produce a medium for cultivation of bacteria and fungi in microbiology.

PREPARATIONS AND DOSE: Liquid Paraffin Emulsion with Agar BPC 1949, dose: 10–30 ml.

SPECIFIC REFERENCES: 1. Yan X *et al* (1998) *Plant Foods Nutr.* 52(3):253. 2.Yoshizawa Y *et al* (1996) *Biosci. Biotechnol. Biochem.* 60(10):1667. 3. Fernandez L *et al* (1989) *Carbohydr. Res.* 190(1):77.

AGARICUS
FOMES OFFICINALIS FAULL.
Fam. Polyporaceae

SYNONYMS: White Agaric, Larch Agaric, Purging Agaric, *Boletus laricis.*

HABITAT: It is a fungus growing in larch forests in Europe and Russia.

DESCRIPTION: Occurs in white, spongy, friable masses. The surface is brownish and the internal structure white and porous. The odour is mealy and the taste sweetish with a bitter acrid aftertaste.

PART USED: Upper part (fruiting body).

CONSTITUENTS: (i) Resin, including agaricin (agaric acid) (ii) Triterpene acids (iii) Polyacetylenes (unspecified) [R4].

MEDICINAL USE: Astringent in small doses, it has been used to alleviate night sweats and diarrhoea and to dry maternal milk after weaning [R1]. Purgative in large doses, and may cause vomiting.

AGNUS CASTUS
VITEX AGNUS-CASTUS L.
Fam. Verbenaceae

SYNONYMS: Chaste Tree, Chaste Berry, Monk's Pepper.

HABITAT: A native shrub of the Mediterranean region and central Asia.

DESCRIPTION: The fruits are small, brownish black, hard round berries about 0.5 cm in diameter with a persistent calyx, containing four seeds. Taste: acrid, peppery; odour: aromatic.

PART USED: Dried, ripe fruits.

CONSTITUENTS: (i) Iridoid glycosides; aucubin, agnoside (ii) Flavonoids, particularly casticin, and orientin, with glycosides of kaempferol and quercetin (iii) Labdane and clerodane diterpenes including vitexilactone and rotundifuran, and others (iv) Volatile oil containing cineole, limonene, sabinene, bornyl acetate, *p*-cymene, camphor, alpha- and beta-pinenes (v) Alkaloids; viticin (vi) Fatty oil composed of alpha-linolenic, caprinic acids and others [R2,R7,R8;1,2].

MEDICINAL USE: Now used mainly as a hormone regulator for disorders of the menstrual cycle, infertility and menopausal symptoms in women, although it has also been used to treat inflammation and acne. Dioscorides described the plant over 2000 years ago and noted that the name 'Agnus castus' means 'chaste lamb', a reference to its reputation for reducing sexual desire in men. This explains the other names 'Chaste Berry' and 'Monk's Pepper', since medieval monks were said to take the plant for this purpose. Many studies have shown that the fruit inhibits the release of various hormones including prolactin, and has a dopaminergic activity in receptor binding studies; the active compounds being the labdane diterpenes. Clinical studies involving over 5000 women have demonstrated efficacy in alleviating premenstrual syndrome and, in combination with other ingredients, for mastalgia. It also displays weak binding to opioid receptors. Not recommended during pregnancy or lactation as it may suppress milk production, however it is generally thought safe. [R2,R7,R8,R17; 2,3,4,5,6,7,8,9,10,11].

PREPARATIONS AND DOSE: Dried berry or equivalent extract, dose: 30–40 mg daily.

SPECIFIC REFERENCES: 1. Hoberg E *et al* (1999) *Phytochemistry* 52(8):1555. 2. American Herbal Pharmacopoeia. 'Chaste Tree Fruit'. Ed. Upton R (2001) 3. Schellenberg R. (2001) *B.M.J.* 4322:134. 4. Halaska M *et al* (1999) *The Breast* 8:175. 5. Lauritzen C *et al* (1997) *Phytomed.* 4:183. 6. Jarry H *et al* (1994) *Exp. Clin. Endocrinol.* 102:448. 7. Berger D *et al* (2000) *Arch. Gynecol. Obstet.* 264:150. 8. Gerhard I *et al* (1998) *Forsch. Komplementamed* 5:272. 9. Hoberg E *et al* (1999) *Z. Phytother.* 20:140. 10. Turner S *et al* (1993) *Comp. Ther. Med.* 1:73. 11. Gorkow C *et al* (1999) Z. *Phytother.* 20:158.

AGRIMONY

AGRIMONIA EUPATORIA L.
Fam. Rosaceae

SYNONYMS: Cocklebur, Stickwort.

HABITAT: Central and northern Europe, North America and temperate Asia, in hedges and fields and by ditches, flowering in July and August.

DESCRIPTION: The leaves, green above and silver-grey underneath, are hairy, 10 cm or longer, with 3–5 pairs of lanceolate, toothed leaflets of different sizes, and half-cordate, toothed stipules. The small flowers are composed of five yellow petals with hairy calices, placed on long, slender spikes. The fruit is small, subconical and ribbed, with hooked bristles. Each contains two seeds. Taste: astringent, slightly bitter.

PART USED: Herb.

CONSTITUENTS: (i) Condensed tannins (catechins) and hydrolysable   *AGRIMONY*

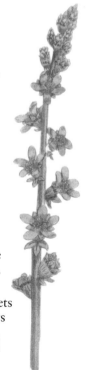

tannins, including ellagitannin, (ii) Flavonoids, e.g. glucosides of luteolin, apigenin and quercetin (iii) Volatile oil (iv) Miscellaneous triterpenes, salicylic acid [R2,R7,R9,1,2,3].

MEDICINAL USE: Mild astringent, diuretic. It is a traditional herb for infantile diarrhoea, urethritis, colitis, cystitis and sore throat [R1]. Extracts have been shown to have anti-diabetic activity [4,5] uricolytic activity [R7] and luteolin 7-glucoside also has a cholegogic action [1]. The infusion has been used clinically with some success in cutaneous porphyria [6]. Aqueous extracts inhibited *Mycobacterium tuberculosis, in vitro* [7] and ethanolic extracts have shown antiviral effects against Colombia SK virus in mice [8]. Other species of *Agrimonia*, such as *A. pilosa*, are used in China for their haemostatic and hypotensive activity. However some of the constituents isolated, such as agrimoniin, and some phloroglucinols, do not occur in *A. eupatoria*. Agrimoniin is an anti-tumour tannin [9] and the phloroglucinols are anti-microbial [10]. *A. pilosa* inhibits HIV-protease [11] and like *A. eupatoria*, has anti-diabetic activity [12].

SPECIFIC REFERENCES: 1. Drozd G *et al* (1983) *Khim. Prir. Soed.* 1:106. 2. Bilia A *et al* (1993) *Fitoterapia* 64:549. 3. Carnat A *et al* (1991) *Plantes Med. Phytother.* 25:202. 4. Gray A *et al* (1998) *Br. J. Nutr.* 80(1):109. 5. Swanston Flatt S *et al* (1990) *Diabetologia* 33(8):462. 6. Patrascu V *et al* (1984) *Ser. Dermato-Venerol.* 29(2):156. 7. Peter-Horvath M *et al* (1964) *Rev. Med.* 10(2):190. 8. Chon S *et al* (1987) *Med. Pharmacol. Exp.* 16(5):407. 9. Muryama T *et al* (1992) *Anticancer Res.* 12:1471. 10. Yamaki M *et al* (1994) *Phytother. Res.* 8:112. 11. Min B *et al* (1999) *Phytother. Res.* 13:680. 12. Hsu F-L *et al* (1992) *Phytother. Res.* 6:108.

AJOWAN
TRACHYSPERMUM AMMI L. SPRAGUE
Fam. Apiaceae

SYNONYMS: Ajwain, Bishop's Weed, Omum, *Carum copticum* Benth. Hook., *Sison ammi* L.

HABITAT: Native to the Mediterranean region but found in many parts of Asia and Africa, and cultivated commercially in India.

DESCRIPTION: An erect, typically umbelliferous annual herb reaching up to 90 cm, either glabrous or with minute, fine, soft hairs. The fruits are small, ovoid, compressed and ridged, grey or brown. The essential oil extracted from the seeds is yellowish or reddish orange, with a strong smell reminiscent of thyme.

PART USED: Seeds, essential oil.

CONSTITUENTS: (i) Volatile oil containing thymol as the major component, with *p*-cymene, dipentene, camphene, myrcene, α- and β- pinene, limonene, carvacrol, α- and γ-terpinene, δ-3-carene and others (ii) Glucopyranosyloxythymol (iii) Fixed oil containing petroselinic, linoleic and oleic acids [R16;1,2].

MEDICINAL USE: Carminative, stimulant, antispasmodic. It is an important herb in Ayurvedic medicine for bronchitis, asthma, and various respiratory and digestive diseases, including colic and diarrhoea, both internally and applied in the form of a poultice. It is used traditionally for cholera, as a liver tonic and for habitual drunkenness [R16]. The active principle is usually considered to be thymol, which is antiseptic, anti-fungal, insecticidal and molluscicidal. Extracts have also shown anti-platelet effects and hypotensive activity [3,4] and the molluscidal and fungitoxic activities have been well-documented [5,6].

PREPARATIONS AND DOSE: Seed, dose: 3–6 g.

SPECIFIC REFERENCES: 1. Garg S *et al* (1998) *Fitoterapia* 69(6):511. 2. Nagalakshmi S *et al* (2000) *J. Food Sci. Technol.* 37(3):277. 3. Srivastava K *et al* (1988) *Prostagland. Leukotrien. Ess. Fatty Acids* 33(1):1. 4. Aftab K *et al* (1995) *Phytomed.* 2(1):35. 5. Singh V *et al* (1999) *Phytother. Res.*13(8):649. 6. Singh J *et al* (1999) *Flav. Frag. J.*14(1):1.

ALDER, BLACK, AMERICAN
PRINOS VERTICILLATUS L.
Fam. Aquifoliaceae

SYNONYMS: Winterberry, Feverbush.

HABITAT: North America and Canada.

DESCRIPTION: Bark: brownish-grey, in quilled thin pieces, with whitish patches surrounded by black margins on outer surface and a greenish or yellowish inner surface. Berries: resemble those of the common Holly. Taste: bitter and acid.

PART USED: Bark, berries.

CONSTITUENTS: Unknown.

MEDICINAL USE: Antiseptic, cathartic [R1].

ALDER, ENGLISH
ALNUS GLUTINOSA (L.) GAERTN.
Fam. Betulaceae

SYNONYMS: *Betula alnus* var *glutinosa* L., Tag Alder, Common Alder.

HABITAT: Grows commonly throughout Europe in damp woods and near water, flowering in April and May.

DESCRIPTION: The bark usually occurs in curved or quilled thin pieces, brownish-grey externally and brownish-orange on the inner surface. The fracture is short and uneven.

PART USED: Bark, leaves.

CONSTITUENTS: Bark: (i) Lignans including dimethoxyisolariciresinol (ii) 10–20% Tannin (iii) Emodin (iv) Phenolic glycosides, e.g. lyonoside (v) Miscellaneous triterpenes, anulin, protanulin, phlobaphene and others. Leaves: Flavonoid glycosides, especially hyperoside [R2,1].

11

MEDICINAL USE: The bark is astringent, and a decoction was used as a gargle for sore throats [R1]. The leaves were used as a poultice for swelling and inflammation, and Pliny recommended that they should be placed in the shoes for tired feet. The wood has been called the Scottish Mahogany; it is resistant to rotting and was used to make troughs and sluices, as well as furniture and clogs in the Lancashire mill towns. The bark and leaves have been used for tanning and to make a dye for leather and wool.

ALFALFA
MEDICAGO SATIVA L.
Fam. Fabaceae

SYNONYMS: Lucerne, Purple Medick.

HABITAT: Native to the Mediterranean region, cultivated widely.

DESCRIPTION: The herb reaches up to about 50 cm. Leaves trifoliate, leaflets obovate, with an acute apex and serrate margin, upper surface glabrous, lower surface with scattered, whitish hairs; stems hollow, ridged. Flowers papilionaceous, blue, in a raceme. Pods loosely spiral, with appressed hairs. Taste and odour: slight.

PART USED: Herb.

CONSTITUENTS: (i) Isoflavones; biochanin A, daidzein, formononetin, genistein and occasionally pterocarpan phytoalexins (ii) Coumarins; coumestrol, daphnoretin, lucernol, medicagol, sativol and trifolial (iii) Alkaloids; stachydrine, homostachydrine, and in the seeds, trigonelline (iv) Nutrients, including pro-vitamin A, vitamins of the B group, C, D, E, and K, folic acid, biotin and others (v) Saponins based on hederagenin, medicagenic acid and soyasapogenols A, B, C, D and E (vi) Porphyrins; phaeophorbide A and chlorophyllide A (vii) Amino acids, including canavanine, and also 4-aminobutyric acid, in the root (viii) Miscellaneous; sterols including campesterol, beta-sitosterol and their esters, hydrocarbons such as triacontane and their corresponding alcohols [R2,R7;1,2,3].

MEDICINAL USE: Nutrient, appetite stimulant. It is used to help patients put on weight during convalescence [R1]. The isoflavones are oestrogenic in animals and the porphyrins have been shown to have the potential to affect liver function and biliary secretion in rats, resulting in photosensitization [4]. The saponins have an anticholesterolaemic effect in monkeys [5] and are anti-fungal against *Candida* and other species [6]. The seeds produced a blood-cholesterol-lowering effect in human patients with hyperlipoproteinemia [7]. Lucerne is a major animal food crop. The young sprouts are used in salads. Generally it is non-toxic, but excessive intake is not recommended due to the oestrogenic effects of the isoflavones, and canavanine can produce a systemic lupus erythematosus (SLE)-like syndrome [R7;8]. Alfalfa may also exacerbate existing SLE [9].

PREPARATIONS AND DOSE: Herb, dose: 5–10 g or equivalent extract.

SPECIFIC REFERENCES: 1. Gestetner B (1974) *Phytochem.* 10:2221. 2. Berrang B (1974) *Phytochem.* 10:2253. 3. Larher F *et al* (1983) *Plant Sci. Lett.* 29(2/3):315. 4. Tapper B *et al* (1975) *J. Sci. Food Agric.* 26:277. 5. Malinow M *et al* (1977) *Steroids* 29:105. 6. Jurzysta M *et al.* (1996) *Adv. Expl. Med. Biol.* 404:565. 7. Molgaard J *et al* (1987) *Atherosclerosis* 65:173. 8. Alcocer-Varela J *et al* (1985) *Arthritis Rheum.* 28:52. 9. Roberts J *et al* (1983) *New Eng. J. Med.* 308:1361.

ALKANET

ALKANNA TINCTORIA (L.) TAUSCH
Fam. Boraginaceae

SYNONYMS: Dyer's Bugloss, Spanish Bugloss, Anchusa, Alkanna, Orchanet.

HABITAT: Indigenous to the Mediterranean and other parts of Europe, and cultivated widely.

DESCRIPTION: Root up to 10 cm long. The root bark is purplish and easily separated from the woody centre, which is yellowish. The leaves are long, narrow and hairy, the flowers blue or purple and trumpet-shaped.

PART USED: Root.

CONSTITUENTS: (i) Alkannins, up to 5%, which are lipophilic isohexenylnaphthazarin red pigments. (ii) Pyrrolizidine alkaloids such as triangularine and derivatives, and 7-angelyl retronecine, have been isolated from the herb [R2;1,2,3] but it is not known whether these hepatotoxic alkaloids occur in extracts used for medicinal or food purposes.

MEDICINAL USE: Rarely used medicinally now and a total extract is not recommended for internal use due to the pyrrolizidine alkaloid content. The herb is astringent [R1] and the alkannins have both anti-microbial and wound-healing properties [4]. It has been used clinically for indolent ulcer [2] and is non-toxic to mice [5]. Dioscorides said that "it helps those bitten by venomous beasts," and that, "to chew the root and spit into the mouth of the serpent will instantly kill the reptile". The alkannins are used nowadays in a much more mundane fashion for colouring sausages and other foodstuffs.

SPECIFIC REFERENCES: 1. Papageorgious V *et al* (1980) *Planta Med.* 39:81 and 39:193. 2. Weidenfeld H *et al* (1985) *Arch. Pharm.* 318:294. 3. Roder E et al (1984) *Phytochemistry.* 23:2125. 4. Papageorgious V (1978) *Experientia* 34:1499. 5. Majlathova L. (1971) *Nahrung* 15:505.

ALLSPICE

PIMENTO DIOICA (MILL.) J W MOORE
Fam. Myrtaceae

SYNONYMS: Pimento, Pimenta, Jamaican Pepper, Clove Pepper, *Pimenta officinalis* Lindl., *Eugenia pimenta* DC.

HABITAT: Native of the West Indies, cultivated in South and Central America; mainly imported from Jamaica and Cuba. Flowers June–August, with berries appearing soon after.

DESCRIPTION: The tree is an evergreen, up to 13 m in height, bearing small white flowers. The fruits are brown, globular, about 0.75 cm in diameter with a rough surface and the remains of the calyx present as a ring of teeth at the apex. There are two kidney-shaped seeds. Odour: aromatic, clove-like.

PART USED: Unripe fruit, occasionally leaves used for oil production.

CONSTITUENTS: (i) Volatile oil, 3–4.5%, the major component of which is eugenol, 60–80%, with cineole, methyleugenol, phellandrene, caryophyllene, cadinols and many others in trace amounts [1]. The leaf oil consists mainly of eugenol (ca. 95%) [R2] (ii) Protein, lipids, vitamins A, C, B_1, B_2 and niacin, minerals.

MEDICINAL USE: Aromatic carminative, often used as an adjunct in the treatment of flatulence, dyspepsia and diarrhoea [R1]. Eugenol has local anaesthetic and antiseptic properties. The oil is anti-microbial [2] larvicidal [3], antioxidant [4], and enhances trypsin activity [5]. It is used mainly as a condiment and spice.

PREPARATIONS AND DOSE: Powdered fruit, dose: 0.5–2 g. Pimento Oil BPC 1949, dose: 0.05 to 0.2 ml.

SPECIFIC REFERENCES: 1. Hogg J *et al* (1974) *Am. Perf. Cosm.* 86:33. 2. Hao Y *et al* (1998) *J. Food Protection.* 61(3):307. 3. Oishi K *et al* (1974) *Nippon Suisan Gakaishi* 40:1241. 4. Saito Y *et al* (1976) *Eiyo To Shokuryo* 29:505. 5. Kato Y *et al* (1975) *Koryo* 113:24.

ALMONDS, BITTER
PRUNUS AMYGDALUS BATSCH VAR AMARA

ALMONDS, SWEET
PRUNUS AMYGDALUS BATSCH VAR *DULCIS*
Fam. Rosaceae

SYNONYMS: Jordan Almonds, *Prunus communis* (L.) Arc. *Amygdalus communis* L.

HABITAT: The almond tree is a native of western Asia but is extensively cultivated.

DESCRIPTION: The fruit is botanically a drupe, the almond is the seed and needs no description.

PART USED: Seed, oil.

CONSTITUENTS: (i) Fixed oil, 35–45%, known as Almond Oil or Sweet Almond Oil, made from both varieties. It consists of triglycerides, mainly triolein and trioleolinolein, with fatty acids including palmitic, lauric, myristic and oleic (ii) Volatile oil, known as Bitter Almond Oil, distilled from Bitter Almonds only, and consisting of about 95% benzaldehyde with 2–3% amygdalin, a cyanogenetic glycoside which is removed before sale (iii) Flavonols including catechins, and oligomeric procyanidins [1] (iv) Other substances such as protein, sterols, prunasin, vitamin E and minerals [R10].

MEDICINAL USE: Almond Oil is used largely as an emollient, alone or as an ingredient of cosmetics. It is also taken internally as a nutrient, demulcent and mild laxative [R1]. Bitter Almond Oil is used mainly as a flavouring agent, in large doses it is toxic, due to the amygdalin content, causing CNS depression and respiratory failure. Almond flour from which the oil has been removed has been used in diabetic food products as it does not contain starch, and has a hypoglycaemic action in rabbits [2]. Recently, a diet supplemented with almonds (36–73g/day) was associated with a lowering of blood LDL-cholesterol levels [3]. Almonds are traditionally given to nursing mothers and invalids in India, and have recently been shown to enhance immune status in mice [4].

BIBLICAL REFERENCES: Genesis 43:11; Exodus 25:33–34; 37:19–20; Numbers 17:8; Ecclesiastes 12:5; Jeremiah 1:11.

SPECIFIC REFERENCES: 1.Santos-Buelga C F *et al* (1998) *Phytochem Anal.* 9 (1):21. 2. Teotia S *et al* (1997) *Indian J. Exp. Biol.* 35(3):295 3. Jenkins D *et al* (2002) *Circulation* 10:1161 4. Puri A *et al* (2000) *J. Ethnopharmacol.* 71(2):89.

ALOE VERA

ALOE VERA (L.) BURM. F.
A. BARBADENSIS MILL
AND OTHERS; SEE ALSO 'ALOES'
Fam. Aloeaceae

SYNONYMS: Aloe Vera Gel.

HABITAT: Cultivated varieties, grown in the tropics, mainly for their reduced anthraquinone content.

DESCRIPTION: Aloe Vera is a mucilaginous gel obtained from the parenchyma tissue in the centre of the leaf, obtained by mechanical or chemical means. This means the product is highly variable in its properties.

CONSTITUENTS: (i) Polysaccharides (known as acemannan) consisting mainly glucomannans (ii) Anthraquinone glycosides (see Aloes) (iii) Glycoproteins such as the aloctins (iv) Others, including enzymes such as carboxypeptidases, sterols, saponins and organic acids [R2,R3,R7,1,2].

MEDICINAL USE: Topically to aid wound healing, relieve burns including sunburn, as an emollient and even for colonic irrigation. Many of these actions have been substantiated by experimental results. Extracts have been shown to be anti-inflammatory, anti-ulcerogenic, anti-tumour, and immunomodulatory and have many other effects. The gel is taken internally as an emollient for ulceration and also as an immunostimulant and aid to treatment of diabetes mellitus.

Enzymes extracted from Aloe Vera gel are analgesic and inhibit thermal damage and vascular permeability in mice. The fresh leaf pulp has been shown to induce carcinogen-metabolizing phase II and antioxidant enzymes, which would help to detoxify reactive metabolites such as those produced by carcinogens and other drugs. It is an ingredient of many cosmetic preparations [R11,R12,1,2,3,4].

SPECIFIC REFERENCES: 1. Winters W (Ed.). Proc. 1991 Int. Cong. Phytotherapy, Seoul, Korea. (1993) *Phytother. Res.* Special Issue Vol 7. 2. Capasso F *et al* (1998) *Phytother. Res.* 12:S124–127. 3. Bunyapraphatsara N *et al* (1996) *Phytomed.* 3:245. 4. Singh R *et al* (2000) *Phytomed.* 7(3):209.

ALOES
(1) *ALOE BARBADENSIS* MILL
(2) *ALOE FEROX* MILL
(3) *ALOE PERRYI* BAKER
OTHER SPECIES AND HYBRIDS
Fam. Aloeaceae

SYNONYMS: (1) Barbados Aloes, Curacao Aloes, *Aloe Vera* Tourn ex L., *A. vera* (L.) Webb. (2) Cape Aloes (3) Socotrine Aloes, Zanzibar Aloes.

HABITAT: (1) West Indies (2) Southern Africa (3) East Africa.

DESCRIPTION: Aloe species are succulent perennials found widely throughout the world in tropical climates. Aloes is an exudate, which drains from the cut leaves, evaporated to dryness. It has a resinous, glassy appearance and very bitter taste. The different species can be distinguished by their appearance and by simple chemical tests: Barbados Aloes is opaque and gives a crimson colour with nitric acid; Cape Aloes is translucent and gives a similar colour reaction; Socotrine Aloes is opaque but gives no colour reaction.

CONSTITUENTS: (i) Anthraquinone glycosides, collectively known as 'Aloin', mainly barbaloin, a C-glycoside of aloe-emodin, with isobarbaloin present in Barbados Aloes only, and other minor C- and O-glycosides such as aloinosides A and B (ii) free aloe-emodin and crysophanol in small amounts (iii) chromones including aloesin, aloeresin E, isoaloeresin D and furoaloesone (iv) resins[R2,R3,R7;1,2,3,4,5].

MEDICINAL USE: Aloes is used internally as a purgative, acting on the lower bowel, and was formerly used as an emmenagogue [R1]. It is a useful laxative but overdose may cause gastritis, diarrhoea and nephritis. The tendency to cause griping is counteracted by taking it in conjunction with antispasmodics such as Belladonna (q.v.) and carminatives. The mechanism of action is thought to be by induction of nitric oxide release [6]. Aloe extracts are reported to have anti-cancer activity *in vitro* and also have hypoglycaemic and antihistamine activity [R7;7,8]. Aloe extracts are described as accelerating the oxidation of ethanol in rats [9], however inhibitors of alcohol metabolism have also been isolated [10]. Aloes is used as a flavouring ingredient in low concentrations and topically as an ingredient of sun creams (see also Aloe Vera), and as a paint to discourage nail-biting, due to its intense bitterness. It may be nephrotoxic in large doses, especially if consumed over a long period. Recently the US Food and Drugs Administration ruled that aloes would not be allowed in over-the-counter (OTC) laxative preparations, due to safety concerns [R2,R3,R7,R8;1,11].

PREPARATIONS AND DOSE: Aloes, dose: 100–300 mg. Aloes Tincture BPC 1949, dose: 2–8 ml.

BIBLICAL REFERENCES: Numbers 24:6; Psalms 45:8; Proverbs 7:17; Song of Solomon 4:14; John 19:39. (These may however refer to *Aquilaria agallochum.*)

SPECIFIC REFERENCES: 1. Capasso F *et al* (1998) *Phytother. Res.* 12:S124. 2. Park M *et al* (1998) *Phytochem. Anal.* 9:186. 3. Van Wyk E-E *et al* (1995) *Planta Med.* 61:250. 4. Rauwald H *et al* (1997) *Pharmazie* 52:962. 5. Speranza G *et al* (1997) *J. Nat. Prod.* 60:692. 6. Izzo A *et al* (1999) *Eur. J. Pharmacol.* 368:43. 7. Al-Awadi F *et al* (1987) *Diabetologia* 28:432. 8. Yamamoto M *et al* (1993) *Japan J. Toxicol. Environ. Health* 39:395. 9. Chung J-H *et al* (1996) *Biochem. Pharmacol.* 52:1461. 10. Shin K *et al* (1997) *J. Nat. Prod.* 60:1180. 11. Luyckx V *et al* (2002) *Am. J. Kidney Dis.* 39(3):E13.

ALSTONIA BARK
ALSTONIA SCHOLARIS (L.) R BR.
ALSTONIA CONSTRICTA F. MUELL
Fam. Apocynaceae

SYNONYMS: A. scholaris = *Echites scholaris* L., Devil Tree, Dita Bark. *A. constricta* = Fever Bark, Australian Quinine, Australian Febrifuge.

HABITAT: A. scholaris is a native of India and the Philippine Islands but is found in many areas of the tropics, *A. constricta* is native to Australia.

DESCRIPTION: A. scholaris occurs in irregular fragments, up to about 1 cm thick, externally rough, brownish-grey, often with darker spots. Inner surface: buff coloured, fracture: short and granular. *A. constricta* occurs in quilled pieces, it has a thick brown cork and is deeply fissured. The inner surface is yellowish-brown and coarsely striated, fracture fibrous. Both taste bitter.

PART USED: Bark.

CONSTITUENTS: Indole alkaloids. *A. scholaris* contains akuammidine and related alkaloids, echitamine, echitenine, echitine, echitamidine, nareline, picrinine, strictamine, scholarine and others. *A. constricta* contains alstonine and derivatives, alstonidine, alstoniline, reserpine, yohimbine, vincamajine and related alkaloids [R2,1,2].

MEDICINAL USE: Febrifuge, anti-malarial, spasmolytic and antihypertensive [R1]. The hypotensive effects of echitamine have been demonstrated and reserpine has a similar effect. *A. scholaris* has produced a fall in temperature in human patients with fevers, however there is conflicting evidence as to whether it is a true anti-malarial. Echitamine has been demonstrated to be devoid of activity against a strain of *Plasmodium berghei* in one report but active in another [3,4]. An extract has protective effects against experimental hepatotoxin-induced liver damage [5] and human lung cancer cell lines [6]. In the past it has been used as a remedy for rheumatism, and as a tonic, although this cannot be recommended. *A. constricta* has a reputation as a uterine stimulant, thought to be due to the reserpine content, and should therefore be avoided in pregnant women.

SPECIFIC REFERENCES: 1. Pelletier S (Ed.) (1983) in: Alkaloids Vol 1. Wiley and Sons. 2. Atta-ur-Rahman *et al* (1985) *Phytochem.* 24:2771. 3. Wright C *et al* (1993) *J. Ethnopharmacol.* 40(1):41. 4. Keawpradub N *et al* (1999) *Planta Med.* 65(8):690. 5. Lin S *et al* (1996) *Am. J. Chin. Med.* 24(2):153. 6. Keawpradub N *et al* (1997) *Planta Med.* 63(2):97.

AMADOU
FOMES FOMENTARIUS (L.) FRIES
Fam. Polyporaceae

SYNONYMS: Surgeon's Agaric, German Tinder, Oak Agaric, *Polyporus fomentarius.*

HABITAT: A fungus growing upon oak and beech trees in Europe and the British Isles.

DESCRIPTION: A hoof-shaped, obliquely triangular, sessile fungus. The inner part is composed of short tubular fibres arranged in layers. It is prepared for use by being sliced, beaten, soaked in a solution of nitre and dried.

CONSTITUENTS: Fomentaric acid, mannofucogalactan and other polysaccharides [R4].

MEDICINAL USE: Amadou was used by the Khanty (Western Siberia) people, mainly for arresting haemorrhages [1], being applied with pressure to the affected part; and for treating ingrown toenails, by inserting between the nail and flesh. Hot water extracts have been shown to have antiviral activity [2].

SPECIFIC REFERENCES: 1. Saar M (1991) *J. Ethnopharmacol.* 31(2):175. 2. Aoki M *et al* (1993) *Biosci. Biotech. Biochem.* 57:278.

AMARANTH
AMARANTHUS HYPOCHONDRIACUS L.
Fam. Amaranthaceae

SYNONYMS: Love-Lies-Bleeding, Red Cockscomb, *Amaranthus melancholicus* L.

HABITAT: A common garden plant, flowering from August until the first frosts.

DESCRIPTION: Rounded tufts of minute flowers, hidden by tapering crimson bracts, are borne on flattened stems.

PART USED: Flowering herb.

CONSTITUENTS: A magenta-red pigment consisting mainly of trisodium 3-hydroxy-4-(4-sulphonaphth-1-ylazo)-naphthalene-2,7-disulphonate (also referred to as Amaranth and E123); unspecified saponins [R2,R14].

MEDICINAL AND OTHER USE: Astringent; used in menorrhagia and diarrhoea as a decoction, and internally as an application in ulcerated conditions of the mouth and throat [R1]. Amaranth is used more often as a colouring for food and medicines. Reports of teratogenicity and carcinogenicity have not been adequately substantiated and Amaranth is presumed to be safe at present. The plant has a long history of use as a pigment for decorative purposes.

AMMONIACUM
DOREMA AMMONIACUM D. DON AND OTHER SPP.
Fam. Apicaeae

SYNONYMS: Gum Ammoniacum.

HABITAT: From the Middle East to northern Russia.

DESCRIPTION: The gum-resin occurs in rounded nodules or, rarely, compacted into masses, which are opaque, whitish becoming brown with age, with a glossy fracture and an acrid taste. It forms an emulsion with water, which is turned orange-red with chlorinated lime.

PART USED: Gum-resin from the flowering and fruiting stems.

CONSTITUENTS: (i) Resin (60–70%), consisting mainly of ammo-resinol (ii) Gum, composed of water soluble polysaccharides (iii) Volatile oil, about 0.5%, containing ferulene as the major component, with linalyl acetate, citronellyl acetate, ferulene, doremyl alcohol and doremone (iv) Free salicylic acid (v) Coumarins; not including umbelliferone which should be absent [R2,R15,1].

MEDICINAL USE: Antispasmodic, expectorant, diaphoretic [R1]. It is useful in chronic conditions of the respiratory tract, in coughs, asthma, bronchitis and catarrh.

SPECIFIC REFERENCES: 1. Ashraf M et al (1977) Pak. J. Sci. Ind. Res. 23(1–2).

ANGELICA
ANGELICA ARCHANGELICA L.
Fam. Apiaceae

SYNONYMS: European Angelica, Angelica officinalis Moench and Hoffm.

HABITAT: Angelica is a common garden plant, and grows wild in many European countries. It flowers in June–July.

DESCRIPTION: The plant grows to a height of up to 2 m, with broad, pointed, serrated leaves which are larger at the base of the plant. The stalk is cylindrical and hollow, and green in colour. The flowers are small and greenish-white, arranged in large, almost spherical umbels. The fruits are whitish, piano-convex, oblong with rounded ends, about 0.5 cm long and 0.25 cm wide, winged at the margins, with three longitudinal ridges on the convex and two on the flat side. The root in commerce is 5–10 cm long, 2–5 cm in diameter, and very hard and fibrous. The fresh root when cut yields a thick yellowish juice. The transverse section shows a brown bark and white inside, with numerous oil cells in the bark. American Angelica is *A. atropurpurea*, which has similar properties and a purplish root.

PART USED: Root, seeds and leaves.

CONSTITUENTS: (i) Volatile oil, obtained mainly from the root and seeds; this has a similar composition, consisting of monoterpenes, mainly alpha-phellandrene, alpha-bisabolene, alpha-caryophyllene, alpha- and beta-pinene, limonene, linalool, borneol, acetaldehyde, menthadienes and nitromenthadienes (ii) Macrocyclic lactones including tridecanolide, 12-methyl-tridecanolide, pentadecanolide (iii) Phthalates such as hexamethylphthalate (iv) Coumarins, especially furocoumarin glycosides such as marmesin, apterin and their dihydro- and hydroxyderivatives; angelicin and byakangelicin derivatives, osthol, umbelliferone, psoralen, bergapten, imperatoren, xanthotoxol, xanthotoxin, oxypeucedanin and more (v) Miscellaneous sugars, plant acids, flavonoids such as archangelenone, and sterols [R2,R7,R9;1,2,3,4].

MEDICINAL USE: Appetite stimulant (in anorexia nervosa), carminative in flatulent dyspepsia, expectorant in respiratory catarrh, anti-asthmatic, diaphoretic, and diuretic [R1]. It has been used to treat coughs and colds as well as indigestion and many other ailments. The spasmolytic activity has been confirmed in isolated ileum preparations [4] and the root also has anti-mutagenic [5] and calcium channel blocking activity [6]. The dry extract has been shown to have anti-inflammatory activity, and the root oil is reported to inhibit bacterial and fungal growth. Xanthotoxol has anti-nicotinic effects [R2,R7]. Many furocoumarins, notably psoralen and 8-methoxypso-ralen, can cause photosensitivity (or phototoxicity) in sensitive individuals; these substances are used in the photochemotherapy of psoriasis and vitiligo. Their biological activity is due to covalent linkages formed with DNA by irradiation with long-wavelength UV light. The coumarins also inhibit cycloxygenase-1 (COX-1) and lipoxygenase enzymes, suggesting anti-inflammatory properties [3]. Angelica is used frequently as a flavouring ingredient in liqueurs such as Chartreuse and Benedictine, in gin and vermouth; the leaves as a garnish or in salads, and the candied stalks in cakes and puddings.

PREPARATIONS: Root, dose: up to 4.5 g daily; or equivalent as extract. Herb, dose: 2–4 g daily.

SPECIFIC REFERENCES: 1. Czygan F-C *et al* (1998) Z. *Phytother.*

19:342. 2. Holm Y *et al* (1997) *Flav. Frag. J.* 12:397. 3. Roos G *et al* (1997) *Pharm. Pharmacol. Lett.* 7:157. 4. Izzo A *et al* (1996) *Phytother. Res.* 10:S107. 5. Salikhova R *et al* (1993) *Bull. Eksp. Biol. Med.* 115(4):371. 6. Harmala P *et al* (1992) *Planta Med.* 58(2):176 and 287.

ANGELICA, CHINESE
ANGELICA SINENSIS L.
Fam. Apiaceae

SYNONYMS: Dong Quai, Danggui.

HABITAT: Angelica is indigenous to China and eastern Asia, found in damp meadows, ravines and coastal areas. It flowers in May to August. Closely related species are common throughout the temperate regions of the world.

DESCRIPTION: A perennial reaching a height of up to 2.5 m. The leaves are large and tripinnate, the leaflets ovate and serrated. The stalks and petioles are cylindrical, grooved and hollow. The flowers are small and greenish-white or yellow, arranged in umbels. The fruits are up to 7 mm long, elliptic and winged. The rhizome is fleshy, short, with fibrous roots, and a sweetish, tangy, aromatic odour and taste.

PART USED: Rhizome, root.

CONSTITUENTS: (i) Phthalates such as ligustilide, angelicide, neph-thalide, butylphthalide and others (ii) Coumarins, including bergapten and 6-methoxy-7-hydroxycoumarin (iii) Volatile oil, containing safrole, isosafrole, carvacrol, verbenone, copaene and others (v) Angelica polysaccharides, brefeldin A, ferulic acid, beta-sitosterol [R5,R13].

MEDICINAL USE: Hormone regulator, but considered to be without hormonal or phytoestrogenic activity itself. It is widely used to treat female complaints such as painful or suppressed menstruation, uterine bleeding and hot flushes (= flashes) associated with the menopause, as well as premenstrual syndrome and mastalgia. It also has antispasmodic, anti-asthmatic, anti-thrombotic, anti-arrhythmic and aphrodisiac activities; and the polysaccharide fraction is immunostimulant and gastroprotective in animals [R2,R5,R17;1,2,3]. The traditional use in the treatment of vitiligo was not substantiated by a melanocyte-stimulating effect, in fact a cytotoxic effect was found *in vitro* instead [4]. Cardioprotective effects were observed in a model of myocardial ischaemia [5] and modulation of migration and proliferation of gastric epithelial cells has been described [6]. Dong quai is generally considered safe although interactions with warfarin may occur [7].

PREPARATIONS AND DOSE: Root, dose: up to 4 g daily, or equivalent as extract.

SPECIFIC REFERENCES: 1. Qi-bing M *et al* (1991) *Chin. Med. J.* 104:776. 2. Choy Y *et al* (1994) *Am. J. Chin. Med.* 22(2):137. 3. Cho C *et al* (2000) *Planta Med.* 66(4):348. 4. Raman A *et al* (1996) *J. Ethnopharmacol.* 54(2–3):165. 5. Chen S *et al* (1995) *Chung Kuo*

Chung Hsi I Chieh Ho Tsa Chih 15(8):486. 6. Ye Y *et al* (2001) *Life Sci.* 68(8):961. 7. Page R *et al* (1999) *Pharmacother.* 19:870.

ANGOSTURA

GALIPEA OFFICINALIS HAN.
Fam. Rutaceae

SYNONYMS: Cusparia Bark, *Cusparia febrifuga*, D.C., *Bonplandia trifoliata* W., *Galipea cusparia* St. Hill. Other species, including *Cusparia trifoliata* Eng. are also used, and may also be called Angostura.

HABITAT: Indigenous to Venezuela, with other species growing in other parts of South America.

DESCRIPTION: The bark is slightly curved or quilled, in pieces about 3 mm thick, with thin laminae on the inner surface, yellowish-grey externally, outer layer sometimes soft and spongy. Transverse section dark brown. Taste: bitter; odour: musty.

PART USED: Bark.

CONSTITUENTS: (i) Bitter principles, known as Angostura bitters I and II, which are unstable glucopyranosyl-cyclopentane derivatives (ii) Quinoline alkaloids, including cusparine, allocusparine, cuspareine, galipine, galipoline, galipolidine, galipidine, quinaldine and others (iii) Volatile oil, about 1–2%, containing galipene and cadinene [R2;1,2].

MEDICINAL USE: Aromatic bitter, tonic, stimulant, and in large doses cathartic and emetic [R1]. It has been used as an anti-diarrhoeal and febrifuge. The alkaloids have been demonstrated to have antispasmodic properties, and are known to be anti-mycobacterial, antiprotozoal and molluscicidal [2,3]. The mixer-drink 'Angostura Bitters' no longer contains Angostura, but is made from Gentian and other bitter herbs.

SPECIFIC REFERENCES: 1. Brieskorn C *et al* (1971) *Phytochemistry* 10:3205. 2. Houghton P *et al* (1999) *Planta Med.* 65(3):250. 3. Gantier J *et al* (1996) *Planta Med.* 62:285.

ANISEED

PIMPINELLA ANISUM L.
Fam. Apiaceae

SYNONYMS: Anise, *Anisum vulgare* Gaertn. *A. officinarum* Moench.

HABITAT: Originally from Egypt and Asia Minor but now widely cultivated in many warmer climates.

DESCRIPTION: Aniseed is an annual herb reaching about 0.5 m. The fruits, sometimes called 'seeds', are greyish or brownish-grey, ovate, hairy and up to 5 mm long with 10 crenate ribs, often with part of the stalk attached. Taste: sweet; odour: characteristic.

PART USED: Fruit.

CONSTITUENTS: (i) Volatile oil, 1–4%, consisting of mainly trans-anethole (70–90%), with estragole (methylchavicol), anise ketone, anisic acid, alpha-caryophyllene, linalool, anisaldehyde, dianethole and photoanethole (polymers of anethole) (ii) Coumarins, such as bergapten, umbelliferone, scopoletin, umbelliprenone (iii) Flavonoid glycosides including rutin, isovitexin and quercetin-, luteolin-, and apigenin-glycosides (iv) Phenylpropanoids, including 1-propenyl-2-hydroxy-5-methoxy-benzene-2-(2-methyl-butyrate) (v) Miscellaneous; lipids, fatty acids, sterols, proteins and carbohydrates [R2,R3,R7,R9].

MEDICINAL USE: Carminative and expectorant, in cough mixtures and lozenges [R1], and as a flavouring and spice. Aniseed has been demonstrated to increase the mucociliary transport *in vitro*, thus supporting its use as an expectorant, and to significantly increase liver regeneration in rats. It has mild oestrogenic effects, thought to be due to the presence of dianethole and photoanethole, which explains the use of this plant in folk medicine to increase milk secretion, facilitate birth and increase libido. Anethole is known to antagonise dopamine receptors, and therefore possibly increase prolactin secretion, and it has anti-inflammatory and anti-carcinogenic effects thought to be due to inhibition of TNF (tumour necrosis factor)-induced cellular responses [R2,R7;1,2,3]. It is generally considered non-toxic [4]. The essential oil exerts anticonvulsant effects in mice and has a relaxant effect on isolated guinea pig trachea [5,6].

PREPARATIONS AND DOSE: Anise Oil BP, dose: 0.05–0.2 ml, Conc. Anise Water BPC, dose: 0.3–1 ml.

BIBLICAL REFERENCES: Matthew 23:23.

SPECIFIC REFERENCES: 1. Mueller-Limmroth W *et al* (1980) *Fortschr. Med.* 98(3):95. 2. Albert-Puleo M (1980) *J. Ethnopharmacol.* 2:337. 3. Chainy G *et al* (2000) *Oncogene* 25:294. 4. Newberne P *et al* (1999) *Food Chem. Toxicol.* 37:789. 5. Pourgholami M *et al* (1999) *J. Ethnopharmacol.* 66(2):211. 6. Boskabady M *et al* (2001) *J. Ethnopharmacol.* 74(1):83.

ANNATTO
BIXA ORELLANA L.
Fam. Bixaceae

SYNONYMS: Annotta, Arnotta, Orellana, Orleana.

HABITAT: Tropical America and cultivated elsewhere.

DESCRIPTION: Commercial product occurs in small circular cakes or cylindrical rolls.

PART USED: Pulp of seeds.

CONSTITUENTS: Carotenoids known as bixins, e.g. trans-bixin and norbixin [R14].

MEDICINAL USE: A traditional remedy for diabetes [R1] especially in the West Indies, but the carotenoids are orange-yellow pigments mainly used as natural colourings for foods, including fish fingers,

23

medicines, fabrics and – reputedly – to dye maggots for fishing, to make them more tempting! The bixins do not possess vitamin A activity, despite being carotenoids. The hypoglycaemic activity has been confirmed experimentally and attributed to trans-bixin [1].

SPECIFIC REFERENCES: 1. Morrison E *et al* (1991) *Trop. Geogr. Med.* 43(1–2) 184.

ARACHIS
ARACHIS HYPOGAEA L.
Fam. Fabaceae

SYNONYMS: Groundnuts, Monkey Nuts, Peanuts.

HABITAT: Tropical Africa, cultivated elsewhere.

DESCRIPTION: The lower flowers develop the fruit (peanuts) which 'bury' themselves in the earth to ripen. They have a well-known, characteristic appearance.

PART USED: Nuts, and oil expressed from the nuts.

CONSTITUENTS: (i) Fixed oil, about 45%, consisting mainly of glycerides of oleic and linoleic acids (ii) Vitamins E, B_1, B_2, and B_3 (iv) Bioflavonoids, in the skins (v) Tannins [R4,R14].

MEDICINAL USE: The oil is an ingredient of emollient creams and bath oils. However its main use is as a food and cooking oil. Peanuts are dangerously allergenic to some individuals.

PREPARATIONS: Arachis Oil BP.

ARBUTUS, TRAILING
EPIGAEA REPENS L.
Fam. Ericaceae

SYNONYMS: Gravel Plant, Ground Laurel, Mountain Pink, Water Pink.

HABITAT: North America.

DESCRIPTION: Leaves broadly ovate, 2.5–4 cm long and about 2 cm broad, leathery, reticulated, with a cordate base and short pointed apex, and short hairs on undersurface.

PART USED: Herb.

CONSTITUENTS: (i) Hydroquinone derivative such as arbutin (ii) Triterpenes based on ursolic acid (iii) Miscellaneous; ericoline, tannins [R4].

MEDICINAL USE: Diuretic, astringent [R1]. Used for urinary tract conditions in the same way as Uva-Ursi and Buchu (q.v.).

ARCHANGEL
LAMIUM ALBUM L.
Fam. Lamiaceae

SYNONYMS: White Deadnettle.

HABITAT: A common wild plant in temperate regions, flowering in early spring and summer.

DESCRIPTION: Stem quadrangular, hairy; leaves opposite, with cordate base, acuminate apex, coarsely serrate, similar to those of the Nettle (q.v.). Flowers; large, white, tubular, two-lipped with two long and two short stamens. Taste: slightly bitter; odour: none.

PART USED: Herb.

CONSTITUENTS: (i) Phenylpropanoids such as lamalboside and acteoside (ii) Iridoids including albosides A and B, lamalbide and caryoptoside (iii)Tannins, mainly catechins (iv) Amines, including histamine, tyramine, choline and methylamine (v) Flavonoids such as tiliroside, quercetin and rutoside (vi) Triterpene saponins (vii) Chlorogenic and rosmarinic acids (viii) An alkaloid, lamiine [R2,R4;1,2].

MEDICINAL USE: Astringent and haemostatic, particularly on the uterus, it has been used for menorrhagia and leucorrhoea [R1]. Other uses are as for Nettle (q.v.).

SPECIFIC REFERENCES: 1. Damtoft S (1992) *Phytochemistry* 31(1):172. 2. Budzianowski J *et al* (1995) *Phytochemistry* 38(4):997.

ARECA NUT
ARECA CATECHU L.
Fam. Arecaceae

SYNONYMS: Betel Nut.

HABITAT: Tropical India, Sri Lanka, Malaysia, Indonesia, the Philippines and parts of East Africa.

DESCRIPTION: The seeds are conical or nearly spherical, about 2.5 cm in diameter, very hard, and with a deep brown testa showing fawn marbling. Taste: slightly acrid, astringent; odour: faint.

PART USED: Seed.

CONSTITUENTS: (i) Pyridine alkaloids, mainly arecoline (0.1–0.5%), with arecaine, guvacine and others (ii) Phlobaphene tannins [R2].

MEDICINAL USE: Previously used as a taenicide in veterinary medicine, to expel tapeworms. It is also astringent, and promotes the flow of saliva, and is used in eastern countries as a masticatory and stimulant [R1]. Due to the increased incidence of some types of oral cancer associated with Betel chewing, this habit is being discouraged. It also appears to cause hyperglycaemia and bronchoconstriction, and the extract has antidepressant effects in an animal model. Arecoline is thought to be the cytotoxic agent and also has parasympathomimetic activity, leading to tachycardia, hypotension, sweating, colic and nausea [1,2,3,4,5,6].

SPECIFIC REFERENCES: 1.Wu M *et al* (2001) *Br. J. Cancer* 85(5):658. 2. Phukan R *et al* (2001) *Br. J. Cancer* 85(5):661. 3. Deng J *et al* (2001) *J. Toxicol. Clin. Toxicol.* 39(4):355. 4. Mannan N *et al* (2000) *J. Nutr.* 83(3):267. 5. Jeng J *et al* (2000) *Carcinogenesis* 21(7):1365. 6. Dar A *et al* (2000) *Pharmacol. Biochem. Behav.* 65(1):1.

ARENARIA RUBRA
SPERGULARIA RUBRA (L.) J & C PRESL.
Fam. Caryophyllaceae

SYNONYMS: Sandwort, Sabline Rouge, S. *rubra* Pers., *Lepigonum rubrum*, Fries., *Tissa rubra* Adans, *Buda rubra* Dum., *Arenaria purpurea* L.

HABITAT: Southern Europe, especially France and Malta, naturalized in North America.

DESCRIPTION: Herb with jointed stems and flat, linear leaves about 1 cm long, with ovate, pointed stipules; flowers small, pink, in spreading panicles. Taste: saline; odour: slightly aromatic.

PART USED: Herb.

CONSTITUENTS: Triterpene glycosides (unspecified). The closely related *Spergularia ramosa* contains oleanane glycosides based on gypsogenin and quillaic acid [R2;1].

MEDICINAL USE: Diuretic; formerly used for diseases of the bladder and venereal disease [R1].

SPECIFIC REFERENCES: 1. De Tommasi N *et al* (1998) *J. Nat. Prod.* 61(3):323.

ARJUNA
TERMINALIA ARJUNA (ROXB.) WIGHT. AND ARN.
Fam. Combretaceae

SYNONYMS: Arjun Myrobalan, *Terminalia cuneata* Roth.

HABITAT: Native to northern Asia, along riversides and streams; cultivated widely elsewhere.

DESCRIPTION: A large evergreen tree, with buttressed trunk and drooping branches. The bark is smooth, pinkish-grey, exfoliating in large thin sheets. The leaves are large and elliptical, the flowers cup-shaped, in spikes, and the fruits are ovoid, up to 5 cm long, glabrous and winged.

PART USED: Bark, occasionally the fruit.

CONSTITUENTS: (i) Triterpenes, the arjunosides I-IV, arjunin, arjunetic, friedelin, arjunctine, arjunic, arjunolic and oleanolic acids, and others (ii) Flavonoids such as arjunolone and arjunone (iii) Polyphenols including gallocatechol, epigallocatechol, catechol [R16;1].

MEDICINAL USE: Traditionally used for heart problems, such as coronary artery disease, congestive heart failure, angina and others, Arjuna is a very important herb in Indian medicine. It is considered sacred and is an important constituent of many herbal formulae in Ayurveda. It has also been used for liver and urogenital diseases and as an antidote to poisoning and to treat infections and staunch bleeding. The powdered bark is mixed with honey for bilious disorders and dysentery, and a decoction used topically to treat ulcers and wounds.

Many of the cardiovascular effects have been confirmed, both pharmacologically in isolated heart preparations, and clinically in heart disease. Anti-arrhythmic activity and a reduction in the number of angina attacks were demonstrated [2,3,4]. Hypotensive and hypocholesterolaemic activity have also been shown [5,6], and antibacterial and antiviral activity against HIV-1 shown *in vitro*, thought to be due to inhibition of HIV-1 protease [7]. The hepatoprotective effect may be mediated via suppression of surface hepatitis B antigen [8].

PREPARATIONS AND DOSE: Powdered bark, dose: 1–3 g or equivalent extract.

SPECIFIC REFERENCES: 1. Dwivedi S *et al* (1989) *Fitoterapia.* 60:413. 2. Radhakrishnan R *et al* (1993) *Phytother. Res.* 7(3):266. 3. Gauthaman K *et al* (2001) *J. Ethnopharmacol.* 75(203):197. 4. Bharani A *et al* (1995) *Int. J. Cardiol.* 49:191. 5. Ram A *et al* (1997) *J. Ethnopharmacol.* 55(3):165. 6. Takahashi S *et al* (1997) *Phytother. Res.* 11(6):424. 7. Ines K *et al* (1995) *Phytother. Res.* 9(3):180. 8. Goto W *et al* (1996) *Phytother. Res.* 10(6):504.

ARNICA

ARNICA MONTANA L.
Fam. Asteraceae

SYNONYMS: Leopard's Bane, European Arnica, Mountain Tobacco.

HABITAT: Native to Europe, from Scandinavia to southern Russia, and central Asia, cultivated elsewhere.

DESCRIPTION: An herbaceous perennial reaching 50 cm, with the leaves in basal rosettes. The terminal flower occurs in the leaf axils of the upper leaf pair. Flower-heads 6–8 cm in diameter, with 10–20 ray florets and up to 100 tubular disc florets, which are bright yellow. The epicalyx and receptacle are hairy.

PART USED: Flowers, occasionally the rhizome.

CONSTITUENTS: (i) Sesquiterpene lactones, including the pseudoguanolides arnifolin, the arnicolides, helenalin and related compounds (ii) Flavonoids such as eupafolin, patuletin, spinacetin, laciniatin, betuletol and hispidulin (iii) Volatile oil, containing thymol and various ethers of thymol (iv) Mucilage and polysaccharides (v) Labdane diterpenes: e.g. labd-13-ene-8-alpha-15-diol (vi) Miscellaneous; resins, bitters (arnicin), tannins, carotenes [R2,R7;1,2,3].

MEDICINAL USE: Anti-inflammatory, analgesic and aid to wound-healing, particularly bruising and muscle pain [R1]. Arnica is usually applied topically rather than internally since it is toxic in high doses, as well as being irritating to mucous membranes. Arnica is an immunostimulant; both helenalin (in high dilutions) and the polysaccharide fraction stimulate phagocytosis *in vitro* when measured by Brandt's granulocyte test. Many sesquiterpene lactones have cytotoxic and anti-inflammatory activity, and their biological effects appear to be mediated through immunological processes.

Helenalin is one of the most active, which would account for the use of Arnica for pain and inflammation. It also has anti-platelet activity, anti-microbial effects and inhibits the rate of lipid peroxidation *in vitro*. [R2,R7,R8,R9,R17;4,5,6,7,8,9].

PREPARATIONS: Arnica Flower Tincture BPC 1949, Arnica Cream.

SPECIFIC REFERENCES: 1. Merfort I (1985) *Planta Med.* 51:136. 2. Merfort I *et al* (1988) *Planta Med.* 54:247. 3. Schmidt T *et al* (1992) *Planta Med.* 58:A713. 4. Puhlmann *et al* (1989) *Planta Med.* 55:99. 5. Lyss G *et al* (1997) *Biol. Chem.* 378:951. 6. Schroder H *et al* (1990) *Thromb. Res.* 57(6):839. 7. Iamemii I *et al* (1998) *Ukr. Biokhim. Zh.* 70(2):78. 8. Woerdenbag H *et al* (1994) *Planta Med.* 60(5):434. 9. Woerdenbag H *et al* (1995) *Phytomedicine* 2(2):434.

ARRACH
CHENOPODIUM VULVARIA L. CURT
Fam. Chenopodiaceae

SYNONYMS: Stinking Arrach, Goosefoot, Dog's Arrach, Goat's Arrach, *Chenopodium olidum* S. Wats.

HABITAT: A European wild plant growing mostly on waste ground, flowering in June and July.

DESCRIPTION: Leaves oval, stalked, about 1 cm long, with entire margin and powdery surface. Odour: strong, fishy.

PART USED: Herb.

CONSTITUENTS: (i) Trimethylamine (in the fresh plant) (ii) Miscellaneous; betaine, tannins [R2,R4].

MEDICINAL USE: Used internally and externally as a spasmolytic to relieve cramps, and as a nervine and emmenagogue. Betaine has been found to improve the degree of steatosis and fibrosis in patients with non-alcoholic steatohepatitis and has been used in the treatment of homocystinuria [R14,1].

SPECIFIC REFERENCES: 1. Abdelmalek F *et al* (2001) *Am. J. Gastroenterol.* 96(9):2711.

ARROWROOT
MARANTA ARUNDINACEAE L.
Fam. Marantaceae

SYNONYMS: Bermuda Arrowroot, Maranta.

HABITAT: Tropical America and the West Indies.

DESCRIPTION: Arrowroot is prepared from the rhizomes of this herbaceous plant, to form a white powder consisting of mainly starch. The grains are about 30–40 μm in diameter, with an irregular oval shape and a visible hilum near the middle.

PART USED: Starch.

CONSTITUENTS: The rhizome contains about 25–27% neutral starch.

MEDICINAL USE: Demulcent, nutritive especially for infants and convalescence [R1]. Usually prepared by boiling in sufficient water to make a thin gruel, which may be flavoured if required.

ARTICHOKE
CYNARA SCOLYMUS L.
Fam. Asteraceae

SYNONYMS: Globe Artichoke, Bur Artichoke, *Cynara cardunculus* Moris.

HABITAT: Indigenous to the Mediterranean region but widely cultivated as a garden vegetable.

DESCRIPTION: A perennial reaching 2 m high, with a characteristic, thistle-like, large globose flower, with overlapping fleshy bracts tapering to a greenish or purplish tip. The petals are bluish-white. Leaves pinnate, prickly, with a glabrous upper surface and grey, pubescent lower suface.

PART USED: Leaf. The flower is used as a vegetable.

CONSTITUENTS: (i) Sesquiterpene lactones, up to 4%, including cynaropicrin, dehydrocynaropicrin, cynaratriol and grossheimin (ii) Caffeic acid derivatives; chlorogenic, neochlorogenic, cryptochlorogenic acid and cynarin (an artefact formed during processing) (iii) Flavonoids; cynaroside, scolymoside and cynarotrioside (iv) Volatile oil containing alpha-selinene, caryophyllene, and eugenol [R2,R7;1,2].

MEDICINAL USE: Choleretic, digestive, anti-emetic, liver protectant, hypolipidaemic, antispasmodic and antioxidant. Traditionally the leaf was used for hepatitis, dropsy, to reduce sweating, and as an aphrodisiac. Artichoke leaf extract is now frequently used to treat dyspepsia, irritable bowel syndrome, liver disorders and certain cardiovascular disorders, especially atherosclerosis. Many of these effects have now been confirmed both pharmacologically and clinically. The leaf extract is known to lower cholesterol and lipid levels in animals, inhibit cholesterol synthesis, protect against experimental liver damage, and show antioxidant effects. Recent clinical studies in human patients have shown that the leaf extract increases bile secretion, lowers blood cholesterol, and has demonstrable efficacy in irritable bowel syndrome and dyspepsia [R2,R7,R8,R17;3,4,5,6,7,8,9].

PREPARATIONS AND DOSE: Extract, dose: usually 640 mg, three times daily with meals.

SPECIFIC REFERENCES: 1. Hammouda F *et al* (1993) *Int. J. Pharmacog.* 31:299. 2. Adzet T *et al* (1987) *J. Nat. Prod.* 50:612. 3. Walker A *et al* (2001) *Phytother. Res.* 15(1):58. 4. Fintelmann V *et al* (1996) *Dtsch. Apot. Ztg.* 136:1405. 5. Fintelmann V *et al* (1998) *Natural Med.* 13:17. 6. Kirchhoff R *et al* (1994) *Phytomedicine* 1(2):107. 7. Kraft K (1997) *Phytomedicine* 4(4):369. 8. Englisch W *et al* (2000) *Arzneim. Forsch.* 50:260. 9. Perez-Garcia F *et al* (2000) *Free Rad. Res.* 33:661. 10. Gebhardt R (1997) *Toxicol. Appl. Pharmacol.*144:279.

ASAFETIDA
FERULA ASSA-FOETIDA L.
FERULA RUBICAULIS BOISS. AND OTHER SPP.
Fam. Apiaceae

SYNONYMS: Gum Asafoetida, Devil's Dung.

HABITAT: Native to south-western Asia, particularly Iran and Afghanistan.

DESCRIPTION: The gum-resin is obtained by incising the roots, which contain a foetid juice. This solidifies to a brownish resin, sometimes with a pinkish tint, in sticky lumps with a pungent, acrid, persistent, alliaceous odour.

PART USED: Oleo-gum-resin.

CONSTITUENTS: (i) Resins, about 40–60%, consisting of asaresinotannols, and their esters, farnesiferols, ferulic acid and other acids (ii) Gum, about 25% composed of polymers of glucose, galactose, L-arabinose, rhamnose and glucuronic acid (iii) Volatile oil, about 6–17%, consisting of polysulphides such as diallyl- and allylpropylsulphides, 2-butylmethyl-, di-, tri-, and tetra-sulphides, propenyl sulphides, sulphated terpenes, pinene, cadinene and vanillin (iv) Coumarins such as assafoetidin, umbelliferone, foetidin, ferocolicin, farnesifol C, gummosin, coniferol, acetylepisamarcadin and umbelliprenin [R2,R7;1,2,3].

MEDICINAL USE: Antispasmodic, expectorant, carminative [R1]. It has been used for nervous disorders as well as for coughs, bronchitis and flatulence. Reports also suggest a hypotensive and anticoagulant effect, similar to that of Garlic (q.v.), and an inhibition of experimental carcinogenesis [4,5,6]. It is mainly used as a flavouring ingredient in Gujerati cooking and for example, in Worcester sauce. It is reputedly non-toxic in doses normally consumed in foods [R7] but is not considered suitable for infants [7].

SPECIFIC REFERENCES: 1. Banerji A *et al* (1988) *Tet. Lett.* 29(3):1557. 2. Nassar M *et al* (1995) *Pharmazie* 50(11):766. 3. Nassar M *et al* (1998) *Fitoterapia* 69(1):41. 4. Buddrus J *et al* (1985) *Phytochemistry* 24(4):869. 5. Kajimoto T *et al* (1989) *Phytochemistry* 28:1761. 6. Unnikrishnan M *et al* (1990) *Cancer Lett.* 51(1)85. 7. Kelly K *et al* (1984) *Paediatrics* 73:717.

ASARABACCA
ASARUM EUROPEAUM L.
Fam. Aristolochiaceae

SYNONYMS: Hazelwort, Wild Nard, *Nardum rusticanum.*

HABITAT: Grows wild in woods in Europe and the Russia, and is cultivated as a garden plant in Britain and America.

DESCRIPTION: A herbaceous perennial, with kidney-shaped, leathery, evergreen leaves; solitary, bell-shaped flowers, with three segments, purplish inside. The rhizome is slender, about 2 mm thick, quadrangular and tortuous, with rootlets at intervals and stem scars on the upper surface.

PART USED: Herb, rhizome.

CONSTITUENTS: (i) Volatile oil, consisting of up to 70% alpha-asarone, with asaraldehyde, methyleugenol, bornyl acetate, trans-isoelemicin and sesquiterpenes (ii) Lipids; including aliphatic alcohols such as n-dodecanol and analogues, alicyclic alcohols, higher aliphatic acids including *n*-hexadecylic and octodecatrienic acids (iii) Caffeic acid derivatives (chlorogenic, etc.), (iv) flavonoids [R2,R4;1,2,3].

MEDICINAL USE: Emetic, purgative, stimulant in small doses. Has been used as an errhine (snuff) in headache; the powder produces intense irritation and mucus flow, which is said to relieve the headache! The root is said to have non-specific immunostimulatory activity *in vitro*, and a product containing the extract was shown to have anti-asthmatic activity in a trial of 90 patients [R2;1,2,3,4]. Alpha-asarone has hypolipidemic activity and anti-thrombotic effects in mice [5,6]. Although not thought to be as toxic as beta-asarone, anti-fertility and teratogenic effects have been observed in rats [7].

SPECIFIC REFERENCES: 1. Gracza L (1987) *Pharmazie* 42(2):141. 2. Gracza L (1980) *Arzneim. Forsch.* 30:767. 3. Gracza L (1991) *Acta Pharm. Hung.* 61(2):86. 4. Rosch A (1984) *Z. Phytother.* 5(6):964. 5. Garduno L *et al* (1997) *J. Ethnopharmacol.* 55(2):161. 6. Poplawski J *et al* (2000) *J. Med. Chem.* 43(20):3671. 7. Jimenez L *et al* (1988) *Ann. Pharm. Francais* 46(3):179.

ASH

FRAXINUS EXELSIOR L.
Fam. Oleaceae

SYNONYMS: Common, European or Weeping Ash.

HABITAT: Great Britain, Europe and North America.

DESCRIPTION: The ash tree is well known, deriving its name from the leaves and bark which are ash-coloured. The bark occurs in thin, greenish-grey pieces about 2 mm thick, with longitudinal furrows and a pale brown inner surface. Taste: faintly bitter; odourless.

PART USED: Bark, leaves.

CONSTITUENTS: (i) Coumarin derivatives including fraxin, fraxetin, fraxidin, fraxinol, isofraxidin, scopoletin (ii) Flavonoids based on aesculetin, including aescin, and others such as rutin and quercetin (iii) Triterpenes including ursolic acid, betulin and betulic acid (iv) Iridoids and secoiridoids such as syringoside, hydroxyligustride and ligstroside (v) Miscellaneous; tannins, sugars, mucilage, volatile oil and resin [R2,R4,1,2,3].

MEDICINAL USE: Laxative, anti-inflammatory, febrifuge; has been used for arthritis and rheumatism [R1]. Anti-inflammatory activity has been confirmed in the rat paw oedema test [4] and the iridoids shown to

31

inhibit complement activation [3]. In a fixed combination with other extracts it has been shown to be anti-rheumatic in human patients [5], and have antioxidant activity [6]. The lipophilic fraction has been found to stimulate phagocytosis in mice inoculated with *Escherichia coli* and an extract has also shown analgesic and anti-exudative effects [7]. The Ash once had a considerable reputation as a cure for snakebite; and as a snake repellent: Pliny is reputed to have said that "if a fire and a serpent be encompassed within a circle of the boughs of an Ash Tree, it will sooner flye into the fire than into them..." [R2;4,5,6].

SPECIFIC REFERENCES: 1. Carnat A *et al* (1990) *Plant. Med. Phytother.* 24:145. 2. Tissut M *et al* (1980) *Phytochemistry* 19:2077. 3. Ivanovska N *et al* (1996) *Phytother. Res.* 10(7):555. 4. El Gazaly M *et al* (1992). *Arzneim. Forsch.* 42(3):333. 5. Klein C (1999) *Wien. Med. Wochenschr.* 149(8-10):248. 6. Schemp H *et al* (2000) *Arzneimitt. Forsch.* 50(4):362. 7. Delaveau P *et al* (1980) *Planta Med.* 40:49.

ASHWAGANDHA
WITHANIA SOMNIFERUM (L.) DUNAL.
Fam. Solanaceae

SYNONYMS: Winter Cherry, *Physalis somnifera* L.

HABITAT: Native to the Mediterranean region, the Middle East, Africa and parts of Asia, growing in stony and semi-arid regions; cultivated widely. It flowers all year round.

DESCRIPTION: A woody shrub, growing from a long tuberous taproot with numerous fibrous roots. The leaves are elliptical with an acute apex, growing in pairs with one larger than the other. The flowers are campanulate, greenish-yellow, in umbellate cymes, and the fruit a red berry enclosed in a papery membrane.

PART USED: Dried root.

CONSTITUENTS: (i) Steroidal lactones, the withanolides A-Y, withaferin A, withasomniferols A-C, and others (ii) Phytosterols including the sitoindosides and others (iii) Alkaloids; ashwagandhine, ashwagandhinine, anahyhygrine, cuscohygrine, withasomnine, withaninine, somniferine and others [R16;1]

MEDICINAL USE: Ashwagandha has been used in Ayurvedic medicine for about 4000 years, as a tonic in debility and for emaciation. It is used to enhance fertility in both men and women and as an aphrodisiac. The name 'Ashwagandha' comes from the Sanskrit 'ashva' meaning horse, and 'gandha', meaning smell, and refers to the odour of the root. The suffix 'somnifera' denotes its sedative properties. It is also widely used for inflammation, colds, asthma and many other disorders, and is considered to be an adaptogen. Many of the effects have been substantiated, both pharmacologically and clinically. The adaptogenic and anti-stress activity was found to be comparable to that of ginseng, and immunomodulatory activity also confirmed. The extract has sedative activity and is reported to be anxiolytic, possibly due to GABA-mimetic activity [R16;1,2,3,4]. Numerous other actions, including antioxidant effects, have been documented [5,6,7], but despite the wealth of information on this herb much of the clinical knowledge is still anecdotal. It does however appear to be safe [R16,R17 and refs therein].

PREPARATIONS AND DOSE: Powdered root, dose: 3–6 g, or equivalent extract.

SPECIFIC REFERENCES: 1. American Herbal Pharmacopoeia 'Ashwagandha'. Ed. Upton R (2000). 2. Karnick C (1991) *Indian Med.* 3(2):1. 3. Bhattacharya S *et al* (1987) *Phytother. Res.* 1(1):32. 4. Mehta A *et al* (1991) *Indian J. Med. Res.* (B) 9:312. 5. Bhattacharya S *et al* (1995) *Phytother. Res.* 9(2):110. 6. Ines K *et al* (1995) *Phytother. Res.* 9(3):180. 7. Goto W *et al* (1996) *Phytother. Res.* 10(6):504.

ASPARAGUS
ASPARAGUS OFFICINALIS L.
Fam. Liliaceae

SYNONYMS: Sparrowgrass.

HABITAT: Native to Europe, North Africa, North America and western Asia, widely cultivated.

DESCRIPTION: Root about 5 cm long, 1–2 cm thick, with a loose, laminate, internal structure. Rootlets long, narrow, compressed; nearly hollow with a central woody cord. Taste: insipid; odourless.

PART USED: Root, herb, the young shoots as food.

CONSTITUENTS: (i) Saponins called asparagosides, at least nine of which have been isolated, and the bitter steroidal glycosides, officinalisnin I and II and aspartic saponin (ii) Asparagusic acid and derivatives (iv) Amino acids including asparagine, arginine and tyrosine (v) Flavonoids, including rutin, kaempferol and quercetin (vi) Polysaccharides, fructans asparagose and asparagosine and inulin [R2;1,2,3].

MEDICINAL USE: Diuretic, laxative, cardiac tonic and sedative [R1]. Has also been used for neuritis and rheumatism, although no clinical or pharmacological work is yet available to support these indications. The crude saponin fraction from the edible shoots has anti-tumour activity against human leukaemia cells *in vitro* [4]. Asparagusic acid has been shown to be nematocidal; this and other sulphur-containing compounds are hydrolysed in the body to form methylmercaptan, which appears in the urine and gives it a characteristic, peculiar smell [R2,R10].

SPECIFIC REFERENCES: 1. Goryanu G *et al* (1976) *Khim. Prir. Soed.* 3:400 and 6:762. 2. Shiomi N *et al* (1976) *Agric. Biol. Chem.* 40:567. 3. Shao Y et al (1997) *Planta Med.* 63:258. 4. Shao Y *et al* (1996) *Cancer Lett.* 104(1):31.

ASPARAGUS, WILD

ASPARAGUS RACEMOSUS WILLD.
Fam. Liliaceae

SYNONYMS: Sparrowgrass, Shatavari.

HABITAT: Grows wild and is cultivated throughout tropical and sub-tropical Asia.

DESCRIPTION: A climber reaching 2 m in height and much branched. The leaves are needle-like soft spines, the flowers numerous, white, minute, fragrant and in racemes. The rootstock is tuberous, and bears many tuberous roots up to 1 m long. The stem is woody and armed with sharp spines. Taste: insipid; odourless.

PART USED: Root, leaves.

Constituents: (i) Steroidal glycosides called shatavarins I-IV, and saponins based on sarosapogenin, arasapogenin and diosgenin (ii) Asparagamine, and alkaloid in the root (iii) Flavonoids, including rutin, hyperoside and quercetin [R16,1,2].

MEDICINAL USE: Traditionally used to promote milk secretion and as a tonic, aphrodisiac and to enhance fertility. It is also used for debility, impotence, dyspepsia and diarrhoea. Shatavari is considered to be an important 'Rasayana' (balancing and rejuvenating herb) in Ayurvedic medicine and the name means 'she who possesses a hundred husbands', referring to its beneficial effects on the female reproductive organs. It has adaptogenic and immunomodulatory activity in experimental conditions [3,4] and a small clinical study demonstrated efficacy in treating gastric ulceration [R16] and reducing gastric emptying time [5]. Other documented effects include antibacterial activity and anti-tussive effects [6,7] and the lactation promoting effects have been shown in buffaloes and rats [R16].

PREPARATIONS AND DOSE: Powdered root, dose: 20–30 g daily, or equivalent extract.

SPECIFIC REFERENCES: 1. Singh J et al (1991) J. Indian Chem. Soc. 68(7):427. 2. Sekirne T et al (1994) Chem. Pharm. Bull. 42(6):1360. 3. Rege N et al (1999) Phytother. Res. 13(4):275. 4. Thatte U et al (1987) Indian Drugs 25(3):95. 5. Dalvi S et al (1990) Postgrad. Med. J. 36(2):91. 6. Mandal S et al (2000) Phytother. Res. 14(2):118. 7. Mandal S et al (2000) Fitoterapia 71(6):686.

ASTRAGALUS

ASTRAGALUS MEMBRANACEUS (FISCH.) BGE.
A. MEMBRANACEUS (FISCH.) BGE. VAR
MONGHOLICUS (BGE.) HSIAO
Fam. Fabaceae

SYNONYMS: Huang qi.

HABITAT: Native to north-eastern China, central Mongolia and Siberia.

DESCRIPTION: A herbaceous perennial reaching 1 m, arising from a taproot. Leaves typically fabaceous, compound pinnate, the leaflets in 18–20 pairs. Flowers dark yellow, campanulate; fruit a legume up to 13 mm long containing dark brown kidney-shaped seeds. The root consists of a long cylindrical taproot, which is internally yellowish in colour and normally found cut in commerce. Rootlets long, twisted, absent from high quality samples.

PART USED: Root.

CONSTITUENTS: (i) Triterpenoid saponins, the astragalosides I-VIII, and their acetyl derivatives, agroastragalosides I-IV, astramembranins I and II and others (ii) Isoflavones, including formononetin and kumatakenin (iii) Polysaccharides known as astragaloglucans [R5;1,2,3,4].

MEDICINAL USE: The use of Astragalus dates back to the legendary Chinese emperor Shen-Nong, who is considered to be the founder of agriculture and even civilization itself. It is important as a general tonic and adaptogen, immunomodulator and is used to treat very many diseases in China. A number of clinical studies confirm its use as an immune stimulant for use in colds and upper respiratory infections, and it is also used as a prophylactic for these same conditions, supported by data from over 1000 patients in China. It is widely used as an adjunctive in the treatment of cancer and appears to potentiate the effects of interferon therapy. Astragalus has antioxidant, hepatoprotective and antiviral activity; and cardio-active effects, mainly relief from angina, have also been found. However the main use is as a general tonic and for immune enhancement. Toxicity does not appear to be a problem. Many clinical and animal studies have been carried out, the results usually published in Chinese, and these are well reviewed in [R17;1].

PREPARATIONS AND DOSE: Powdered root, dose: 9–30 g daily (up to 60 g in serious cases) or equivalent extract.

SPECIFIC REFERENCES: 1. Upton R (Ed.) 'Astragalus' American Herbal Pharmacopoeia. Pub: AHP. Sacramento, US (1999). 2. He Q *et al* (1991) *J. Nat. Prod.* 54(3):810. 3. Toda S *et al* (1998) *Phytother. Res.* 12(1):59. 4. Tomoda M *et al* (1992) *Phytochemistry* 31(1):63.

AVENS
GEUM URBANUM L.
Fam. Rosaceae

SYNONYMS: Colewort, Herb Bennet, Benedict's Herb, *Radix caryophyllata.*

HABITAT: A hedgerow plant growing wild in most parts of Europe, including Great Britain, flowering in May or June.

DESCRIPTION: A perennial, erect herb reaching 20–60 cm, with stem leaves occurring as two leaflets and one terminal, toothed lobe; insignificant small yellow flowers occurring in cymes, and distinctive fruits appearing as a brown ball of awned seeds which are covered in hooked bristles.

PART USED: Herb, root.

CONSTITUENTS: (i) Tannins, approximately 15%, consisting of gallotannins and ellagitannins including sanguiin H-6, casuarictin, pendunculagin, potentillin and tellimagrandin (ii) Phenolics such as vicianose and eugenol and sugars [R2,1,2,3].

MEDICINAL USE: Astringent, styptic, tonic, febrifuge, stomachic [R1]. It has also been used for diarrhoea, and leucorrhoea, taken as an infusion, as a gargle for sore throats, and as a bath additive for haemorrhoids. Anti-inflammatory activity has been shown by inhibition of prostaglandin synthesis via cyclooxygenase, and platelet activating factor induced exocytosis *in vitro* [4].

SPECIFIC REFERENCES: 1. Psenak M *et al* (1970) *Planta Med.* 19:154. 2. Vollman C (1991) *Dtsch Apot. Ztg.* 131:2081. 3. Vollman C *et al* (1995) *Dtsch Apot. Ztg.* 135:1238. 4. Tunon H *et al* (1995) *J. Ethnopharmacol.* 48(2):61.

AVOCADO
PERSEA AMERICANUM P. MILL.
Fam. Lauraceae

SYNONYMS: Avocado Pear, Aguacarte.

HABITAT: A native of Mexico now cultivated widely in the tropics and subtropics, particularly South Africa, California, Florida, Australia and South America for its fruit.

DESCRIPTION: A tall tree with straggling branches, with narrow, pointed, dark green leaves arranged spirally, especially at the ends of branches. Flowers greenish-yellow occurring in panicles, giving rise to the distinctive pear-shaped fruits which may be green and smooth, or wrinkled and purplish-brown, with a soft oily flesh and a single large stone.

PART USED: Leaf, fruit.

CONSTITUENTS: Leaf: (i) Essential oil, composed of alpha-terpinene, alpha-cubebene, alpha-pinene, alpha-myrcene, alpha-ocimene, estragole, sabinene and others (ii) Flavonoids such as afzelin, cynaroside, luteolin and quercetin (iii) Tannins and procyanidins. [R12,1]. Fruit: (i) Fatty acids and oils, based on linoleic, linolenic, palmitic, stearic and many others, both saturated and unsaturated (ii) Phenolics such as caffeic, chlorogenic and *p*-coumaric acids (iii) Vitamins, minerals, sterols, amino acids and sugars. The fruit is a rich source of nutrients [R12].

MEDICINAL USE: The fruits are eaten widely and the seed oil is prized for use in cosmetics. The leaf has been used as an abortifacient, emmenagogue, contraceptive, anti-diarrhoeal, anti-hypertensive, and diuretic. Many of these uses have not yet been substantiated. Anti-hypertensive, antiviral and anti-inflammatory activity of the leaf extract has been shown in animals [1,2,3]. The fruit is safe to eat although it may induce allergic reactions in sensitive individuals.

The oil in combination with vitamin B12 has been found to be effective in treating psoriasis [4]. For review see [R12].

SPECIFIC REFERENCES: 1. De Almeida P *et al* (1998) *Phytother. Res.* 12(8):562. 2. Yasukawa K *et al* (1993) *Phytother. Res.* 7(2):185. 3. De A Ribeiro R (1988) *J. Ethnopharmacol.* 24(1):19. 4. Stucker M *et al* (2001) *Dermatology* 203(2):141.

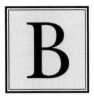

BACOPA MONNIERA

BACOPA MONNIERA L.
Fam. Scrophulariaceae

SYNONYMS: Thyme leaved Gratiola, Brahmi, *Herpestris monniera* (L.) Penn., *Lysimachia monniera* L. *Gratiola monniera* L., *Monniera cunefolia* Michx.

HABITAT: India and many other Asian countries.

DESCRIPTION: A small, glabrous, prostrate herb. The leaves are small, fleshy, sessile and kidney-shaped, the flowers solitary, blue or white with purple veins. Fruits are ovoid capsules within a persistent calyx.

PART USED: Dried whole plant.

CONSTITUENTS: (i) Saponins and triterpenes, based on bacogenins and jujubogenins, and known as bacosides A-C and bacosaponins A-E, hersaponin, monnierin, betulinic acid, bacosine and others [R16;1,2,3,4] (ii) Alkaloids; brahmine and herpestine [R16] (iii) Flavonoids based on luteolin and apigenin [5].

MEDICINAL USE: Traditionally used in India to promote the intellect, and as a nervine, it is an important herb in Ayurveda. It is also used as a bitter, coolant and astringent, and for asthma and bronchitis, and is also given to children with diarrhoea. In combination with Bael (q.v.), a clinical trial alleviated some symptoms of irritable bowel syndrome [6]. An extract significantly improved cognitive processes in human volunteers [7] and also protected against phenytoin-induced cognitive dysfunction in rats [8]. It has been shown to possess antioxidant activity [9], anxiolytic [10], bronchodilatory [11], calcium antagonistic [12] and analgesic effects in animals. For further detail, see [R16].

PREPARATIONS AND DOSE: Dried herb, dose: 5–10 g, or equivalent extract.

SPECIFIC REFERENCES: 1. Mahato S *et al* (2000) *Phytochem.* 53(6):711. 2. Garai S *et al* (1996) *Phytochem.* 43(2):447. 3. Rastogi S *et al* (1994) *Phytochem.* 36(1):133. 4. Chakravarty A *et al* (2001) *Phytochem.* 58(4):553. 5. Proliac A *et al* (1991) *Pharm. Acta Helv.* 66(5–6):153. 6. Yadav S *et al* (1989) *Indian J. Med. Res.* 90:496. 7. Stough C A *et* (2001) *Psychopharmacol.* 156(4):481. 8. Vohora D *et al* (2000) *J. Ethnopharmacol.* 71(3):383. 9. Bhattacharya S *et al* (2000) *Phytother. Res.* 14(3):174. 10. Bhattacharya S *et al* (1998) *Phytomedicine* 5(2):77. 11. Dar A *et al* (1997) *Phytomedicine* 4(4):319. 12. Dar A *et al* (1999) *J. Ethnopharmacol.* 66(2):167.

BAEL

AEGLE MARMELOS CORR.
Fam. Rutaceae

SYNONYMS: Bel, Indian Bael, Bengal Quince.

HABITAT: India and many parts of Southeast Asia.

DESCRIPTION: A medium-sized deciduous tree, armed with sharp spines. The fruits are large, globular or ovoid, with a hard outer coat, and divided internally like an orange. The flesh is reddish, with numerous seeds covered in a gummy layer. Taste: sweet, mucilaginous, slightly acid.

PART USED: Ripe and unripe fruit, fresh and dried, other parts used less frequently.

CONSTITUENTS: Fruit: (i) Coumarins, including xanthotoxol, alloimperatorin, marmesin, marmelide, marmelosin and psoralen (ii) Flavonoids including rutin (iii) Alkaloids including allocryptopine, O-isopentenylhalfordinol and O-methylhalfordinol (iv) Tannic acid [R16;1,2]. Leaf: (i) Alkaloids; aegeline and aegelanine (ii) Essential oil (iii) Flavonoids including luvangetin (iv) Tannins, condensed [R16].

MEDICINAL USE: Stomachic, digestive, astringent [R1]. In India, it is almost a specific for dysentry and diarrhoea. The fruit is eaten fresh, or the pulp combined with sugar and tamarind to produce a refreshing drink. Both the ripe and unripe fruits are astringent and are used for diarrhoea and dysentery, and the ripe fruits are also used as a tonic. The roots have been used to treat palpitations and depression and the leaves may be made into a poultice for ulcers. A clinical trial has shown benefits (in combination with *Bacopa monneri*) in irritable bowel syndrome and many other uses are supported by experimental results [3]. The leaves have antiulcer, cardiotonic, immunomodulatory and hypoglycaemic effects, and the essential oil obtained from them was anti-microbial [4,5,6,7]. There are many other uses of the plant; for further detail, see [R16].

PREPARATIONS AND DOSE: Dried fruit powder, dose: 2–12 g.

SPECIFIC REFERENCES: 1. Sharma B *et al* (1981) *Planta Med.* 43:102. 2. Barthakur N *et al* (1989) *Trop. Agr.* 66(1):65. 3. Yadav S *et al* (1989) *Indian J. Med. Res.* 90:496. 4. Rana K *et al* (1997) *J. Ethnopharmacol.* 57(1):29. 5. Abeysekera A *et al* (1996) *Fitoterapia* 67(4):367. 6. Das A *et* (1996) *Indian J. Exp. Biol.* 34(4):341. 7. Arul V *et al* (1999) *J. Pharm. Pharmcol.* 51:S252.

BALM
MELISSA OFFICINALIS L.
Fam. Lamiaceae

SYNONYMS: Sweet Balm, Lemon Balm, Cure-all.

HABITAT: A common plant in Britain, Europe, western Asia and North Africa, widely cultivated, flowering in spring and early summer.

DESCRIPTION: A perennial herb with an odour of lemon; leaves opposite, stalked, about 3–4 cm long, ovate, wrinkled, with a coarsely serrate margin and a rounded base. Flowers small, insignificant, white or cream.

PART USED: Herb.

CONSTITUENTS: (i) Volatile oil, 0.1–0.2%, consisting mainly of alpha- and beta citral (= neral and geranial), with caryophyllene oxide, and in smaller quantities terpenes such as linalool, citronellal, germacrene-D, alpha-caryophyllene, nerol, geraniol, traces of eugenyl acetate, cis- and trans-beta-ocimene, copaene, alpha-cubebene and others (ii) Flavonoids in low concentrations; cynaroside, cosmosiin, isoquercitrin, luteolin-7-glucoside and rhamnazin (iii) Polyphenolics, including protocatechuic acid, caffeic acid, rosmarinic acid and tannins (iv) Triterpenic acids such as ursolic and pomolic acids [R2,R9;1,2,3].

MEDICINAL USE: Carminative, sedative, diaphoretic and febrifuge [R1]. Hot water extracts have antiviral properties, mainly due to the rosmarinic acid and other polyphenolics. Topical formulations containing extracts of Balm are used for the treatment of cutaneous lesions of Herpes Simplex virus, the antiviral activity having been confirmed *in vitro* and by clinical trial [R2;2,4,5]. Aqueous extracts also inhibit division of tumour cells, and tannin-free extracts inhibit protein biosynthesis in cell-free systems of rat liver [6]. The sedative effects are widely investigated and the herb is used as an ingredient of herbal teas, often with other herbs, for nervous disorders and insomnia. The sedative effects have been demonstrated in numerous studies [R8;7,8]. The anti-hormonal effects of Balm, mainly anti-thyroid, are also well-documented. Freeze-dried aqueous extracts inhibit many of the effects of exogenous and endogenous thyroid-stimulating hormone (TSH) on bovine thyroid gland by interfering with the binding of TSH to plasma membranes and by inhibiting the enzyme iodothyronine deiodinase *in vitro*. It also inhibits the receptor binding and biological activity of immunoglobulins in the blood of patients with Graves disease, a condition which results in hyperthyroidism [9,10]. Recently, cholinergic activity has been found for extracts using human cerebral cortical cell membrane homogenates [11]. For further information see [R2,R8,R17] and references therein.

PREPARATIONS AND DOSE: Dried herb, dose: 2–4 g, or equivalent extract, three times daily.

SPECIFIC REFERENCES: 1. Enjalbert F *et al* (1983) *Fitoterapia* 2:59. 2. Yamasaki K E *et al* (1998) *Biol. Pharm. Bull.* 21(8):829. 3. Hermann E C *et al* (1995) *Proc. Soc. Exp. Biol. Med.*124:869. 4. Mohrig A (1996) *Dtsch. Apot. Ztg.* 136:4575. 5. Koytchev R *et al* (1999) *Phytomedicine* 6(4):225. 6. Chlabicz J *et al* (1984) *Pharmazie* 39(11):770. 7. Volk S *et al* (1999) *Z. Phytother.* 20:337. 8. Orth-Wagner S *et al* (1995) *Z. Phytother.* 16:147. 9. Auf'mkolk M *et al* (1985) *Endocrinology* 116:1687. 10. Auf'mkolk M *et al* (1984) *Horm. Metab. Res.* 16:183. 11. Wake G. *et al* (2000) *J. Ethnopharmacol.* 69(2):105.

BALM OF GILEAD
POPULUS CANDICANS AIT
P. GILEADENSIS ROULEAU
P. TACAMAHACCA MILL
P. BALSAMIFERA L.
P. NIGRA L. AND OTHERS
Fam. Salicaceae

SYNONYMS: Poplar buds, Gileadensis, Mecca balsam, Balsam Poplar, *P. balsamifera* Du Rol is a synonym of *P. tacamahacca*; there is some confusion as to whether *P. balsamifera* L. and *P. tacamahacca* Mill. are the same species or not.

HABITAT: *P. candicans* is a native of Arabia; *P. gileadensis* and *P. nigra* are cultivated in Europe; the others are North American.

DESCRIPTION: *P. candicans* is a small tree or shrub, the others are larger trees. The buds are similar, being about 2 cm long and 0.5 cm wide, with brown scales; these are narrow, ovate, closely overlapping and polished-looking; the inner scales are sticky and resinous. Taste: slightly bitter; odour: balsamic.

PART USED: Leaf buds, collected in the spring before they open. The bark of these species is also used.

CONSTITUENTS: (i) Phenolic glycosides; salicin, (salicyl alcohol glucoside), populin (benzoyl salicin), cinnamrutinosides (in *P. tremula*) (ii) Volatile oil, 0.5–2%, the major constituent of which is a-caryophyl-lene, with cineole, arcurcumene, bisabolene, farnesene, acetophenone and others (iii) Flavonoids; apigenin, chrysin (phloroglucin benzoate), galengine, pinocembrin, pinobanksin and others (iv) *P. nigra* contains lignans, such as isolariciresinol mono-beta-D-glucopyranoside [R2;1,2,3].

MEDICINAL USE: Expectorant, stimulant, antipyretic and analgesic [R1]. It is a common ingredient of cough mixtures and ointments used for rheumatic and other muscular pains and for skin diseases. The phenolic glycosides such as salicin have antioxidant activity and the anti-inflammatory and antipyretic effects of the salicylates (see Willow). Flavonoids from *P. nigra* have been shown to have 5-alpha-reductase activity [3] and the volatile oil constituents have the usual antiseptic and expectorant activity [R2;4].

PREPARATIONS AND DOSE: Dried leaf buds, dose: 4 g, as an infusion, or equivalent extract, three times daily.

BIBLICAL REFERENCES: Genesis 37:25; 43:11; Jeremiah 8:22; 46:11; 51:8; Ezekiel 27:17.

SPECIFIC REFERENCES: 1. Picar S *et al* (1994) *J. Nat. Prod.* 57:808. 2. Jossang A *et al* (1994) *Phytochemistry* 35:547. 3. Komoda Y (1989) *Chem. Pharm. Bull.* 37(11):3128. 4. Vonkruedener S *et al* (1996) *Arzneim. Forsch.* 46:809.

BALMONY
CHELONE GLABRA L.
Fam. Scrophulariaceae

SYNONYMS: Bitter Herb, Snake Head, Turtle Head or Turtle Bloom.

HABITAT: North America.

DESCRIPTION: Leaves opposite, oblong-lanceolate, shortly stalked; flowers/fruits crowded in a short spike; seeds almost circular, winged, with a dark centre. Taste: very bitter; odour: slightly tea-like.

PART USED: Aerial parts collected during flowering and fruiting period.

CONSTITUENTS: (i) Iridoids including catalpol (ii) Resin [R2;1].

MEDICINAL USE: Anti-emetic, cholagogue, laxative, antidepressant [R1]. No clinical or pharmacological work available.

PREPARATIONS AND DOSE: Powdered herb, dose: 0.5–1 g.

SPECIFIC REFERENCES: 1. Belofsky G et al (1989) Phytochemistry 28:1601.

BANANA
MUSA SAPIENTUM L.
M. SAPIENTUM VAR *PARADISIACA* L.
Fam. Musaceae

SYNONYMS: Banana: *M. sapientum*; Plantain: *M.sapientum* var *paradisiaca.*

HABITAT: A herbaceous perennial, indigenous to the Indomalayan area, and naturalized and cultivated extensively throughout the tropics for the fruit, which is used as a food in most parts of the world.

DESCRIPTION: Bananas occur in various sizes and need no description. Plantains, *M. sapientum* var *paradisiaca*, are much larger.

PART USED: Fruits, both ripe and unripe. Bananas are eaten raw, and plantain is cooked as a vegetable. Medicinally, the leaf, root and flower are sometimes used.

CONSTITUENTS: Fruit pulp: (i) Phytosterols including the sito-indosterols I-III, campesterol and others (ii) Amino acids including 5-hydroxytryptamine (serotonin), tryptamine and dopamine (iii) Fatty acids; palmitic, linoleic, linolenic [R2;1]. For the constituents of other parts of the plant, see [R2].

MEDICINAL USE: The fruit is traditionally used for gastrointestinal disorders, particularly for preventing and treating ulcers. The sweet banana, *M. sapientum*, has both types of activity whereas the plantain seems to be mainly preventative in effect. Different varieties have varying potency [R2;2,3,4]. Banana powder is a traditional Indian remedy for non-ulcer dyspepsia and a small trial in human patients found it beneficial [5].

SPECIFIC REFERENCES: 1. Ghosal S (1985) Phytochemistry 24:1807. 2. Best R et al (1984) Br. J. Pharmacol. 82:107. 3. Pannangpetch P et al (2001) Phytother. Res. 15(5):407. 4. Goel R et al (1989) J. Pharm. Pharmacol. 41:747. 5. Arora A et al (1989) Lancet 335(8689):612.

BARBERRY
BERBERIS VULGARIS L.
Fam. Berberidaceae

SYNONYMS: Barbery, Berberidis, Pipperidge Bush, *Berberis dumetorum* Gouan.

HABITAT: A common garden bush, native to Europe and the British Isles, naturalized in parts of North America, flowering in April and May.

DESCRIPTION: A spiny, deciduous bush, reaching about 2.5 m, and bearing yellow flowers, followed by red berries, among the leaves. The stem bark is thin, externally yellowish-grey; the root bark dark brown; both with an orange-yellow inner surface. Taste: very bitter.

PART USED: Bark of stem and root, root and berries.

CONSTITUENTS: (i) Alkaloids of the isoquinoline type, mainly berberine, berbamine and derivatives, berberrubine (unique to *B. vulgaris*), bervulcine, columbamine, isotetrandrine, jatrorrhizine, magnoflorine, oxyacanthine and vulvracine (ii) Miscellaneous; including chelidonic acid, resin, tannins etc. [1,2].

MEDICINAL USE: Antipyretic, anti-haemorrhagic, anti-inflammatory and antiseptic [R1]. In the Far East, berberine-containing plants are specifically used for bacillary dysentery and diarrhoea. The root extract was found to have a greater anti-inflammatory effect in an acute model of inflammation than the isolated alkaloids berbamine nd protoberberine [3] and the fruit extract was anticholinergic and antihistaminic *in vitro* [4]. Berberine has well-documented pharmacological actions; it is highly bactericidal, amoebicidal and trypanocidal. The mechanism of its anti-diarrhoeal activity has been partially investigated: berberine enters into the cytosol or binds to the cell membrane and inhibits the catalytic unit of adenylate cyclase. It is active *in vitro* and in animals against cholera, and in humans against diarrhoea [R16,R17;5]. Berberine has some anticonvulsant and uterine-stimulant activity; it stimulates bile secretion and has sedative and hypotensive effects in animals as well as anti-tumour promoting and hepatoprotective effects [R2,R11,R17;6]. Berbamine is also antibacterial. The other alkaloids are also active: palmatine is hypotensive in a similar manner to berberine, it is a uterine stimulant. Jatrorrhizine has a sedative effect in animals, is hypotensive, and anti-fungal; isotetrandrine is anti-tubercular in animals and has significant anti-inflammatory action *in vitro*; oxycanthine and magnoflorine are hypotensive [R2,R11,R17]. Many of the alkaloids are anti-neoplastic in a variety of *in vitro* systems, and although no toxicity problems have so far been observed, it would be wise to avoid these preparations during pregnancy.

PREPARATIONS AND DOSE: Powdered bark, dose: 1–2 g, or equivalent extract, three times daily.

SPECIFIC REFERENCES: 1. Willaman J *et al* (1970) *Lloydia* 33(3A):1. 2. Ikram M (1975) *Planta Med.* 28:253. 3. Ivanovska N *et al* (1996) *Int. J. Immunopharmacol.* 18(10):553. 4. Shamsa F *et al* (1999) *J. Ethnopharmacol.* 64(2):161. 5. Khin-Maung U *et al* (1985) *Br. Med. J.* 291:1601. 6. Fukuda K *et al* (1999) *J. Ethnopharmacol.* 66(2):227.

BARBERRY, INDIAN
BERBERIS ARISTATA DC
Fam. Berberidaceae

SYNONYMS: Berberis, *B. chitria* Lindl., *B. floribunda* Wall.

HABITAT: India and other parts of Asia.

DESCRIPTION: A small, erect, spiny and glabrous shrub, with elliptical leaves and yellow flowers in racemes, followed by bright red berries. Strips of the dried stem, externally greyish-brown, internally greenish-yellow, often covered with moss or lichen, and with conspicuous yellow medullary rays.

PART USED: Stem, root bark.

CONSTITUENTS: (i) Alkaloids; berberine, berbamine, aromaline, karachine, palmatine, oxyacanthine, oxyberberine, taxilamine, jatrorrhizine and others (ii) Chitrianines A,B and C have been isolated from the root [R16;1,2].

MEDICINAL USE: Used in India for intermittent fevers, and the debility caused by them, especially when accompanied by diarrhoea and bilious symptoms [R1]. It is used to treat enlargement of the spleen and liver, in jaundice, dysentery and for various infections. A decoction may be applied topically to ulcers and sores, and for eye infections. Anti-microbial effects against *Leishmania, Entamoeba, Giardia* and *Trichomonas* have been shown *in vitro* and clinically, and anti-platelet and anti-inflammatory activity described [R16,R17;1,2,3]. For further details and references see [R16].

PREPARATIONS AND DOSE: Powder, dose: 0.5–4 g, or equivalent extract.

SPECIFIC REFERENCES: 1. Hussaini F *et al* (1985) *Phytochemistry* 24(3):633. 2. Chauhan A *et al* (1989) *Pharmazie* 44(7):510. 3. Shah B *et al* (1998) *Phytother. Res.* 12:S60-62. 4. Tripathi Y *et al* (1995) *Phytother. Res.* 10:628. 5. Kaneda Y *et al* (1991) *Ann. Trop. Med. Parasitol.* 85(4)417.

BARLEY
HORDEUM DISTICHON L.
H. VULGARE L.
Fam. Graminae

SYNONYMS: Pearl Barley, Perlatum, *Hordeum sativum* Pers.

HABITAT: Widely cultivated throughout the world.

PART USED: Decorticated seeds, germinating seeds.

CONSTITUENTS: (i) Nutrients; proteins, and prolamines such as hordein, edestin and the albumin leusosin among others, sugars, starch, fats (ii) Vitamins of the B group (iii) Germinating radicle and leaves contain the alkaloids hordenine and gramine (iv) Leaves and husks contain hemicelluloses and glycosylflavones including tricin [R2].

MEDICINAL USE: Nutritive and demulcent during convalescence and in cases of diarrhoea, bowel inflammation etc. [R1]. Barley water is prepared from the grains; so is malted barley, which is used to prepare extract of malt, used as a source of nutrients, beer and whisky.

BASIL
OCIMUM BASILICUM L.
Fam. Lamiaceae

SYNONYMS: Sweet or Garden Basil.

HABITAT: Cultivated worldwide.

DESCRIPTION: An annual herb reaching about 20 cm, with an erect stem and numerous branches. The leaves are opposite, stalked, broadly ovate and pointed; usually pale green and dotted with oil glands, however purple varieties occur as ornamentals. The flowers, which appear in summer, are small and whitish, sometimes with a purple tinge, in long loose spikes. This plant should not be confused with Wild Basil, which is *Calamintha clinopodium* and has clusters of small red flowers.

PART USED: Herb.

CONSTITUENTS: Volatile oil, up to about 1%, the major constituents of which are linalool (up to 55%) and estragole (methyl chavicol), with, in widely varying proportions, methyl cinnamate, cineole, beta-caryophyllene, alpha-phellandrene and derivatives, ocimene, borneol, eugenol, methyl eugenol, geraniol, anethole, cadinols, sabinene, myrcene, limonene, *p*-cymene, and camphor. The constitution depends on chemotype and variety. 'Reunion' or 'Exotic' basil oil contains more camphor and very little linalool, and is considered to be of an inferior quality [1].

MEDICINAL USE: Aromatic, carminative, vermifuge, antibacterial, analgesic [R1]. Basil has also been used for diseases of the kidney. The vermicidal activity has been substantiated, and the antibacterial effects demonstrated both *in vitro* and clinically in acne sufferers in India [2]. Basil leaves were found to increase levels of enzymes responsible for detoxifying carcinogens, indicating a role in chemoprevention [4] and the oil has a preservative effect against food-borne bacteria [5], which is relevant given that the herb is used often as a flavouring in foods. An extract of the leaves showed antiviral activity *in vitro* [6]. The oil is reportedly non-toxic; however estragole is a known hepato-carcinogen in animals.

SPECIFIC REFERENCES: 1. Grayer R *et al* (1996) *Phytochemistry* 43(5):1033. 2. Balambal R *et al* (1985) *J. Assoc. Phys.* (India) 33(8):507. 3. Kusamran W *et al* (1998) *Food Chem. Toxicol.* 36(6):475. 4. Lachowicz K *et al* (1998) *Lett. Appl. Microbiol.* 26(3):209. 5. Basil. Eds: Holm Y and Hiltunen R (1999). *Medicinal and Aromatic Plants – Industrial Profiles.* Pub: Taylor and Francis, London, UK.

BASIL, HOLY
OCIMUM SANCTUM L.
Fam. Lamiaceae

SYNONYMS: Sacred Basil, Tulsi.

HABITAT: Cultivated throughout the tropics, especially India.

DESCRIPTION: An erect, annual herb reaching about 1.5 m. The leaves are opposite, elliptical or oblong, pubescent on both sides. The flowers are very small and purplish or crimson in long close spikes.

PART USED: Leaves, root and seeds.

CONSTITUENTS: Leaf: (i) Volatile oil, composed of linalool, beta-caryophyllene, elemene, eugenol, eugenal, carvacrol, methyl chavicol and others (ii) Sterols including ursolic acid, campesterol, cholesterol, beta-sitosterol and stigmasterol (iii) Flavonoids such as vicenin-2, galuteolin, cirsilineol, cirsimaritin, isothymusin, isothymonin, apigenin (iv) Polyphenols; caffeic, gallic, rosmarinic, chlorogenic and other acids, vanillin and gallic acid esters [R16;1,2,3,4].

MEDICINAL USE: Holy basil is a very important herb in Ayurvedic medicine, as an expectorant in bronchitis, and for coughs and colds. It is also considered to purify the mind and body. Traditionally it is valued for its insecticidal, vermicidal and deodorant properties, and is used both internally and topically as an anti-inflammatory. This has been substantiated in various *in vitro* tests, and antioxidant activity also described [4,5]. Extracts of the leaves have been found to have immunomodulatory and anti-stress activity and protect against certain types of carcinogenesis, lipid peroxidation and radiation, indicating a chemopreventative role [R16;6,7]. Administration of the fresh leaves to rabbits reduced serum cholesterol and lipid levels [8] and produced hypoglycaemia in human patients with type II diabetes mellitus [9].

SPECIFIC REFERENCES: 1. Skaltsa-Diamantidis H *et al* (1990) *Plantes Med. Phytother.* 24(2):79. 2. Skaltsa M *et al* (1987) *Fitoterapia* 58(4):286. 3. Norr H *et al* (1992) *Planta Med.* 58(6):547. 4. Godwhani S *et al* (1987) *J. Ethnopharmacol.* 21(2):153. 5. Kelm M *et al* (2000) *Phytomedicine* 7(1):7. 6. Karthikeyan K *et al* (1999) *Oral Oncol.* 35(1):112. 7. Sarkar A *et al* (1994) *Indian J. Physiol. Pharmacol.* 38(4):311. 8. Agrawal P *et al* (1996) *Int. J. Pharmacol. Ther.* 34(9):406. 9. Ganasoundari A *et al* (1997) *Br. J. Radiol.* 70:599.

BAYBERRY
MYRICA CERIFERA L.
Fam. Myricaceae

SYNONYMS: Candleberry, Waxberry, Wax Myrtle.

HABITAT: Native to North America but widely cultivated in Europe and the British Isles.

DESCRIPTION: An evergreen shrub or small tree. The bark occurs in short quilled pieces about 2 mm thick, with a white, peeling outer layer, covering a red-brown, hard inner layer. The fracture is granular. Taste: astringent and bitter; odour: slightly aromatic.

PART USED: Bark.

CONSTITUENTS: (i) Triterpenes, including taraxerol, taraxerone, myricadiol, myriceric acid A, and myriceron caffeoyl ester (ii) Flavonoids, such as myricitrin (iii) Miscellaneous tannins, phenols, resins and gums [R7;1,2,3].

MEDICINAL USE: Stimulant, astringent, diaphoretic, and an ingredient of many composite remedies for a wide range of ailments, especially coughs and colds [R1]. An infusion of the bark is taken internally, and powdered bark used externally in poultices for ulcers and sores. Myricadiol has some mineralo-corticoid activity, and myricitrin is bactericidal and spermatocidal [1]. Myriceric acid A and myriceron caffeoyl ester are specific endothelin receptor antagonists [2,3]. The wax from the berries has been used for making candles, and it is an ingredient of Bay Rum, a traditional dressing for the hair.

PREPARATIONS: Powdered bark, dose: 1–4 g, or equivalent extract.

SPECIFIC REFERENCES: 1. Paul B D *et al* (1974) *J. Pharm. Sci.* 63:958. 2. Sakurawi K *et al* (1996) *Chem. Pharm. Bull.* 44(2):343. 3. Mihara S *et al* (1993) *Eur. J. Pharmacol.* 246(1):33.

BEARSFOOT
POLYMNIA UVEDALIA L.
Fam. Asteraceae

SYNONYMS: Uvedalia, Leaf Cup, Yellow Leaf Cup.

HABITAT: North America.

DESCRIPTION: The root is greyish-brown, finely furrowed longitudinally, about 0.5–1 cm diameter with a tough, coarsely fibrous fracture and a thin, brittle bark. Taste: saline, faintly bitter; odour: none. This is a North American plant and must not be confused with English Bearsfoot, which is *Helleborus foetidus.*

PART USED: Root.

CONSTITUENTS: Unknown.

MEDICINAL USE: Stimulant, laxative, anodyne [R1]. Has been used as a hair tonic in the form of an ointment.

BEEBEERU BARK
NECTANDRA RODIOEI HOOK.
Fam. Lauraceae

SYNONYMS: Greenheart Bark, Bibiru Bark, Bebeeru Bark.

HABITAT: Guyana.

DESCRIPTION: Flat, heavy, hard pieces, 5–10 mm thick, grey-brown in colour with shallow depressions on the outer portions, the inner portions coarsely striated. Fracture: granular.

PART USED: Bark.

CONSTITUENTS: Alkaloids including bibirine, tannins [R4].

MEDICINAL USE: Stomachic, tonic and febrifuge [R1]. Rarely used now.

PREPARATIONS: Powdered bark, dose: 1–2 g.

BELLADONNA
ATROPA BELLADONNA L.
Fam. Solanaceae

SYNONYMS: Deadly Nightshade.

HABITAT: Native to central and southern Europe, cultivated worldwide. Sometimes found on waste ground and in gardens in England.

DESCRIPTION: The herb is a perennial, reaching 1 m high. The leaves are ovate, up to 25 cm long, with an entire margin; the flowers campanulate, greenish to purplish in colour, followed by shiny black berries. All parts of the plant contain alkaloids, the leaves and root are most often used medicinally. The root in commerce is usually up to 10 cm long, 2 cm diameter, pale brown with short transverse scars and a whitish transverse section. The plant is collected when in flower.

PART USED: Herb, root.

CONSTITUENTS: (i) Tropane alkaloids, up to 0.5% in both leaves and roots, consisting mainly of (–)-hyoscyamine, atropine (racemic hyoscyamine), hyoscine (scopolamine), belladonnine, their N-oxides, and other minor alkaloids, including cuscohygrine (in the root only) (ii) Volatile pyridine and pyrrolidine bases (iii) Flavonoids such as scopoletin, scopolin, and kaempferol and quercetin derivatives [R3,R9,R14].

MEDICINAL USE: Narcotic, sedative, mydriatic [R1]. The major alkaloids have anticholinergic activity, causing central nervous system stimulation followed by depression. Peripheral anticholinergic (anti-muscarinic) effects including the reduction of secretions and decreasing motility of the gastrointestinal tract. For these reasons Belladonna is used in stomach mixtures and powders as a sedative, in bronchial conditions as an antispasmodic, for colds and fevers to reduce nasal secretions, and externally as a liniment or plaster for rheumatic and muscular pains. Side effects include palpitations, elevated blood pressure, intense thirst and a rise in intra-ocular pressure. Overdose is dangerous, causing the effects already mentioned together with dizziness, flushing, photophobia caused by mydriasis, constipation, confusion, hallucinations, delirium and death. For more details of individual alkaloids see [R14]. Atropine is still widely used as an anti-muscarinic agent in pharmacological research and occasionally paradoxical effects are reported. For example, although disruption of the cholinergic system produces impairment of cognitive processes, under certain conditions atropine will actually facilitate memory, and also amplify cholinergic transmission. These effects have been shown experimentally and doses used are much lower than the normal anticholinergic doses [1,2].

PREPARATIONS AND DOSE: From the leaf: Belladonna Dry Extract BP, dose: 15–60 mg; Belladonna Tincture BP, dose: 0.5–2 ml. From the root: Belladonna Liquid Extract BPC 1968; Belladonna Adhesive Plaster.

SPECIFIC REFERENCES: 1. Ghelardini C *et al* (1990) *Br. J. Pharmacol.* 101:49. 2. Ghelardini C *et al* (1998) *Phytother. Res.* 12:S7.

BENZOIN
STYRAX BENZOIN DRY.
S. PARALLELONEURUS PERKINS
Fam. Styraceae

SYNONYMS: Gum Benzoin, Gum Benjamin, Sumatra Benzoin, Palembang Benzoin.

HABITAT: Sumatra and Java.

DESCRIPTION: Benzoin is obtained by making triangular wounds in the tree, from which the sap exudes and hardens on exposure to the air. The first exudate forms the 'almonds' of benzoin, followed by greyish-brown resinous lumps; these are compressed together into a solid mass. (The greyish-brown resin alone is known as Palembang Benzoin and is considered to be of inferior quality.) Siam benzoin is obtained from *Styrax tonkinense* (Pierre) Craib ex Hartwich, it occurs in separate 'tears' coated with reddish-brown resin and has an odour of vanilla.

PART USED: Gum.

CONSTITUENTS: (i) Cinnamic, benzoic and sumaresinolic acid esters, mainly coniferyl cinnamate, cinnamyl cinnamate (= styracin), coniferyl benzoate, accounting for up to 90% (ii) Free acids, benzoic acid 10–20%, cinnamic acid up to 30%, and sumaresinolic acid (iii) Benzaldehyde (iv) Vanillin, up to about 1%. All are variable in proportion depending on source. Siam benzoin contains mainly coniferyl benzoate (ca. 70%), with cinnamyl benzoate, free benzoic acid, sumaresinolic acid and vanillin [R14].

MEDICINAL USE: Antiseptic, expectorant and astringent [R1]. Sumatra benzoin is an ingredient of Friar's Balsam, which is used topically on wounds and ulcers to protect and disinfect the skin and to treat mouth ulcers; and as an inhalation in coughs, colds and bronchitis. Preliminary studies have shown that the lipophilic fraction of benzoin stimulates phagocytosis [1] and the cinnamic acid derivatives to be antimutagenic [2]. Benzoin is used in perfumery as an antioxidant and fixative.

PREPARATIONS AND DOSE: Benzoin Inhalation BP; Benzoin Tincture BPC; Compound Benzoin Tincture BP (Friar's Balsam).

SPECIFIC REFERENCES: 1. Delaveau P *et al* (1980) *Planta Med.* 40:49. 2. Mitscher L *et al* (1992) *Mutat. Res.* 267(2):229–41.

BERGAMOT
CITRUS BERGAMIA RISSO.
Fam. Rutaceae

HABITAT: Indigenous to tropical Asia, cultivated widely.

SYNONYMS: Citrus aurantium subsp. *bergamia* Wright et Arn.

DESCRIPTION: A small tree with a typical citrus fruit, greenish-yellow; oil extracted from the fresh rind just before ripening.

PART USED: Fruit rind.

CONSTITUENTS: (i) Essential oil, containing terpenes and sesquiterpenes including linalyl acetate (up to 60%), with linalool, limonene, phellandrene, β-farnesene, alpha-*trans* bergamotene, beta-bisabolene, alpha- and beta-pinenes (ii) Furocoumarins; bergapten, bergamottine, citropten, bergaptol, xanthotoxin, 5-methoxypsoralen and others [R18,R19].

MEDICINAL USE: Has been used for upper respiratory tract disorders, but the main use is in perfumery and as a flavouring agent, for example in Earl Grey tea. The furanocoumarins are photosensitising, and bergamot oil has been found to be carcinogenic when applied to mouse skin and subsequently irradiated with UV light; however in its absence it is not phototoxic [R18]. Bergamottine is anti-arrhythmic and anti-anginal in experimental *in vivo* and *in vitro* tests, possibly acting as a calcium antagonist [1,2].

SPECIFIC REFERENCES: 1. Occhiuto F *et al* (1996) *Phytother. Res.* 10(6):491. 2. Occhiuto F *et al* (1997) *Phytother. Res.* 11(6):451.

BETEL
PIPER BETLE L.
Fam. Piperaceae

SYNONYMS: Chavica betle Miq.

HABITAT: Indigenous to the Indian subcontinent and Malaysia, cultivated elsewhere.

DESCRIPTION: Leaves cordate, 6–8 cm long, about 5 cm wide, with 5–7 radiating ribs and a paler green under surface.

PART USED: Leaf.

CONSTITUENTS: (i) Volatile oil, containing cadinene, chavicol, cineole, eugenol, caryophyllene, carvacrol, safrole, anethole, estragole and others (ii) Triterpenes; ursolic acid, beta-sitosterol etc. (iii) Polyphenolics; piperbetol, methylpiperbetol, piperol A and B [1,2,3].

MEDICINAL USE: Rarely used medicinally but chewed with Areca Nut (q.v.) and lime in the form of a betel 'quid' as a stimulant in India, Sri Lanka, Pakistan, Malaysia and other parts of the world. It increases the flow of saliva and is thought to improve the voice and prevent worm infestation. A liquid extract of the root has been used to treat infections and inflammation of the respiratory tract, and for debility and impotence. The roots are thought to be contraceptive. Numerous diverse pharmacological activities have been described, including calcium channel blocking and cholinomimetic effects; promotion of wound-healing, platelet-activating factor antagonism, anti-fertility and antihypertensive activity; for further detail and references see [2]. It has been suggested that the well-documented antimutagenic and carcinogenic effects [2,4,5] mitigate against the carcinogenicity of arecoline in Areca nut (Betel nut, *Areca catechu, qv.*) and even tobacco, however as yet this needs to be demonstrated clinically. Antioxidant activity has been described for the leaf extract, and no toxic effects were observed when fed to mice at high doses over two weeks [6].

SPECIFIC REFERENCES: 1. Garg S *et al* (1996) *Indian J. Chem.* 35:874. 2. Gilani A *et al* (2000) *Phytother. Res.* 14(6):436. 3. Saeed S *et al* (1993) *Biochem. Soc. Trans.* 21:462S. 4. Zeng H *et al* (1997) *Planta Med.* 63:296. 5. Bhide S *et al* (1991) *J. Ethnopharmacol.* 34(2-3):207. 6. Chaudhary D *et al* (2003) *Phytother. Res.* 17 *in press.*

BETH ROOT

TRILLIUM ERECTUM L.
T. PENDULUM WILLD. AND OTHER SPP.
Fam. Liliaceae

SYNONYMS: Birthroot, Wake Robin.

HABITAT: North America.

DESCRIPTION: The rhizome is dull brown, sub-conical, more or less compressed, 3–5 cm long and 2–3 cm diameter, often ringed with oblique lines and with numerous wrinkled rootlets on the lower surface. Taste: sweetish then acrid; odour: characteristic.

PART USED: Rhizome.

CONSTITUENTS: Saponin glycosides such as trillin (diosgenin monoglucoside) and trillarin (diosgenin diglucoside), diosgenin, cryptogenin, nologenin and others [R2;1,2].

MEDICINAL USE: Astringent, anti-haemorrhagic and expectorant [R1]. Used internally for menorrhagia and haematuria as an infusion, for leucorrhoea as a douche, and for varicose and other ulcers as a poultice, with Slippery Elm and a small amount of Lobelia seed (q.v.). The American Indians used this plant as an aid to parturition, hence the name Birthroot.

PREPARATIONS AND DOSE: Powdered root, dose: 0.5–1 g, or equivalent extract.

SPECIFIC REFERENCES: 1. Fukuda N *et al* (1981) *Chem. Pharm. Bull.* 29:325. 2. Nakano K *et al* (1983) *Phytochemistry* 22:325. 3. Nakano K *et al* (1982) *Yakugaku Zasshi* 102:1249.

BILBERRY
VACCINIUM MYRTILLUS L.
Fam. Vacciniaceae

SYNONYMS: Huckleberry, Whortleberry, Hurtleberry, Blueberry.

HABITAT: Grows chiefly in hilly and mountainous regions of Europe, Asia and North America, on moorland, heaths and on acid soil. It is cultivated extensively. It flowers in May–June, and the berries ripen in July–September.

DESCRIPTION: Fruits blue-black, globular, about 0.5–1 cm in diameter with the calyx ring at the apex and containing numerous small oval seeds.

PART USED: Ripe fruit, leaves.

CONSTITUENTS: Fruit: (i) Anthocyanosides, at least 0.3%, consisting of cyanidin, delphidin and malvidin glucosides (ii) Vitamin C (iii) Volatiles such as trans-2-hexenal, ethyl 2- and 3-methyl butyrates (iv) Catechins and other polyphenols, especially in unripe fruit. Unlike other *Vaccinium* species, bilberry fruit does not contain arbutin, or other hydroquinone derivatives [1]. Leaves: (i) Flavonoids including quercetin derivatives; hyperoside, quercitrin (ii) Caffeic acid derivatives, catechins and iridoids (iii) Quinolizidine alkaloids; myrtine and epimyrtine. For review, see [1].

MEDICINAL USE: Traditionally used as an astringent, antiseptic, diuretic and refrigerant; and particularly for diarrhoea, as a decoction. These include haemorrhoids and vision disorders such as retinopathy caused by diabetes or hypertension, and other forms of venous insufficiency. The anthocyanosides are mainly responsible for activity, due to their antioxidant and free radical-scavenging properties, particularly for the ophthalmic and vascular systems and their spasmolytic action on the gut. These effects are mediated in part by stimulation of vasodilatory prostaglandin production. The anthocyanoside fraction has anti-platelet effects and inhibits some proteolytic enzymes. They are also anti-inflammatory, anti-ulcer, and anti-atherosclerotic and have numerous other beneficial effects on the body, including reducing fluid retention, many of which have been supported by clinical studies [R7,R17; 1,2,3,4,5,6,7,8]. Bilberries are a popular food, especially in desserts. The leaves and anthocyanosides have anti-diabetic activity [2,3].

PREPARATIONS AND DOSE: Dried extract (standardised to an anthocyanin content of 25%), dose: 160–480 mg daily.

SPECIFIC REFERENCES: 1. Morazzoni P *et al* (1996) *Fitoterapia* 62:3. 2. Cignarella A *et al* (1996) *Thromb. Res.* 84(5):311. 3. Cohen B *et al* (2000) *Metabolism* 49(7):880. 4. Martin-Aragon (1998) *Phytother. Res.* 12:S1045. 5. Christie S *et al* (2001) *Phytother. Res.* 15(6):467. 6. Joseph J *et al* (1999) *J. Neurosci.* 19:8114. 7. Neef H *et al* (1995) *Phytother. Res.* 9:45. 8. Bomser J *et al* (1996) *Planta Med.* 62:212.

BIRCH

BETULA PENDULA ROTH
B. PUBESCENS EHRH.
AND OTHER SPECIES AND HYBRIDS
Fam. Betulaceae

SYNONYMS: Silver Birch, White Birch, *B. alba* L., *B. verrucosa* Ehrh.

HABITAT: COMMONLY found in woods in Britain and Europe as far as Siberia.

DESCRIPTION: A fairly large tree, producing catkins of male and female flowers. The leaves are rhomboidal or oval, pointed, shiny, stalked, with a serrate margin, about 2.5–3.5 cm long and 2–3 cm broad. The young bark has a silvery, papery, layered external surface marked with linear brown lenticels; older bark is rough, blackish-brown outside with white lines showing in transverse section. Fracture: short; taste: astringent and bitter.

PART USED: Bark and leaves.

CONSTITUENTS: Bark: (i) Betulinic acid, a pentacyclic triterpenoid [1]. Leaves: (i) Flavonoids, mainly hyperoside, with luteolin and quercetin glycosides (ii) Caffeic acid derivatives, including chlorogenic acid (iii) Monoterpene glucosides, the betula alboisides and roseoside (iv) Volatile oil, containing caryophyllenes and methyl salicylate (v) Betulenols and their acetates (vi) Betula triterpene saponins 1-3 (vii) Anthocyanins [R2,R9;2,3,4,5].

MEDICINAL USE: The bark is a source of betulinic acid, an anti-tumour agent being developed for use in skin cancers and other tumours. It has activity in several carcinoma cell lines including human melanoma, brain tumour cells including medulloblastoma and neuroblastoma, and prevents tumour promotion in a two-stage carcinogenesis model [1,6,7,8]. Betulinic acid is also a specific inhibitor of human immunodeficiency virus [9]. The bark is also used for the preparation of Birch Tar Oil, by destructive distillation, which has been used to treat psoriasis and eczema. This should not be confused with Sweet Birch Oil, which is produced from *Betula lenta* L. and consists almost entirely of methyl salicylate. The leaves are bitter and astringent, and are used to treat infections of the kidney, bladder and urethra, such as cystitis, and kidney and bladder stones [R1]. They are also used for rheumatic conditions [R2,R9].

PREPARATIONS: Birch Tar Oil BPC 1949.

SPECIFIC REFERENCES: 1. Pisha E *et al* (1995) *Nature Med.* 1(10):1046. 2. Carnat A *et al* (1996) *Ann. Pharm. Fr.* 175:231. 3. Lee M *et al* (1992) *Pharm. Res.*15(3):211. 4. Rickling B *et al* (1993) *Planta Med.* 59:77. 5. Demirchi B *et al* (2000) *Planta Med.* 66(5):490. 6. Fulder S *et al* (1999) *Int. J. Cancer* 82(3):435. 7. Selzer E *et al* (2000) *J. Invest. Dermatol.* 114(5):935. 8. Yasukawa K *et al* (1991) *Oncology* 48(1):72. 9. Soler F *et al* (1996) *J. Med. Chem.* 39(5):1069.

BIRTHWORT
ARISTOLOCHIA CLEMATIS L.

LONG BIRTHWORT
ARISTOLOCHIA LONGA L.

INDIAN BIRTHWORT
ARISTOLOCHIA LONGA L.
Fam. Aristolochiaceae

HABITAT: *A. clematis* is European, *A. longa* from North America, and *A. indica* from India.

DESCRIPTION: *A. clematis*: the root is sub-cylindrical, 2 cm or more in diameter, externally pale brown, smooth, striated or warty. Transverse fracture whitish with brown dots due to vascular bundles containing oleo-resin.

PART USED: Root.

CONSTITUENTS: (i) All contain aristolochic acids and aristolactams, which are non-basic aporphinoids. *A. clematis* contains aristolochic acids I, II, III, IV and D; *A. longa* contains aristolochic acid I and aristored, and *A. indica* contains aristolochic acids I, D, D methyl ether lactam, methyl aristolochate, aristolactam, aristolactam II, aristolactam N-beta-D-glucoside, and aristolactam C N-beta-D-glucoside. *A. indica* also contains (ii) 12-secoishwaran-12-ol (iii) savinin (iv) naphthaquinones such as aristolindoquinone (v) the alkaloids magnoflorine and aristolochinine (vi) p-coumaric acid [R16;1,2,3].

MEDICINAL USE: Treatment of wounds, aromatic and stimulant. It is taken internally as well as applied topically. Extracts are anti-inflammatory, immunostimulant and have other effects, and the plant has been well investigated; see [R16]. *A. indica* especially is used as an abortifacient, with aristolochic acid acting as an anti-fertility agent in several ways including anti-implantation and anti-oestrogenic. It is also is cytotoxic, carcinogenic and nephrotoxic. Aristolochic acid I forms a toxic DNA adduct, aristolactam I, *in vivo*, and has caused numerous deaths in women taking a related herb *A. fangchi* as part of a weight-reducing product [3,4]. In view of this, there is no justification for using these plants medicinally. All species are banned from sale in many countries.

SPECIFIC REFERENCES: 1. Mix D *et al* (1982) *J. Nat. Prod.* 45(6):657. 2. Che C-T *et al* (1984) *J. Nat. Prod.* 47(2):331. 3. Stiborova M *et al* (1999) *Exp. Toxicol. Pathol.* 51(4–5) 421. 4. Nortier J *et al* (2000) *New. Eng. J. Med.* 342(23):1686.

BISTORT

POLYGONUM BISTORTA L.
Fam. Polygonaceae

SYNONYMS: Snakeweed, Adderwort, English Serpentary,
Dragonwort, Osterick.

HABITAT: It grows in shaded places in the north of England, Europe
and Asia, flowering in May and June.

DESCRIPTION: The rhizome is reddish-brown, about 5 cm long and
1.5 cm broad, bent twice into an S-shape (hence the synonyms). It is
channelled on the upper surface and transversely striated, with root
scars on the lower surface. Fracture: short, showing a pinkish pith,
white-grey cortex, and thick bark; taste: astringent; odourless.

PART USED: Root and rhizome.

CONSTITUENTS: (i) Polyphenolic compounds such as ellagic acid,
tannins, (about 15–20%, mainly catechins) and traces of emodin (ii)
Phlobaphene, a red-brown pigment (iii) Triterpenes; friedelanol and
5-glutinen-3-one [1,2].

MEDICINAL USE: Astringent, anti-diarrhoeal, anti-catarrhal, anti-
haemorrhagic. Anti-inflammatory activity has been observed and traced
to the triterpenes [2]. Interferon-inducing activity has also been seen in
cultured kidney cells [4]. It is used as a mouthwash and gargle, douche
and ointment, as well as being taken internally as a decoction or infusion.

PREPARATIONS AND DOSE: Powdered rhizome, dose: 1–2 g, or
equivalent extract.

SPECIFIC REFERENCES: 1. Rao P *et al* (1977) *Curr. Sci.* 48(18):640.
2. Duwiejua M *et al* (1999) *Planta Med.* 65(4):371. 3. Duwiejua M
et al (1994). *J. Pharm. Pharmacol.* 46(4):286. 4. Smolarz H *et al* (1999)
Acta Pol. Pharm. 56(6) 459.

BITTER APPLE

CITRULLUS COLOCYNTHIS SCHRAD.
Fam. Cucurbitaceae

SYNONYMS: Colocynth Pulp, Bitter Cucumber.

HABITAT: Arabian Gulf, Sri Lanka, Egypt and Syria.

DESCRIPTION: Occurs in commerce as light, whitish balls, about 5 cm
diameter, often broken. The seeds, which are oval and dark green, are
usually removed before use.

PART USED: Pulp of the peeled fruit.

CONSTITUENTS: (i) Cucurbitacins, including cucurbitacins I and L
(= elatericin B and dihydroelateracin B) which are glycosides of
cucurbitacin E (= elaterin) (ii) Miscellaneous; citrullol, flavonoids
and an unnamed alkaloid [1,2.3]. The rind contains uncharacterised
alkaloids and saponins [3].

MEDICINAL USE: Cathartic, irritant, drastic purgative. It has been used

55

for constipation and painful menstruation. It is seldom used alone because of the griping effects, and its use can no longer be recommended. Toxic effects after chronic use include hypokalaemia, oliguria and oedema, similar to acute nephritis, and symptoms resembling Crohn's disease and Addisons Disease. The drug should never be taken by nursing mothers since the active constituents appear in breast milk [R14]. The rind is a traditional treatment for diabetes in some Mediterranean countries, and both insulinotropic and hypoglycaemic activity have been demonstrated [5].

PREPARATIONS AND DOSE: Compound Colocynth and Jalap Tablets BPC 1963, dose: 1–3 tablets.

SPECIFIC REFERENCES: 1. Lavie D *et al* (1964) *Phytochemistry* 3:52. 2. Abdel Hassan I *et al* (2000) *J. Ethnopharmacol.* 71(1-2):325. 3. Rawson M (1966) *Lancet* 1:1121. 4. Hatam N *et al* (1988) *Phytochem.* 28(4):1268. 5. Nmila R *et al* (2000) *Planta Med.* 66(5):418.

BITTER ROOT
APOCYNUM ANDROSAEMIFOLIUM L.
Fam. Apocynaceae

SYNONYMS: Dogsbane, Milkweed, Wild Cotton.

HABITAT: Mountainous regions of Europe, flowering in June and July.

DESCRIPTION: The root is 3–6 mm thick, with a pale brown, transversely wrinkled and cracked bark which is about half as thick as the whitish centre. Groups of stone cells are visible in the outer bark. Taste: bitter and astringent. *Apocynum cannabinum* (Canadian Hemp, q.v.) is often substituted; however it has a yellowish wood and no stone cells in the outer bark.

PART USED: Root.

CONSTITUENTS: (i) Cardiac glycosides, including strophanthin, androsin, apocynin, cymarin, apocymarin and apobioside [R4]. *A. cannabinum* contains similar compounds (ii) Essential oil containing acetovanillin [R4].

MEDICINAL USE: Emetic, cathartic, diuretic and cardiac stimulant [R1]. For further information on these glycosides see *Strophanthus.* An alcoholic extract of the plant at a sub-toxic dose has been shown to damage transplanted tumours in mice [1]. The herbalist John Parkinson, in the 16th century, wrote that it was a "soveraine remedy against all poysons ... and against the biting of a mad dogge", hence the name Dogsbane. In the light of present knowledge it would be better to give it to the mad dog than its victim.

SPECIFIC REFERENCES: 1. Belkin M *et al* (1952) *J. Nat. Sci. Inst.* 13:742.

BITTERSWEET
SOLANUM DULCAMARA L.
Fam. Solanaceae

SYNONYMS: Woody Nightshade, Felonwood, Felonwort, Dulcamara.

HABITAT: Found widely in hedges and on waste ground in the British Isles, Europe, Asia and North Africa.

DESCRIPTION: The plant is a climber, bearing distinctive purple and yellow flowers in July, followed by oval red berries. The shoots are greenish-brown, nearly cylindrical, about 0.5 cm thick, slightly furrowed longitudinally or sometimes warty. The pith is often hollowed. The transverse section shows a green layer in the bark and a radiate ring of wood (more in older stems). Taste: bitter then sweet. Odour: unpleasant when fresh, this is lost on drying. The root bark is thin and tough, blackish-grey internally, with groups of fibres of the inner bark forming pale brown wedges. Taste: astringent, slightly bitter; odourless.

PART USED: Twigs, root bark.

CONSTITUENTS: (i) Steroidal alkaloids, including soladulcamaridine, soladulcidine, solanidine, solasodine, tomatidine, their hydroxy derivatives, and beta-solamarine (ii) Steroidal saponins: the solamayocinosides A-F, soladulcine A and B, soladulcosides A and B, and others [1,2,3].

MEDICINAL USE: Anti-rheumatic, diuretic; used as a decoction and taken with milk. Bittersweet also has a long history of use as a folklore treatment for warts, tumours and skin infections. Anti-inflammatory activity has been shown in prostaglandin biosynthesis and PAF inhibition assays [4] and the steroidal saponins have anti-fungal activity [5]. The alkaloids however are teratogenic [1] so must be avoided by pregnant women.

BIBLICAL REFERENCES: Exodus 12:8

SPECIFIC REFERENCES: 1. Keeler R *et al* (1990) *Toxicon* 28(8):873. 2. Yamashita T *et al* (1991) *Chem. Pharm. Bull.* 39(6):1626. 3. Lee Y *et al* (1994) *Chem. Pharm. Bull.* 42(3):707. 4. Tunon H *et al* (1995) *J. Ethnopharmacol.* 48(2):61. 5. Wolters B (1965) *Planta Med.* 13:139.

BITTERSWEET, AMERICAN
CELASTRUS SCANDENS L.
Fam. Celastraceae

SYNONYMS: Waxwork, False Bittersweet.

HABITAT: North America.

DESCRIPTION: Root, bark.

CONSTITUENTS: Unknown, apart from a pigment celastrol [R4].

MEDICINAL USE: Alterative, diuretic and diaphoretic [R1]. Has been used for leucorrhoea, rheumatism and menstrual and liver disorders, but rarely used nowadays.

BLACKBERRY
RUBUS FRUTICOSUS L.
RUBUS VILLOSUS AIT.
Fam. Rosaceae

SYNONYMS: Bramble. *R. villosus* = American blackberry or Dewberry.

HABITAT: R. fructicosus is native to temperate Europe, *R. villosus* to the northern United States, both cultivated elsewhere.

DESCRIPTION: A low-growing plant bearing stout prickles on the stem, the leaves are divided into equal lobes in *R. fructicosus*, but unequally in *R. villosus.*

PART USED: Root, root bark, leaves. The fruits are a popular food.

CONSTITUENTS: Both contain tannins and gallic acid. *R. fruticosus* leaves contain (i) Flavonoid glycosides of kaempferol and quercetin (ii) Tannins; dimeric ellagitannins and gallotannins [R2;1,2]. The fruits contain (i) Anthocyanosides and flavonoids [3,4] (ii) Volatile oil containing limonene, *p*-methylacetophenone, beta-myrcene, *m*-cymene, pinenes and others [5].

MEDICINAL USE: Astringent, and tonic, mainly used for diarrhoea. The fruits have antioxidant effects and can be used in a similar way to Bilberry (q.v.).

SPECIFIC REFERENCES: 1. Henning W (1981) *Z. Lebens. Unters. Forsch.* 173:180. 2. Mukherjee M *et al* (1984) *Phytochemistry* 23:2882. 3. Jiao H *et al* (2000) *J. Agric. Food. Chem.* 48(11):5672. 4. Nikitina V *et al* (2000) *Pharm. Chem. J.* 34(11):596. 5. Weilin L *et al* (2000) *Chin. Pharm. J.* 33(6):335.

BLACK CUMIN
NIGELLA SATIVA L.
Fam. Ranunculaceae

SYNONYMS: Small Fennel, Kalonji.

HABITAT: Indigenous to the Mediterranean region but cultivated widely in India and many other parts of the world.

DESCRIPTION: A small annual herb reaching about 45 cm. The leaves are finely pinnate and segmented, up to 4 cm long. Seed three-sided, small and black.

PART USED: Seeds.

CONSTITUENTS: (i) Alkaloids; nigellidine, nigellicine, nigellamine (ii) Flavonoid glycosides of kaempferol and quercetin (iii) Sterols cholesterol, campesterol, stigmasterol and others (iii) Volatile oil composed of thymoquinone, thymol, 2-(2-methoxypropyl)-5-methyl-1,4-benzenediol, limonene, citronellol, carvone, dithymoquinone and others [R16;1,2,3,4].

MEDICINAL USE: Anti-microbial, hepatoprotective, anti-diabetic, anti-fertility, anti-inflammatory, cytotoxic and anthelmintic. Kalonji seeds are important in Ayurvedic medicine. The essential oil inhibits platelet aggregation [4] and has antioxidant activity [5].

SPECIFIC REFERENCES: 1. Attar-ur-Rahman A, *et al* (1993) *J. Nat. Prod.* 55(5):676. 2. Merfot I *et al* (1997) *Phytochemistry* 46(2):359. 3. Akbar A *et al* (1988) *Phytochemistry* 27(12):3977. 4. Enomoto S *et al* (2001) *Biol. Pharm. Bull.* 24(3):307. 5. Burits M *et al* (2000) *Phytother. Res.* 14(5): 323.

BLACKCURRANT
RIBES NIGRUM L.
Fam. Saxifragaceae

HABITAT: A well-known garden plant grown for its fruit.

DESCRIPTION: Leaves palmate, stalked, about 5 cm diameter, with three to five pointed, serrate angular lobes, and yellow glands scattered on the under surface. The fruits are shiny, purplish-black berries, about 0.5–1 cm diameter, with the calyx ring visible at the apex. Odour: very characteristic.

PART USED: Leaves, fruit.

CONSTITUENTS: Leaves: (i) Volatile oil, a small amount, containing mainly terpenes (ii) Flavonoids including rutin and isoquercitrin [1]. Fruit: (i) Anthocyanosides, about 0.3%, concentrated mainly in the skin, consisting mainly of glycosides of cyanidol and delphinidol [2,3] (ii) Vitamin C, about 120 mg per 100 g fresh weight (iii) Tannins [R4]. Seed oil: Polyunsaturated fatty acids including gamma linolenic and cis-octadecatetraenoic acid [4,5].

MEDICINAL USE: The leaves are reputedly diuretic, hypotensive and refrigerant and have been used as an infusion for inflammatory conditions, sore throats and hoarseness [R1]. The fruits are useful in diarrhoea and as a source of Vitamin C. The anthocyanosides are reportedly bacteriostatic, and have vasoprotective and anti-inflammatory effects including inhibition of prostaglandin biosynthesis [1,5]. They are mildly spasmolytic, and anti-secretory against cholera toxin-induced intestinal fluid secretion *in vitro* [R4]. Fruit extracts have anti-viral activity against the influenza virus *in vitro*, due to inhibition of virus release from infected cells [6]. The seed oil is a source of unsaturated fatty acids, particularly gamma-linolenic acid, and has shown beneficial effects in patients with rheumatoid arthritis and mild hypertension [7,8]. Blackcurrants are widely used as a food and flavouring.

SPECIFIC REFERENCES: 1. Chanh P *et al* (1986) *Prostagland. Leukotr. Med.* 22(3):295. 2. Kyerematen G *et al* (1986) *Acta Pharm. Sueca* 23:101. 3. Constantino L *et al* (1992) *Planta Med.* 58(4):342. 4. Moine G *et al* (1992) *Chem. Phys. Lip.* 60(3):273. 5. Declume C (1989) *J. Ethnopharmacol.* 27(1-2):91. 6. Knox Y *et al* (2003) *Phytotherapy Res.*17 *in press.* 7. Watson J *et al* (1993) *Br. J. Rheumatol.* 32(12):1055. 8. Deferne J *et al* (1996) *J. Hum. Hypertension* 10(8):531.

BLACK HAW
VIBURNUM PRUNIFOLIUM L.
Fam. Caprifoliaceae

SYNONYMS: Stagbush, American Sloe.

HABITAT: Eastern and central parts of North America.

DESCRIPTION: The young bark occurs in thin quilled pieces, with a glossy purplish-brown outer surface with scattered warts. Older bark has a greyish brown outer surface and whitish inner surface, with the thin corky layer separating away easily. Fracture: short; taste: astringent and bitter; odour: slightly valerianic. The root bark is reddish-brown and very bitter.

PART USED: Stem and root bark.

CONSTITUENTS: (i) Iridoid glycosides; 2'-O-acetyl-dihydropenstemide, 2'-O-*p*-coumaroyl-dihydropenstemide, patrinoside and others (ii) Coumarins, including scopoletin, aesculetin and 1-methyl-2,3-dibutyl hemimellitate (iii) Triterpenes such as ursolic and oleanolic acids (iv) Miscellaneous; chlorogenic and caffeic acids, arbutin, plant acids and traces of volatile oil [1,2].

MEDICINAL USE: Uterine tonic, sedative, nervine, antispasmodic, anti-diarrhoeal [R1]. Used particularly for preventing miscarriage in the last four or five weeks of pregnancy, although the advisability of this has not been established. It is used in dysmenorrhoea and after childbirth to check pain and bleeding. The iridoids have an *in vitro* spasmolytic effect on the uterus and intestines [2,3] and some of the sedative effects may be due to the presence of scopoletin, which has a number of pharmacological actions thought to be mediated via autonomic transmission blockade [4].

PREPARATIONS AND DOSE: Dried bark, dose: 2.5–5 g as a decoction, or equivalent extract, three times daily.

SPECIFIC REFERENCES: 1. Upton, R (ed.) 'Black Haw' *American Herbal Pharmacopoeia.* Pub: AHP, Sacramento, USA (2000). 2. Tomassini L *et al* (1999) *Planta Med.* 65(2):195. 3. Cometa M *et al* (1998) Fitoterapia 69(5):23. 4. Ojewole J (1984) *J. Crude Drug Res.* 22(2):81.

BLACK NIGHTSHADE
SOLANUM NIGRUM L.
Fam. Solanaceae

SYNONYMS: Garden Nightshade, *S. americanum* Mill.

HABITAT: Found in drier areas of Asia, Africa, America and other parts of the world, on waste ground and roadsides, also cultivated widely.

DESCRIPTION: An erect annual herb reaching about 45 cm. The leaves are ovate or lanceolate, with an acute apex. Flowers small, violet, typically Solanaceous, borne in umbellate cymes. Berries shiny, green when unripe and becoming purplish-black when ripe, containing many small yellow seeds.

PART USED: Whole plant, fruit.

CONSTITUENTS: (i) Steroidal glycoalkaloids; solanine, solamargine, solasoline, solanigrine, especially in the unripe fruit (ii) Steroidal saponins; nigrumnins I and II, and others based on diosgenin and trigogenin [R16;1].

MEDICINAL USE: Hepato-protective, used for hepatitis and other liver disorders. This has been substantiated experimentally [2]. It is widely used in Ayurveda for this purpose, and for inflammation of the spleen and digestive system. Extracts have shown anti-ulcerogenic effects in rats [3] and a cytoprotective role against gentamicin-induced kidney cell damage *in vitro* [4]. The leaves have been applied to wounds and burns in the form of a poultice, and a decoction used as a gargle for sore throats [R16].

SPECIFIC REFERENCES: 1. Ikeda T *et al* (2000) *Chem. Pharm. Bull.* 48(7):1062. 2. Nadeem, M *et al* (1997) *Fitoterapia* 68(3):245. 3. Akhtar A *et al* (1989) *J. Ethnopharmacol.* 27(1-2):163. 4. Kumar V *et al* (2001) *Fitoterapia* 72:481.

BLACK ROOT
VERONICASTRUM VIRGINICA (L.) FARW.
Fam. Scrophulariaceae

SYNONYMS: Culver's Root, Culver's Physic, Physic Root, *Leptandra virginica* (L.) Nutt., *Veronica virginica* Tourn.

HABITAT: Eastern parts of North America.

DESCRIPTION: Rhizome about 0.5 cm in diameter, showing stem bases at intervals of 1–2 cm, blackish-brown, with transverse scars in rings 0.25–0.5 cm apart, chiefly on the lower surface. Rootlets wiry, brittle, with a horny fracture showing a paler core of wood and a thick brown cortex.

PART USED: Rhizome, root.

CONSTITUENTS: Active constituents largely unknown: (i) Volatile oil containing esters of cinnamic acid, methoxycinnamic acid, and dimethoxycinnamic acid (ii) Saponins (unspecified) [R2,R4].

MEDICINAL USE: Mild cathartic, diaphoretic, spasmolytic and cholagogue [R1]. It is used especially for chronic constipation associated with liver dysfunction.

PREPARATIONS AND DOSE: Powdered root, dose: 1–4 g

BLADDERWRACK
FUCUS VESICULOSUS L.
Fam. Fucaceae

SYNONYMS: Kelp, Seawrack, Black Tang, Bladder Fucus, Rockweed, Cutweed.

HABITAT: A seaweed found very commonly in colder waters.

DESCRIPTION: The fronds are flat, forked, greenish-black, about 1–2 cm broad and up to 30 cm long, with a distinct midrib and oval bladders, usually in pairs. *Fucus serratus* has no bladders and a serrate margin. Taste: mucilaginous, saline; odour: seaweed-like.

PART USED: Whole plant.

CONSTITUENTS: (i) Phenolic compounds, including free phloroglucinol and its dehydropolymerization products the fucols, the fucophorethols (which are polyhydroxyoligophenylethers) and high molecular weight phlorotannin derivatives [1,2,3] (ii) Mucopolysaccharides, including alginic acid (algin) [R7] (iii) Sulphated polysaccharides such as fucoidan and laminarin (iv) Trace metals; iodine, up to 0.4% [R7].

MEDICINAL USE: Anti-obesity agent, nutritive and source of trace elements [R1]. A beneficial effect has been demonstrated on obese patients in a small study carried out in Italy. Bladderwrack has been shown to have antibiotic activity [1,3]. The lectin-like mucopolysaccharides are immunomodulatory and induce lymphocyte transformation; they have been shown to react with several *Candida* species and are bioadhesive to mucus membranes [3,4]. Polysaccharide fractions have been shown to reduce serum lipids and blood glucose in rats [5,6] and fucoidan promotes contraction of collagen gels, which is a property important in promoting wound-healing [7]. Seaweeds are a good source of iodine; however they tend to accumulate toxic waste metals such as cadmium and strontium when grown in a polluted environment and should be avoided in these circumstances.

PREPARATIONS AND DOSE: Dried thallus, dose: 5–10 g as an infusion, three times daily.

SPECIFIC REFERENCES: 1. Glombitza K *et al* (1981) *Tetrahedron* 37(22):3861. 2. Glombitza K *et al* (1977) *Planta Med.* 32(1):33. 3. Criedo M *et al* (1983) *I.R.C.S. Med. Sci.* 11(3):286. 4. Schmidgall J *et al* (2000) *Planta Med.* 66(1):48. 5. Vasquez-Freire M *et al* (1996) *Phytother. Res.* 10:647. 6. Vasquez-Freire M *et al* (1996) *Phytother. Res.* 10:S184. 7. Fujimura T *et al* (2000) *Biol. Pharm. Bull.* 23(10):1180.

BLOODROOT
SANGUINARIA CANADENSIS L.
Fam. Papaveraceae

SYNONYMS: Sanguinaria, Red Root, Red Indian Paint, Tetterwort.

HABITAT: North America and Canada.

DESCRIPTION: The rhizome is about 1 cm in diameter, 5 cm or more in length, reddish brown and longitudinally wrinkled. The fracture is short and shows a whitish transverse section with numerous red latex vessels. Rootlets are about 1 mm thick, brittle and wiry. Taste: bitter and acrid; odour: slight.

PART USED: Rhizome.

CONSTITUENTS: Isoquinoline alkaloids, including sanguinarine (about

1%), chelerythrine, sanguidaridine, oxysanguinaridine, sanguilutine, berberine, coptisine, chelilutine, chelirubine, protopine, sanguidimerine, sanguirubine, alpha- and beta-allocryptopine and others [R2,R7].

MEDICINAL USE: An ingredient of many cough preparations, since sanguinarine is expectorant, anti-microbial and has local anaesthetic properties. It has also been used as a tonic and to treat fevers, and externally for all kinds of skin infections and burns [R1]. Ointments containing bloodroot have been used to treat epithelial tumours and skin infections, and dentifrices containing the extract are widely used [R2,R7;1,2,3].

PREPARATIONS AND DOSE: Powdered root, dose: 0.5–2 g, or equivalent extract.

SPECIFIC REFERENCES: 1. Becci P *et al* (1987) *J. Toxicol. Environ. Health* 20:199. 2. Godowki K *et al* (1989) *J. Clin. Dent.* 1:96. 3. Karlowsky J. (1991) *Can. J. Pharm.* 124:262.

BLUE FLAG
IRIS VERSICOLOR L.
I. CAROLINIANA WATSON
Fam. Iridaceae

HABITAT: Eastern and central North America and northern Asia, growing in marshy places, producing distinctive blue flowers in spring. Commonly grown in Britain as an ornamental.

DESCRIPTION: The rhizome is sub-cylindrical, about 2 cm in diameter, becoming flattened at the larger end where the cup-shaped stem scar can be seen. The outer surface is annulate, with numerous stem and root scars. Fracture: short, resinous, showing a reddish-brown transverse section with a yellow endodermis and whitish vascular bundles. Taste: acrid; odour: slight, aromatic. Blue flag should not be confused with either Orris or Acorus calamus (q.v.).

PART USED: Rhizome.

CONSTITUENTS: (i) Volatile oil, containing furfural (ii) Triterpenoids including iriversical and beta-sitosterol (iii) Iridin (irisin), a bitter glycoside (iv) Acids such as salicylic, lauric and isophthalic (v) Miscellaneous sterols, gums and tannins [R7;1,2].

MEDICINAL USE: Alterative, anti-inflammatory, cathartic, diuretic, stimulant and anti-obesity agent [R1]. It is also used externally as a poultice or ointment, for skin diseases of various kinds. It was used in traditional Indian medicine to treat obesity and in one study Blue Flag was shown to reduce food intake in rats [3]; however it is toxic, irritant and emetic in large doses.

PREPARATIONS AND DOSE: Powdered rhizome, dose: 1 g; or equivalent extract.

SPECIFIC REFERENCES: 1. J A Duke (1985) Handbook of Medicinal Herbs. CRC Press. 2. Krick W *et al* (1983) *Z. Naturforschung* 38:689. 3. Bambhole V *et al* (1985) *Sach. Ayurveda* 37(9):557.

BLUE MALLOW
MALVA SYLVESTRIS L.
Fam. Malvaceae

SYNONYMS: Common Mallow, Mauls, *M. vulgare* F. Gray.

HABITAT: A wild plant indigenous to southern Europe and naturalized worldwide.

DESCRIPTION: Leaves stalked, with five to seven lobes, hairy and with prominent veins on the under surface. Flowers mauve, with darker veins. Taste: mucilaginous; odourless.

PART USED: Herb, flowers.

CONSTITUENTS: (i) Sulphated flavonol glycosides; gossypin-3-sulphate, hypolaetin-8-O-beta-D-glucoside-3'-sulphate, gossypetin-8-O-beta-D-glucuronide-3-sulphate (ii) Mucilage (iii) Anthocyanins (in the flowers) (iv) Malvin, the diglucoside of malvidin, and delphinidin (v) Scopoletin (vi) Miscellaneous; tannins, carotene and ascorbic acid [R2;R9,1,2,3].

MEDICINAL USE: Demulcent, pectoral. The infusion is used for colds and coughs, and a poultice of the leaves applied to insect stings and bites [R1]. The mucilage from the leaves has anti-complement activity [4].

SPECIFIC REFERENCES: 1. Classen B *et al* (1993) *Planta Med.* 59:A614. 2. Pourrat H *et al* (1990) *Pharm. Act. Helv.* 65(3):93. 3. Tosi B *et al* (1995) *Int. J. Pharmacog.* 33(4):353. 4. Tomoda M *et al* (1989) *Chem. Pharm. Bull.* 37(11):3029.

BOGBEAN
MENYANTHES TRIFOLIATA L.
Fam. Menyanthaceae

SYNONYMS: Buckbean, Marsh Trefoil.

HABITAT: Marshy ground and Europe, Asia and America.

DESCRIPTION: An aquatic or creeping perennial, with trefoil leaves and spikes of pink and white flowers, each with a five lobed petal-tube and fringed with long white hairs. Flowers April–June.

PART USED: Herb.

CONSTITUENTS: (i) Iridoid glycosides; foliamenthin, dihydrofoliamenthin, menthiafolin and loganin (ii) Pyridine alkaloids, including gentianine (iii) Lactones, such as scopoletin, scoparone, loliolide and braylin (iv) Flavonoids including rutin, hyperoside and trifoliin (v) Triterpenes; lupeol, betulin, betulinic acid (vi) Phenolic acids including caffeic and protocatechuic [R2,R7,R9;1,2,3,4].

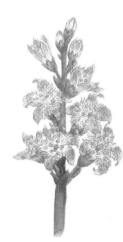

BOGBEAN

MEDICINAL USE: Bitter tonic, deobstruent, used also for rheumatism [R1]. Caffeic and ferulic acids have known choleretic action and it has been suggested that they may act as synergists to the iridoids [5]. The extract has a beneficial effect on renal failure, thought to be due to inhibition of platelet activating factor (PAF) [6]. It is laxative in doses larger than those given below [4].

PREPARATIONS AND DOSE: Dried herb, dose: 1–2 g, or equivalent extract, three times daily.

SPECIFIC REFERENCES: 1. Adamczyk U *et al* (1990) *Plantes Med. Phytother.* 24(2):73. 2. Swiatek L *et al* (1986) *Planta Med.* 52:530. 3. Junior P *et al* (1989) *Planta Med.* 32:112. 4. Janeczko Z *et al* (1990) *Phytochemistry* 29:3885. 5. Swiatek L *et al* (1986) *Planta Med.* 52:60P. 6. Tumon H *et al* (1994) *Phytomedicine* 1:39.

BOLDO
PEUMUS BOLDO MOL.
Fam. Monimiaceae

SYNONYMS: Boldu boldus Lyons, *Boldea fragrans* Gay.

HABITAT: Indigenous to Chile, naturalized in mountainous parts of the Mediterranean.

DESCRIPTION: Leaves oval, up to about 7 cm long, 3 cm broad, rather thick and brittle with an entire, slightly revolute margin and a short stalk. The upper surface is papillose, both surfaces slightly pubescent. Taste: bitter, aromatic; odour: camphoraceous, lemony.

PART USED: Leaves; bark for extraction of alkaloids.

CONSTITUENTS: (i) Alkaloids, of the isoquinoline type, including boldine, isoboldine, isocorydine, norisocorydine, N-methyllaurotetanine, laurolitsine, reticuline and others (ii) Volatile oil, containing mainly *p*-cymene, 1,8-cineole, ascaridole and linalool (iii) Flavonoid glycosides based on isorhamnetin [R2,R7,R9;1,2].

MEDICINAL USE: Cholagogue, liver stimulant and diuretic; used for the treatment of gallstones and cystitis and as an aid to slimming [R1]. Animal studies have shown that the total alkaloid extract has a greater choleretic activity than boldine alone [3]. Boldine has a number of different pharmacological activities such as inhibiting rat liver microsomal enzymes [4] and various antioxidant effects [5,6]. It sensitizes the ryanodine receptor and induces release of calcium ions from skeletal muscle sites [7] and protects against oxidative damage in experimentally diabetic mice [8]. Boldine does not appear to be genotoxic [9] nor cause histological damage [10].

PREPARATIONS AND DOSE: Dried leaf, dose: 60–200 mg, or equivalent extract, three times daily.

SPECIFIC REFERENCES: 1. Vogel H *et al* (1999) *Planta Med.* 65(1):90. 2. Urzua A *et al* (1983) *Fitoterapia* 4:174. 3. Bombardelli P *et al* (1976) *Fitoterapia* 47:3. 4. Cederbaum A *et al* (1992) *Biochem. Pharmacol.* 44(9):1765. 5. Kringstein P *et al* (1995) *Free Rad. Biol. Med.* 18(3):559. 6. Jiminez I *et al* (2000) *Phytother. Res.* 14(5):339. 7. Kang J-J *et al* (1998) *Planta Med.* 64(1):18. 8. Yoon Y *et al* (2000) *Pharm. Res.* 42(4):361. 9. Tavares D *et al* (1994) *Mutat. Res.* 321(3):139. 10. Almeida E *et al* (2000) *Phytother. Res.* 14(1):99.

BONDUC

CAESALPINIA BONDUCELLA FLEMING.
Fam. Caesalpiniaceae

SYNONYMS: Nikkar Nut, Fever Nut, *C. crista* L, *C. bonduc* Roxb.

HABITAT: West Indies, India and elsewhere.

DESCRIPTION: The plant is an extensive climber armed with prickles. Leaves bipinnate, up to 60 cm long, with 6–8 pairs of small leaflets on each and a pair of hooked spines at the base. Flowers yellow, small, in dense terminal racemes. The pods are covered with prickles and contain the hard, polished grey seeds, which are said to resemble eyeballs.

PART USED: Seeds, roots, bark and leaves.

CONSTITUENTS: Root: (i) Diterpenes such as the caesaldekarins C, F and G, bonducellpins A, B, C and D, and caesalpinin are present in the root (ii) Diosgenin. Seed: (i) Diterpenes; a series of caesalpins (ii) Bonducellin, an isoflavone (iii) Fatty acids; lignoceric, oleic, linolenic and others, phytosterols etc. [R16,1,2,3].

MEDICINAL USE: Febrifuge, tonic [R1]. The seeds are a traditional remedy for diabetes and this effect has been supported by several studies showing anti-hyperglycaemic and hypolipidaemic effects in animals [4], as well as anti-filarial activity [3]. It also has uterine-stimulating [5] and anti-inflammatory properties, and antimalarial, antibacterial [6], antiviral and anti-estrogenic effects [R16].

PREPARATIONS AND DOSE: Seeds, dose: 1–2 g, root, dose: 1–2 g, or equivalent extract.

SPECIFIC REFERENCES: 1. Peter S *et al* (1998) *Phytochemistry* 47(6):1153. 2. Sonia R *et al* (1997) *J. Nat. Prod.* 60(12):1219. 3. Rastoggi S *et al* (1996) *Fitoterapia* 67(1):63. 4. Sharma S *et al* (1997) *J. Ethnopharmacol.* 58:39. 5. Datte J *et al* (1998) *J. Ethnopharmacol.* 60:149. 6. Saeed A *et al* (2001) *Fitoterapia* 72:807.

BONESET

EUPATORIUM PERFOLIATUM L.
Fam. Asteraceae

SYNONYMS: Feverwort, Thoroughwort.

HABITAT: North America.

DESCRIPTION: A perennial herb with opposite leaves, 10–15 cm long, lanceolate, tapering to a narrow point and united at the base. The margin is crenate and shiny yellow points due to the resin glands visible on the under surface. Taste: astringent and persistently bitter. The flowers are small and inconspicuous and occur in cymose-paniculate inflorescences.

PART USED: Herb.

CONSTITUENTS: (i) Sesquiterpene lactones; eupafolin, euperfolitin, eufoliatin, eufoliatorin, euperfolide, eucannabinolide and helenalin (ii)

Immunostimulatory polysaccharides, mainly 4-*O*-methylglucuroxylans (iii) Flavonoids; quercetin, kaempferol, hyperoside, astragalin, rutin, eupatorin and others (iv) Miscellaneous; diterpenes such as dendroidinic acid, hebenolide; sterols and a small amount of volatile oil [R2,R7;1,2,3].

MEDICINAL USE: Febrifuge, expectorant, diaphoretic, tonic and laxative [R1]. Used particularly for catarrh, bronchitis and skin diseases. Both the polysaccharides and the sesquiterpene lactones are immunostimulatory in low concentrations; they enhance phagocytosis *in vitro* [1,2,3]. An extract of the plant has been shown to be weakly anti-inflammatory in rats [4]. Some of the sesquiterpene lactones, and also eupatorin, are known to exhibit cytotoxic activity *in vitro* [1].

PREPARATIONS AND DOSE: Powdered herb, dose: 0.5–1 g as an infusion, three times daily.

SPECIFIC REFERENCES: 1. Vollmar A *et al* (1986) *Phytochemistry* 25:377. 2. Wagner H *et al* (1972) *Phytochemistry* 11:1505. 3. Woerdenbag H *et al* (1992) *Z. Phytother.* 13(4):134. 4. Benoit P *et al* (1976) *Lloydia* 39:160.

BONESETTER
CISSUS QUADRANGULARIS L.
Fam. Vitaceae

SYNONYMS: Vitis quadrangularis (L.) Wallich.

HABITAT: Drier parts of Asia, Arabia and Africa.

DESCRIPTION: A rambling shrub with a thick, fleshy, ridged quadrangular stem, constricted at the nodes. The leaves are simple, fleshy, alternate, ovate with a serrate margin. Tendrils arise from the stem nodes. Flowers are small and greenish-yellow in umbellate cymes.

PART USED: Leaves, stem, root.

CONSTITUENTS: (i) Stilbene derivatives; quadrangularins A, B and C, with resveratrol, piceatannol and others (ii) Phytosterols and lipids; mainly triacontanol, onocerol, friedelin and taraxerol derivatives [R16;1,2,3].

MEDICINAL USE: The herb is known for its bone-healing activity, applied as a poultice, hence the name. It is an important herb in Ayurvedic medicine for this purpose and for gastrointestinal and other disorders. The phytosterol fraction enhanced the rate of healing in experimental fractures in numerous tests [R16 and refs therein].

SPECIFIC REFERENCES: 1. Adesanya S *et al* (1999) *J. Nat. Prod.* 62(12):1694. 2. Gupta M *et al* (1990) *Phytochemistry* 29:336. 3. Gupta M *et al* (1991) *Phytochemistry* 30:336.

BORAGE
BORAGO OFFICINALIS L.
Fam. Boraginaceae

SYNONYMS: Burrage, Bee Plant, Starflower.

67

HABITAT: Indigenous to Great Britain, Europe and North Africa, naturalized in North America and elsewhere.

DESCRIPTION: A large annual. The leaves are oval, pointed, with bristles on both surfaces, about 7 cm or more in length, about 3 cm broad, and a slightly sinuous margin. The stem is robust, ridged and bristly; the flowers blue, star-shaped with the anthers forming a cone in the middle. Taste: cucumber-like, saline; odourless.

PART USED: Leaves.

CONSTITUENTS: Leaf: (i) Pyrrolizidine alkaloids, including lycopsamine, intermedine and their acetyl derivatives, amabiline and supinine (ii) Choline [R2,R7;1]. Seed: (i) Fixed oil containing gamma-linolenic acid (GLA), up to 25%. The oil does not contain the toxic alkaloids [2].

MEDICINAL USE: Diuretic, demulcent, emollient, refrigerant [R1]. It is used for fevers and pulmonary disease taken as an infusion, and externally as a poultice. Although the pyrrolizidine alkaloids are present in very small amounts (2–10 ppm) in commercial samples [1], it would be advisable not to use this plant internally, especially when fresh (see Comfrey). The seed oil is used as a source of GLA in a similar way to Evening Primrose oil (q.v.). Clinical studies with atopic eczema and infantile seborrhoeic dermatitis have demonstrated some success [3,4] and the oil was also found to improve skin function in elderly people [5]. Animal studies showed the oil reduced body fat accumulation [6] and reduced arrhythmias in aged rats [7].

SPECIFIC REFERENCES: 1. Luthry J *et al* (1984) *Pharm. Act. Helv.* 59:242. 2. Langer T *et al* (1997) *Sci. Pharm.* 65(4):321. 3. Tolleson A *et al* (1993) *Br. J. Dermatol.* 129(1):95. 4. Henz B *et al* (1999) *Br. J. Dermatol.* 140(4):685. 5. Brische T *et al* (2000) *Arch. Geront. Geriatr.* 30(2):139. 6. Takahashi Y *et al* (2000) *Comp. Biochem. Physiol.* (B) 127(2):213. 7. Charnock J *et al* (2001) *Nutr. Res.* 14(7):1089.

BOX

BUXUS SEMPERVIRENS L.
Fam. Buxaceae

HABITAT: A native of Europe and Asia, cultivated elsewhere as an ornamental shrub.

DESCRIPTION: A well-known evergreen shrub or tree, with small, thick leaves and waxy yellow flowers.

PART USED: Leaves.

CONSTITUENTS: (i) Steroidal alkaloids and amines: buxadine and derivatives, buxamines A-F, buxaminol, buxanine, buxarine, buxatine, buxazidine B, buxazine, buxenone, buxeridine, buxetine, buxpsiine, cyclobuxine B and D, cyclovirobuxine D, spirofornabuxine, cyclobuxaphylamine and derivatives, semperviroxazolidine, semperviraminol, cyclomicrobuxine, osnanine and many others [1,2,3,4] (ii) 4-Mercapto-4-methylpentan-2-one, a volatile thiol responsible for the odour of Box [5].

MEDICINAL USE: Formerly used for 'purifying the blood' and for rheumatism [R1], but far too toxic to recommend. Symptoms of poisoning are severe abdominal pain, vomiting, convulsions and death. Cyclobuxine is anti-inflammatory and hypotensive, and has been shown to protect the isolated rat heart from ischaemic injury [6].

BIBLICAL REFERENCES: Isaiah 41:19 and 60:13.

SPECIFIC REFERENCES: 1. Rahman A-U *et al* (1997) *J. Nat. Prod.* 60(8):770. 2. Rahman A-U *et al* (1998) *Nat. Prod. Lett.* 12(4):299. 3. Rahman A-U *et al* (1999) *J. Nat. Prod.* 62(5):665. 4. Fourneau C *et al* (1997) *Tetrahedron Lett.* 38(17):2965. 5. Tominaga T *et al* (1997) *Flav. Frag. J.* 12(6):373. 6. Lee J-H *et al* (1993) *Planta Med.* 59(4):296.

BOXWOOD, AMERICAN
CORNUS FLORIDA L.
Fam. Cornaceae

SYNONYMS: American Dogwood, Flowering Cornel or Boxwood, Dog Tree.

HABITAT: Eastern and central North America.

DESCRIPTION: The bark occurs in slightly curved pieces, greyish and scaly or, where the outer layer is removed, pale brown and irregularly cracked longitudinally; inner surface pinkish-brown, rough, with small raised lines. Transverse fracture shows faint medullary rays and raised groups of stone cells. Taste: astringent and bitter.

PART USED: Bark, root-bark.

CONSTITUENTS: (i) Steroidal saponins based on sarsapogenin (ii) Verbenalin, an iridoid glycoside (iii) Phenolic acids and tannins [R2,1].

MEDICINAL USE: Tonic, astringent, stimulant [R1]; formerly used by native Americans in a similar way to quinine for malaria and also headaches and exhaustion. Preliminary studies have revealed an anti-plasmodial activity and also a molluscicidal effect against the snail host of *Leishmania* [1].

SPECIFIC REFERENCES: 1. Hostettman K *et al* (1978) *Helv. Chim. Acta* 61:1990.

BROMELAIN
ANANAS COMOSUS L., AND OTHER SPECIES OF BROMELIAD.
Fam. Bromeliaceae

SYNONYMS: Pineapple, Ananase.

HABITAT: Pineapples are native to the tropical Americas but are widely cultivated for food.

DESCRIPTION: A terrestrial stem with a terminal flower, which becomes a fleshy syncarp, topped with a tuft of leaves. The pineapple is well-known as a fruit and has a characteristic pleasant taste and odour. The enzymes are extracted from the fruit and stem.

PART USED: Proteolytic enzymes extracted from stem. The juice and fruit are
common foods.

CONSTITUENTS: Protease inhibiting enzymes known as bromelain, having molecular weights between 5000 and 6000 [1]. The juice contains carbohydrates, anthocyanins, sugars and various other nutritional ingredients [R13,1].

MEDICINAL USE: Anti-inflammatory, anti-oedematous, anti-arthritic, analgesic, wound-healing. The use of bromelain has also been proposed for atherosclerosis, dysmenorrhea, scleroderma, infection and sports injuries [2]. Bromelain is anti-inflammatory in animal studies [3] and recently, purified bromelain has been used orally to treat successfully bruising, arthritis, joint stiffness and pain, and is considered to be an effective alternative to non-steroidal inflammatory drugs, as shown by a number of clinical trials [2,4,5,6]. It also has immunomodulatory effects [7] and can be used post-operatively to improve healing [1]. For other uses of the juice, fruit and leaf, see [R13].

PREPARATIONS AND DOSE: Isolated enzymes (Bromelain), 200 mg tablets.

SPECIFIC REFERENCES: 1. Cooreman W *et al* (1976) *Pharm. Acta Helv.* 51(4):73. 2. Werbach M *et al* (1994) Botanical Influences on Illness: a source book of clinical research. *Third Line Press, USA.* 3. Emancipator S *et al* (1997) *Int. J. Immunother.* 13:67. 4. Klein G *et al* (2000) *Clin. Drug Invest.* 19(1):15. 5. Klein G *et al* (1997) *Arzt Praxis* 51:879. 6. Lehmann V (1996) *Nephrol. Dial. Transplant.* 11:953. 7. Taussig S *et al* (1988) *J. Ethnopharmacol.* 22:191.

BROOKLIME
VERONICA BECCABUNGA L.
Fam. Scrophulariaceae

SYNONYMS: Water Pimpernel.

HABITAT: Common in Europe in wet places.

DESCRIPTION: A low creeping hairless perennial, with oval stalked leaves and small (7–8 mm) blue flowers occurring in loose spikes at the base of the upper leaves.

PART USED: Herb.

CONSTITUENTS: (i) Iridoid glycosides including aucubin (ii) Miscellaneous bitters and tannins [R4]. Brooklime accumulates chromium when grown in polluted water so care should be taken if used medicinally [1].

MEDICINAL USE: Alterative and diuretic [R1], but rarely used. Culpeper said it would "provoke the urine and break away the stone and pass it away". Aucubin has been reported to stimulate the uric acid secretion of the kidneys, and to have a mild laxative effect in animals. The aglycone, aucubigenin, is antimicrobial [2]; however very little is known of this plant.

SPECIFIC REFERENCES: 1. Zurayk R *et al* (2001) *Water, Air, Soil Pollut.* 127(1–4):373. 2. Phytochemical Dictionary, 1993 Eds Baxter and Harborne; Pub Taylor and Francis. 572.

BROOM
CYTISUS SCOPARIUS (L.) LINK.
Fam. Fabaceae

SYNONYMS: *Sarothamnus scoparius* (L.) Koch., *S. vulgaris* Wim., *Spartium scoparium* L. Scotch Broom, Irish Broom, Broomtops, Besom, Scoparium.

HABITAT: British Isles, Europe, and naturalized in North America, South Africa and parts of Asia.

DESCRIPTION: A tall deciduous shrub with ridged stems, bearing small trefoil, lanceolate leaves and yellow, two-lipped (papilionaceous) flowers, followed by greenish-black pods, about 3 cm long and 0.5 cm broad. Taste: bitter; odourless.

PART USED: Flowering tops.

CONSTITUENTS: (i) Quinolizidine alkaloids; sparteine, lupanine, 13-hydroxylupanine, isosparteine, ammodendrine, N-methylangustifoline, dihydrolupanine and derivatives. (ii) Isoflavone glycosides including genistein, 3'-O-methylorobol, 7-glucosyl-3-O-methylorobol, scoparin (= scoparoside) and sarothamnoside (iii) Flavonoids; quercetin, isoquercetin and spiraeoside (iv) Phenethylamines; tyramine, epinine and salsolidine (v) Essential oil, containing eugenol, benzylalcohol, phenol, cresols, guaiacol, isovaleric acid and benzoic acid (vi) Miscellaneous: caffeic and p-coumaric acids, tannins and pigments [R2,R7,R9;1,2].

MEDICINAL USE: Cardiac insufficiency, palpitations, cardiac arrhythmias [R1]. Broom is also diuretic and cathartic. The effects are mainly due to sparteine, which has a number of pharmacological effects. It reduces the conductivity of cardiac muscle and has been used clinically to treat tachycardia, although should only be used under medical supervision. Sparteine also causes respiratory depression and has an oxytocic (but unpredictable) effect in inducing labour. Small doses stimulate, and large doses paralyse, autonomic ganglia [R2,R7,R14;3]. Broom tops have also been abused by smoking the herb for a perceived stimulant effect, which may be attributable to the eugenol content of the oil, but this is neither proven nor advisable.

PREPARATIONS AND DOSE: Concentrated Decoction of Broom BPC 1949, dose: 8–15 ml.

SPECIFIC REFERENCES: 1. Murakoshi I *et al* (1986) *Phytochem.* 25(2):252. 2. Brum-Bousquet M *et al* (1981) *Planta Med.* 43(4):367. 3. Gesser G (1996) *Z. Phytother.* 17(5):320.

BROOMCORN

SORGHUM VULGARE PERS., *SORGHUM BICOLOR* (L.)
MOENCH, AND OTHER SPECIES
Fam. Graminae

SYNONYMS: Sorghum Seeds, Guineacorn, Millet, Durri.

HABITAT: Domesticated throughout the world.

DESCRIPTION: Seeds white, about 3 mm in diameter, rounded and slightly compressed.

PART USED: Seeds.

CONSTITUENTS: Mainly protein, mucilage.

MEDICINAL USE: Demulcent, taken as a decoction [R1]. More often used as a food, and as a cereal grain, production of sorghum is ranked fourth in the world. *S. bicolor* seeds are used medicinally in Africa for chickenpox and hepatitis, and the leaf for anaemia and jaundice [1].

SPECIFIC REFERENCES: 1. African Traditional Medicine. Neuwinger H D (2000). Pub. MedPharm, Stuttgart.

BRYONY, BLACK

TAMUS COMMUNIS L.
Fam. Dioscoreaceae

SYNONYMS: Blackeye Root.

HABITAT: Lanes and hedgerows in Britain and Europe.

DESCRIPTION: A hairless perennial climber with heart-shaped leaves, bearing green, six-petalled flowers in May, followed by crimson, egg-shaped berries. The root is nearly cylindrical, 2–3 cm diameter, 6–8 cm long, with scattered, wiry, rootlets. The outside is blackish-brown, the inside whitish and yielding a slimy paste when scraped. Taste: acrid; odour: slightly earthy.

PART USED: Root.

CONSTITUENTS: (i) Steroidal spirostane glycosides, such as dioscin and gracillin [205] (ii) Phenanthrene derivatives, including the phenolic batatasin, and several substituted dihydrophenanthrenes (iii) Mucilage, composed of glucans, in the root [1,2,3,4].

MEDICINAL USE: Rubifacient, diuretic [R1]. The fresh root is scraped and the pulp rubbed into the parts affected by gout, rheumatism etc. The mucilage from the stem and berries can produce dermatitis, and the skin-irritant properties were investigated and found to be due to calcium oxalate crystals [5]. It is reputed to be a diuretic and the extract has shown antiviral properties [6].

SPECIFIC REFERENCES: 1. Aquino R *et al* (1985) *J. Nat. Prod.* 48(3):502. 2. Aquino R *et al* (1985) *J. Nat. Prod.* 48(5):811. 3. Ireland C *et al* (1981) *Phytochem.* 20:1569. 4. Barbakadze V *et al* (1996) *Planta Med.* 62:A275. 5. Schmidt R *et al* (1983) *Contact Dermatitis* 9(5):390. 6. Aquino R *et al* (1991) *J. Chemother.* 3:305.

BRYONY, WHITE
BRYONIA ALBA L.
B. DIOICA JACQ.
Fam. Cucurbitaceae

SYNONYMS: English Mandrake, Bryonia, Wild Vine.

HABITAT: Central and southern Europe, northern Asia.

DESCRIPTION: Both are perennial, dioecious vines, climbing by means of tendrils (unlike Black Bryony), with large, palmate, 5-lobed leaves. The flowers are greenish-white, in small clusters, followed by red berries in the case of *B. dioica*, and black berries in *B. alba*. The root is large, up to 6 cm in diameter, and normally occurs in commerce cut transversely. The section shows concentric rings and radiating lines of medullary rays.

PART USED: Root.

CONSTITUENTS: (i) Cucurbitacins, including cucurbitacins B, D, E, I, J, K, L, together with dihydro-, tetrahydro- and deoxy derivatives; bryodulcigenin, cucurbitacin glycosides including bryonin, elaterinide and bryonoside (ii) Triterpenes including bryonolic acid (iii) Polyhydroxyunsaturated fatty acids (mainly trihydroxyoctadecadienic acids) (iv) Miscellaneous; a small amount of volatile oil, tannins and lectins [R2,1,2,3,4,5,6].

MEDICINAL USE: Cathartic, counter-irritant, hydrogogue, anti-rheumatic [R1]. White Bryony has been used internally in small doses for intestinal ulcers, asthma, hypertension and as an adjunct in parturition; and externally as a rubifacient for myalgia. It is used widely in homoeopathic preparations. The polyhydroxy acids from *B. alba* have been shown to have prostaglandin-like activity in several biological systems such as platelet aggregation and isolated smooth-muscle preparations [1], and induce hypoglycaemia under experimental conditions [2]. They also restored disordered lipid metabolism in alloxan diabetic rats [6]. The cucurbitacins are cytotoxic *in vitro* and *in vivo*, with anti-tumour effects. The most active are cucurbitacins B, D and E [5]. An ethanolic extract of *B. dioica* has an antiviral effect *in vitro* [7]. White Bryony may precipitate menstruation and is highly toxic, especially in large doses, so should be avoided at least during pregnancy.

SPECIFIC REFERENCES: 1. Panosyan A *et al* (1983) *Planta Med.* 47(1):17. 2. Panosyan A *et al* (1981) *Dok. Biochem.* 256(1):72. 3. Akihisa T *et al* (1996) *Chem. Pharm. Bull.* 44(6):1202. 4. Pohlmann J (1980) *Planta Med.* 47:17. 5. Suganda A *et al* (1983) *J. Nat. Prod.* 46:646. 6. Karageuzyan K *et al* (1998) *Planta Med.* 64:417. 7. Vartanian G *et al* (1984) *Byull. Eksp. Biol. Med.* 97(3):295.

BUCHU
AGATHOSMA BETULINA (BERG) PILLANS
Fam. Rutaceae

SYNONYMS: Round or short Buchu, Bucco, Diosma, *Barosma betulina* Bart. et Wendl. Oval Buchu is *A. crenulata* (L.) Pillans.

(= *B. crenulata* (L.) Hook.) Long Buchu is *A. serratifolia* (Curt.)
Spreeth (= *B. serratifolia* (Curt) Willd)

HABITAT: South Africa.

DESCRIPTION: Small, greenish-yellow leaves with a short petiole and
visible oil glands. Round or 'short' buchu leaves are rhomboidal in
shape, 12 cm long and 0.5–1.5 cm broad. The margin is serrate near
the base; the apex blunt and recurved. Oval buchu leaves are oval and
slightly longer, up to 3 cm long, with a blunt apex, not recurved. Long
buchu leaves have a serrate margin, a truncate apex and are lanceolate
in shape, up to 4 cm long. All have a large oil gland at the apex and at
marginal indentations, with smaller glands scattered throughout the
lamina. Taste and odour: very characteristic.

PART USED: Leaves.

CONSTITUENTS: (i) Volatile oil, up to about 3% (less in long buchu),
of very variable composition. The main constituents are diosphenol
(= buchu camphor), up to about 12%; however in long buchu there
may be little or none; pulegone, (+)- and (−)-isopulegone, up to 10%
and 3% each respectively, with more in long buchu; 8-mercapto-*p*-
menthan-3-one (two isomers), responsible for the blackcurrant-type
odour; 8-acetylthiomenthone, piperitone epoxide, which has been
disputed, (+)menthone, (−)-isomenthone, *p*-cymol, limonene, terpineol
and others (ii) Flavonoids; rutin, diosmin, hesperidin, quercetin and
derivatives (iii) Miscellaneous; vitamins of the B group, tannin and
mucilage [R17;1,2,3].

MEDICINAL USE: Diuretic, diaphoretic, stimulant [R1]. The diuretic
activity is attributed to the diosphenol content. Buchu is also used
particularly as a urinary antiseptic, however no *in vitro* effect against
urinary pathogens and only weak activity against other bacteria have
yet been observed. The essential oil has spasmolytic effects on isolated
smooth muscle of guinea pig ileum and the results suggested the
involvement of cyclic AMP [4]. For inflammation of the bladder it is
taken as an infusion.

PREPARATIONS AND DOSE: Concentrated Buchu Infusion BPC 1954,
dose: 4–8 ml.

SPECIFIC REFERENCES: 1. Didry N *et al* (1982) *Plantes. Med.
Phytother.* 16(4):249. 2. Kaiser R *et al* (1975) *J. Agric. Food Chem.*
23:943. 3. Wellenweber E *et al* (1992) *Fitoterapia* 63(1):86. 4.
Lis-Balchin M *et al* (2001) *J. Pharm. Pharmacol.* 53(4):579.

BUCKTHORN
RHAMNUS CATHARTICUS L.
Fam. Rhamnaceae

SYNONYMS: Common Buckthorn, *Baccae spinae-cervinae.*

HABITAT: Britain and parts of Europe.

DESCRIPTION: A deciduous shrub or small tree, often thorny, with
elliptical, finely toothed leaves. The berries are globular, 8–10 mm

diameter, black. The bark has a glossy reddish or greenish-brown cork.

PART USED: Berries, occasionally bark.

CONSTITUENTS: (i) Anthraquinone derivatives, including emodin, aloe-emodin, chrysophanol and rhein glycosides, frangula-emodin, rhamnicoside, alaterin and physcion [R2,R9;1] (ii) In the bark: naphlolide glycosides of the sorigenin type [R3] (iii) Flavonoid glycosides [R4].

MEDICINAL USE: The berries are used to make Syrup of Buckthorn, which is a laxative [R1]. It is used particularly in veterinary practice. The bark may be found as an adulterant of other *Rhamnus* species (q.v.). Hepatic damage has been reported in mice fed with the extract but no other signs of toxicity were observed [2].

PREPARATIONS AND DOSE: Buckthorn Syrup (for veterinary use), dose: 2–4 ml.

SPECIFIC REFERENCES: 1. Rauwald H *et al* (1981) *Planta Med.* 42:244. 2. Lichtensteiger C *et al* (1997) *Toxicol. Pathol.* 25(5):449.

BUGLE

AJUGA REPTANS L.
Fam. Lamiaceae

SYNONYMS: Common Bugle, Bugula, Middle Comfrey or Confound, Sicklewort, Herb Carpenter.

HABITAT: Europe, including the British Isles, North Africa and parts of Asia.

DESCRIPTION: Leaves opposite, ovate, with a slightly toothed margin. Stems quadrangular; flowers tubular, bluish or ash-coloured.

PART USED: Herb.

CONSTITUENTS: (i) Iridoid glycosides, including harpagide and acetyl harpagide, ajureptoside [1,2] (ii) Phytoecdysterones such as ajuga lactone and cyasterone and others [3,4] (iii) Neo-clerodane diterpenes named the ajugatansins, and ajugavensin A and ajugareptansone A [5] (iv) Miscellaneous hydroxycinnamic acid derivatives including ros-marinic acid, and anthocyanins based on delphidin and cyanidin [6,7].

MEDICINAL USE: Internally as an astringent, particularly in mouth and throat infections, and as a choleretic [R1]. Externally it has been used as an analgesic, for bruising and other wounds, and as a mild laxative. These actions are probably due to the iridoid content. Harpagide and deacetyl harpagide have vasoconstrictor activity on isolated smooth muscle preparations [8]. The ecdysterones are insect anti-feedant compounds. In 1640, the herbalist Parkinson recommended an ointment made "of the leaves of Bugle two parts; of Self-heal, Sanicle and Scabious, of each one part, bruised and boiled in Hog's Lard or in a mixture of Sheep's Suet and Olive Oil until the herbs are crisp and then strained forth and kept for use".

SPECIFIC REFERENCES: 1. Elbrecht A *et al* (1996) *Biochem. Mol. Biol.*

26:519. 2. Shoji N *et al* (1992) *J. Nat. Prod.* 55(7):1004. 3. Calagno M *et al* (1995) *Tetrahedron* 51(44):12119. 4. Camps F *et al* (1993) *Phytochemistry* 32:1361. 5. Carbonell P *et al* (2001) *Phytochem. Anal.* 12(1):73. 6. Lamaison C *et al* (1991) *Fitoterapia* 62(2):166. 7. Terahara N *et al* (1996) *Phytochemistry* 55:199. 8. Breschi M *et al* (1992) *J. Nat. Prod.* 55(8):1145.

BUGLEWEED

LYCOPUS VIRGINICUS L.
Fam. Lamiaceae

SYNONYMS: Sweet Bugle, Water Bugle. Gypsywort. The closely related *L. europaeus* is also called Gypsywort.

HABITAT: Eastern North America. *L. europaeus* is the European species.

DESCRIPTION: Leaves glabrous, elliptical-lanceolate, toothed above but entire near the base. Stem quadrangular; flowers in axillary clusters with a purplish four-lobed corolla and only two fertile stamens. Taste: bitter; odour: mint-like.

PART USED: Herb.

CONSTITUENTS: (i) Phenolic acid derivatives; caffeic, rosmarinic, chlorogenic, ellagic and other acids. The active constituents are thought to be adducts of these formed by autoxidation [1] (ii) Flavonoids based on apigenin and luteolin, including cosmosiin, genkwanin and pillion [2] (iii) Isopimarane diterpenoids [3]. Iridoids are reputed to be absent although they are present in other *Lycopus* species, including *L. europeus.* [R2].

MEDICINAL USE: Sedative, astringent, cough remedy [R1]. Anti-hormonal, particularly anti-thyrotropic, activity, has been described for the freeze-dried extract of *L. virginicus*, which induces pituitary thyroid stimulating hormone (TSH) repletion in hypothyroid rats, and reduction of TSH levels in euthyroid rats [4]. This may account for the sedative effects. Extracts of both *L. virginicus* and *L. europaeus* also prevent bovine TSH binding to and stimulating adenyl cyclase in human thyroid membranes. Bugleweed extracts have been used empirically in the treatment of Graves disease, which is a condition in which a thyroid-stimulating antibody is found in the blood; this has been shown to bind to and be inhibited by the plant extract [5]. Anti-gonadotrophic activity has been demonstrated in rats; the active constituents are thought to be quinones formed from the autoxidation of the phenolic acids [6,7,8].

PREPARATIONS AND DOSE: Dried herb, dose: 1–3 g as an infusion, or equivalent extract, three times daily.

SPECIFIC REFERENCES: 1. Jeremic D *et al* (1985) *Tetrahedron* 41(2):357. 2. Bucar F *et al* (1995) *Planta Med.* 61:489. 3. Hussein A *et al* (2000) *J. Nat. Prod.* 63(3):419. 4. Sourgens H *et al* (1982) *Planta Med.* 45:78. 5. Auf'mkolk M *et al* (1985) *Endocrinology* 116(5):1687. 6. Gumbinger H *et al* (1981) *Contraception* 23(6):661. 7. Winterhoff

H *et al* (1988) *Planta Med.* 54:101. 8. John M *et al* (1993) *Planta Med.* 59:195.

BUGLOSS
ECHIUM VULGARE L.
Fam. Boraginaceae

SYNONYMS: Viper's Bugloss, Blueweed.

HABITAT: A common European plant.

DESCRIPTION: Stems up to about 60 cm, with stiff, bulbous hairs, bearing alternate, lanceolate, bristly leaves. Flowers blue, funnel-shaped, irregularly tubular, in curved clusters. The fruit consists of four seed-like 'pyrenes', shaped like the head of a snake (hence the synonym). Taste: mucilaginous; odourless. The common Bugloss, *Anchusa arvensis* L. has smaller, wheel-shaped blue flowers and wavy, toothed leaves.

PART USED: Herb.

CONSTITUENTS: Pyrrolizidine alkaloids; asperumine, echimidine, echiminine and heliosupine [1,2].

MEDICINAL USE: Formerly used as a diuretic, demulcent, expectorant and anti-inflammatory [R1]; however due to the presence of the alkaloids it should not be taken internally. It would however probably be safe (if not effective) to do as Dioscorides advised, "If the leaves be held in the hand, no venomous creatures will come near the holder to sting him for that day."

SPECIFIC REFERENCES: 1. Delorme P *et al* (1977) *Plantes. Med. Phytother.* 11:5. 2. El-Shazly A *et al* (1996) *J. Nat. Prod.* 59(3):310.

BUPLEURUM
BUPLEURUM FALCATUM L.
B. CHINENSIS DC.
AND OTHER SPECIES.
Fam. Apiaceae

SYNONYMS: Hare's Ear, Chai Hui (Chinese), Saiko (Japanese).

HABITAT: Northern Europe and Asia, including the Far East, China, Japan and Korea.

DESCRIPTION: The leaves are entire, elliptical and parallel-veined, hence the name 'Hare's Ear', and the yellow flowers are present in composite umbels, both axillary and terminal. The root is tuberous, with a few small rootlets.

PART USED: Root.

CONSTITUENTS: (i) Triterpene saponins, known as saikosaponins a, b1, b2, b3, b4, c, d, e, and f, and their sapogenins, the saikogenins A, B, C, D etc. (ii) Polysaccharides known as bupleurans (iii) Phytosterols [R5,R17,R20;1,2,3].

MEDICINAL USE: Anti-inflammatory, hepatoprotective, antitussive. Bupleurum is used in Traditional Chinese medicine for fever, liver disorders, irregular menstruation and prolapse of the womb and rectum. It is frequently combined with Astragalus (q.v.) for debility and prolapse. The saikosaponins are anti-inflammatory; they increase circulating levels of endogenous corticosterone and also potentiate its effects when given concurrently [2,3,4]. Their site of action is thought to be the hypothalamus and or/ pituitary [5,6] and it has been suggested that they may have a potential use in decreasing the dose of glucocorticoid drugs and reduce adrenal suppression [5]. Anti-inflammatory effects have also been demonstrated in various models including the pouch granuloma, and the rat paw oedema tests, and inhibition of prostaglandin synthesis observed [R17,R20;6]. The saikosaponins also raise blood sugar levels and increase liver glycogen stores [R20]. Immunomodulatory activity is exhibited by saikosaponins a and d, and saikogenin D, measured as an increase in number and activation of macrophages [7] and increase antibody response after immunization with sheep red blood cells [8]. The extract, and saikosaponins a and d, are hepatoprotective in several models of liver injury, and although they increase protein synthesis mechanism is unknown [9,10,11]. The effect on the kidney is shown by the reduction of urinary protein excretion in rats given an experimental form of nephrotic syndrome and the activity ascribed at least in part to the elevation of corticosterone levels in the blood, and anti-platelet activity [12,13]. The bupleurans and the saikosaponins have anti-ulcer activity [14] but the saikosaponins can produce nausea and gastric irritation in large doses [R17,R20]. Other effects documented include sedation, lowering blood cholesterol levels, antipyretic and antitussive properties but, despite the pharmacological studies, good clinical trial evidence is lacking. It is generally well-tolerated, although a traditional Chinese formulation (Minor Bupleurum Combination) containing Bupleurum with other herbs, has induced pneumonitis in some patients. However the causative agent was not positively identified [15]. For more detail see [R17].

PREPARATIONS AND DOSE: Dried root, dose: 3–12 g as a decoction, or equivalent extract, daily.

SPECIFIC REFERENCES: 1. Yamada S *et al* (1991) *Planta Med.* 57(6):555. 2. Yokoyama H *et al* (1981) *Chem. Pharm. Bull.* 29(2):500. 3. Nose M *et al* (1989) *Chem. Pharm. Bull.* 37(10):2736. 4. Hashimoto M *et al* (1985) *Planta Med.* 51(5):401. 5. Hiai S *et al* (1981) *Chem. Pharm. Bull.* 29(2):495 and (1986) 34(3):1195. 6. Ohuchi K *et al* (1985) *Planta Med.* 51(3):208. 7. Kumazawa Y *et al* (1989) *Int. J. Immunopharmacol.* 11(1):21 and (1990) 12(5):531. 8. Ushio Y *et al* (1991) *Int. J. Immunopharmacol.* 13(5):493 and 501. 9. Abe H *et al* (1982) *Naunyn Schmied. Arch. Pharmacol.* 320(3):266. 10. Abe H *et al* (1985) *J. Pharm. Pharmacol.* 37(8):555. 11. Lin C *et al* (1990) *Am. J. Chin. Med.* 18(3–4):105. 12. Abe H *et al* (1986) *Eur. J. Pharmacol.* 120(2):171. 13. Hattori T *et al* (1991) *Nippon Yakurigaku Zasshi* 97(1):13. 14. Sun X *et al* (1991) *J. Pharm. Pharmacol.* 43(10):699. 15. Mizushima Y *et al* (1997) *Phytother. Res.* 11:295.

BURDOCK
ARCTIUM LAPPA L.
Fam. Asteraceae

SYNONYMS: Lappa, Bardane, Great or Thorny Burr, Beggar's Buttons, *Arctium majus* Bernh.

HABITAT: Grows in hedges and ditches in Europe, parts of Asia, North America; cultivated in Japan. Flowers in June and July.

DESCRIPTION: A large biennial with broad, blunt, cordate leaves up to about 40 cm long; flower-heads purple, globular, with hooked bracts forming burrs. The root is usually found in commerce cut or split; externally longitudinally furrowed, internally whitish or buff-coloured. The fruits are brownish-grey, wrinkled, about 6 mm long by 4 mm broad. *Arctium minus* Bernh. is also used; it is rather similar but smaller. Taste: herb, bitter; root, sweetish and mucilaginous.

PART USED: Herb, root, fruits ('seeds').

CONSTITUENTS: (i) Lignans, including arctigenin, its glycoside arctiin, and matairesinol, and in the fruits, a series of sesqui- and di-lignans known as the lappaols A, B, C etc. (ii) Polyacetylenes, in the root, mainly tridecadienetetraynes and tridecatrienetriynes, with the sulphurcontaining arctic acid (iii) Sesquiterpenes, in the leaves, including arctiol, (= 8-hydroxyeudesmol), beta-eudesmol, fukinone, fukinanolide and derivatives, petasitolone and eremophilene (iv) Inulin (up to 50%) in the roots (v) Miscellaneous organic acids, fatty acids and phenolic acids; including, isovaleric, lauric, myristic, caffeic and chlorogenic acids [1,2,3,4,5].

MEDICINAL USE: Alterative, diuretic, diaphoretic, orexigenic, anti-rheumatic, antiseptic [R1]. It is usually taken as a tea or a decoction; and for skin problems such as eczema and psoriasis in the same way or as a poultice. Burdock has also been used to treat tumours, particularly in Chinese medicine, and in fact arctigenin and arctiin have been shown to induce differentiation and inhibit proliferation of leukaemia cell lines [6,7,8]. This is at least partly attributable to arctiin [8]. Other cytotoxic effects have also been reported [9] and arctigenin also regulates immune responses and inhibits TNF production under certain conditions [10]. The lignans inhibit the binding of platelet activating factor to rabbit platelets, indicating an anti-allergic effect [11]. The antimicrobial properties are thought to be due to the polyacetylenes [2]. The root is eaten as a food in parts of Asia, and the fibre from it is refered to as 'gobo'. Antimutagenic activity has been described and numerous other properties including anti-diabetic, hepato-protective and antioxidant effects, see [12 and refs therein].

PREPARATIONS AND DOSE: Dried root, dose: 2–6 g as an infusion, or equivalent extract, three times daily.

SPECIFIC REFERENCES: 1. Ichihara A *et al* (1978) *Tet. Lett.* 33:305. 2. Schulte K *et al* (1967) *Arzneim. Forsch.* 17:829. 3. Umehara K *et al* (1996) *Chem. Pharm. Bull.* 44(12):2300. 4. Moritani S *et al* (1996)

Biol. Pharm. Bull. 19(11):1515. 5. Umehara K *et al* (1993) *Chem. Pharm. Bull.* 41(10):1779. 6. Hirano T *et al* (1994) *Life Sci.* 55(13):1061. 7. Ryu S *et al* (1995) *Arch. Pharm. Res.* 16(6):462. 8. Hirose M *et al* (2000) *Cancer Lett.* 155(1):79. 9. Boik J In: Natural Compounds in Cancer Therapy, Oregon Med. Press. 2001, p.280. 10. Cho J *et al* (1999) *J. Pharm. Pharmacol.* 51(11):1267. 11. Iwakami S *et al* (1992) *Chem. Pharm. Bull.* 40(5):1196. 12. Tamayo C *et al* (2000) *Phytother. Res.* 14(1):1.

BURNET, GREATER
SANGUISORBA OFFICINALIS L.
Fam. Rosaceae

SYNONYMS: Garden Burnet, Diyu (Chinese).

HABITAT: Common in damp grassland in temperate regions throughout the world.

DESCRIPTION: Leaves pinnate, with about thirteen opposite leaflets, rounded at the ends and sharply serrate. Flower-heads are deep red, oblong or globose, consisting of two or three fertile flowers at the top with protruding crimson stamens and twenty or thirty barren flowers below. Taste: astringent; odourless.

PART USED: Herb, root and rhizome (often roasted in Chinese medicine).

CONSTITUENTS: (i) Tannins and related compounds; sanguisorbic acid dilactone, a series of ellagitannins named sanguiins H1 to H6 (at present), methyl glucoside gallates, galloyl catechins, and hamameloses, sanguinarine H, casuarinin, 3,3'4-tri-*O*-methylellagic acid and others [1,2,3,4,5] (ii) Triterpenes glycosides, particularly in the root, based on ursolic acid, known as sanguisorbins A-E, ziyu glycosides I and II and betulinic acid [R2;6] (iii) Flavonoids including rutin [R2].

MEDICINAL USE: Anti-haemorrhagic, astringent [R1]. Both leaves and root are used internally for ulcerative colitis and diarrhoea, in the form of an infusion or tincture, or applied topically as a poultice for bleeding and haemorrhoids. The anti-haemorrhagic effect has been demonstrated in animals, and has been shown to be due at least in part to the 3,3'4-tri-*O*-methylellagic acid [5]. Burnet is also used to reduce exudation and decrease tissue oedema in burns and scalds. It also has a mild anti-emetic action and antimicrobial activity against a variety of common pathogens. Clinical studies have confirmed its usefulness in bacillary dysentery, and topically for skin diseases such as eczema and *Tinea pedis* [R20]. Sanguiin H6 inhibits DNA topisomerase [7] and the extract has demonstrated antiviral effects against hepatitis B virus [8,9,10]. Sanguiin H-11 inhibited chemotaxis of neutrophils induced by platelet-activating factor and other inflammatory mediators [11]. Recently, an extract of *Sanguisorba* was shown to inhibit pigmentation induced by ultraviolet light in human keratinocytes [12]. The leaves may be used as a spring vegetable or in a salad.

PREPARATIONS AND DOSE: Dried herb, dose: 2–6 g as an infusion, or equivalent extract, three times daily.

SPECIFIC REFERENCES: 1. Nonoka G *et al* (1982) *J. Chem. Soc. Perkin Trans.* 10(4)1067. 2. Tanaka T *et al* (1984) *Chem. Pharm. Bull.* 32(1)117. 3. Tanaka T *et al* (1983) *Phytochem.* 22:2575. 4. Nonoka G *et al* (1984) *Chem. Pharm. Bull.* 32(1)483. 5. Kosuga *et al* (1984) *Chem. Pharm. Bull.* 32:488. 6. Reher G *et al* (1993) *Phytochem.* 32:3909. 7. Bascow K *et al* (1993) *Planta Med.* 59:240. 8. Kim T *et al* (2003) *Phytother. Res.* 16 *in press.* 9. Chung T *et al* (1995) *Phytother. Res.* 9:429. 10. Chung T *et al* (1997) *Phytother. Res.* 11:179. 11. Konishi K *et al* (2000) *Biol. Pharm. Bull.* 23(2):213. 12. Hachiya A *et al* (2000) *Biol. Pharm. Bull.* 24(6):688.

BURNET SAXIFRAGE

PIMPINELLA SAXIFRAGA L.
Fam. Apicaeae

SYNONYMS: Lesser Burnet.

HABITAT: Dry grassland, particularly on lime, throughout Europe.

DESCRIPTION: Root spindle-shaped, brownish, up to 15 cm long, often crowned with several hollow stem bases. Fracture: short, showing a thick bark dotted with resin canals and a whitish central porous woody pith. Leaves pinnate with oval serrate leaflets; flower-heads white, globular umbels. Taste: cucumber-like; odourless.

PART USED: Root, less frequently, herb.

CONSTITUENTS: (i) Volatile oil, about 0.4% in the root, composed of pseudo-isoeugenol tigliate (major ingredient), pregeijerene, geigerene, betabisabolene, germacrenes A-D, azulenes and others (ii) Coumarins such as umbelliferone, bergapten, pimpinellin and isopimpinellin (iii) Caffeic acid derivatives including chlorogenic acid (iv) Polyynes in the root (v) Flavonoids in the leaf [R2,1,2].

MEDICINAL USE: Aromatic, carminative, stimulant [R1]. Used in lung ailments and to increase gastrointestinal motility; externally for varicose veins.

SPECIFIC REFERENCES: 1. Martin R *et al* (1985) *Planta Med.* 51:198. 2. Bohn I (1991) *Z. Phytother.* 12:98.

BURRA GOKEROO

PEDALIUM MUREX L.
Fam. Pedaliaceae

SYNONYMS: Barra Gokhru, Bada Gokrhu.

HABITAT: India.

PART USED: Seeds.

CONSTITUENTS: (i) Sapogenins based on diosgenin (ii) Flavones [1,2].

MEDICINAL USE: Antispasmodic, demulcent, diuretic [R1]. Has been used for incontinence, impotence and irritation of urinary organs as an infusion.

SPECIFIC REFERENCES: 1. Zafar R *et al* (1989) *Indian Drugs* 27(3):202. 2. Mangle M *et al* (1998) *Indian Drugs* 35(4):189.

BURR MARIGOLD
BIDENS TRIPARTITA L.
Fam. Asteraceae.

SYNONYMS: Water Agrimony.

HABITAT: Damp places throughout Europe.

DESCRIPTION: Flower-heads yellow, button-like, consisting solely of disc florets; leaves lanceolate, toothed, opposite, trifid.

PART USED: Herb, root.

CONSTITUENTS: (i) Flavonoids, isocoreopsin and iso-okanin (ii) Polyacetylenes (iii) Volatile oil, containing eugenol, ocimene and cosmene (iv) Hydroxycoumarins such as umbelliferone and scopletin (v) Polysaccharides (vi) Miscellaneous compounds including vitamins (tocopherol, ascorbic acid) sterols and tannins [R2;1,2,3,4,5].

Medicinal Use: Astringent, diaphoretic, diuretic [R1]. Used in the treatment of gout, ulcerative colitis and haematuria; and in Russia for treating alopecia. Immunomodulatory activity has been shown in the polysaccharide fraction [3] and antimalarial activity ascribed to the acetylenes and flavonoids [R2;4,5].

PREPARATIONS AND DOSE: Dried herb, dose: 2–4 g as an infusion, or equivalent extract, three times daily.

SPECIFIC REFERENCES: 1. Alvarez L *et al* (1991) *Acta Pharm. Hung.* 62:317. 2. Alvarez L *et al* (1996) *Planta Med.* 62:3555. 3. Bauer R (1993) *Z. Phytother.* 14:23. 4. Brandao M *et al* (1997) *J. Ethnopharmacol.* 57:137. 5. Geissberger P *et al* (1991) *Acta Trop.* 57:251.

BUSH TEA
CYCLOPIA GENISTOIDES L.
Fam. Fabaceae

SYNONYMS: Rooibosch, Boschori-Busch. Honeybush tea is *Cyclopia intermedia* E. Mey.

HABITAT: South Africa.

DESCRIPTION: Reddish-brown stalks 1–2.5 cm long with the aroma and taste of tea.

PART USED: Leaves, twigs and flowers.

CONSTITUENTS: Cyclopine, oxycyclopine, tannin and volatile oil [R4]. Honeybush tea contains mangiferin and flavonoids based on hesperitin and iso-kuranetin [R2]. Neither contains caffeine.

MEDICINAL USE: Both are used as a substitute for tea where caffeine is not advisable and for liver and kidney complaints [R1]. Honeybush tea is used to enhance digestion.

BUTCHER'S BROOM
RUSCUS ACULEATUS **L.**
Fam. Ruscaceae

SYNONYMS: Kneeholm, Kneeholy, Pettigree, Sweet Broom.

HABITAT: Europe, in dry woods and among rocks, often cultivated.

DESCRIPTION: Evergreen shrub with leaves reduced to small scales; stems flattened at the ends into oval cladodes each bearing a small whitish flower in the centre, followed by a round scarlet berry, and ending in a sharp spine.

PART USED: Herb.

CONSTITUENTS: (i) Saponin glycosides including ruscine and ruscoside, based on ruscogenin (1-beta-hydroxydiosgenin) and neoruscogenin. The roots contain similar compounds, including the aculeosides A and B (ii) Benzofuranes such as euparone and ruscodibenzofurane [R2;1,2,3,4,5].

BUTCHER'S BROOM

MEDICINAL USE: Anti-inflammatory, diaphoretic, aperient. Particularly used in venous insufficiency, for which a considerable body of supporting evidence is available. The alcoholic extract and the ruscogenins have been shown to have anti-inflammatory activity and diminish vascular permeability. A beneficial effect on retinopathy and lipid profiles of diabetic patients has also been described [6]. The extract may be taken internally as a decoction, topically in the form of an ointment, or as a suppository for haemorrhoids. Venous constriction has been recorded with patients applying an extract of Butcher's Broom topically [7] and beneficial effects have been seen in both patients with chronic venous insufficiency [8] and pregnant women with varicose veins [9]. These actions are thought to be mediated by calcium and alpha-adrenergic blockade at a microcirculatory level [10], but do not involve endothelin A receptors [11]. The saponins exhibit significant anti-elastase activity *in vitro* [12]. A use in alleviating orthostatic hypotension has recently been suggested [13]. Extracts are widely used in cosmetic preparations.

PREPARATIONS AND DOSE: Dried extract equivalent to 7–11 mg glycosides, calculated as ruscogenin.

SPECIFIC REFERENCES: 1. Bombardelli E (1976) *Fitoterapia* 47:3. 2. Dunaouau C *et al* (1996) *Planta Med.* 62(2):189. 3. Mimaki Y *et al* (1998) *Chem. Pharm. Bull.* 46(2):298 and (5):879. 4. Mimaki Y *et al* (1998) *J. Nat. Prod.* 61(10):1279. 5. Van Rensen (2000) *Z. Phytother.* 21(5):271. 6. Adamek B *et al* (1996) *Phytother. Res.* 10:659. 7. Berg D (1990) *Fortschr. Med.* 108(24):41. 8. Parrado F *et al* (1999) *Clin. Drug Invest.* 18(4):255. 9. Berg D (1992) *Fortschr. Med.* 110(3):67. 10. Bouskela E *et al* (1994) *Clin. Hemorheology* 14(S1):S23. 11. Miller V *et al* (1994) *Clin. Hemorheology* 14(S1):S37. 12. Facino R *et al* (1995) *Arch. Pharm.* 328(10):720. 13. *Redman D* (2000) *J. Alt. Compl. Med.* 6(6):539.

BUTTERBURR
PETASITES HYBRIDUS L.
Fam. Asteraceae

SYNONYMS: P. *vulgaris* Desf., *Tussilago petasites.*

HABITAT: In low, wet ground throughout Europe and the British Isles.

DESCRIPTION: A downy perennial, with very large heart-shaped leaves and lilac-pink brush-like flowers which occur in spikes in March before the leaves appear.

PART USED: Root, herb.

CONSTITUENTS: (i) Sesquiterpene lactones (eremophinolides) including a series of petasins and isopetasins, neopetasin, petasalbin, furanopetasin, petasinolides A and B and furoeremophilone (ii) Pyrrolizidine alkaloids; the major one being senecionine, with integerrrimine, senkirkine, petasitine, neopetasitine. These are present in higher concentrations in the root (iii) Volatile oil with dodecanal as the main constituent (iv) Flavonoids including isoquercetin glycosides (v) Pectin, mucilage; and inulin in the root [R2;1,2,3,4,5].

MEDICINAL USE: Tonic, stimulant, diuretic. Traditionally used as a remedy for asthma, fevers, colds and urinary complaints [R1]. Extracts inhibit leukotriene synthesis and are spasmolytic [5,6] and the anti-inflammatory activity is considered to be due mainly to the petasin content [7]. Butterburr has been suggested as a prophylactic treatment for migraine and a recent randomized, double-blind comparative study using 125 patients over two weeks of treatment, has shown that butterburr extract is as potent an antihistamine for use in seasonal allergic rhinitis as cetirizine [8]. Internal use is recommended only if the alkaloids are present in negligible amounts or have been removed from preparations.

PREPARATIONS AND DOSE: Dried root 4.5–7 g daily, in the form of a characterised extract (not suitable for use as an infusion or tea). Maximum daily intake of pyrrolizidine alkaloids: 0.1 microgram (internal); 10 mcg (external).

SPECIFIC REFERENCES: 1. Roder E (1992) *Deutsche Apot. Ztg.* 132:2427. 2. Chizola R (1992) *Planta Med.* 58:A693. 3. Wildi E *et al* (1998) *Planta Med.* 64(3):264. 4. Brune K (1993) *Deutsche Apot. Ztg.* 133:3296. 5. Ko W *et al* (2000) *Planta Med.* 66(7):650. 6. Novotny L *et al* (1961) *Tet. Lett.* 20:697. 7. Thomet O *et al* (2000) *Biochem. Pharmacol.* 61(8):1041. 8. Schapowal A. (2002) *Br. Med. J.* 324(7330):144.

BUTTERNUT
JUGLANS CINERARIA L.
Fam. Juglandaceae

SYNONYMS: White Walnut, Lemon Walnut, Oilnut.

HABITAT: North America.

DESCRIPTION: The inner bark occurs in flat or curved pieces 0.5–2 cm thick. Fracture: short, having a chequered appearance due to the brown fibres alternating with the white medullary rays. Taste: bitter and slightly acrid; odour: faint, rancid.

PART USED: Inner bark.

CONSTITUENTS: (i) Naphthaquinones, including juglone, juglandin and juglandic acid (ii) Fixed and essential oil, tannins [R2].

MEDICINAL USE: Laxative, tonic vermifuge. Butternut has been used as a dermatological agent, anti-haemorrhoidal and cholagogue. Juglone has antimicrobial, anti-neoplastic and anti-parasitic activity and is a mild purgative.

BUTTON SNAKEROOT
LIATRIS SPICATA (L.) WILLD.
Fam. Asteraceae

SYNONYMS: Gay-feather, Backache Root.

HABITAT: North America.

DESCRIPTION: Rhizome 1 cm or more in diameter, somewhat tuberculate, with several cup-shaped scars. Externally brownish and slightly wrinkled; internally whitish, speckled with dark grey dots, very tough. Taste: bitter; odour: faintly aromatic, resembling cedar.

PART USED: Rhizome.

CONSTITUENTS: (i) Sesquiterpene lactones; spicatin, euparin and desacetyl-4'-desoxyprovincalin and its epimers [1,2] (ii) Flavonoids; quercetin-3-glucoside, the 3-rutinoside and others (iii) Volatile oil, in trace amounts. Little recent information is available.

MEDICINAL USE: Has been used in kidney diseases and for menstrual disorders [R1], often in conjunction with Unicorn Root, as an infusion.

SPECIFIC REFERENCES: 1. Seshadri T (1972) *Phytochem.* 11:881. 2. Lowry B (1973) *Nature* 241:61.

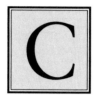

CABBAGE TREE
ANDIRA INERMIS (Sw) KUNTH.
Fam. Fabaceae

SYNONYMS: Jamaica Cabbage Tree, Yellow Cabbage Tree, Worm Bark, *Geoffraeya inermis* Sw.

HABITAT: West Indies.

DESCRIPTION: The bark occurs in long flat pieces about 3 mm thick, greyish-white and fissured externally, the inner surface brownish and striated. Fracture laminated with yellow fibres. Taste: mucilaginous and bitter; odour: slight but disagreeable.

PART USED: Bark.

CONSTITUENTS: (i) Isoflavones, including biochanin A, genistein, pratensein, calycosin, formononetin, lanceolarin, and their glucosides [1,2] (ii) Alkaloids; andirine, berberine and N-methyltyrosine [3].

MEDICINAL USE: Febrifuge, cathartic, vermifuge [R1]. Usually taken as an infusion. The isoflavones are oestrogenic and have anti-fungal activity, and the extract has also been shown to be active against several fungi [4].

SPECIFIC REFERENCES: 1. Kraft C *et al* (2000) *J. Ethnopharmacol.* 73(1–2):131. 2. Da Silva P *et al* (2000) *Fitoterapia* 71(6):663. 3. Kreitmar H (1952) *Pharmazie* 7:507. 4. Freixa B *et al* (1998) *Phytother. Res.* 12(6):427.

CAJUPUT
MELALEUCA LEUCADENDRON L.
Fam. Myrtaceae

SYNONYMS: Cajeput, White Tea Tree, Swamp Tea Tree, Paperbark Tree, *M. cajuputi* Roxb.

HABITAT: Southeast Asia, Australia, cultivated elsewhere.

DESCRIPTION: The tree, from which the oil is distilled, is large with a distinctive crooked trunk. The oil is distilled from the fresh leaves and twigs and redistilled until colourless or pale yellow; it has an odour recalling that of camphor and eucalyptus.

PART USED: Oil, leaves.

CONSTITUENTS: (i) Essential oil, composed of cineole, (usually 50–65%, but variable) is the major component, with alpha-pinene, alpha-terpineol, nerolidol, limonene, benzaldehyde, valeraldehyde, dipentene, various sesquiterpenes and 3,5-dimethyl-4,6-di-O-methylphloroacetophenone [R14;1] (ii) Triterpenes, in the leaves, such as farnesol, squalene, betulinic acid, platanic acid and others [2] and in the heartwood, oleanane and taraxesterol derivatives [2] (ii) Flavonoids in the leaves, including the novel leucadenones A-D [3] and the more common myricetin, kaempferol and quercetin derivatives, with ledol, palustrol, viridflorol and others [4].

MEDICINAL USE: The oil is used as a stimulant, antispasmodic, diaphoretic and expectorant [R1]. Used internally as an ingredient of remedies for colds, headaches and toothaches; carminative mixtures; and externally as a rubefacient in rheumatism and muscle stiffness. Cineole (see *Eucalyptus*) has antiseptic properties [R14].

PREPARATIONS AND DOSE: Cajuput Oil BPC, dose: 0.05–0.2 ml; Compound Methyl Salicylate Ointment BPC.

SPECIFIC REFERENCES: 1. Lee C *et al* (1998) *J. Nat. Prod.* 61(3):375. 2. Lee C *et al* (1999) *J. Nat. Prod.* 62(7):1003. 3. Lee C *et al* (1998) *Tet. Lett.* 40:7255. 4. Kitanov G *et al* (1992) *Fitoterapia* 63(4):379.

CALABAR BEAN
PHYSOSTIGMA VENENOSUM BALF.
Fam. Caesalpiniaceae

SYNONYMS: Ordeal bean, Chopnut.

HABITAT: West Africa.

DESCRIPTION: The plant is a woody climber, bearing Papilionaceous flowers, followed by pods containing two or three dark brown or blackish seeds. The seeds are kidney-shaped, up to about 3 cm long, 1.5 cm broad and 1.5 cm thick, with the hilum extending along the whole convex side. The cotyledons are whitish.

PART USED: Ripe seeds.

CONSTITUENTS: Alkaloids; mainly physostigmine (eserine), with eseramine, isophysostigmine, physovenine, geneserine, calabatine, calabacine and others [R3;1,2].

MEDICINAL USE: Rarely used medicinally nowadays, except as a source of physostigmine. This alkaloid is an anticholinesterase, and therefore prevents breakdown of acetylcholine, increasing neuromuscular transmission. Physostigmine is still used occasionally in ophthalmology, to decrease intra-ocular pressure in glaucoma (for short periods only) and as an antidote to anticholinergics such as atropine, baclofen and tricyclic antidepressants. Physostigmine derivatives are under investigation for treating Alzheimer's disease (for example rivastigmine). The alkaloids have reported analgesic activity [1] and the beans were originally used as an ordeal poison by tribes in West Africa, for those accused of witchcraft [R14;2]. They are extremely poisonous.

PREPARATIONS AND DOSE: Physostigmine sulphate eye drops, dose: up to 1%.

SPECIFIC REFERENCES: 1. Sampson J *et al* (2000) *Phytother. Res.* 14(1):24. 2. Robinson B (1988) *W. Afr. J. Pharmacol. Drug Res.* 8(1):1.

CALAMINT
CALAMINTHA NEPETA (L.) Savi.
Fam. Lamiaceae

SYNONYMS: Common Calamint, Basil Thyme, Mountain Mint, C. officinalis Moench., C. menthifolia Host. C. ascendens Jord. C. montana Lam.

HABITAT: Occurs on dry, often calcareous banks in Europe and North Africa.

DESCRIPTION: Leaves broadly ovate, slightly serrate, stalked. Flowers pale purple; calyx with upper teeth triangular, erect, fringed with hairs, lower teeth longer, awl-shaped. Taste and odour: mint-like.

PART USED: Herb.

CONSTITUENTS: (i) Volatile oil, about 0.35%, of which the major constituents are piperitone oxide, piperitone, pulegone, menthol, thymol, beta-bisabolene and cineole [1,2] (ii) Triterpenes such as ursolic acid and calaminthadiol [R2;3,4] (iii) Rosmarinic acid [5].

MEDICINAL USE: Diaphoretic, expectorant [R1]. The oil has shown antimicrobial activity, which was ascribed to the pulegone content [2].

SPECIFIC REFERENCES: 1. Kokkalo E et al (1990) Flav. Frag. J. 5:23. 2. Flamini G et al (1999) Phytother. Res. 13(4):349. 3. de Pooter H et al (1987) Phytochem. 26:3355. 4. Baldovinin N et al (2000) Flav. Frag. J. 15:50. 5. Lamaison C et al (1991) Fitoterapia 62(2):166.

CALAMUS
ACORUS CALAMUS L.
Type I = var AMERICANUS
Type II = var VULGARIS L. (= VAR CALAMUS)
Type III = var AUGUSTATUS BESS.
Type IV = var VERSUS L.
Fam. Araceae

SYNONYMS: Sweet Flag, Sweet Sedge, Myrtle Flag, Shuichangpu (Chinese), Vacha (Hindi), Calamus aromaticus.

HABITAT: Thought to originate in Europe but now found throughout the world. Type I is a diploid American variety, type II is a European triploid, and types III and IV are subtropical tetraploids. The plant is semi-aquatic, growing on riverbanks and in marshy places.

DESCRIPTION: The rhizome is pale fawn-coloured, longitudinally wrinkled, with numerous oblique transverse leaf scars above, particularly near the stem, and small circular root scars underneath. Fracture: short, showing a whitish, porous interior, with scattered vascular bundles visible when wetted. Taste: aromatic, pungent and bitter; odour: sweet and aromatic. In commerce the peeled rhizome is usually angular and often split.

PART USED: Rhizome.

CONSTITUENTS: Volatile oil of variable composition. In types II,

III and IV the major constituent is usually beta-asarone (isoasarone). In type I, beta-asarone is absent, and the main constituents are alpha-asarone, the shyobunones and isoshyobunones, isoacorone, acorone, acorenone, calamendiols [1]. Other constituents of the oil include acoragermacrone, acolamone, isoacolamone, pinene, azulene, methyleugenol, methylisoeugenol, camphor, galangin, asaraldehyde, and acoric acid [2,3].

MEDICINAL USE: Aromatic, spasmolytic, carminative, it is used mainly for flatulence, colic and dyspepsia [R1]. The rhizome ('root') has been used candied and in the form of an infusion since ancient times. In parts of Asia it is used to enhance memory, and given ritually to newborn babies in India to promote speech development and intellect. In China it is used after stroke. The oil has spasmolytic, cyto-protective and anti-ulcer activity in rats [4]. It has been known for some time that beta-asarone is carcinogenic in animals; however recent studies have demonstrated that type I (the American variety), which does not contain beta-asarone, is in fact superior in spasmolytic activity to the other types [1]. Therefore, although absolute safety has not been proven, it would be preferable to use this variety for internal use. The oil has anticonvulsant activity [5], anti-inflammatory, analgesic and antibacterial activity [6]. Preparations containing beta-asarone are banned from sale in the US [R16,R7].

PREPARATIONS AND DOSE: Powdered root, dose: 1–4 g, or equivalent extract.

BIBLICAL REFERENCES: Exodus 30:23; Song of Solomon 4:14; Ezekiel 27:19. As Sweet Cane in Isaiah 43:24 and Jeremiah 6:20.

SPECIFIC REFERENCES: 1. Keller K *et al* (1985) *Planta Med.* 51(1):6. 2. Rohr M (1979) *Phytochem.* 18(2) 279 and 328. 3. Mazza G (1985) *J. Chrom.* 328:179. 4. Rafatullah S *et al* (1994) *Fitoterapia* 65(1):19. 5. Martis G *et al* (1991) *Fitoterapia* 62(4):331. 6. Vohora S *et al* (1989) *Ann. Nat. Acad. Med. Sci.* 25(1):13.

CALOTROPIS

CALOTROPIS PROCERA BROWN.
Fam. Asclepiadaceae

SYNONYMS: Mudar Bark, *Asclepias procera* Willd.

HABITAT: India.

DESCRIPTION: The bark occurs in irregular short pieces, slightly quilled or curved, about 0.3–0.5 cm thick. Externally greyish-yellow, soft and spongy; internally yellowish-white. Fracture: short; taste: acrid and bitter.

PART USED: Bark, root bark, latex.

CONSTITUENTS: (i) Cardiac glycosides; cardenolides based on calotropagenin with cyclic sugars [1] (ii) Triterpenes; calotropursenyl acetate and calotropfriedelenyl acetate [2] (iii) a norditerpene ester, calotropterpenyl ester [2].

89

MEDICINAL USE: Used in many tropical countries, such as India, as a remedy for dysentery, diarrhoea and other conditions, and topically for eczema [R1]. The latex has been reported to be anti-inflammatory and anti-diarrhoeal when given to rats [3], although when injected in the rat hind paw it induces inflammation [4]. Analgesic activity has been demonstrated in mice [5]. It has anti-plasmodial activity but causes haemolysis of erythrocytes [6] and is anthelmintic in sheep [7]. Antimicrobial effects of the flowers [8] and wound-healing activities of the latex in guinea pigs have also been reported [9].

SPECIFIC REFERENCES: 1. Seiber J *et al* (1982) *Phytochem.* 21(9):2343. 2. Ansari S *et al* (2001) *Pharmazie* 56(2):175. 3. Kumar S *et al* (2001) *J. Ethnopharmacol.* 76(1):115. 4. Singh H *et al* (2000) *J. Pharmacol. Toxicol. Methods* (43(3):219. 5. Dewan S *et al* (2000) *J. Ethnopharmacol.* 73(1–2):307. 6. Sharma P *et al* (2001) *J. Ethnopharmacol.* 74(3):239. 7.Al-Qarawi A *et al* (2001) *Vet. Res. Comm.* 25(1):61. 8. Larhsini M *et al* (2001) *Phytother. Res.* 15(3):250. 9. Rasik A *et al* (1999) *J. Ethnopharmacol.* 68(1–3):261.

CALTROPS
TRIBULUS TERRESTRIS L.
Fam. Zygophyllaceae

SYNONYMS: Gokhru (India).

HABITAT: Wastelands of China, India, other Asian countries and parts of Europe and South Africa.

DESCRIPTION: A thorny, perennial creeper with solitary pale yellow flowers and pinnate leaves. The fruits are globose, each with two pairs of spines, one pair being longer than the other. The fruits have five locculi, each containing several seeds, and are said to resemble the cloven hoof of a cow.

PART USED: Fruit, root, flowers.

CONSTITUENTS: (i) Saponins, in the fruits, including protodioscin, terrestrosins A-E, gitonin, desglucolanatigonin and tigogenin and furostanol glycosides [1,2]. The flowers contain saponins based on ruscogenin, hecogenin and diosgenin [3] (ii) Lignans; tribulusamides A and B in the fruit and flowers.

MEDICINAL USE: Used for many different purposes, including digestive disorders, inflammation, and as an emmenagogue and aphrodisiac. It has a particular use in kidney and bladder stones and this has been substantiated in metabolic studies in rats [4,5]. It has pro-erectile activity on the *corpus cavernosum* in rabbits [6] and is a cardiac stimulant (as would be expected from the glycosides). Antibacterial, cytotoxic and other effects have been reported [R16;7].

PREPARATIONS AND DOSE: Powdered root, dose: 0.5–1 g, or equivalent extract.

SPECIFIC REFERENCES: 1. Bedir E *et al* (2000) *J. Nat. Prod.* 63(12):1699. 2. Yan W *et al* (1996) *Phytochem.* 42(5) 1414. 3. Zafar R *et al* (1992) *Fitoterapia* 63(1):90. 4. Sangheeta D *et al* (1993) *Phytother. Res.* 7(2):116. 5. Sangheeta D *et al* (1994) *J. Ethnopharmacol.* 44(2):61. 6. Adakain P *et al* (2000) *Ann. Acad. Med. Singapore* 29(1):22. 7. Ali N *et al* (2001) *J. Ethnopharmacol.* 74(2):173.

CALUMBA

JATEORHIZA PALMATA MIERS.
Fam. Menispermaceae

SYNONYMS: Colombo, *Cocculus palmatus* D.C.

HABITAT: East Africa and Madagascar, cultivated in Europe.

DESCRIPTION: The root occurs in circular sections about 3–8 cm diameter with a depressed centre and a thick bark. Transverse section yellowish, with vascular bundles in radiating lines. The outer surface is greyish-brown and the fracture short and mealy. Taste: mucilaginous, very bitter; odour: slight.

PART USED: Root.

CONSTITUENTS: (i) Isoquinoline alkaloids, 2–3%; palmatine, jatrorrhizine and its dimer bisjatrorrhizine, columbamine (ii) Bitters including calumbin, a di-lactone (iii) Dihydronaphthalenes such as chasmanthin and palmanin (iv) Volatile oil containing thymol. Tannins are reportedly absent. [R2,R3].

MEDICINAL USE: Bitter tonic, orexigenic, carminative [R1]. For effects of palmatine and jatrorrhizine, see Barberry.

PREPARATIONS AND DOSE: Powdered root, dose: 0.5–2 g, or equivalent extract.

CAMPHOR

CINNAMOMUM CAMPHORA (L.) NEES & EBERM.
Fam. Lauraceae

SYNONYMS: Gum Camphor, Laurel Camphor, Camphire, *Laurus camphora* L., *Camphora officinarum* Nees.

HABITAT: Central China, Japan, India and others.

DESCRIPTION: A colourless, crystalline, translucent mass with a characteristic odour, often imported in small square pieces. It is obtained by passing steam through the chipped wood; the distillate contains camphor, which is resublimed, leaving an essential oil.

PART USED: Distillate from the wood.

CONSTITUENTS: Camphor of natural origin is a dextro-rotatory ketone (unlike synthetic camphor which is optically inactive). Other constituents include (i) Volatile oil, containing some residual camphor, safrole, borneol, heliotropin, terpineol and vanillin (ii) Lignans, of which at least five have been isolated, including secoisosolariciresinol dimethyl ether [1] and kusunokiol [2].

MEDICINAL USE: Topically as a rubifacient and mild analgesic; and

91

as an ingredient of lip balms, chilblain ointments, cold sore lotions and liniments for muscle pain and stiffness [R1]. Large quantities should not be applied externally since camphor may be absorbed through the skin causing systemic toxicity. Small doses can be taken internally for colds, diarrhoea and other complaints; but overdosing causes vomiting, convulsions, palpitations and can be fatal. Camphor is highly mycostatic against *Aspergillus flavus* [3]. Ngai camphor is from *Blumea balsamifera* (Compositae) and Borneo camphor from *Dryobalanops aromatica* (Dipterocarpaceae). Both have similar uses.

BIBLICAL REFERENCES: Song of Solomon 1:14 and 4:13.

SPECIFIC REFERENCES: 1. Takaoka D *et al* (1975) *Nippon Kagaku Kaishi* 12:2192. 2. Stone J *et al* (1951) *Anal. Chem.* 23:771. 3. Mishra A *et al* (1991) *Int. J. Pharmacog.* 29(4):259.

CAMPTOTHECA

CAMPTOTHECA ACUMINATA DECNE
Fam. Nyssaceae

SYNONYMS: Happy Tree, Xi-Shu.

HABITAT: China.

DESCRIPTION: A tropical, slow-growing tree, which produces seeds only after six to 10 years.

PART USED: Seeds.

CONSTITUENTS: (i) Pyroloquinoline alkaloids, referred to as the campthothecins, such as camptothecin itself, together with hydroxycamptothecin, methoxycamptothecin methylangustoline and others [R3,R14;1].

MEDICINAL USE: A source of alkaloids, particularly the camptothecins, which are used to prepare irinotecan (11-hydroxycamptothecin), topotecan and others used for the treatment of solid tumours such as those of the colon, rectum, lung and ovaries [R14]. Camptothecin derivatives are topoisomerase I inhibitors which inhibit DNA synthesis [R3,R14;2].

SPECIFIC REFERENCES: 1. Lin L *et al* (1989) *Phytochem.* 28:1295. 2. Wiseman R *et al* (1996) *Drugs* 52:606.

CANADIAN HEMP

APOCYNUM CANNABINUM L.
Fam. Apocynaceae

SYNONYMS: Black Indian Hemp, *Apocynum pubescens* Brown.

HABITAT: North America and Canada.

DESCRIPTION: The root is about 0.5 cm or more in diameter, rarely branched, longitudinally wrinkled, fissured transversely, pale brown externally. The bark is thick, whitish, with a central, porous, radiate wood, and a small, central pith. Fracture: short; taste: bitter and disagreeable; odourless.

PART USED: Root, rhizome.

CONSTITUENTS: (i) Cardiac glycosides, including strophanthin, strophanthin, cannogenin, cannogenol glycosides, cymaroside, oleadroside, digitoxoside and digitaloside (ii) Pregnane derivatives: neridienone and 6,7-didehydrocortexone [1].

MEDICINAL USE: Diaphoretic, diuretic, emetic, expectorant [R1]. Formerly used for cardiac dropsy, as the actions are similar to Strophanthus (q.v.) [R2].

SPECIFIC REFERENCES: 1. Abe F et al (1994) Chem. Pharm. Bull. 42(10):2028.

CANCHALAGUA
CENTAURIUM CHILENSIS (WILLD) DRUCE.
Fam. Gentianaceae

SYNONYMS: Erythraea chilensis Pers.

HABITAT: Pacific coast of America.

DESCRIPTION: Closely resembles Centaury, but is more branched, with linear leaves and stalked flowers.

PART USED: Herb.

CONSTITUENTS: Erythrocentaurin, a bitter, and tannins. Not well investigated [R4].

MEDICINAL USE: Bitter, tonic, stimulant [R1]; used in a similar way to Centaury (q.v.).

CANELLA
CANELLA WINTERANA (L.) GAERTN.
Fam. Canellaceae

SYNONYMS: White Cinnamon, West Indian Wild Cinnamon, Canella alba Murr.

HABITAT: The West Indies and Florida.

DESCRIPTION: The bark occurs in quilled pieces, fawn-coloured externally, the ash-grey cork having been removed by gentle beating; chalky white on inner surface. Transverse fracture short, with numerous bright orange-yellow oleo-resin cells. Taste: biting, aromatic; odour: reminiscent of cinnamon.

PART USED: Bark.

CONSTITUENTS: (i) Volatile oil, up to 1.25%, containing a-pinene, eugenol, caryophyllene, canellal (= muzigadial, a sesquiterpene dialdehyde), 4,13-epoxymuzigadial, dihydroxycinnamolide, 3-methoxy-4,5-methylenedioxy-cinnamaldehyde and others [1,2,3].

MEDICINAL USE: Aromatic, stimulant, tonic, usually in combination with other drugs [R1]. Canella bark has actions similar to those of Cinnamon (q.v.). Canellal has been shown to be antimicrobial and anti-feedant in insects [3]. It is more often used as a condiment [R2].

93

SPECIFIC REFERENCES: 1. El Feraly M *et al* (1980) *J. Nat. Prod.*
43:407. 2. Kioy D *et al* (1990) *J. Nat. Prod.* 53(5):1372. 3. Al-Said M
et al (1988) *Phytochem.* 28(1):297.

CARAWAY
CARUM CARVI L.
Fam. Apiaceae

SYNONYMS: Caraway Seed or Fruit, *Apium carvi* Crantz.

HABITAT: Native to Europe, Asia and North Africa, widely cultivated.

DESCRIPTION: The fruits are small, brown and slightly curved, about
4–8 mm long and 1–2 mm wide. They are tapered at both ends with
five longitudinal ridges. Odour: pleasant, aromatic and characteristic.

PART USED: Fruit.

CONSTITUENTS: (i) Volatile oil, consisting of carvone (40–60%)
and limonene, with dihydrocarvone, carveol, dihydrocarveol, pinene,
thujone, anethofuran, and other minor constituents [R2,1] (ii) A series
of *p*-menthane triols and their glucosides [2] (iii) Flavonoids: mainly
quercetin derivatives [3].

MEDICINAL USE: Antispasmodic, carminative, stimulant and
expectorant [R1]. It is used mainly for stomach complaints in both
adults and children. The antispasmodic and carminative effects in
dyspepsia have been confirmed using a combination of caraway with
peppermint oil [4] and caraway oil shown to reduce foaming of
gastrointestinal fluids *in vitro* [5]. Carvone, anethofuran and limonene
induce glutathione S-transferase enzymes, suggesting a chemopreventative effect [1] and the oil inhibited croton oil-induced skin tumours
in mice, especially when applied topically [6]. The oil has been
shown to be hypoglycaemic in rats [7]. For full review, see [8].

PREPARATIONS AND DOSE: Powdered seeds, dose: 0.5–2 g; Caraway
Oil, dose: 0.05–0.2 ml.

SPECIFIC REFERENCES: 1. Zheng G *et al* (1992) *Planta Med.*
58(4):338. 2. Matsumura T *et al* (2001) *Tetrahedron* 57(38)8067. 3.
Hopf H *et al* (1977) *Phytochem.* 16:1715. 4. Micklefield G *et al* (2000)
Phytother. Res. 14(1):20. 5. Harries N *et al* (1978) *J. Clin. Pharm.*
2:171. 6. Schwaireb M (1993) *Nutr. Cancer* 19(3):321. 7. Kalia A *et al*
(1994) *Indian J. Clin. Biochem.* 9(2):79. 8. Caraway. Ed: Nemeth E
(1999) *Medicinal and Aromatic Plants – Industrial Profiles.* Pub: Taylor
and Francis, London, UK.

CARDAMON
ELETTARIA CARDAMOMUM (L.) MATON.
Fam. Zingiberaceae

SYNONYMS: Cardamom Seed.

HABITAT: Indigenous to the Malabar Coast of India and Sri Lanka,
but now cultivated widely in the tropics.

DESCRIPTION: Ovoid or oblong fruit, somewhat triangular in cross-section and longitudinally finely striated. Mysore and Malabar cardamoms are usually bleached to a cream or pale buff colour, they have a smoother surface but are found less often in commerce now than the smaller, greener Alleppy or Ceylon varieties. All samples should be whole, containing seeds which are about 4 mm diameter and dark reddish-brown. Taste: aromatic and pungent; odour: highly aromatic, pleasant.

PART USED: Fruits, seeds.

CONSTITUENTS: Volatile oil, the major components of which are 1,8-cineole and alpha-terpinylacetate, with limonene, alpha-terpineol, sabinene, linalool, nerolidol, farnesol, and 3-methyl-pentan-2-ol [R2;1].

MEDICINAL USE: Carminative, stomachic, stimulant [R1]. The oil has antispasmodic activity in rabbits, acting via muscarinic receptor blockage, and analgesic activity in mice [2], and increases gastric acid secretion in rats [3]. The oil increases glutathione-S-transferase activity and reduces levels of cytochrome P450 enzymes [4]. It acts as a penetration enhancer for indomethacin through the skin [5]. For full review, see [6]. Cardamom is most often used as food flavouring.

PREPARATIONS AND DOSE: Powdered fruit, dose: 0.5–2 g; Aromatic Cardamom Tincture BP, dose: 2–4 ml; Compound Cardamom Tincture BP, dose: 2–4 ml.

SPECIFIC REFERENCES: 1. Menon A *et al* (1999) *Flav. Frag. J.* 14(1):65. 2. Al-Zuhair H *et al* (1996) *Pharmacol. Res.* 34(1-2):79. 3. Vasudevan K *et al* (2000) *Indian J. Gastroenterol.* 19(2):53. 4. Banerjee S *et al* (1994) *Nutr. Cancer* 21(3):263. 5. Tsai Y-H *et al* (1999) *Biol. Pharm. Bull.* 22(6):642. 6. Cardamom. Ed. Ravindran P (2002) *Medicinal and Aromatic Plants – Industrial Profiles.* Pub: Taylor and Francis, London, UK.

CAROB
CERATONIA SILIQUA L.
Fam. Caesalpiniaceae

SYNONYMS: St John's Bread, Locust Bean.

HABITAT: Native to southeastern Europe and western Asia, cultivated elsewhere.

DESCRIPTION: Pods about 10–30 cm long and 3–5 cm broad, containing flattish, oval, dark brown seeds in a light-brown fleshy pulp.

PART USED: Seed pulp.

CONSTITUENTS: (i) Mucilages, about 30%, consisting of glucomannans, especially carubine (ii) Tannins and polyphenols including the flavonoids schaftoside, neoschaftoside and isoschaftoside (iii) Tannins and (iv) Protein [R2,R19;1].

MEDICINAL USE: Anti-diarrhoeal, as a decoction for catarrh and to improve the voice [R1]. Carob is used as a substitute for cocoa as it

95

contains no stimulants such as theobromine or caffeine, and in fact has been shown to contain compounds which bind to the benzodiazepine receptor and may therefore have potential sedative or anxiolytic activity [2]. This plant should not be confused with the Carob Tree, *Jacaranda procera* or *J. caroba*, natives of South America and South Africa, the leaves of which are reputed to be diuretic and sedative. Carob (*Ceratonia*) reduces blood cholesterol, glucose and insulin levels in the rat [1]. Carob flour is now widely used for thickening feeds in the treatment of infantile diarrhoea and sickness [3,4].

PREPARATIONS AND DOSE: Carob flour, dose: 0.5–1% of feeds, for infants.

SPECIFIC REFERENCES: 1. Forestieri A *et al* (1989) *Phytother. Res.* 3(1):1. 2. Avallone R *et al* (2002) *Fitoterapia* 73(5):390. 3. Loeb H *et al* (1989) *J. Ped. Gastroenterol. Nutr.* 8(4):480. 4. Greally P *et al* (1992) *Arch. Dis. Childhood* 67(5):618.

CARROT, WILD

DAUCUS CAROTA L., SUBSP. *CAROTA*
Fam. Apiaceae

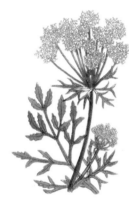

WILD CARROT

SYNONYMS: Queen Anne's Lace.

HABITAT: Europe, Asia and North Africa. This is the wild form of the garden carrot.

DESCRIPTION: The aerial parts resemble those of the garden carrot, but the root is small and white. The fruits are typically umbelliferous, composed of small double achenes, ridged, with numerous bristles arranged in five rows.

PART USED: Herb, fruit.

CONSTITUENTS: Fruit: (i) Volatile oil consisting of asarone, *cis*-beta-bergamotene, beta-bisabolene, carotol, caryophyllene and its oxide, coumarin, daucol, beta-elemene, geraniol, geranyl acetate, limonene, alpha-pinene, beta-selinene, alpha-terpineol, terpinen-4-ol and others (ii) Flavonoids; apigenin-4'-*O*-beta-D-glucoside, kaempferol-3-*O*-beta-D-glucoside and apigenin-7-*O*-beta-D-galactomannoside [R2,R7;1,2,3]. Herb (i) Volatile oil containing the terpenes carotol and geranyl acetate (ii) Flavonoids; 3-*O*-methyl-kaempferol, apigenin, quercetin, myricetin and sakuranetin [3] (iii) Miscellaneous; petroselinic acid, tannins.

MEDICINAL USE: The herb is used as a diuretic, carminative and anti-lithic, particularly for kidney stone, cystitis and gout [R1]. The seed is used for similar purposes but is usually considered to be more potent, being diuretic, emmenagogue, carminative and anti-flatulent. Diuretic activity has been described for the fruits [4] and anti-tumour activity for the extract *in vitro* has been reported [5]. Other properties include spasmolytic and liver protectant effects [R7;6]; anti-fertility (oestrogenic) and other actions in animals [R7;3,7].

PREPARATIONS AND DOSE: Herb, dose: 2–4 g, or equivalent extract.

SPECIFIC REFERENCES: 1. El-Moghazi *et al* (1980) *Planta Med.* 40:382.
2. Ceska O *et al* (1986) *Phytochem.* 25:81. 3. Dhar V *et al* (1990)
Fitoterapia 61:255. 4. Mahran G *et al* (1991) *Phytother. Res.* 5(4):169. 5.
Majumder P *et al* (1998) *Phytother. Res.* 12(8):584. 6. Handa S (1986)
Fitoterapia 57:307. 7. Lal R *et al* (1986) *Fitoterapia* 57:243.

CASCARA AMARGA
PICRAMNIA ANTIDESMA SW.
P. PENTANDRA SW.
P. PARVIFOLIA ENGLER
P. SELLOWI AND OTHER SPP.
Fam. Simaroubaceae

SYNONYMS: West Indian Snakewood (*P. antidesma*), Bitter Bush
(*P. pentandra*).

HABITAT: West Indies and Central America.

DESCRIPTION: Bark usually found in small fragments about 2–3 mm
thick, externally greyish, internally deep brown, inner surface nearly
smooth. Fracture: short, showing numerous dots due to stone cells.
Taste: astringent then bitter and earthy.

PART USED: Bark.

CONSTITUENTS: (i) Anthaquinone glycosides based on chrysophanol,
emodin, physcion and aloe-emodin (ii) Triterpenes including betulinic
acid and epibetulinic acid [1,2].

MEDICINAL USE: Bitter tonic, alterative, laxative [R1]. For the typical
effects of the anthraquinone glycosides, see Senna.

SPECIFIC REFERENCES: 1. Propinigis I *et al* (1980) *Trib. Farm.*
48(1–2):24. 2. Cam J (1975) *Bol. Soc. Quim. Peru* 39(4):204. 3. Herz W
et al (1972) *Phytochem.* 11:3061.

CASCARA SAGRADA
RHAMNUS PURSHIANUS D.C.
Fam. Rhamnaceae

SYNONYMS: Sacred Bark, Chittem Bark, Cascara, *Rhamnus purshiana*
L., *Frangula purshiana* (D.C.) A. Gray ex J C Cooper.

HABITAT: Native to the Pacific coast of North America.

DESCRIPTION: In commerce, the bark is usually supplied in curved
pieces or quills, about 1 mm or more thick, purplish-brown, furrowed
longitudinally, with transverse lenticels, and lichens and mosses visible
as silver-grey or greenish patches. The inner surface is reddish-brown,
longitudinally striated and transversely wrinkled. Fracture: pale to dark
brown, darkening with age. Taste: bitter and nauseous; odour: leathery.

PART USED: Bark, collected in the spring and early summer and stored for
at least a year before use, to eliminate constituents causing griping pain.

CONSTITUENTS: Up to 10% anthraquinone glycosides, consisting of the cascarosides A and B (which are stereoisomeric aloin-8-gluco-sides), C and D (stereoisomeric 11-deoxy-aloin-8-glucosides) and E and F (C-glucosyl aloin-8-glucosides) [1,2,3,4,5]; with other minor glycosides including barbaloin, frangulin, chrysaloin, the heterodi-anthrones palmidin A, B and C (see Rhubarb) and the free aglycones [R3,R7].

MEDICINAL USE: Stimulant laxative [R1]. The cascarosides act on the large intestine; they inhibit water and electrolyte re-absorption from the colon, thought to be by involving inducible nitric oxide synthase, and thus stimulating peristalsis [6]. The glycosides are more effective than the hydrolyzed aloins [R3,R7]. Genotoxicity *in vitro* has been reported [7], and the US Food and Drugs Administration have ruled that cascara will not be allowed in over-the-counter laxative preparations, due to safety concerns. However, fears that anthranoid laxative use is a risk factor for colorectal cancer were shown to be unfounded in a prospective case control study [8], and Cascara was shown not to induce colonic tumours and aberrant crypt foci in an experimental model of colon cancer in rats, unlike bisacodyl [9].
It is used for habitual constipation, although excessive use should be avoided to prevent undue loss of electrolytes, and should not be taken during pregnancy or lactation. Cascara often forms a part of herbal formulae for dyspepsia, digestive complaints and haemorrhoids.

PREPARATIONS AND DOSE: Powdered bark, dose: 1–2.5 g; Cascara Dry Extract BP, dose: 100–300 mg; Cascara tablets BP, dose: 1 or 2 tablets.

SPECIFIC REFERENCES: 1. Evans F *et al* (1975) *J. Pharm. Pharmacol.* 27:91P. 2. Fairbairn J *et al* (1977) *J. Pharm. Sci.* 66:1300. 3. Manitto P *et al* (1995) *J. Nat. Prod.* 58:419. 4. Griffini A *et al* (1992) *Planta Med.* 58:S7:A593. 5. DeWitte P *et al* (1991) *Planta Med.* 57:440. 6. Izzo A *et al* (1997) *Eur. J. Pharmacol.* 323(1):93. 7. Helmholz H *et al* (1993) *Pharm. Zeit.* 138:3478. 8. Nusko G *et al* (2000) *Gut* 46(5):651. 9. Borrelli F *et al* (2001) *Life Sci.* 69(16)1871.

CASCARILLA
CROTON ELEUTERIA BENNETT.
Fam. Euphorbiaceae

SYNONYMS: Sweet Wood Bark.

HABITAT: Native to the West Indies; grows also in tropical America.

DESCRIPTION: The bark occurs in short quilled pieces, usually with a chalky, more or less cracked, white surface, with black dots due to the fruit of lichens. The transverse fracture is reddish-brown. Taste: aromatic, bitter; odour: aromatic, particularly when burnt, hence its use in flavouring tobacco.

PART USED: Bark.

CONSTITUENTS: (i) Volatile oil, 1.5–3%, containing limonene, *p*-cymene, eugenol, beta-caryophyllene, dipentene, cineole, methyl thymol, cascarilladiene, cascarillone and cascarillic acid (ii) Diterpenes including cascarillin A (iii) Miscellaneous; vanillin, betaine, cuparophenol, [R2;1].

MEDICINAL USE: Stimulant, aromatic, tonic [R1]. Used in dyspepsia, flatulence and diarrhoea and as an anti-emetic, usually taken as an infusion.

SPECIFIC REFERENCES: 1. Hagedorn M et al (1991) *Flav. Frag. J.* 6(3):193.

CASHEW NUT
ANACARDIUM OCCIDENTALE L.
Fam. Anacardiaceae.

SYNONYMS: East Indian Almond, *Cassuvium pomiferum.*

HABITAT: Cultivated extensively in the tropics.

DESCRIPTION: Fruit kidney-shaped, smooth, pale greyish-brown, about 23 cm long and 1 cm broad and thick.

PART USED: Seeds, leaves, bark, liquid from shell (as a pesticide).

CONSTITUENTS: Seeds (nuts): (i) Fatty oil, mainly oleic and linoleic esters, anacardoside and others [R2;1,2]. The caustic liquid in the shell surrounding the seed contains (ii) anacardic acids, cardols, methyl cardols and cardanols, which are alkyl phenols [3]. The bark yields a resin containing similar compounds. Leaves: (i) Flavonoids, mainly
glycosides of quercetin and kaempferol and hydroxybenzoic acid [4].

MEDICINAL USE: Leaves and bark are used as an infusion for toothache and sore gums in West Africa, and as a febrifuge in malaria [R1]. Anacardic acids are bactericidal against *Staphylococcus aureus* as well as being fungicidal, vermicidal and protozoicidal [5,6]. The liquid containing them, from the shell of cashew, is being investigated as an alternative molluscicidal agent, to control snail vectors of schistosomiasis [3,7] and it is also larvicidal against the *Aedes aegypti* mosquito [7]. It inhibits alpha-glucosidase, invertase and aldose reductase [3], has a weak tumour-promoting effect in experimental skin carcinogenesis [8] and is mutagenic [9].

SPECIFIC REFERENCES: 1. Gil R *et al* (1995) *Phytochem.* 58:405. 2. Nagaraja K *et al* (1987) *Pl. Foods Hum. Nutr.* 37:307. 3. Toyomizu M *et al* (1993) *Phytother. Res.* 7(3):252. 4. Laurens A *et al* (1976) *Plantes. Med. Phytother.* 27:354. 5. Ogunlana E *et al* (1975) *Planta Med.* 27:354. 6. Sullivan J *et al* (1982) *Planta Med.* 44:175. 7. Laurens A *et al* (1997) *Phytother. Res.* 11(2):145. 8. Banerjee S *et al* (1992) *Cancer Lett.* 62(2):149. 9. George J *et al* (1997) *Cancer Lett.* 67(2):149.

CASSIA
CINNAMOMUM CASSIA BLUME
Fam. Lauraceae

SYNONYMS: Chinese Cinnamon, False Cinnamon, *Cinnamomum aromaticum* Nees, *Cassia lignea,* Rougui (Chinese).

HABITAT: Southeast Asia, China.

DESCRIPTION: The bark is brown, in quilled pieces, sometimes with the remains of the outer layer present. The quills are rarely found inserted inside one another as in Cinnamon (q.v.). Taste and odour: reminiscent of cinnamon, but distinctive.

PART USED: Bark. Cassia Oil BPC is distilled from the leaves and twigs.

CONSTITUENTS: (i) Volatile oil, consisting mainly of trans-cinnamaldehyde, with hydroxycinnamaldehyde (HCA), 2'-benzoyloxycinnamaldehyde (BCA), cinnamylacetate, phenylpropylacetate and numerous trace constituents including salicylaldehyde and methyleugenol (ii) Glycosides and polyphenols, such as the cassiosides, cinnamosides, procyanidins B_2, B_4, B_5, B_7, B_{10}, C_1, and others; the cinnamonols D_1 and D_4, cinnamtannins I, II, and III; the cinncassiols A–E and their glucosides [1,2,3,4,5,6].

MEDICINAL USE: Aromatic, stomachic, tonic, antipyretic, diaphoretic and analgesic [R1]. It is widely used in Chinese medicine, for vascular disorders particularly. The volatile oil is carminative and antiseptic; cinnamaldehyde and extracts of the bark are anti-thrombotic [8]. Cinnamaldehyde is however very volatile and easily lost from the crude drug and its preparations. Aqueous extracts show potent anti-allergic properties in mice [9] and the cinncassiols are thought to be responsible for at least some of these effects [1,2]. Cassioside and cinnamoside are anti-ulcerogenic [4]. Other activities exhibited by extracts of the bark include inhibition of human tumour growth (using xenografts on nude mice) [3], antipyretic and interleukin-1-alpha regulating effects [10], prevention of glutamate-induce neuronal death in cultured cerebellar granule cells [11] and inhibition of mutagenesis in the Ames test, attributed to modulation of xenobiotic bioactivation and detoxification processes [12]. The oil is used mainly for flavouring medicines, cosmetics, toothpastes, mouthwashes and foods [R7].

PREPARATIONS AND DOSE: Powdered bark, dose: 0.5–1 g or equivalent extract; Cassia oil BPC 1949, dose: 0.05–0.2 ml.

BIBLICAL REFERENCES: Exodus 30:24; Psalm 45:8; Ezekiel 27:19.

SPECIFIC REFERENCES: 1. Nohara T *et al* (1982) *Phytochem.* 21(8):2130. 2. Nohara T *et al* (1985) *Phytochem.* 24(8):1849. 3. Lee C-W *et al* (1999) *Planta Med.* 65(3):263. 4. Shiraga Y *et al* (1988) *Tetrahedron* 44(15):4703. 5. Morimoto S *et al* (1986) *Chem. Pharm. Bull.* 34(2):643. 6. Otsuka H *et al* (1982) *Yakugaku Zasshi* 102:162.

7. Lockwood G (1979) *Planta Med.* 36:380. 8. Matsuda H *et al* (1987) *Chem. Pharm. Bull.* 35(3):1275. 9. Lee E (2000) *Nat. Prod. Sci.* 6(1):49. 10. Shiraki K *et al* (1998) *Eur. J. Pharmacol.* 348(1):45. 11. Shimada Y *et al* (2000) *Phytother. Res.* 14(6):466. 12. Sharma N *et al* (2001) *Mut. Res.* 480–481:179.

CASSIA PODS
CASSIA FISTULA L.
Fam. Caesalpiniaceae

SYNONYMS: Pudding Stick.

HABITAT: Cultivated in the tropics.

DESCRIPTION: The pods are up to 50 cm long, with the interior divided into compartments containing the seeds and a thin layer of black fruit pulp.

PART USED: Pulp.

CONSTITUENTS: (i) Anthraquinone glycosides, sennosides A and B (ii) Sugars, mainly saccharose (iii) In the seeds, fatty oil and sterols [R2].

MEDICINAL USE: A pleasant fruit laxative [R1], acting in a similar way to Senna (q.v.), but rather milder. The seeds are reported to reduce blood cholesterol levels in rats [1].

PREPARATIONS AND DOSE: Cassia Pulp BPC 1959, dose: 4–8 g.

SPECIFIC REFERENCES: 1. El-Saadany S *et al* (1991) *Nahrung* 35:807.

CASTOR OIL PLANT
RICINUS COMMUNIS L.
Fam. Euphorbiaceae

SYNONYMS: Castor Bean, Palma Christi.

HABITAT: Probably native to eastern Africa, but naturalized and cultivated worldwide in warmer climates.

DESCRIPTION: A tall, branched shrub, with large, palmate leaves and irregular serrate margins, often with a bluish or reddish tinge. The flowers are monoecious, in terminal racemes. The fruit capsules are spiny and soft, or smooth and grooved, containing the large oval seeds. These are cream or greyish-brown and often mottled or speckled with brown or black markings.

PART USED: Oil expressed from seed, leaves.

CONSTITUENTS: Seeds: (i) Fixed oil, consisting mainly of glycerides of ricinoleic, isoricinoleic acids, and to a lesser extent stearic, linoleic, dihydroxystearic and other acids [R16]. The seeds are highly poisonous, but the toxin, ricin, is left behind in the cake after pressing and steam treatment: it is a mixture of proteins, called ricins A, B, C, D and E, and alpha-, beta, and gamma-ricins [R16;1]. The seed cake also contains an alkaloid, ricinine [2]. Leaves: (i) Flavonoids, coumarins and phenolic

101

acids including corilagic, epicatechin, ellagic, gallic and chlorogenic acids; hyperoside, rutin and others [R16;3] (ii) Alkaloids; ricinine and N-demethylricinine [3] (iii) Sterols including brassicasterol, campesterol, lupeol and others [R16].

MEDICINAL USE: Castor oil has been used since ancient times as a laxative and purgative [R1], the activity being due mainly to the ricinoleic acid content. Ricinoleic acid has multiple effects on the intestinal mucosa, including release of prostanoids, nitric oxide and platelet-activating factor. Castor oil decreases fluid reabsorption and increases secretion in the small intestine and colon; it also causes histological abnormalities [4,5] and so should not be used regularly or for long periods. It has been used to expel worms after treatment but should not be used for this purpose since it may facilitate absorption of some anthelmintics. The oil has a folklore reputation for inducing labour and as an emmenagogue; and a processed seed extract has contraceptive activity [6]. Castor oil is emollient and soothing to the skin and eye and is an ingredient of many cosmetic and ophthalmic preparations. Ricinine is goitrogenic [2] and a central nervous system stimulant [7]. The leaves are hepatoprotective [8], antimicrobial [9] and have various other effects [R16]

PREPARATIONS AND DOSE: Castor Oil BP, dose: 5–20 ml.

SPECIFIC REFERENCES: 1. Lin J *et al* (1986) *Toxicon* 24(8):757. 2. Pahuja D N *et al* (1979) *Biochem. Pharmacol.* 28:461. 3. Kang, S *et al* (1985) *J. Nat. Prod.* 48(1):155. 4. Izzo A *et al* (1996) *Phytother. Res.* 10:S109. 5. Gaginella T *et al* (1998) *Phytother. Res.* 12:S128. 6. Okwuasaba F *et al* (1997) *Phytother. Res.* 11(8):547. 7. Ferraz A *et al* (1999) *Pharmacol. Biochem. Behav.* 63(3):367. 8. Visen P *et al* (1992) *Int. J. Pharmacog.* 30(4):241. 9. Verpoorte R *et al* (1987) *J. Ethnopharmacol.* 21(3):315.

CAT'S CLAW
UNCARIA TOMENTOSA (WILLD.) D.C.
U. GUIANENSIS (AUBL.) GMEL.
Fam. Rubiaceae

SYNONYMS: Una de Gato.

HABITAT: The Amazon River basin, South America.

DESCRIPTION: A large vine bearing climbing hooks, which are said to resemble the claws of a cat.

PART USED: Aerial parts.

CONSTITUENTS: (i) Alkaloids, both tetracyclic and pentacyclic oxindoles, including uncarines C and E, mitraphylline, rhynchophylline, isorhynchophylline [1,2,3,4]. There are two chemotypes, one containing pentacyclics and the other tetracyclic alkaloids [1] (ii) Triterpenes based on 19-hydroxyursolic acid [5], stigmasterol, campesterol and others (iii) Miscellaneous; quinovic acid glycosides, epicatechin etc. [R7].

MEDICINAL USE: Traditionally used by the people of the Peruvian rainforest for inflammatory disorders such as arthritis and rheumatism, and for asthma, gastric ulcer, skin diseases and cancer, it is now being widely used elsewhere in the world. Anti-inflammatory activity has been confirmed in clinical studies using patients with osteoarthritis of the knee, and no deleterious effects on haematological parameters were observed [6]. Inhibition of NF-kappa-B has been proposed as at least part of the mechanism [7], together with antioxidant and immunomodulation via suppression of TNF-alpha synthesis [8]. Immune enhancement was also noted in male volunteers, as measured by an elevation in the lymphocytes/neutrophil ratios of peripheral blood after pneumococcal vaccination [9]. Toxicity studies *in vitro* using Chinese hamster ovary and bacterial cells showed no adverse effects [10]. Commercial preparations of Cat's Claw inhibited human cytochrome P450 3A4 enzymes *in vitro* [11]. The tetracyclic alkaloids are active on the nervous system, whereas the pentacyclics affect the cellular immune system and their effects are thought to be antagonistic to each other [1]. However, a total alkaloid extract exerted a beneficial effect on memory impairment in mice with experimental amnesia induced by dysfunction of the cholinergic system. In the case of uncarine E, glutamate involvement was also implicated [3]. Other therapeutic activities ascribed to Cat's Claw include antioxidant properties [12], anti-tumour activity [13] and an interaction with oestrogen receptors [14]. In general it is non-toxic although renal failure was reported in a patient who added a large dose of Cat's Claw to her existing multi-drug regimen [15].

PREPARATIONS AND DOSE: Powdered herb, dose: 0.5–5 g daily, or equivalent extract.

SPECIFIC REFERENCES: 1. Rheinhard K-H (1997) *Z. Phytother.* 18(2):112. 2. Keplinger K *et al* (1999) *J. Ethnopharmacol.* 64:23. 3. Abdel-Fattah M *et al* (2000) *J. Pharm. Pharmacol.* 52:1553. 4. Ganzera M *et al* (2001) *Planta Med.* 67(5):447. 5. Kitajima M *et al* (2000) *Tetrahedron* 56(4):547. 6. Sandoval M *et al* (2001) *Inflammation Res.* 50(9):442. 7. Sandoval M *et al* (1998) *Aliment. Pharmacol. Therapeut.* 12(12):1279. 8 Sandoval M *et al* (2000) *Free Rad. Biol. Med.* 29(1):71. 9. Lamm S *et al* (2001) *Phytomedicine* 8(4):267. 10. Maria A *et al* (1997) *J. Ethnopharmacol.* 57(3):183. 11. Budzinski J *et al* (2000) *Phytomedicine* 7(4):273. 12. Desmarchelier C *et al* (1997) *Phytother. Res.* 11:254. 13. Lee K *et al* (1999) *Planta Med.* 65:759. 14. Salazar E *et al* (1997) *Proc. Western Pharmacol. Soc.* 41:123. 15. Hilepo J *et al* (1997) *Nephron* 77:361.

CATECHU, BLACK

ACACIA CATECHU WILLD.
Fam. Mimosaceae

SYNONYMS: Cutch, Dark Catechu, Terra Japonicum, Khadira, *Catechu nigrum.*

HABITAT: India, China, Japan; now commonly found elsewhere.

DESCRIPTION: The extract occurs in commerce as black shining pieces or cakes, sometimes with the remains of leaf on the outside. Taste: very astringent then bitter and sweetish; odourless.

PART USED: Extract from leaves and young shoots.

CONSTITUENTS: (i) Tannins; mainly catechutannic acid, with acacatechin and others (ii) Flavonoids and anthocyanins, including quercetin, quercitrin, fisetin, cyanidanol and others [R16,1].

MEDICINAL USE: Astringent [R1]. It is used in chronic diarrhoea, dysentery and chronic catarrh, to arrest excessive mucous discharges and check haemorrhage, among other activities. It has also been shown to be hypotensive *in vivo* and *in vitro*; its mechansim of action is thought to be bradykinin-related and due to vasodilatation [2]. The ethyl acetate activity demonstrated hepatoprotective activity in an animal model [3].

SPECIFIC REFERENCES: 1. Despande V *et al* (1981) *Indian J. Chem.* 20B:658. 2. Sham J *et al* (1984) *Planta Med.* 42:177. 3. Jayasekhar P *et al* (1997) *Indian J. Pharmacol.* 29:246.

CATECHU, PALE
UNCARIA GAMBIER ROXB.
Fam. Rubiaceae

SYNONYMS: Gambir, Gambier, *Terra japonica, Ourouparia gambir* Baill.

HABITAT: Southeast Asia.

DESCRIPTION: Occurs as pale reddish to dark brownish-black cubes or lozenges, with a dull, powdery fracture. Taste similar to Black Catechu (q.v.).

PART USED: Extract of leaves and shoots.

CONSTITUENTS: (i) Tannins; mainly catechins, up to 35%, and catechutannic acid up to 50% (ii) Indole alkaloids including gambirine gambiridine and others (iii) Flavonoids such as quercetin (iv) Pigments and gambirfluorescin [R2,R19;1,2].

MEDICINAL USE: Astringent [R1]. Uses are similar to those of Black Catechu (q.v.). Gambirine is reported to be hypotensive and d-catechu to constrict blood vessels [R19].

PREPARATIONS AND DOSE: Powder, dose: 0.3–1 g; Pale Catechu BP (Vet) 2000; Tincture of Catechu BP 1989.

SPECIFIC REFERENCES: 1. Merlini L *et al* (1967) *Tetrahedron* 23:3129. 2. Phillipson J *et al* (1978) *Lloydia* 41:503.

CATNIP
NEPETA CATARIA L.
Fam. Labiatae

SYNONYMS: Catnep, Catmint.

HABITAT: A common European herb, cultivated in Britain and North America.

DESCRIPTION: Leaves stalked, cordate-ovate, pointed, with a serrate margin and a whitish, hairy undersurface. The stem is quadrangular and hairy. Flowers tubular, two-lipped, white with crimson dots, arranged in short, dense, spikes. Taste and odour: mint-like but characteristic.

PART USED: Herb.

CONSTITUENTS: (i) Volatile oil, containing the monoterpenes alpha- and beta-nepetalactone, epi-nepetalactone, 5,9-dehydronepeta-lactone, carvacrol, citronellal, nerol, geraniol, pulegone, thymol, caryophyllene and nepetalic acid [R2;1] (ii) Iridoids, including epideoxyloganic acid and 7-deoxyloganic acid [2] (iii) Rosmarinic acid [3].

MEDICINAL USE: Diaphoretic, refrigerant, febrifuge, spasmolytic, anti-diarrhoeal, sedative [R1]. Used particularly for colds and colic in the form of a tea. It has a folklore reputation as a hallucinogen, however this is usually disputed. A case has however been described where a young child showed central nervous system depression after consuming a large quantity of catnip [4] and administration to mice produced an amphetamine-like effect [5]. Other studies have shown behavioural effects, although weak, in young chicks [6] as well as the well-known intoxicating effect on cats [7]. Nepetalactone is thought to be the active principle and has specific receptor sub-type agonist activity [8]. The oil is an effective insect repellant, again due to the nepetalactone content, paticularly against mosquitos [9].

CATNIP

PREPARATIONS AND DOSE: Dried herb, dose: 2–4 g or equivalent extract.

SPECIFIC REFERENCES: 1. Sastry S *et al* (1972) *Phytochem.* 11:453. 2. Tagawa M *et al* (1983) *Planta Med.* 47:109. 3. Lamaison C *et al* (1991) *Fitoterapia* 62(2):166. 4. Osterhoudt K *et al* (1997). *Vet Hum. Toxicol.* 39(6):373. 5. Massoco C *et al* (1995) *Vet. Hum. Toxicol.* 37(6):530. 6. Sherry C *et al* (1981) *Quart. J. Crude Drug Res.* 19(1):31. 7. Hatch R (1972) *Am. J. Vet. Res.* 33:143. 8. Aydin S *et al* (1998) *J. Pharm. Pharmacol.* 50(7):813. 9. Peterson C *et al* (2001) *Pesticide Outlook* 12(4):154.

CEDRON
SIMABA CEDRON PLANCH.
Fam. Simaroubaceae

HABITAT: Central and South America.

DESCRIPTION: Commercial samples of the seed usually consist of the separated cotyledons; these are flattened on one side and convex on the other, are of a greyish-yellow tint and are about 4 cm long and 1–1.5 cm wide. Taste: very bitter; odour: recalling that of coconut.

PART USED: Seeds, less often the wood.

CONSTITUENTS: Quassinoids and protolimonoids, including chapparin, chaparrinone, glaucarubol, glaucarubalone, ailaquassin A, samaderine Z, guanepolide, polyandrol, simalikalactone D, cedronolactones A-D, and cedronin [1,2,3].

MEDICINAL USE: Febrifuge, bitter, tonic [R1]. The seeds have been employed in the treatment of malaria: it is now known that these quassinoids have antimalarial and anti-inflammatory properties *in vivo* and *in vitro*. Cedronin is active against chloroquine sensitive and resistant strains of types of *Plasmodium* [1] and shows *in vitro* cytotoxicity [1], as does cedronolactone A [3].

PREPARATIONS AND DOSE: Powder, dose: 0.05–0.5 g or equivalent extract.

SPECIFIC REFERENCES: 1. Moretti C *et al* (1994) *J. Ethnopharmacol.* 43(1):57. 2. Vieira L *et al* (1998) *Fitoterapia* 69(1):88. 3. Ozeki A *et al* (1998) *J. Nat. Prod.* 61(6)776.

CELANDINE
CHELIDONIUM MAJUS L.
Fam. Papaveraceae

SYNONYMS: Greater Celandine. Not related to the Lesser Celandine, also known as Pilewort (q.v.).

HABITAT: A common garden plant in Europe, flowering in May.

DESCRIPTION: Leaves pinnate, green above, greyish below, 15–30 cm long and 5–8 cm wide. Leaflets opposite, deeply cut, with rounded teeth. Stems have recurved hairs and exude a saffron yellow juice when fresh and broken. The flowers are yellow, consisting of four small petals, and are followed by narrow pods containing the black shiny seeds. Taste: bitter and acrid; odour: disagreeable.

PART USED: Herb.

CONSTITUENTS: (i) Alkaloids, including allocryptopine, berberine, chelamine, chelerythrine, chelidonine, coptisine, magnoflorine, protopine, sanguinarine, sparteine, stylopine and others [R7,R17;1,2,3] (ii) Poly-phenolic acids including chelidonic acid and caffeic acid derivatives [4].

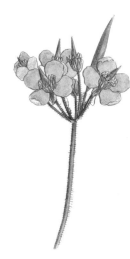

GREAT CELANDINE

MEDICINAL USE: Alterative, diuretic [R1]. Has been used in the treatment of jaundice, eczema, and the fresh juice as an application for corns and warts [R17]. In Chinese medicine this herb is also highly regarded and used as an analgesic, anti-tussive, anti-inflammatory and detoxicant. The alkaloids have reputed sedative activity, and have been shown to have an affinity for GABA-A receptors *in vitro* [4]; they also inhibit 5- and 12-lipoxygenase activity [2]. Chelidonium extracts increase choleresis in isolated perfused rat liver [5] and improve the parameters of experimental hepatic injury in animals [6]. They also inhibit acetylcholine-induced contractions of rat isolated ileum [7]. Extracts have anti-tumour effects in animals and are antimicrobial [R17] as well as anti-inflammatory [2]. Chelerythrine is a protein kinase

C inhibitor and extracts inhibit proliferation of keratinocytes [8]. These results go some way towards substantiating the therapeutic use of the herb, and spasmolytic and cholagogue effects have been demonstrated clinically [R17]; however clinical results are meagre at present.

PREPARATIONS AND DOSE: Powder, dose: 2–4 g, or equivalent extract, three times daily.

SPECIFIC REFERENCES: 1. Dostal J et al (1995) *J. Nat. Prod.* 58:723. 2. Colombo M et al (1995) *Pharm. Res.* 33(2):127. 3. Hahn R et al (1993) *Planta Med.* 59:71. 4. Haberlain H et al (1996) *Planta Med.* 62:227. 5. Vahlenisiek U et al (1995) *Planta Med.* 61:267. 6. Mitra S et al (1996) *Phytother. Res.* 10:354. 7. Boegge S et al (1996) *Planta Med.* 62:173. 8. Vavreckova C et al (1996) *Planta Med.* 62:491.

CELERY

APIUM GRAVEOLENS L.
Fam. Apiaceae

SYNONYMS: Smallage, Qincai (Chinese).

HABITAT: Cultivated widely. The wild variety grows in marshy places and has an unpleasant odour.

DESCRIPTION: Celery is a well-known plant needing no description. The seeds are very small, about 1 mm long, plano-convex, brown, with five paler, longitudinal ribs. Taste and odour: characteristic.

PART USED: Seeds. Stems of *A. graveolens* var *dulce* (Mill) Pers. are used as a vegetable.

CONSTITUENTS: (i) Volatile oil containing terpenes including *d*-limonene (major) with alpha-selinene, santalol, alpha- and beta-eudesmol, dihydrocarvone, menthadienols, others [1,2] (ii) Phthalides; mainly 3-*n*-butylphthalide, ligustilide, sedanolide, and sedanenolide [1,3,4] (iii) Coumarins; bergapten, isoimperatorin, isopimpinellin, osthenol and celeroside [5] (iv) Flavonoids; apiin and apigenin [R2,R7].

MEDICINAL USE: Anti-inflammatory, carminative, diuretic, sedative, tonic, reputed aphrodisiac [R1]. Some of these actions have been substantiated by experimentation; for example the aqueous extract has been shown to reduce adjuvant-induced arthritis in rats [6] and the ethanolic extract is anti-inflammatory in mice [7]. The extract can also protect against gastric damage in rats induced by NSAID's (non-steroidal anti-inflammatory agents) [8] and reduce lipid levels in rats fed a high fat diet [9]. The phthalides are sedative and exhibit anti-epileptic activity in mice [10]. Diuretic activity has also been described [11].

PREPARATIONS AND DOSE: Powdered seeds, dose: 1–4 g, or equivalent extract.

SPECIFIC REFERENCES: 1. Zheng G-Q et al (1993) *Nutr. Cancer* 19(1):77. 2. Macleod G et al (1989) *Phytochem.* 28:1817. 3. Uhlig J J. *Food Sci.* 52:658. 4. Fehr D (1987) *Pharmazie* (1979) 34:658. 5. Garg

107

S *et al* (1980) *Planta Med.* 38:363. 6. Lewis D *et al* (1985) *Int. J. Crude Drug Res.* 28(1):27. 7. Atta A *et al* (1998) *J. Ethnopharmacol.* 60(2):117. 8. Whitehouse M *et al* (2001) *Inflammopharmacology* 9 (1-2):201. 9. Tsi D *et al* (1995) *Planta Med.* 61(1):18. 10. Yu R *et al* (1985) *Acta Pharm. Sinica* (1987):566. 11. Mahran G *et al* (1991) *Phytother. Res.* 5(4):169.

CENTAURY

CENTAURIUM ERYTHRAEA RAFIN.
Fam. Gentianaceae

SYNONYMS: Century, Feverwort, *Centaurium minus* Moench, *C. umbellatum* Gilib., *Erythraea centaurium* Pers.

HABITAT: Native to Europe, including the British Isles, western Asia, North Africa and naturalized in North America.

DESCRIPTION: Stem up to 30 cm high, bearing opposite, lanceolate-ovate leaves having 3–5 longitudinal ribs, hairless, and entire at margins. Flowers pink, with twisted anthers. Taste: bitter; odour: slight.

PART USED: Herb.

CONSTITUENTS: (i) Secoiridoids. These glycosides are the so-called 'bitter principles' and include sweroside, its m-hydroxybenzoyl esters centapicrin and desacetylcentapicrin, the related glucosides decentapicrin A, B and C, gentiopicroside (= gentiopicrin), and swertiamarin [1,2] (ii) Alkaloids; gentianine, gentianidine, gentioflavine [R2] (iii) Xanthone derivatives such as eustomin, demethyleustomin, 1,8-dihydroxy-3,5,6,7-tetramethoxyxanthone, hydroxylated trimethoxyxanthones [3,4,5] (iv) Phenolic acids including protocatechuic, m- and p-hydroxybenzoic, vanillic, syringic, p-coumaric, ferulic and caffeic [6] (v) Triterpenes; beta-sitosterol, campesterol, brassicasterol, stigmasterol, alpha- and beta-amyrin, erythrodiol and others [6].

MEDICINAL USE: Aromatic, bitter, stomachic, tonic [R1]. Centaury is widely used in disorders of the upper digestive tract, in dyspepsia, for liver and gall bladder complaints and to stimulate the appetite in a similar manner to Gentian (q.v.). The xanthones are antimutagenic *in vitro* [5] and exhibit diuretic activity in rats [7]. Analgesic and antipyretic properties have also been observed for the aqueous extract [8]. For review see [6] and for information on the pharmacology of gentianin, gentianidine, gentiopicroside and swertiamarin, see Gentian.

PREPARATIONS AND DOSE: Powder, dose: 2–4 g, or equivalent extract, three times daily.

SPECIFIC REFERENCES: 1. Van der Sluis W *et al* (1980) *Planta Med.* 39:268. 2. Neshta N *et al* (1983) *Khim. Prir. Soed.* 1:106. 3. Bishay D *et al* (1978) *Planta Med.* 33:422. 4. Valentao P *et al* (2000) *Nat. Prod. Lett.* 14(5):319. 5. Schimmer O *et al* (1996) *Planta Med.* 62(6):561. 6. Schimmer O *et al* (1994) *Zeit. Fur Phytother.* 15(5):299. 7. Haloui M *et al* (2000) *J. Ethnopharmacol.* 71(3):465. 8. Berkan T *et al.* (1991) *Planta Med.* 57:34.

CHAMOMILE, ROMAN
CHAMAEMELUM NOBILE (L) ALL.
Fam. Asteraceae

SYNONYMS: English Chamomile, Roman Chamomile, Double Chamomile, Manzanilla, *Anthemis nobilis* L.

HABITAT: Indigenous to most of Europe, widely cultivated.

DESCRIPTION: Flowers mainly double, consisting of ligulate florets only, with a conical, solid receptacle, covered with lanceolate, membranous scales (known as palae). Leaves pinnately divided into short and hairy leaflets. Taste: aromatic and very bitter; odour: pleasant, characteristic. Wild chamomiles, with only an outer row of ligulate florets, are sometimes known as 'Scotch' chamomiles.

PART USED: Flowers, herb.

CONSTITUENTS: (i) Volatile oil, up to 1.75%, consisting mainly of esters of tiglic and angelic acids, with chamazulene, pinocarvone, 1, 8-cineole, alpha-pinene, isobutyrate esters, cyclododecane, pinen-3-one and others (ii) Sesquiterpene lactones of the germacranolide type, including nobilin, 1,10-epoxynobilin and 3-dihydronobilin (iii) Flavonoids such as anthemoside, cosmioside, chamaemeloside, luteolin and apigenin and their 7-glucosides (iv) Coumarins including scopoletin and its glucoside (v) Phenolic acids; trans-caffeic and ferulic acids and their glucosides (v) Polyynes such as cis- and trans- dehydromatricaria esters [R2,R7,1,2,3 and refs therein].

CHAMOMILE

MEDICINAL USE: Stomachic, anti-emetic, antispasmodic, mild sedative [R1]. Taken internally and applied externally as a lotion. It is used as a soothing and analgesic application in toothache, earache and neuralgia, and as a cream or ointment for wounds, sore nipples and nappy rash. The sesquiterpene lactones have anti-tumour activity *in vitro* and the flavonoid apigenin is sedative. For details of biological activities of individual components, see German Chamomile. Chamaemeloside has hypoglycaemic activity [3]. It is an ingredient of many shampoos and hair rinses for blonde hair. There are surprisingly few studies on Roman Chamomile. For further information, see [R7].

SPECIFIC REFERENCES: 1. Isaac O (1993) *Zeit. Phytother.* 14:212. 2. Damiani P *et al* (1983) *Fitoterapia* 54(5):213. 3. Konig G *et al* (1998) *Planta Med.* 64(7):612.

CHAMOMILE, GERMAN
MATRICARIA RECUTITA L.
Fam. Asteraceae

SYNONYMS: Single Chamomile, Hungarian Chamomile, *M. chamomilla* L., *Chamomilla vulgaris* S F Gray, *C. recutita*. Any of the above names may be found in the literature.

HABITAT: Native to Europe and north-western Asia, naturalized in North America, and extensively cultivated.

DESCRIPTION: The flowerheads are much smaller than those of Roman Chamomile, and have only one row of ligulate florets, which are usually bent backwards when dried. The receptacle is conical and hollow, and has no membranous bracts. Taste: bitter and aromatic; odour: characteristic.

PART USED: Flowers.

CONSTITUENTS: (i) Volatile oil (about 2%), containing alpha-bisabolol up to 50%; azulenes including chamazulene, guaiazulene and matricine, alpha-bisabolol oxides A and B, alpha-bisabolone oxide A, farnesene and others (ii) Flavonoids including apigenin and luteolin, and their glycosides and acetylglucosides, patuletin and quercetin (iii) Spiroethers, such as cis- and trans-en-yn-dicycloether (iv) Coumarins; e.g. umbelliferone and herniarin (v) Polysaccharides: xyloglucurans [R7,R8,R17 and refs therein].

MEDICINAL USE: Sedative, carminative, antispasmodic, analgesic, anti-inflammatory and antiseptic [R1]. Chamomile has been extensively investigated; see review refs [R7, R8, R9, R17]. It is frequently used as a tea, often in the form of tea bags, for insomnia, gout, sciatica, indigestion and diarrhoea, and topically in the same way as Roman Chamomile (q.v.). It has a particular place in the treatment of children's ailments, for colic, teething pains and infantile convulsions [1]. Matricine and (–)-alpha-bisabolol have significant anti-inflammatory and analgesic activity; chamazulene, guaiazulene and the oxides of alpha-bisabolol less (as measured by a number of *in vivo* and *in vitro* systems). Natural (–)-alpha-bisabolol has been shown to be more effective than synthetic racemic bisabolol in healing burns, and chamomile extract helps to alleviate radiation burns resulting from radiotherapy as well as soothing eczema. Bisabolol also has an ulceroprotective and antispasmodic effect; it prevents the formation of ulcers induced by indomethacin and alcohol and also reduces the healing time. Chamazulene is antioxidant and inhibits leukotriene B4 synthesis. The flavonoids, especially apigenin, are also spasmolytic, anti-inflammatory and sedative [2,3]. German Chamomile is considered non-toxic and tests done on alpha-bisabolol at least have shown no problems, and no teratogenicity. See reviews [R2,R7,R8,R9,R17;4,5,6, and refs therein].

PREPARATIONS AND DOSE: Powdered flowers, dose: 2–8 g, or equivalent extract.

SPECIFIC REFERENCES: 1. Weizman Z *et al* (1993) *J. Pediatrics* 122(4):650. 2. Viola H *et al* (1995) *Planta Med.* 62:213. 3.

Yamada K *et al* (1996) *Biol. Pharm. Bull.* 16(9):1244. 4. Fuller E *et al* (1993) *Deutsche Apot. Zeit.* 133:4224. 5. Maiche A *et al* (1991) *Acta Oncol.* 30:395 62. 6. Miller T *et al* (1996) *Planta Med.* 62:60.

CHAPARRAL
LARREA TRIDENTATA CAV.
Fam. Zygophyllaceae

SYNONYMS: Creosote Bush.

HABITAT: South America, Mexico, southern North America.

DESCRIPTION: A scrubby desert shrub with resinous leaves, hence the synonym 'creosote bush'.

PART USED: Leaves, twigs.

CONSTITUENTS: (i) Lignans, nordihydroguaiaretic acid (NDGA) being the major, with dihydroguaiaretic acid, norisoguaiacin, and demethylated derivatives of these (ii) Volatile oil, containing calamene, eudesmol, limonene and others (iii) Flavonoids, including kaempferol, quercetin and isorhamnetic glycosides, gossypetin, herbacetin, and various ethers and acetylated derivatives (iv) Miscellaneous triterpenes, saponins, resins and amino acids [R7;1,2,3,4].

MEDICINAL USE: A traditional remedy for cancer, rheumatism and inflammation of all types. Most of the actions of the herb are thought to be due to the content of NDGA, which is also antioxidant and antimicrobial. The leaf extract has anti-proliferative activity against a T-lymphoma cell line without affecting viability of normal lympho-cytes [5] and *in vivo* anti-tumour activity on some types of mammary carcinomas [6,7]. However, the NDGA is not solely responsible for this action although it may contribute to the overall effect [8]. NDGA is an immunomodulator [9]. Hepatitis has been reported for chaparral in several cases [10], but the safety or toxicity of NDGA remains uncertain.

SPECIFIC REFERENCES: 1. Fronczek F *et al* (1988) *J. Nat. Prod.* 50:497. 2. Sakakibara M *et al* (1977) *Phytochem.* 16:1113. 3. Sakakibara M *et al* (1975) *Phytochem.* 14:849 and 2079. 4. Xue H-Z *et al* (1988) *Phytochem.* 27:233. 5. Anesini C *et al* (1996) *Fitoterapia* 67:329. 6. Anesini C *et al* (1997) *Phytother. Res.* 11:521. 7. Anesini C *et al* (2001) *Phytomedicine* 8(1):1. 8. Pavani M *et al* (1994) *Biochem. Pharmacol.* 48:1935. 9. Tang D *et al* (1996) *Proc. Natl. Acad. Sci. USA* 93:5241. 10. Gordon D *et al* (1995) *JAMA* 273:489.

CHAULMOOGRA
HYDNOCARPUS KURZII (KING) WARB.
H. WIGHTIANA BLUME AND OTHER SPP.
Fam. Flacourtaceae

SYNONYMS: Hydnocarpus, *Taraktogenos kurzii = H. kurzii.* Various species of *Chaulmoogra* have been used, however the botanical origin is not always apparent.

111

HABITAT: Indian subcontinent, southern Asia.

DESCRIPTION: Seeds greyish, about 2–3 cm long and 1.5 cm diameter, irregularly angular with rounded ends. Kernel oily, enclosing two thin, heart-shaped, three-veined cotyledons and a straight radicle. Taste: acrid; odour: disagreeable.

PART USED: Seeds, oil expressed from the seeds.

CONSTITUENTS: Fixed oil, constituting about 50–60% of the kernel. The oil is composed of cyclopentenic acids including hydnocarpic, dihydrohydnocarpic, gorlic, chaulmoogric, dihydrochaulmoogric, taraktogenic, isogaleic and arachnic acids, and their esters, and 5'-methylhydnocarpin [1,2,3].

MEDICINAL USE: Anti-leprotic, dermatic, febrifuge, sedative [R1]. The oil is applied topically, particularly for skin diseases, such as eczema and psoriasis, as an ointment, and has been used in the form of injections for leprosy [R2;1,2]. Compounds isolated from the oil may be used as lead compounds in the development of new anti-leprotic agents [2]. 5'-Methyl hydnocarpin is a multi-drug pump inhibitor, and potentiates, for example, the antibiotic activity of berberine against *Staphylococcus aureus* [3]. The seeds may be taken powdered in the form of pills.

PREPARATIONS AND DOSE: Oil, dose: 0.3–1 ml.

SPECIFIC REFERENCES: 1. Lefort D *et al* (1969) *Planta Med.* 17:261. 2. Hooper M (1985) *Leprosy Rev.* 56(1):57. 3. Stermitz F *et al* (2000) *Proc. Natl. Acad. Sci.* 97(4):1433.

CHEKEN
EUGENIA CHEQUEN MOL.
Fam. Myrtaceae

SYNONYMS: Myrtus cheken Spreng.

HABITAT: Chile.

DESCRIPTION: Leaves leathery, ovate, about 1–1.5 cm long, 0.5–1 cm wide, entire margins, very shortly stalked with numerous minute, round, translucent oil cells. Taste: astringent, aromatic and bitter, recalling that of bay leaves; odour: slight.

PART USED: Leaves.

CONSTITUENTS: (i) Volatile oil, about 1% (ii) Bitters, including chekenone, chekenetin, chekenine (iii) Tannins [R4].

MEDICINAL USE: Diuretic, expectorant, tonic [R1]. Very little information is available.

CHERRY LAUREL
PRUNUS LAUROCERASUS L.
Fam. Rosaceae

SYNONYMS: Cherry-bay.

HABITAT: Native to Russia but cultivated in many temperate countries.

DESCRIPTION: Leaves leathery, glossy, about 10–15 cm long by 3–5 cm wide, oblong, lanceolate, serrate with a recurved margin and pointed apex. On the undersurface there are two or three punctate glands close to the midrib near the base. Odour: when the fresh leaves are bruised, reminiscent of oil of bitter almonds.

PART USED: Leaves.

Constituents: (i) Cyanogenetic glycosides, about 1.5%, mainly mandelonitrile glucosides, the *d*-isomer of which is prunasin and the *l*-isomer sambunigrin. The racemic mixture of these is referred to as prulaurasin (ii) Volatile oil, composed of benzaldehyde, benzyl alcohol and traces of hydrocyanic acid (iii) Miscellaneous; ursolic acid, tannin etc. Flavonoids are reported to be absent from this species [R3,R19;1].

MEDICINAL USE: Sedative, anti-tussive, stomachic. Mostly used to produce cherry-laurel water for medicinal use in cough medicines. The oil, with the hydrocyanic acid removed, has been used as a flavouring agent.

PREPARATIONS AND DOSE: Cherry-laurel Water BPC 1949, dose: 2–8 ml.

SPECIFIC REFERENCES: 1. Mimaki, Y *et al* (1994) *Nat. Med.* 48(1):86.

CHERRY STALKS
PRUNUS AVIUM L. (AND OTHER SPECIES).
Fam. Rosaceae

DESCRIPTION: Fruit stalks about 4 cm long and 1 mm thick, enlarged at one end.

MEDICINAL USE: Rarely used nowadays but at one time considered to be an astringent tonic [R1]. Anti-inflammatory effects were reported for the extract when evaluated in the rat paw oedema test [1].

SPECIFIC REFERENCES: 1. Blazso G *et al* (1994) *Pharmazie* 49(7):540.

CHERRY, WILD
PRUNUS SEROTINA EHRH.
Fam. Rosaceae

SYNONYMS: Virginian Prune Bark.

HABITAT: Widely distributed throughout Canada and North America.

DESCRIPTION: The bark occurs in flat, curved or channelled pieces, up to about 4 mm in thickness; larger pieces are considered to be of inferior quality. The external surface in the young bark is covered with a smooth, glossy, red-brown cork with white lenticels, often exfoliating to reveal the greenish brown cortex. The older bark is rougher and darker. The inner surface is brownish, longitudinally striated, often with adherent patches of yellowish wood. Taste: astringent and bitter; odour: similar to benzaldehyde (when damp).

113

PART USED: Bark.

CONSTITUENTS: (i) Prunasin, a cyanogenetic glycoside which is hydrolyzed by the enzyme prunase to hydrocyanic acid, amygdalin (ii) Benzaldehyde (iii) Miscellaneous; 3,4,5-trimethoxybenzoic acid (= eudesmic acid), *p*-coumaric acid, trimethyl gallate, scopoletin, tannins, sugars etc [R2,R3,R19;1,2].

MEDICINAL USE: Anti-tussive, sedative, astringent [R1]. Wild cherry bark has been used for centuries in cough syrups, particularly for irritable and persistent coughs such as those due to bronchitis and whooping cough. It is also used for nervous dyspepsia and as an astringent in diarrhoea.

SPECIFIC REFERENCES: 1. Santamour F (1998) *Phytochem.* 47:1537. 2. Nahrstedt S (1992) *Proc. Phytocem. Soc. Eur.* 33:249.

CHESTNUT

CASTANEA SATIVA MILL.
Fam. Fagaceae

SYNONYMS: Sweet Chestnut, Spanish Chestnut, C. *vulgaris* Lam., C. *vesca, Fagus castanea.* American Chestnut leaves are from C. *dentata* Borkh, (= C. *americana* Michx.).

HABITAT: Europe.

DESCRIPTION: Leaves leathery, about 15–20 cm long, 6–8 cm broad, oblong-lanceolate with sharply dentate margin. In the American Chestnut, the teeth on the margin are curved forward.

PART USED: Leaves.

CONSTITUENTS: (i) Tannins, including the ellagitannins pedunculatin, casuarictin, tellimagrandin I and II, potentillin, castalagin and vescalagin (ii) Flavonoids such as rutin, quercetin, myricetin, hesperetin, kaempferol and apigenin [R2,R9,1,2].

MEDICINAL USE: Anti-tussive, astringent, anti-rheumatic. Used especially for paroxysmal coughs, catarrh and whooping cough, and for diarrhoea. The infusion may be used as a gargle in pharyngitis. The ethyl acetate fraction is antimicrobial against both Gram negative and Gram positive bacteria, including *Pseudomonas aeruginosa, Proteus vulgaris* and *Staphylococcus aureus* [2], and cough suppression by the extract has been reported [3].

PREPARATIONS AND DOSE: Powdered leaf, dose: 2–4 g or equivalent extract.

BIBLICAL REFERENCES: Genesis 30:37; Ezekiel 31:8, as the 'Oriental Plane'.

SPECIFIC REFERENCES: 1. Haddock E *et al* (1982) *Phytochem.* 21:1049. 2. Basile A *et al* (2000) *Fitoterapia* 71:S110. 3. Ferrara L *et al* (1999) Int. Symposium on *Castanea sativa* Lugano, Switzerland, 19–18 Sept. 1999.

CHICKWEED
STELLARIA MEDIA (L.) VILL.
Fam. Caryophyllaceae

SYNONYMS: Starweed, *Alsine media* L.

HABITAT: A common weed. As Joseph Miller says, "it grows everywhere in moist places and in gardens too frequently."

DESCRIPTION: Stem jointed, with a line of hairs down one side only, leaves ovate, about 1 cm long by 0.5 cm broad. Flowers singly in the axils of the upper leaves, petals white and narrow, equal in length to the sepals. Taste: slightly saline; odourless.

PART USED: Herb.

CONSTITUENTS: (i) C-glycosylflavones and other flavonoids such as rutin [R2;1,2] (ii) Phenolic acids such as benzoic, ferulic and ascorbic acids [3] (iii) Monoacylgalactolipids [4].

CHICKWEED

MEDICINAL USE: Antipruritic, vulnerary, emollient, anti-rheumatic [R1]. Most often used in the form of an ointment. Culpeper writes of an ointment made by boiling "in oil of trotters or sheep's fat". Chickweed is still used as an ointment (although presumably not in the same base), and as a poultice for eczema, psoriasis, ulcers and boils. It is used internally for rheumatism, and was formerly used as a source of vitamin C. The flavones are antioxidants [1] and an extract was found to inhibit glucosyl transferase from *Streptococcus sobrinus,* which is implicated in the development of dental caries.

PREPARATIONS AND DOSE: Dried herb, dose: 1–5 g or equivalent extract, three times daily.

SPECIFIC REFERENCES: 1. Budzianowski J *et al* (1991) *Planta Med.* 57(3):290. 2. Budzianowski J *et al* (1991) *Pol. J. Pharmacol. Pharm.* 43:395. 3. Kitanov G (1992) *Pharmazie* 47(6):470. 4. Hohmann J *et al* (1996) *Fitoterapia* 67(4):381. 5. Yasuda H *et al* (1991) *Jap. J. Pharmacog.* 45(2):128.

CHICORY
CICHORIUM INTYBUS L.
Fam. Asteraceae

SYNONYMS: Succory.

HABITAT: Native to Europe and parts of Asia, naturalized in North America and cultivated extensively.

DESCRIPTION: Root brownish, with tough, loose, reticulated white layers surrounding a radiate woody column. Often crowned with remains of the stem.

PART USED: Root, leaves.

CONSTITUENTS: (i) Sesquiterpene lactones; lactucin and lactupicrin (= intybin), 8-desoxylactucin, magnolialide, artesin, the chicorosides B and C and sonchoside C [R2;1,2,3] (ii) Coumarins; chiconin, esculetin,

115

umbelliferone and scopoletin, in the herb [4] (iii) Polyphenolic acids and flavonoids, in the aerial parts: chicoric, chlorogenic, monocaffeoyl and hydroxycinnamic acids; luteolin and quercetin glucosides and glucuronides [R2;5] (iv) Polyyines, in the root [R2].

MEDICINAL USE: Diuretic, tonic, laxative [R1]. A decoction has been used for liver complaints, gout and rheumatism. Some of the sesquiterpene lactones are cytotoxic [1,3] and magnolialide appeared to induce differentiation of a human leukaemia cell line *in vitro* [1]. Preliminary screening has shown anti-inflammatory, hepatoprotective, choleretic and hypoglycaemic activity in rats [6] and an inhibitory effect on mast cell mediated allergic reactions in mice [7]. Immunostimulatory effects were also observed in an *in vitro* study measuring proliferation of lymphocytes [8]. The root had a cholesterol and triglyceride lowering effect when incorporated into the feed of rats fed with atherosclerotic diets [9]. The roasted root is used in coffee mixtures and substitutes.

SPECIFIC REFERENCES: 1. Lee K-T *et al* (2000) *Biol. Pharm. Bull.* 23(8):1005. 2. Park H-J *et al* (2000) *Nat. Prod. Sci.* 6(2):86. 3. Seto M *et al* (1988) *Chem. Pharm. Bull.* 36(7):2423. 4. Wagner H in 'Biology and Chemistry of the Compositae' eds V Heywood *et al* Acad. Press (1977). 5. Mulinacci N *et al* (2001) *Chromatographia* 54(7–8):455. 6. Ki S-Y *et al* (1999) *Nat. Prod. Sci.* 5(4):155. 7. Kim H *et al* (1999) *Pharmacol. Res.* 40(1):61. 8. Amirghofran Z *et al* (2000) *J. Ethnopharmacol.* 72(1–2):167. 9. Kaur N *et al* (1991) *Med. Sci. Res.* 19(19):643.

CHILLI PEPPER
CAPSICUM FRUTESCENS L.
C. ANNUUM L. AND VARIETIES
Fam. Solanaceae

SYNONYMS: Capsicum, Chili or Cayenne Pepper, Hot Pepper, Tabasco Pepper. The botanical classification tends to be confused in the literature. Green and Red (or Bell) Peppers and Paprika are produced by milder varieties.

HABITAT: Indigenous to tropical America and Africa, and widely cultivated.

DESCRIPTION: The fruit is so common it needs little description. Capsicums vary widely in colour, size and pungency. The pods may reach 10 cm or more in length; they are conical, with the colour ranging from green in the unripe fruit to yellow and red, depending on variety.

PART USED: Fruit, oleo-resin of the fruit (= capsicin), isolated capsaicin, the pungent principle.

CONSTITUENTS: (i) Capsaicinoids, which are esters of vanillyl amine with C8-C13 fatty acids; the major component being capsaicin itself (8-methyl-*N*-vanillylnon-6-enamide), with dihydrocapsaicin, nordihydrocapsaicin, homodihydrocapsaicin and others (ii) Carotenoids; capxanthin, capsorubin, alpha-carotene [R2,R7,1 and refs therein].

116

MEDICINAL USE: Stimulant, tonic, carminative, spasmolytic, diaphoretic, antiseptic, rubefacient and counter-irritant [R1]; this is one of the most widely used of all natural remedies. It is taken internally to improve peripheral circulation, alleviate flatulence and colic and stimulate the digestive system; as a gargle in laryngitis; and topically in the form of an ointment for muscle pain and stiffness, lumbago and unbroken chilblains. Capsaicin has a large number of pharmacological actions, including effects on the circulatory system, smooth muscle, and heat regulation of the body. It acts on vanilloid receptors, causing inflammation, but also desensitizes sensory nerve endings to pain stimulation by deleting the neuropeptide substance P from local C-type nerve fibres. It is used as a local analgesic in the treatment of post-herpetic neuralgia, diabetic neuropathy and osteoarthritis, and other forms of intractable pain, and for pruritis. The effects of capsicum on the gastrointestinal system are also complex; for a full account of the scientific literature see [R14,1,2,3 and references therein]. Recently capsaicin has been investigated for the treatment of pre-malignant and squamous cell lesions of the epithelium [4]. Chilli peppers are used widely in cooking to give a hot, pungent flavour; they are non-toxic at normal doses but should be used carefully.

PREPARATIONS AND DOSE: Tincture of Capsicum BPC 1973, dose: 0.3–1 ml; Capsicum Oleoresin BPC, dose: 0.6–2 mg; Strong Capsicum Tincture 1934, dose 0.06–0.2ml; capsaicin cream 0.025%, 0.075% and 0.75%.

SPECIFIC REFERENCES: 1. Cordell G *et al* (1993) *Ann. Pharmacother.* 27:330. 2. Fusco B *et al* (1997) Drugs: 7:909. 3. Winter J *et al* (1995) *Br. J. Anaesth.* 75:157. 4. Terry J *et al* (2001) *US Patent* 6,235,788.

CHINA
SMILAX CHINA L.
Fam. Smilacaceae

HABITAT: Native to Japan but grows elsewhere in the Far East.

DESCRIPTION: Tubers cylindrical, often somewhat flattened, 10–15 cm long and 2–5 cm diameter, with short, knotty branches and a rusty, shiny bark. Internally, pale fawn coloured. Taste: insipid; odourless.

PART USED: Tuber.

CONSTITUENTS: Steroidal saponins, based on diosgenin [1].

MEDICINAL USE: Alterative [R1]. Has been used occasionally as a substitute for Sarsaparilla (q.v.) and a source of diosgenin. A boiling water extract, made to mimic the preparation of the plant as it is normally used as a food, was found to inhibit mutagenesis induced by benzo[a]pyrene [2].

SPECIFIC REFERENCES: 1. Kim C *et al* (1991) *Arch. Pharm. Res.* 14(4):305 2. Lee H *et al* (1988) *Mutat. Res.* 204(2):229.

CHIRETTA

SWERTIA CHIRATA BUCH.-HAM.
Fam. Gentianaceae

SYNONYMS: Brown Chirata, White Chirata, Chirayta, *Ophelia chirata.*

HABITAT: Northern India.

DESCRIPTION: Stems brown or purplish, 2–4 mm thick, cylindrical below and becoming quadrangular upwards, containing a wide, yellowish pith, leaves opposite, lanceolate or ovate, entire with three to seven longitudinal ribs. Flowers: small and panicled; fruit: a two-valved capsule. Taste: intensely bitter; virtually odourless.

PART USED: Herb.

CONSTITUENTS: (i) Iridoids, including amarogentin (= chiratin), amarogenin, chiratinin, gentiopicrin, gentiorucin, swertiomarin, amaroswerin, sweroside and others [R16;1] (ii) Xanthone derivatives, including decussatin, mangiferin, swerchirin, swertianin, isobellidifolin, chiratol and others [R2,R16,1,2] (iii) Triterpenes, including beta-amyrin, lupeol and kairatenol [3] (iv) Alkaloids: gentianine, gentiocrucine, enicoflavine [4].

MEDICINAL USE: Bitter tonic, orexigenic, stomachic, febrifuge and antimalarial [R1]. It is mainly used as a traditional remedy for biliousness and liver disorders. Several of the constituents including amarogentin are hepato-protective against various toxins *in vivo* [5] and *in vitro* [6]. Amarogentin is an inhibitor of topoisomerase of *Leishmania donovani* [1] and swerchirin has *in vivo* antimalarial activity in rodents [7], thus substantiating the reputed anti-protozoal activity. The total extract is anti-leprotic *in vitro* [8] and antioxidant [9]. Other properties including anti-inflammatory, hypoglycaemic and anti-ulcerogenic activities have been described [R16 and refs therein].

PREPARATIONS AND DOSE: Dried herb, dose: 0.3–2 g or equivalent extract, three times daily.

SPECIFIC REFERENCES: 1. Ray S *et al* (1996) *J. Nat. Prod.* 59(1):27. 2. Banerjee S *et al* (2000) *Indian J. Pharmacol.* 32(1):21. 3. Chakravarty K *et al* (1992) *Tet. Lett.* 33(1):125. 4. Sharma P (1982) *Indian J. Pharm. Sci.* 44(2):36. 5. Karan M *et al* (1999) *Phytother. Res.* 13(1): 24 and (2):95. 6. Reen R *et al* (2001) *J. Ethnopharmacol.* 75(2–3):239. 7. Goyal H *et al* (1981) *J. Res. Ayur. Siddha* 2(3):286. 8. Asthana J *et al* (2001) *Indian Drugs* 38(2):82. 9. Scartezzini P *et al* (2000) *J. Ethnopharmacol.* 71(1–2):23.

CHIRETTA, GREEN

ANDROGRAPHIS PANICULATA NEES.
Fam. Acanthaceae

SYNONYMS: Kalmegh, Bhunimba.

HABITAT: The Indian subcontinent.

DESCRIPTION: An erect, branched, annual herb reaching 1 m in height. It has broadly lanceolate, glabrous leaves, small white or pale pink flowers with brown or purple blotches in loose panicle. The capsules are oblong and contain numerous yellowish-brown seeds.

PART USED: Whole plant, roots.

CONSTITUENTS: (i) Diterpenes called andrographolides, consisting of andrographolide, neoandrographolide, deoxyandrographolide, andrographiside, andropanoside and others. The roots contain andrographin and panicolin [R16;1,2,3] (ii) Flavonoids; apigenin derivatives and various hydroxyflavones have been isolated [R16,1].

MEDICINAL USE: A traditional Ayurvedic remedy for jaundice and liver disorders, it is also used as a bitter tonic, stomachic, anti-diarrhoeal, anti-inflammatory and antimalarial. Hepatoprotective, as well as choleretic effects, have been confirmed and are attributed to the andrographolides [3,4]. Antiviral activity has been reported *in vitro* [5] and immunomodulatory effects [6], and to support these results clinical studies have indicated a potential use in the treatment of the common cold [7]. Antimalarial activity *in vitro*, and protection from the associated hepatic damage, has been described [8,9]. Andrographolide-induced cell differentiation [2] and inhibited tumour necrosis factor alpha-induced upregulation of endothelial adhesion, which is implicated in inflammation [10]. Other activities including anti-platelet, anti-filarial, anti-atherosclerotic and anti-diarrhoeal activities have been described; see [R16, and refs therein].

PREPARATIONS AND DOSE: Dose: 20–40 g three times daily, as an infusion or decoction.

SPECIFIC REFERENCES: 1. Abeysekara A *et al* (1990) *Fitoterapia* 61(5):473. 2. Matsuda T *et al* (1994) *Chem. Pharm. Bull.* 42(6):1216. 3. Kapil A *et al* (1993) *Biochem. Pharmacol.* 46(1):1216. 4. Tripathi G *et al* (1991) *Phytother. Res.* 5(4):176. 5. Otake T *et al* (1995) *Phytother. Res.* 9(1):6. 6. Puri A *et al* (1993) *J. Nat. Prod.* 56(7):995. 7. Hancke J *et al* (1995) *Phytother. Res.* 9(8):559. 8. Misra P *et al* (1992) *Int. J. Pharmacog.* 30(4):263. 9. Chander R *et al* (1995) *Int. J. Pharmacog.* 33(2):135. 10. Habtermariam S (1998) *Phytother. Res.* 12(7):37.

CICELY, SWEET
MYRRHIS ODORATA (L.) SCOP.
Fam. Apiaceae

SYNONYMS: Sweet Chervil, Great Chervil.

HABITAT: Southern Europe, cultivated as a garden plant elsewhere.

DESCRIPTION: Leaves large, tripinnate, leaflets ovate-lanceolate, usually with white splashes near the base, hairy on the veins below and on the margins. Root whitish, 1–4 cm broad, with a radiate structure. Taste and odour: sweet and anise-like. American Sweet Cicely is from *Osmorhiza longistylis* D.C.

PART USED: Root, herb.

119

CONSTITUENTS: (i) Volatile oil, containing trans-anethole, germacrene-D, beta-caryophyllene, limonene, chavicol methyl ether, alpha-pinene, alpha-farnesene, and myrcene (ii) Flavonoids such as luteolin and apigenin glucosides [R2].

MEDICINAL USE: Carminative, stomachic, expectorant[R1]. The dried root is used as a decoction for coughs and flatulence, and the herb as an infusion for anaemia and as a tonic. Cicely Root and Angelica were used to 'prevent' infection in the time of the Great Plague.

CINCHONA
CINCHONA PUBESCENS VAHL. AND OTHER VARIETIES
AND HYBRIDS OF THE GENUS *CINCHONA*
Fam. Rubiaceae

SYNONYMS: Peruvian Bark, Jesuit's Bark. Red Cinchona, 'cinchona rubra', is *C. pubescens* (= *C. succirubra* Pavon) and Yellow Cinchona 'cinchona flava' is *C. calisaya* Wedd. or *C. ledgeriana* Moens et Trim.

HABITAT: Native to mountainous regions of tropical America, cultivated in Southeast Asia and parts of Africa.

DESCRIPTION: The bark occurs in quills or flat pieces up to 30 cm long, and 36 mm thick. The external surface is brownish-grey, usually fissured with an exfoliating cork, and lichens and mosses may be seen as greyish-white or greenish patches. Inner surface: yellowish to reddish-brown, fracture: fibrous; taste: very bitter and astringent; odour: slight.

PART USED: Bark of stem and root.

CONSTITUENTS: (i) Quinoline alkaloids, consisting mainly of quinine, with quinidine, cinchonine and cinchonidine. Other alkaloids include epi- and hydro-derivatives of these, quinamine and many others (ii) Triterpene glycosides such as chinovic acid-3-*O*-chinovoside and chinovic acid-3-*O*-glucoside (iii) Miscellaneous; tannins, including the phlobatannin cinchotannic acid, quinic acid, resin, wax etc. [R2,R9,R19 and refs therein].

MEDICINAL USE: Antimalarial, febrifuge, tonic, orexigenic, spasmolytic and astringent [R1]. The bark is used for the extraction of the alkaloids quinine and its isomer quinidine. Both have antimalarial activity although quinine is more widely used. The natural alkaloids have been the basis for the development of newer semi-synthetic drugs. Both quinine, and even more so quinidine, are cardiac antiarrhythmic agents, and quinidine is still used clinically for this purpose. Quinine salts are used in the prevention of night cramps and are also an ingredient of many analgesic and cold and flu remedies. Chronic overdose can result in the condition known as cinchonism, which is characterized by headache, abdominal pain, rashes and visual disturbances. Cinchona and quinine should not be taken in large doses during pregnancy except by patients suffering from malaria [R14].

PREPARATIONS AND DOSE: Powdered Bark, dose: 0.3–1 g or equivalent extract; quinine (as sulphate) for night cramps, dose: 200–300 mg.

CINERARIA MARITIMA

SENECIO CINERARIA DC
Fam. Asteraceae

SYNONYMS: Dusty Miller, *S. maritimus* L.

HABITAT: Native to the West Indies but introduced into Britain, North America and elsewhere as a garden plant.

DESCRIPTION: Leaves 15–20 cm long and about 5–6 cm wide, pinnate, each segment three-lobed, white with a dense white covering of hairs beneath. Flower-heads yellow, about 1 cm across.

PART USED: Juice of the plant.

CONSTITUENTS: Pyrrolizidine alkaloids including jacobine, jacodine and senecionine [1].

MEDICINAL USE: The sterilized juice of the plant was once employed for the treatment of capsular and lenticular cataract of the eye [R1], and was applied to the eye by means of a medicine dropper.

SPECIFIC REFERENCES: 1. Willaman J *et al* (1970) *Lloydia* 33(3A):1.

CINNAMON

CINNAMOMUM VERUM J S PRESL.
AND ITS VARIETIES
Fam. Lauraceae

SYNONYMS: Ceylon cinnamon, *C. zeylanicum* Nees. *C. zeylanicum* Blume, *Laurius cinnamomum* L. Saigon cinnamon is from *C. laureirii* Nees., Batavian or Padang cinnamon is from *C. burmanii* (Nees.) Bl., and Chinese Cinnamon, more commonly known as Cassia (q.v.), is from *C. aromaticum.*

HABITAT: Native to southern India and Sri Lanka, but cultivated elsewhere.

DESCRIPTION: Cinnamon in commerce consists of the inner bark, in the form of pale brown, thin quills, several rolled inside one another. Quills usually 0.5–1 cm wide, not exceeding 1 mm in thickness. Taste: sweet pungent and aromatic; odour: characteristic.

PART USED: Inner (peeled) bark; oil distilled from bark and leaves.

CONSTITUENTS: (i) Essential oil (up to about 4%) in the bark, consisting of cinnamaldehyde, (up to 75%), with cinnamyl acetate, cinnamyl alcohol, cuminaldehyde, eugenol and methyleugenol, and many others. The leaf oil has a much greater proportion of eugenol, up to 80%, with linalool and piperitone [1] (ii) Diterpenes; cinnzelanin and cinnzelanol [2] (iii) Tannins, consisting of polymeric tetrahydroxyflavandiols [3], possibly similar to those found in Cassia (q.v.).

MEDICINAL USE: Aromatic, astringent, stimulant, carminative [R1]. Cinnamon has been used for thousands of years to treat nausea and vomiting, diarrhoea, rheumatism, colds, hypertension, female complaints and many other disorders, with some justification.

121

Cinnamon bark has analgesic, anti-inflammatory, antioxidant, antibacterial, anti-protozoal and fungitoxic properties [4,5,6,7] (see also Cassia). Cinnamon leaf oil is antiseptic and anaesthetic, due to the eugenol content. It is not interchangeable with the bark oil and is more usually used as an industrial source of eugenol. Cinnamon is non-toxic in normal usage although mutagenic and embryotoxic effects have been noted with high doses in animals [8,9]. Cinnamon bark and oil are used widely as a flavouring agent in food, as well as in mouthwashes, cosmetics, tonics and other pharmaceuticals.

PREPARATIONS AND DOSE: Powdered Bark, dose: 0.3–1.2 g; Cinnamon Oil BP, dose: 0.05–0.2 ml.

BIBLICAL REFERENCES: Exodus 30:23; Proverbs 7:17; Song of Solomon 4:14; Revelation 18:13.

SPECIFIC REFERENCES: 1. Raina V *et al* (2001) *Flav. Frag. J.* 16(5):374. 2. Isogai A *et al* (1977) *Agric. Biol. Chem.* 41:1779. 3. Buchalter L (1971) *J. Pharm. Sci.* 60:144. 4. Atta A *et al* (1998) *J. Ethnopharmacol.* I60(2):117. 5. Dhuley J (1999) *Indian J. Exp. Biol.* 37(3):238. 6. Singh H *et al* (1995) *Allergy* 50(12):995. 7. Viollon C *et al* (1996) *Fitoterapia* 67(3):279. 8. Ungsurungsi M *et al* (1984) *Food Chem. Toxicol.* 22(2):109. 9. Pellagatti L *et al* (1994) *Fitoterapia* 65(5):431.

CITRONELLA
CYMBOPOGON NARDUS (L.) RENDLE
C. WINTERANUS (L.) JOWITT
Fam. Poaceae

SYNONYMS: Mana grass; Ceylon (or Lenabatu) citronella is *C. nardus*; Java (or Maha Pengiri) citronella is *C. winteranus.*

HABITAT: Native to tropical Asia, particularly India and Sri Lanka.

DESCRIPTION: A perennial grass, with typically linear leaves. The volatile oil extracted from citronella is pale yellow, with a characteristic lemony fragrance.

PART USED: Volatile oil.

CONSTITUENTS: Citronellal, citronellol and geranial, are the major components, and are higher in Java citronella; together with geranyl citronellal and other acetates, linalool, beta-pinene, caryophyllene, limonene and others [R14,R19;1].

MEDICINAL USE: The oil is an insect repellent and is antibacterial and anti-fungal. It is also used in aromatherapy and has recently been shown to activate both the parasympathetic and sympathetic nervous systems when inhaled by human volunteers, measured as a change in heart rate, blood flow, electrocardiogram and galvanic skin conductance [2]. A herbal tea made from the leaves has been used as an antispasmodic in digestive disorders and as a vermifuge. The oil is used as a fragrance ingredient in soaps and cosmetic products but can cause sensitization in some individuals [R19].

SPECIFIC REFERENCES: 1. Naqvi A *et al* (2002) *Flav. Frag. J.* 17(2):109. 2. Saeki Y *et al* (2001) *Int. J. Aromather.* 11(3):118.

CLARY
SALVIA SCLAREA L.
Fam. Lamiaceae

SYNONYMS: Clary Sage, Clary Wort, Clarry, Cleareye, Muscatel Sage.

HABITAT: Native to southern Europe; cultivated worldwide.

DESCRIPTION: Leaves large, heart-shaped, pointed, wrinkled, covered with velvety hairs. Flowers, appearing from June to August, are blue or white, with large membranous bracts longer than the calyx. Taste: warm and aromatic, slightly bitter; odour: aromatic, recalling that of Tolu balsam.

PART USED: Herb, and at one time the seeds.

CONSTITUENTS: Volatile oil, about 0.1%, consisting mainly of linalyl acetate; with linalool, beta-pinene, beta-myrcene, phellandrene, and the labdane diterpene alcohols sclareol and manool [R19;1].

MEDICINAL USE: Antispasmodic, used in digestive disorders and for kidney diseases [R1]. The oil has previously been reported to be anticonvulsant in animals and to potentiate the effects of some hypnotics; however more recent toxicity screening in rats showed no untoward central nervous system or other effects [2]. Sclareol is antibacterial [3], a fungal growth regulator and plant growth inhibitor [4,5]. The oil is used as a flavouring component in food and cosmetic products, and especially in tobacco.

SPECIFIC REFERENCES: 1. Allured S (1975) *Cosmet. Perfum.* 900(4):69. 2. Malone M *et al* (1991) *Fitoterapia* 62(2):123. 3. Ulubelen A *et al* (1985) *Phytochem.* 2:1386. 4. Bailey J *et al* (1974) *J. Gen. Microbiol.* 85:57. 5. Bailey J *et al* (1975) *Nature* 255:328.

CLIVERS
GALIUM APARINE L.
Fam. Rubiaceae

SYNONYMS: Cleavers, Goosegrass, Burweed, Goosebill.

HABITAT: A common wild plant in temperate regions. Culpeper says, "It is also an inhabitant in gardens that it ramps upon and is ready to choak what ever grows near it", a statement that is still true today.

DESCRIPTION: Leaves lanceolate, about 1–2 cm long and 0.5 cm broad, in whorls of six, with backward pointing bristly hairs at the margins. Stem quadrangular. Flowers small, insignificant, dull white; fruits nearly globular, about 3 mm in diameter, covered with hooked bristles. Taste: slightly saline; odourless.

PART USED: Herb.

CONSTITUENTS: (i) Iridoids, including asperuloside, asperulosidic acid, 10-deacetylasperulosidic acid and monotropein [R2;R7;1,2] (ii) Polyphenolic acids, such as *p*-coumaric, *p*-hydroxybenzoic, gallic and caffeic acids [R2,R7] (iii) Alkaloids, such as protopine, 1-hydroxydes-oxypeganine, harmine, and others [R2,R7;3] (iv) Flavonoids, such as luteolin [4] (v) Fatty acids and sterols including linolenic, linoleic and lauric acids; stigmasterol, lanosterol and campesterol [5] (vi) Anthraquinone derivatives: alizarin, xanthopurpurin, galiosin and derivatives, in the roots but not the herb [R7].

MEDICINAL USE: Diuretic, aperient, tonic, alterative, mild astringent [R1]. It is used particularly for enlarged lymph glands and in cystitis and psoriasis. Asperuloside in common with other iridoids is a mild laxative in animals. Pharmacological and clinical results are sparse; however asperuloside can be chemically converted to prostanoid intermediates and may find an important use here [6].

PREPARATIONS AND DOSE: Powdered herb, dose: 2–4 g, or equivalent extract, three times daily.

SPECIFIC REFERENCES: 1. Corrigan D *et al* (1978) *Phytochem.* 17:1131. 2. Deliorman D *et al* (2001) *Pharm. Biol.* 39(3):234. 3. Sener B *et al* (1991) *Gaz. Uni. Ecz. Fakultasi Dergisi* 8(1):13. 4. Bhan M *et al* (1976) *Indian J. Chem.* 14:475. 5. Tzakou O *et al* (1990) *Fitoterapia* 61(1):93. 6. Berkowitz W *et al* (1982) *J. Org. Chem.* (47):824.

CLOVE

SYZYGIUM AROMATICUM (L.) MERR. ET PERRY
Fam. Myrtaceae

SYNONYMS: *Eugenia caryophyllus* Spreng., E. *caryophyllata* Thunb., E. *aromatica* (L.) Baill.

HABITAT: Native to the Molucca Islands, Indonesia; introduced into East Africa, Madagascar, Malaysia, Brazil and other tropical parts.

DESCRIPTION: The cloves, or flower-buds, are brown, about 1–1.5 cm long, the lower portion consisting of the calyx tube enclosing in its upper half the ovary filled with minute ovules. There are numerous stamens and four calyx teeth, surrounded by the unopened, globular corolla of four concave, overlapping petals. Taste and odour: characteristic. On pressing with the fingernail, oil should exude.

PART USED: Unexpanded flower buds; the oil distilled from them.

CONSTITUENTS: (i) Volatile oil, about 15–20%, consisting mainly of eugenol (usually 85–90% but variable), with acetyl eugenol, alpha- and beta-caryophyllene and their oxides, methyl salicylate, benzaldehyde; the sesquiterpenes alpha-copaene, gamma- and delta-cadinene and alpha-cubebene, alpha-humulene and its epoxide and others [R7;1] (ii) Tannins; eugeniin, casuarictin, tellimagrandin I, 1,3-di-O-galloyl-4,6-hexahydroxydiphenyl-beta-D-glucopyranoside [2] (iii) Chromones; bifiorin and isobifiorin [2] (iv) Miscellaneous; flavonoids (kaempferol, rhamnetin etc.), sterols (sitosterol, campesterol and stigmasterol), crategolic acid methyl ester, lipids etc. [R7,R19].

MEDICINAL USE: Stimulant, aromatic, carminative, anti-emetic [R1].
Clove oil particularly is used as an anodyne in toothache and is a
constituent of many dental preparations. It has antiseptic, antispasmodic,
antihistaminic and anthelmintic properties, many of which are due to
the eugenol content. Eugenol inhibits prostaglandin synthesis and the
metabolism of arachidonic acid by human polymorphonuclear
leukocytes, inhibits smooth muscle activity *in vitro* and is anti-inflammatory [3,4]. It protects the gastric mucosa against platelet-activating
factor and ethanol-induced damage in rats [5] and, along with the
caryophyllene and humulene derivatives, induces detoxifying enzymes
such as glutathione-S-transferase, suggesting an anti-carcinogenic effect
[1]. Tellimagrandin shows antiviral activity by inhibiting virus-cell
fusion (syncytia formation) [2]. Extracts are larvicidal to the mosquito
Culex pipiens [6]. Cloves and clove oils are used in the preparation of
certain types of cigarette, such as Indian 'beedis' and Indonesian
'kretaks', for their stimulant action, and in cookery. Clove extracts
are used in cosmetics and perfumery for their antioxidant [7] and
antibacterial effects [8], as well as for their pleasant odour.

PREPARATIONS AND DOSE: Clove powder, dose: 120–300 mg; Conc.
Clove Infusion BPC 1954, dose: 2–4 ml; Clove Oil BP, dose: 0.05–0.2 ml.

SPECIFIC REFERENCES: 1. Zheng G-Q *et al* (1992) *J. Nat. Prod.*
55(7):999. 2. Hyoung J *et al* (2001) *Planta Med.* 67(3):277. 3. Bennett A
et al (1988) *Phytother. Res.* 3:124. 4. Srivastava K (1990) *Planta Med.*
56(6):501. 5. Capasso R *et al* (2000) *Fitoterapia* 71:S131. 6. El Hag E
et al (1999) *Phytother. Res.* 13(5):388. 7. Kim B *et al* (1997) *Int. J.
Cosmet. Sci.* 19(6):299. 8. Larhsini M *et al* (2001) *Phytother. Res.*
15(3):250.

CLUBMOSS
LYCOPODIUM CLAVATUM L.
Fam. Lycopodiaceae

SYNONYMS: Lycopodium Seed, Vegetable Sulphur.

HABITAT: Central and northern Europe and many other places.

DESCRIPTION: Stem woody, slender, elongated, with a few lateral,
forked branches, and a few scattered, whitish roots below. Leaves
crowded and scale-like, hair-tipped. Spore cases in spikes borne on
erect forked, club-shaped branches, at right angles to the prostrate
stem. Spores yellow, somewhat triangular, forming a mobile powder,
which floats on water without being wetted.

PART USED: Plant and spores.

CONSTITUENTS: Alkaloids, about 0.1–0.2%, of which the major
one is lycopodine; with dihydrolycopodine, clavatine, clavatoxine,
nicotine and many others [1] (ii) Triterpenes and sterols including
alpha-onocerin, lycoclavatol, serratendionol beta-sitosterol,
campesterol and others [R2,R9] (iii) Flavonoids including apigenin

125

and luteolin glycosides, and chrysoreriol [R2,R7].

MEDICINAL USE: Sedative [R1]. It has been used for urinary disorders, in the treatment of spasmodic retention of urine, catarrhal cystitis and chronic kidney disorders, and as a gastric sedative in indigestion and gastritis. However, the alkaloids can be toxic and should be used with care.

SPECIFIC REFERENCES: 1. Ayer W (1991) Nat. Prod. Rep. 8:455 (and refs therein).

COCA

ERYTHROXYLUM COCA LAM.
E. NOVOGRANATENSE (MORRIS) HIERON
Fam. Erythroxylaceae

SYNONYMS: Bolivian Coca is *E. coca*; Peruvian Coca is *E. novogranatense* (= *E. truxillense* Rusby).

HABITAT: Native to the South American Andes, cultivated there and elsewhere at altitudes above 450 m.

DESCRIPTION: *E. coca* leaves are brownish green, oval, thin but tough, up to 5 cm long and 2.5 cm wide, with two lines on the undersurface parallel to the midrib, margins entire, apex rounded, and a faint projecting line occurring on the upper surface of the midrib. *E. novogranatense* leaves are green, oblanceolate, and very brittle, about 4 cm long and 1.5 cm broad without any projecting line on the midrib.

PART USED: Leaves.

CONSTITUENTS: (i) Tropane alkaloids, up to 2.5%, mainly cocaine, with other derivatives of ecgonine; hygrine, cuscohygrine, alpha-truxilline, nicotine, and others (ii) Volatile oil, containing methyl salicylate, *trans*-2-hexenal, *cis*-3-hexenal, 1-hexanol, N-methylpyrrole and dihydrobenzaldehyde (iii) Flavonoids including rutin [R3;1,2]

MEDICINAL USE: Central nervous system stimulant, local anaesthetic [R1]. The pharmacological effects are due almost entirely to the presence of cocaine, which is increasingly being used illicitly as a stimulant. It causes dependence and social problems with frequent use, especially when taken in a form of solid 'free base', with sodium bicarbonate, known as 'crack' cocaine. Heart disease has recently been found to be more prevalent in chronic cocaine users than in age-matched controls [3]. The medical indications of cocaine are now restricted to its use as a local anaesthetic, mainly in ophthalmic surgery. The leaf is still chewed by the people of the Andes to relieve hunger, fatigue and altitude sickness. Coca leaf extract (with the cocaine removed!) is used to flavour soft drinks.

SPECIFIC REFERENCES: 1. Novak M *et al* (1987) *Planta Med.* I53(1):113. 2. Homstedt B *et al* (1977) *Phytochem.* 16:1753. 3. Roldan D *et al* (2001) *Cardiol.* 95(1):25.

COCCULUS INDICUS

ANAMIRTA COCCULUS (L.) WIGHT ET ARNOTT.
Fam. Menispermaceae

SYNONYMS: Fish Berries, Levant Berries, *Anamirta paniculata* Colebr.

HABITAT: Indonesia.

DESCRIPTION: Fruits: kidney-shaped, about 1 cm long, blackish, containing a horseshoe-shaped seed. Fruit shell: tasteless, seed: bitter and oily.

PART USED: Berries or seeds.

CONSTITUENTS: Picrotoxin, which is a mixture of oxygenated sesquiterpenes including picrotoxinin, picrotin, methyl picrotoxate [R3;1,2].

MEDICINAL USE: Stimulant, parasiticide, anti-fungal [R1]. Though very poisonous, picrotoxin is a powerful central nervous system stimulant and was formerly used to counteract barbiturate poisoning. Now used in neuroscience and pesticide research to investigate GABA receptor ion channels. Anti-fungal activity against various plant and other pathogens has been described [2]. Cocculus berries have been used as a fish poison [R3].

SPECIFIC REFERENCES: 1. Pradhan P *et al* (1990) *Indian J. Chem.* (B.) 29(7):676. 2. Agarwal S *et al* (1999) *Indian Drugs* 36(12):754.

COCILLANA

GUAREA RUSBYI (BRITON) RUSBY
Fam. Meliaceae

SYNONYMS: Guapi Bark, Huapi Bark, Grape Bark, *Sycocarpus rusbyi* (Britt).

HABITAT: Eastern Andes.

DESCRIPTION: The bark occurs as flat or curved pieces; the outer surface is fissured and grey-brown in colour with orange-brown patches where the cork has been removed. Inner surface: brown, and longitudinally striated. Taste: astringent, slightly nauseous; odour: characteristic. Other species are being used, however these have not been specified [1].

PART USED: Bark.

CONSTITUENTS: (i) Alkaloids reported, but unspecified (ii) Volatile oil (iii) Miscellaneous; tannins, flavonols, anthraquinones etc. [R2;1]. The closely related *Guarea cedrata* and *G. thompsoni* have yielded limonoids, such as dreagenin and methyl acetoxyangolensate [2].

MEDICINAL USE: Expectorant [R1]. Used in cough syrups in a similar way to Ipecacuanha (q.v.). Little information is available, however *G. guidonia,* which is used in Brazil as an anti-inflammatory agent, has shown *in vivo* activity [3].

PREPARATIONS AND DOSE: Powdered Bark, dose: 0.5–1 g; Cocillana Liquid Extract BPC, dose: 0.5–1 ml.

SPECIFIC REFERENCES: 1. Novak M *et al* (1987) *Planta Med.*
53(1):113. 2. Connolly J *et al* (1972) *J. Chem. Soc.* P:1145. 3. Oga S
et al (1981) *Planta Med.* 42(3):310.

COCOA

THEOBROMA CACAO L.
Fam. Sterculiaceae

SYNONYMS: Cacao, Theobroma, Chocolate Tree.

HABITAT: Indigenous to Mexico and South America, but now
cultivated extensively in many tropical countries.

DESCRIPTION: Oval seeds, oblong compressed about 2 cm long,
with a thin, papery husk. When roasted and powdered they are
known as cocoa, and the oil when removed is known as cocoa
butter. The flavoured confection made from them is of course
chocolate, and the taste and odour need no description.

PART USED: Seeds, seed oil, husks.

CONSTITUENTS: (i) Xanthine derivatives and amines; mainly
theobromine with some caffeine and tyramine (ii) Alkaloids;
trigonelline and salsoladine, a tetrahydroisoquinoline, and others
[1,2] (iii) Catechins, mainly catechin and epicatechin [3] (iv) Fixed
oil, known as cocoa butter or theobroma oil, about 50% of the 'nibs'
(cotyledons) (iii) Many flavour ingredients; for full account and
references see [R3,R14,R19,1].

MEDICINAL USE: Nutritive, stimulant, diuretic [R1]. The name
'Theobroma', means 'food of the gods', and was given by Linnaeus
(from the Greek '*theos*' meaning 'god' and '*broma*' meaning food),
a sentiment many will agree with. The pharmacological effects are
mainly due to theobromine and caffeine, which have similar properties
although theobromine is weaker than caffeine in most respects. The
catechins are antioxidants, similar to those found in Tea (q.v.), and in
fact dark chocolate is a very rich source of these, containing over 50
mg per 100 g. They may therefore protect against heart disease and
other disorders although more research is needed. The alkaloid
salsoladine has psychoactivity, and binds to dopaminergic D2
receptors [2]. For a summary of the biological activity of cocoa,
see [1]. Cocoa butter is an emollient and is used in cosmetic creams,
but the main use of cocoa is as a food.

SPECIFIC REFERENCES: 1. Duke J (2000) *J. Med. Food* 3(2):115. 2.
Melzig M *et al* (2000) *J. Ethnopharmacol.* 73(1–2):153. 3. Arts I *et al*
(1999) *Lancet* 354:488.

COFFEE
COFFEA ARABICA L.
C. CANEPHORA PIERRE EX FROEHNER
C. LIBERICA
AND OTHER SPECIES AND HYBRIDS
Fam. Rubiaceae

SYNONYMS: Arabian Coffee is from *C. arabica*; Robusta Coffee is from *C. canephora* (syn. *C. robusta* Linden ex De Wild.).

HABITAT: Indigenous to Ethiopia, but cultivated in most tropical countries.

DESCRIPTION: The beans are oval-concave on one side, flat on the other, with a central longitudinal groove, grey-green when fresh and brown when roasted. Odour and taste: very aromatic and characteristic.

PART USED: Kernel of the dried, ripe seed, roasted.

CONSTITUENTS: (i) Xanthine derivatives, the main one being caffeine, with some theobromine and theophylline (ii) Chlorogenic and related polyphenolic acids (iii) Diterpenes including kahweol, cafestrol in the oil, and norditerpene glycosides known as atractylosides (iv) Miscellaneous; trigonelline, polyamines, tannins, carbohydrates; for a full account and references see [R2,R19,1].

MEDICINAL USE: Stimulant and diuretic [R1]. Most of these effects are due to the caffeine content. As a beverage coffee is well-known, and if taken in excess it results in unpleasant side effects such as tachycardia and wakefulness. Coffee is rarely used medicinally but caffeine is an ingredient of many analgesic preparations as it potentiates the effect of paracetamol (acetominophen) and aspirin, and produces a feeling of well-being. Studies have indicated that boiled coffee made from whole beans may increase blood lipid levels to detrimental effect, but the more usual filter coffee does not. This was ascribed to the lipids and diterpenes of the oil [1,2]. Regular consumption of coffee (2–3 cups per day) also lowered the risk of gallstone disease in men. Coffee promotes bile flow and stimulates the release of cholecystokinin, which increases gall bladder and large bowel motility [3]. A recent prospective study in women showed no association between coffee consumption (more than 4 cups per day) and colorectal cancer [4].

SPECIFIC REFERENCES: 1. Mensinck R *et al* (1995) *J. Intern. Med.* 237:543. 2. Zock P *et al* (1990) *Lancet* 335(8700):1235. 3. Leitzmann M *et al* (1999) *JAMA* 281(22):2106. 4. Terry P *et al* (2001) *Gut* 49:87.

COHOSH, BLACK
CIMICIFUGA RACEMOSA NUTT.
Fam. Ranunculaceae

SYNONYMS: Black Snakeroot, Bugbane, Rattleroot, Rattleweed, Squawroot, *Actaea racemosa* L., *Macrotys actaeoides* Rafin.

HABITAT: North America and Canada.

DESCRIPTION: Rhizome thick, hard and knotty, with short lateral branches, cylindrical, compressed, marked with transverse leaf scars. Transverse section: horny with a hard, thick, bark. Rootlets, when present, show a 'Maltese Cross' effect in transverse section. Taste: bitter and acrid; odour: disagreeable.

PART USED: Rhizome, root.

CONSTITUENTS: (i) Triterpene glycosides, based on acetylacteol and cimegenol, including actein, 27-deoxyactein, cimigoside, cimicifugodes H-1, H-2 and H-3, and racemoside (ii) Isoflavones such as formononetin (disputed) and others (iii) Isoferulic and salicylic acids (iv) Alkaloids; cytisine and methyl cytosine [R2;R7;1,2,3,4,5].

MEDICINAL USE: Black Cohosh is widely employed now for premenstrual disorders and menopausal ailments, although it was formerly used as a sedative, anti-inflammatory, anti-tussive and diuretic [R1]. Most of the research has been done on its hormone-regulating effects, but pharmacological studies have shown conflicting results. For example, the methanol extract was found to bind to oestrogen receptors *in vitro* and in rat uteri, which was originally ascribed to the presence of isoflavones [6], and it produced a selective reduction in luteinizing hormone (LH) [7]. However other studies have disputed these effects as being important clinically [R8;1]. Several human studies have demonstrated efficacy in alleviating menopausal symptoms although some of the results and mechanisms are controversial, particularly regarding the possible oestrogenic effects and use in women who have received primary treatment for breast cancer [8,9]. Mutagenicity, teratogenicity and other toxicity studies have proved negative, and it is now considered to be safe in women for whom conventional hormone-replacement therapy is contra-indicated [R17]. Adverse effects are minor and include gastrointestinal disturbance and lowering of blood pressure with high doses, and it should be avoided in pregnancy and lactation because of insufficient data. For a full account of the therapeutic use of Black Cohosh see [R7,R8,R17;1,2,9 and refs therein].

PREPARATIONS AND DOSE: Powdered Root, dose: 0.3–2 g; or equivalent extract

SPECIFIC REFERENCES: 1. Foster S (1999) *HerbalGram* 45:35. 2. Upton R (ed.) *'Black Cohosh'. American Herbal Pharmacopeia*. Pub: AHP, Sacramento, USA (2002). 3. Struck D *et al* (1997) *Planta Med.* 63:289. 4. Koeda M *et al* (1997) *Chem. Pharm. Bull.* 42:2205. 5. He K *et al* (2000) *Planta Med.* 66(7):635. 6. Jarry H *et al* (1985) *Planta Med.* 4:316. 7. Jarry H *et al* (1985) *Planta Med.* 51:1:46. 8. Liske E *et al* (1998) *Menopause* 5:520. 9. Jacobson J *et al* (2001) *J. Clin. Oncol.* 19(10):2739.

COHOSH, BLUE

CAULOPHYLLUM THALICTROIDES MICH.
Fam. Berberidaceae

SYNONYMS: Papoose Root, Squawroot, *Leontice thalictroides* L.

HABITAT: North America.

DESCRIPTION: Rhizome brownish grey, about 10 cm long and
0.5–1 cm thick, knotty with short branches; with numerous, crowded,
concave stem scars on the upper surface, and long, paler brown,
tough rootlets about 1 mm thick underneath. Internally it whitish
with narrow, woody rays. Taste: sweetish, then bitter and acrid;
nearly odourless.

PART USED: Rhizome.

CONSTITUENTS: (i) Alkaloids, including methylcytisine (= caulo-
phylline), anagyrine, baptifoline, magnoflorine, taspine, thalictroidine,
lupanine, sparteine, isolupanine and others (ii) Triterpene saponins;
caulosaponins and cauloside D, based on hederagenin [R2,R7,1,2,3,4].

MEDICINAL USE: Anti-inflammatory, antispasmodic, diuretic,
vermifuge and emmenagogue [R1]. Used particularly for rheumatism,
and for female complaints such as amenorrhoea and threatened
miscarriage, but should be avoided during the first trimester of
pregnancy. The North American Indians used the rhizome to facilitate
childbirth, hence the synonyms. The alkaloids however, particularly N-
methyl cytisine, are implicated as teratogens, and taspine is embryotoxic
[3]. Extracts are anti-inflammatory in the rat paw oedema test [2].

PREPARATIONS AND DOSE: Powdered root, dose: 0.3–2 g, or
equivalent extract.

SPECIFIC REFERENCES: 1. Strigina L *et al* (1975) *Phytochem.* 15:1583.
2. Benoit P *et al* (1976) *Lloydia* 39:160. 3. Kennelly E *et al* (1999)
J. Nat. Prod. 62(1):1385. 4. Betz J *et al* (1998) *Phytochem. Anal.*
9(5):232. 5. Woldemariam T *et al* (1997) *J. Pharm. Biomed. Anal.*
15(6):839.

COLA

COLA ACUMINATA (BEAUV.) SCHOTT ET ENDL.
C. NITIDA (VENT.) SCHOTT ET ENDL.
Fam. Sterculiaceae

SYNONYMS: Kola, Guru Nut, *Sterculia acuminata* Beauv. *Garcinia kola*
Heckel (Guttiferae) is also known as Cola.

HABITAT: Native to West Africa and extensively cultivated in the
tropics, particularly Nigeria, Brazil and Indonesia.

DESCRIPTION: The seed is found in commerce as the dried, fleshy
cotyledons with the testa removed. They are red-brown, often irregular
in shape, usually oblong, convex on one side and flattened on the
other, up to 5 cm long and about 2.5 cm in diameter.

PART USED: Seed.

131

CONSTITUENTS: (i) Xanthine derivatives, mainly caffeine, with traces of theobromine and theophylline (ii) Tannins and phenolics; *d*-catechin, *l*-epicatechin, kolatin, kolatein, kolanin, and in the fresh nut, catechol and (–)-epicatechol (iii) Amines including dimethylamine, methylamine, ethylamine and isopentylamine (iv) Miscellaneous; phlobaphene, an anthocyanin pigment known as 'kola red', betaine etc [R2,R19,1,2,3]. *Garcinia kola* also contains xanthones, together with volatiles including 6-methylhept-5-en-6-one, farnesol lavender lactone and linalool, hydroxybiflavonols and a polyisoprenyl benzophenone, kolanone [4,5].

MEDICINAL USE: Stimulant, diuretic, cardiac tonic, astringent and anti-diarrhoeal [R1]. Cola extracts are an ingredient of many tonics for depression, tiredness and to stimulate the appetite; the main stimulant and diuretic ingredient is caffeine. A preparation of cola nut with Ephedra (q.v.) decreased body weight and fat, and increased HDL-cholesterol levels in a randomized double-blind placebo-controlled study of 167 people [6]. One of the major uses is as flavouring in the manufacture of soft drinks. Ingestion of cola nuts causes an increase in arterial blood pressure in rats [7], and an increase in exploratory locomotor activity [8]. *Garcinia cola* has anti-microbial properties [5] as well as anti-ulcer and gastric acid lowering effects in rats [9].

PREPARATIONS AND DOSE: Powder, dose: 1–3 g, or equivalent extract.

SPECIFIC REFERENCES: 1. Morton J (1992) *Basic Life Sci.* 59:739. 2. Oliver-Bever B (1986) in Medicinal Plants of Tropical West Africa, Cambridge University Press, UK. 3. Atawodi S *et al* (1995) *Food Chem Toxicol.* 33(8):625. 4. Onayade O *et al* (1998) *Flav. Frag. J.* 13(6):409. 5. Madabunyi I (1995) *Int. J. Pharmacog.* 33(3):232. 6. Boozer C *et al* (2002) *Int. J. Obes.* 26(5):593. 7. Osim R *et al* (1993) *Int. J. Pharmacog.* 31(3):193. 8. Ettarh R *et al* (2000) *Pharm. Biol.* 38(4):281. 9. Ibironke G *et al* (1997) *Phytother. Res.*11(4):312.

COLCHICUM
COLCHICUM AUTUMNALE L.
Fam. Colchicaceae

SYNONYMS: Meadow Saffron, Naked Ladies.

HABITAT: North Africa and Europe, including parts of the British Isles.

DESCRIPTION: The plant produces a crocus-like pale purple flower in the autumn. The corm is usually found in transverse slices, notched on one side, kidney-shaped in outline and white and starchy internally. Taste: sweetish at first then bitter and acrid. The seeds are dull brown, nearly spherical, very hard, finely pitted, with a crest-like projection at the hilum. Taste: bitter and acrid, odourless.

PART USED: Corm, seeds.

CONSTITUENTS: (i) Alkaloids, the most important of which is colchicine, with demecolcine, 2-demethyl colchicine, colchiceine,

N-formyl-N-desacetyl colchicine, lumicolchicine and many others
(ii) Miscellaneous; flavonoids, including apigenin, 6-methoxy benzoic
and salicyclic acids, a glycoside, colchiside [R3;1,2,3,4].

MEDICINAL USE: Isolated colchicine alkaloid is now used specifically
for the relief of pain in acute gout, usually when other methods have
failed [5]. Historically, the corm was recommended in Arabian texts
for use in gout, and it has been used (rarely) as an anti-rheumatic
preparation. However, the highly toxic properties were well-known,
and it was rarely deemed suitable for herbal use. Colchicine is a
mitotic poison, which inhibits microtubule formation during cell
division. For this reason it is employed in plant breeding to induce
polyploidy, which is the multiplication of the chromosomes in a cell
nucleus [R3]. Side effects include severe gastrointestinal pain, nausea
and diarrhoea, which have even been noted after ingestion of the
flowers [6]. Larger doses cause renal damage and alopecia and
colchicine may cause foetal abnormalities. The fatal dose can be
as little as 7 mg [R14].

PREPARATIONS AND DOSE: Colchicine: for acute gout; dose:
500 mcg when required, up to a maximum of 6 mg over three days.

SPECIFIC REFERENCES: 1. Santavy F *et al* (1981) *Planta Med.* 43:153.
2. Ulrichova J *et al* (1993) *Planta Med.* 59:144. 3. Gasisc O *et al*
(1976) *Planta Med.* 30:75. 4. Fell K *et al* (1976) *Lloydia* 30:123.
5. Lettello C (2000) *The Alkaloids* 53:287. 6. Danel V *et al* (2001)
J. Toxicol. Clin. Toxicol. 39(4):409.

COLEUS
COLEUS FORSKOHLII BRIQ.
Fam. Lamiaceae

HABITAT: India.

DESCRIPTION: A typical herbaceous Labiate plant with serrated leaf
margins; not normally found in commerce.

PART USED: Herb.

CONSTITUENTS: (i) Labdane diterpenes, including colforsin
(forskolin), and various analogues including epi-deoxycoleonol (ii)
Phenolic glycosides including coleoside B (iii) Triterpene glycosides,
such as coleonolic acid, based on ursolic acid [1,2,3,4].

MEDICINAL USE: Used as a source of colforsin rather than as a herbal
remedy. Forskolin is cardiotonic, antihypertensive and vasodilatory,
with a positive cardiac inotropic effect [5]. It also relaxes tracheal
smooth muscle [6] and inhibits platelet aggregation [7], due to its
specific inhibition of adenylate cyclase. It is used for this purpose
in pharmacological research. An extract of the plant showed
anti-secretory activity against *Escherichia coli* endotoxin *in vitro* [8].

SPECIFIC REFERENCES: 1. Gabetta B *et al* (1988) *Phytochem.*
28(3):859. 2. Tandon J *et al* (1992) *Bioorg. Med. Chem. Lett.* 2(3):249.
3. Ahmed B *et al* (1991) *Pharmazie* 46(2):157. 4. Roy R *et al* (1990)

Tet. Lett. 31(24):3467. 5. Baumann G *et al* (1990) *J. Cardiovasc. Pharmacol.* 16(1):93. 6. Tsukawaki M *et al* (1987) *Lung* 165(4):225. 7. Agarwal K *et al* (1989) *Thromb. Haemostasis* 61(1):106. 8. Gupta S *et al* (1993) *Int. J. Pharmacog.* 31(3):198.

COLOPHONY

PINUS PALUSTRIS MILL.
P. PINASTER AND OTHER SPECIES
Fam. Pinaceae

SYNONYMS: Rosin.

HABITAT: Worldwide.

DESCRIPTION: Colophony resin is the residue left after the distillation of turpentine. It varies in colour from pale yellow to brown, and appears in brittle masses. For medicinal use the paler resin is preferred.

PART USED: Resin.

CONSTITUENTS: (i) Diterpene resin acids including abietic, dihydroabietic, neoabietic, palustric, pimaric and isopimaric acids and others (ii) Diterpene alcohols and aldehydes (iii) Miscellaneous sterols and phenolic acids [1].

MEDICINAL USE: Formerly used as an adhesive in dressings. but may cause allergic reactions. The ointment is used for boils and ulcers [R1]. In Chinese medicine colophony from oriental *Pinus* species is used to treat rheumatism, ringworm, bronchitis and other conditions, and is taken internally as well as applied externally. Colophony has many other uses in the printing and adhesives industries.

PREPARATIONS AND DOSE: Colophony Ointment BPC 1959.

SPECIFIC REFERENCES: 1. Zinkel D (1975) *Chem. Tech.* 5(4):235.

COLTSFOOT

TUSSILAGO FARFARA L.
Fam. Asteraceae

SYNONYMS: Coughwort, Horsehoof, Foal's Foot, Bull's Foot.

HABITAT: A common wild plant in Britain and Europe, growing in damp places. The flowers appear in early spring before the leaves.

DESCRIPTION: Leaves hoof-shaped, with angular teeth on the margins, about 10 cm in diameter, long-stalked, green above and coated with matted, long white hairs on the lower surface and on the upper surface when young. The flowers are bright yellow, up to 2 cm diameter, with a scaly pedicel. Taste: mucilaginous, slightly bitter, astringent; odourless.

PART USED: Leaves, flowers.

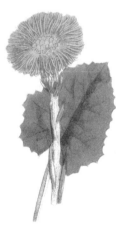

COLTSFOOT

CONSTITUENTS: (i) Mucilage, composed of acidic polysaccharides (ii) Flavonoids; rutin, hyperoside and isoquercetin (iii) Pyrrolizidine alkaloids, including senkirkine, tussilagine and isotussilagine, in variable amounts, very small (about 0.015%) or absent, depending on source (iv) Triterpenes and sterols; alpha- and beta-amyrin, campesterol etc. (v) Acids including isomeric tussilaginic acids and 2-pyrrolidine acetic acid [R2,R71,2,3,].

MEDICINAL USE: Expectorant, demulcent, anti-tussive, anti-catarrhal [R1]. Coltsfoot is used for pulmonary complaints, irritating or spasmodic coughs, whooping cough, bronchitis, laryngitis and asthma. The polysaccharides are anti-inflammatory and immunostimulating, as well as demulcent, and the flavonoids also have anti-inflammatory and antispasmodic action, which supports the use of Coltsfoot in coughs and colds [R7;1]. The pyrrolizidine alkaloids have caused hepatotoxicity in rats fed daily on high doses, but not on daily low-dose regimes, and appear not to cause damage to human chromosomes *in vitro* [4]; however samples containing significant quantities of them should not be used.

PREPARATIONS AND DOSE: Powdered root, dose: 0.6–2 g, three times daily by decoction, or equivalent extract.

SPECIFIC REFERENCES: 1. Berry M (1996) *Pharm. J.* 256:234. 2. Roder E (1992) *Deutsche Apot. Ztg.* 132:2427. 3. Passreiter C (1992) *Planta Med.* 58:A694. 4. Kraus C *et al* (1985) *Planta Med.* 51(2):89.

COLUMBO, AMERICAN

FRASERA CAROLINENSIS WALT.
Fam. Gentianaceae

SYNONYMS: F. walteri, F. canadensis.

HABITAT: North America and Canada.

DESCRIPTION: Root usually occurs in pieces 8–10 cm long and about 1–2.5 cm thick, often split longitudinally. The thick bark is pale brownish-grey and wrinkled transversely above and longitudinally below. Fracture: short and rather spongy; taste: resembling that of Gentian (q.v.).

PART USED: Root.

CONSTITUENTS: Methoxyxanthones including gentiopicroside (= gentiopicrin) [R4].

MEDICINAL USE: Tonic, stimulant [R1]. Little is known of the plant but it has been used in a similar way to Gentian (q.v.).

COMBRETUM

COMBRETUM SUNDAICUM MIG.
Fam. Combretaceae

SYNONYMS: Opium Antidote, Jungle Weed. *Combretum caffrum* is much more important now.

HABITAT: China.

DESCRIPTION: Leaves 10–13 cm long and about 6 cm broad, with 8–10 lateral spreading veins, perforated in the axils, surface minutely scaly on the young leaves. Taste: slightly astringent and tea-like.

PART USED: Herb.

CONSTITUENTS: Unknown. The related *C. caffrum* contains stilbenes, the combretastatins.

MEDICINAL USE: Reported to have been used in China for the treatment of the opium habit [R1]. The combretastatins, particularly combretastatin A-4, are anti-cancer drugs, now being clinically tested. They act as mitosis inhibitors [R3].

COMFREY
SYMPHYTUM OFFICINALE L.
Fam. Boraginaceae

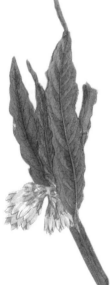

COMFREY

SYNONYMS: Blackwort, Nipbone, Knitbone, Consolida. Tuberous Comfrey is *S. tuberosum* L., and Russian Comfrey is *Symphytum* x *uplandicum*.

HABITAT: Common in moist places in Britain, Europe and the North Americas.

DESCRIPTION: The plant grows up to 1 m in height, bearing large, bristly obovate or lanceolate leaves, which may reach up to 25 cm long and 10 cm broad. The stem is hollow and also bristly. The flowers are bell-like, occurring in forked spikes; they are white or mauve or, in the case of S. *tuberosum*, white only, and S. *x uplandicum*, purple only. The root is brownish-black, deeply wrinkled. Fracture: short, showing in transverse section a thick bark and broad medullary rays. Taste: sweetish, mucilaginous; odourless.

PART USED: Root, leaves.

CONSTITUENTS: (i) Allantoin [1] (ii) Phenolic acids; cinnamic, salicylic, rosmarinic, chlorogenic, caffeic, lithospermic and many other acids [2,4] (iii) Mucilage, about 29%, composed of a polysaccharide containing glucose and fructose [4] (iv) Steroidal saponins (in the root), including cauloside and leontoside [5], and symphytoxin-A, a glycoside of hederogenin [6] (v) A glycopeptide of approximately 9000 daltons molecular weight [7] (vi) Pyrrolizidine alkaloids, including echimidine, symphytine, lycopsamine, symlandine, their acetyl and other derivatives and their N-oxides are often cited as present [8], and they can be found in significant quantities in the fresh herb and root. However in practice they were found to be absent in all commercial samples of the dried herb tested, as they are labile [9]. *S. tuberosum* has a much lower alkaloid content than the others [1].

MEDICINAL USE: Demulcent, astringent, anti-inflammatory, vulnerary, anti-psoriatic [R1]. Comfrey has been used for hundreds of years for pulmonary complaints, as a gastric sedative, and for rheumatism and painful joints. It is also used in the form of an ointment, oil or poultice for psoriasis, eczema, ulcers and to promote wound-healing. The anti-inflammatory activity of extracts of Comfrey has been demonstrated *in vitro* and *in vivo* using alkaloid-free extracts [10,11]. The glycopeptide is anti-inflammatory [7] and other isolated high molecular weight compounds were found to inhibit complement activity [12]. A recent clinical study showed efficacy of a Comfrey extract applied topically in the management of soft-tissue injury [13]. The presence of rosmarinic acid may also contribute to the effect [2]. The soothing and wound-healing properties are probably due to the allantoin, a well-known dermatological agent. An aqueous extract (comparable to a herbal tea) stimulates the release of a prostaglandin-like material from rat gastric mucosa [14], possibly explaining its usefulness as a gastric sedative. The pyrrolizidine alkaloids are undoubtably hepatotoxic and Comfrey has been implicated in causing hepatic veno-occlusive disease after chronic use [1,15]. However they are not part of the therapeutic effect and not usually found in commercial samples of the herb [9], so only samples from which they have been removed should be used. See also [R7].

PREPARATIONS AND DOSE: Powdered root, dose: 2–4 g, powdered leaf, dose: 2–8 g three times daily, or equivalent extract. Comfrey ointment: 10–15% extractive in a suitable base.

SPECIFIC REFERENCES: 1. Bhandari P *et al* (1985) *J. Pharm. Pharmacol.* 37:50P. 2. Gracza L *et al* (1985) *Arch. Pharm.* 312(12):1090. 3. Grabias B *et al* (1998) *Pharm. Pharmacol. Letters* 8(2):81. 4. Franz G (1969) *Planta Med.* 17:217. 5. Vali M *et al* (1995) *Planta Med.* 61(1):94. 6. Petersen G *et al* (1994) *Fitoterapia* 65(4):333. 7. Hiermann A *et al* (1998) *Pharm. Pharmacol. Letters* 8(4):154. 8. Stickel F *et al* (2000) *Pub. Health Nutr.* 3(4A):510. 9. Gray A *et al* (1983) *J. Pharm. Pharmacol.* 35:13P. 10. Andres R *et al* (1990) *Planta Med.* 56(6):664. 11. Petersen G *et al* (1993) *Planta Med.* 59(7S):A703. 12. Van den Dungen F *et al* (1991) *Planta Med.* 57(2S):A62. 13. Koll R *et al* (2000) *Z. Phytother.* 21:127. 14. Stamford I *et al* (1983) *J. Pharm. Pharmacol.* 35:816. 15. Weston C *et al* (1987) *Br. Med. J.* 295:183.

CONDURANGO
MARSDENIA CONDURANGO NICH.
Fam. Asclepiadaceae

SYNONYMS: Eagle Vine, *Gonolobus condurango* (Nick.) Triana.

HABITAT: Ecuador and Peru.

DESCRIPTION: Occurs in quilled pieces, 5–10 cm long, about 1–2 cm in diameter, and 2–6 mm thick. Outer surface: brownish-grey, often warty, with patches of lichen; inner surface paler in colour, striated. Transverse fracture: granular, yellowish-white, with scattered, fine, silky fibres. Taste: bitter and somewhat acrid; odour: faintly aromatic.

PART USED: Bark.

CONSTITUENTS: (i) Glycosides based on condurangogenins, which are esterified polyoxypregnanes; known as Condurango glycosides A, A_1, C, C_1, A_0, C_0 and B_0; and D_0 and its 20-O-methyl and 20-iso-O-methyl derivatives [1,2,3].

MEDICINAL USE: Alterative, stomachic, orexigenic [R1]. Used specifically for nervous dyspepsia, anorexia and as a gastric sedative. Condurango glycosides A_0, B_0, C_0 and D_0 are anti-tumour in several *in vitro* systems [1,2].

PREPARATIONS AND DOSE: Powdered bark, dose: 1–4 g, or equivalent extract.

SPECIFIC REFERENCES: 1. Hayashi K *et al* (1980) *Chem. Pharm. Bull.* 28:1954. 2. Hayashi K *et al* (1981) *Chem. Pharm. Bull.* 29:2725. 3. Hayashi K *et al* (1982) *Chem. Pharm. Bull.* 30:2429.

CONTRAYERVA
DORSTENIA CONTRAYERVA L.
AND OTHER SPECIES OF *DORSTENIA*
Fam. Moraceae

SYNONYMS: Contrajerva.

HABITAT: Moist thickets and forests of Mexico, Guatemala, Venezuela, Peru, West Indies.

DESCRIPTION: Rhizome about 2–4 cm long, 1 cm thick, reddish-brown, rough with leaf scars, nearly cylindrical, tapering suddenly at the end into a tail-like root with numerous curled, wiry rootlets. Taste: slightly aromatic, then acrid.

PART USED: Rhizome.

CONSTITUENTS: (i) Furanocoumarins including bergapten, bergaptol and its rhamnopyranosyl –beta-D-glucopyranosyl glycoside [1,2] (ii) Catechin and epicatechin [2].

MEDICINAL USE: Used as a febrifuge, emmenagogue, anti-diarrhoeal and for snakebite by indigenous people [R1]. The root is normally taken by infusion, and was said by the herbalist Joseph Miller in 1722 to "resist the bites of venomous creatures". The name in Spanish means antidote; however no further information on this usage is available. The extract is antimicrobial and weakly larvicidal [1].

SPECIFIC REFERENCES: 1. Terreaux P *et al* (1995) *Phytochem.* 39:645. 2. Caceres A *et al* (2001) *Fitoterapia* 72:376.

COOLWORT
TIARELLA CORDIFOLIA L.
Fam. Saxifragaceae

SYNONYMS: Mitrewort.

HABITAT: America.

DESCRIPTION: Leaves heart-shaped, 6–12 cm wide, with radiate veins and five to 12 pointed, irregularly toothed lobes. Taste: faintly astringent; odourless.

PART USED: Herb.

CONSTITUENTS: Unknown.

MEDICINAL USE: Diuretic, tonic [R1]. It has been used for most complaints of the urinary organs and for dyspepsia, taken mainly as an infusion.

COPAIBA
COPAIFERA LANGSDORFFII DESF.
AND OTHER SPECIES OF *COPAIFERA*
Fam. Leguminosae

SYNONYMS: Copaiva or Copaiba Balsam.

HABITAT: Tropical South America.

DESCRIPTION: The oleoresin (= oil) is tapped from cavities in the tree-trunk, where it accumulates, by drilling holes in the wood. It varies considerably in viscosity and colour, from relatively fluid and pale yellowish in colour to a more resinous material with a red or fluorescent tint. Taste: unpleasant; odour: characteristic.

PART USED: Oil or oleoresin.

CONSTITUENTS: (i) Volatile oil, containing alpha- and beta-caryophyllene as the major components, with copaene, *l*-cadinene, gamma-humulene, beta-bisabolol, bergamotene, aromadendrene, curcumene and many others (ii) Diterpenes such as copalic, copaiferic, copaiferolic acids, their methyl esters and others [R19;1,2,3].

MEDICINAL USE: Carminative, antiseptic, stimulant, diuretic, used mainly for cystitis, bronchitis and leucorrhoea [R1]. The oil is antibacterial and anti-inflammatory [3].

PREPARATIONS AND DOSE: Copaiba Oil BPC 1934, dose: 0.3–1.2 ml.

SPECIFIC REFERENCES: 1. Delle Monache G *et al* (1971) *Tet. Lett.* 8:659. 2. Ferrari M *et al* (1971) *Phytochem.* 10:905. 3. Viega V *et al* (2001) *Phytother. Res.* 15(6):476.

CORIANDER
CORIANDRUM SATIVUM L.
Fam. Apiaceae

HABITAT: Native to Europe, Africa, Asia, and naturalized in North America.

DESCRIPTION: The fruits are globular, about 0.5 cm diameter, with fine longitudinal ridges, separable into two halves, each of which is concave internally and shows two brown, longitudinal oil glands or vittae. Taste: aromatic; odour: characteristic. Unripe fruits have an unpleasant, fetid odour, resembling rubber.

PART USED: Fruits.

CONSTITUENTS: (i) Volatile oil, the major component being d-linalool (= coriandrol), with anethole, borneol, camphor, carvone, decyl acetate, elemol, geraniol, geranyl acetate, limonene and gamma-terpinene (ii) Flavonoids including quercetin, 3-*O*-methyl kaempferol, rhamnetin, apigenin and homoeriodictyol (iii) Coumarins including psoralen, angelicin, scopoletin, umbelliferone (iv) Phthalides such as neocnidilide (v) Phenolic acids including caffeic and chlorogenic [R2,R19;1,2].

MEDICINAL USE: Aromatic, carminative, antispasmodic [R1]. Experiments have shown that Coriander is hypoglycaemic and anti-inflammatory in animals [3,4] and the oil is reported to be larvicidal and bactericidal [R19]. Coriander seeds and the fresh leaves are used widely in cookery.

PREPARATIONS AND DOSE: Coriander Oil BP, dose: 0.05–2 ml.

BIBLICAL REFERENCES: Exodus 16:31; Numbers 11:7.

SPECIFIC REFERENCES: 1. Diedrreichsen A et al (1996) Planta Med. 862S:A82. 2. Gijbels M et al (1982) Fitoterapia 53(1–2):17. 3. Mascolo N et al (1987) Phytother. Res. 1(1):28. 4. Swanston-Flatt S et al (1990) Diabetologia 33(8):462.

CORN ERGOT
USTILAGO ZEAE (BECKM.) UNGER
Fam. Ustilaginaceae

SYNONYMS: Cornsmut, Cornbrand, Ustilago, U. maydis Leveille.

HABITAT: Wherever corn (maize) is grown.

DESCRIPTION: A blackish powder in irregular, globose masses, consisting of fungal spores with portions of the enclosing membrane. Taste and odour: unpleasant.

PART USED: Fungus.

CONSTITUENTS: (i) Quinones such as gunacin [1] (ii) Viral toxins, e.g. 'KP4' [2] (iii) Indole alkaloids (unspecified) (iv) Ustilagin, a choline sulphonic acid ester [R4].

MEDICINAL USE: Has been used in the same way as Ergot (q.v.) after childbirth, for post-partum and other types of haemorrhage [R1]. Gunacin has antibiotic activity [1] and KP4, a viral toxin or 'killer peptide', is also toxic to similar species of fungus [2].

SPECIFIC REFERENCES: 1. Werner R et al (1979) J. Antibiotics 32(11):1104. 2. Park C et al (1994) J. Molec. Microbiol. 11(1):155.

CORNFLOWER
CENTAUREA CYANUS L.
Fam. Asteraceae

SYNONYMS: Bluebottle. According to Culpeper it was also called Hurtsickle as "it turns the edges of the sickles that reap the corn".

HABITAT: Grows wild throughout Europe, especially in cornfields, naturalized elsewhere and cultivated in gardens.

DESCRIPTION: The flower-heads are globular with closely overlapping fringed scales and florets. The florets are usually bright blue, but other colours have been cultivated. They are tubular, and the outer ones trumpet-shaped and seven-lobed.

PART USED: Flowers.

CONSTITUENTS: (i) Flavonoids, including quercimetrin, and the anthocyanins pelargonin and cyanin (ii) Sesquiterpene lactones including cnicin (iii) Di- and ter-thiophenes such as 5-(3-butenyl-1-ynyl)-2,2'-bithienyl (BBT) and its acetoxy derivative (iv) Acetylenic compounds (v) Coumarins, e.g. cichonin (= esculetin-7-glucoside) (vi) Polysaccharides composed mainly of galacturonic acid, arabinose, glucose, rhamnose and galactose [1,2,3,4].

MEDICINAL USE: Less frequently used in medicine today, but formerly used as a tonic and stimulant, and for inflammation of the eye [R1]. The polysaccharides are anti-inflammatory in a number of systems such as carrageenan, zymosan and croton oil-induced oedema, and also interfere with complement [4]. Cnicin is anti-fungal and antibiotic [5,6,7]. Nowadays Cornflower extracts are used as an ingredient of cosmetics such as hair shampoos and rinses and eye lotions.

SPECIFIC REFERENCES: 1. Bandyukova V *et al* (1967) *Khim. Prir. Soedin.* 3:57. 2. Wagner H *et al* (eds) 'Plant Drug Analysis' (1984) *Springer-Verlag, Berlin.* 3. Tosi B *et al* (1991) *Phytother. Res.* 5(2):59. 4. Garbacki N *et al* (1999) *J. Ethnopharmacol.* 68(1–3):235. 5. Barrero A *et al* (2000) *Fitoterapia* 71(1):60. 6. Barrero A *et al* (1995) *Fitoterapia* 66(3):227. 7. Vanhaelen-Fastre R *et al* (1976) *Planta Med.* 29:179.

CORN SILK
ZEA MAYS L.
Fam. Graminae

SYNONYMS: Stigmata maydis.

DESCRIPTION: Fine, silky, yellowish threads, up to 20 cm long, consisting of the styles and stigmas from the female flowers of unripe maize. Taste: sweetish; odourless.

PART USED: Flower pistils.

CONSTITUENTS: (i) Volatile oil, containing carvacrol, alpha-terpineol, menthol and thymol (ii) Sterols; beta-sitosterol, ergosterol and stigmasterol (iii) Flavonoids including maysin and its 3'-methyl ether (iv) 6-methoxybenzoxazolinone (v) Miscellaneous; unspecified saponins, plant acids, the alkaloid hordenine, cryptoxanthin, vitamins and others [R2,R4,R7,R19,R20].

MEDICINAL USE: Demulcent, diuretic [R1]. Used mainly for urinary tract complaints such as cystitis, urethritis and prostatitis. The diuretic and choleretic activity has been demonstrated in animal tests [1], and clinically to some extent. Hypoglycaemic and hypotensive effects have also been described. In China it is used for oedema and hepato-biliary disease [R19,R20].

SPECIFIC REFERENCES: 1. Grases E *et al* (1993) *Phytother. Res.* 7(2):146.

CORSICAN MOSS
ALSIDIUM HELMINTHOCORTON KUTZ.
Fam. Rhodomelaceae

SYNONYMS: Fucus helminthocorton L.

HABITAT: North Atlantic Ocean.

DESCRIPTION: Occurs in tangled tufts of slender, brownish-white, cylindrical threads with a striated appearance. Taste and odour: typically seaweed-like.

CONSTITUENTS: Active constituents unknown.

MEDICINAL USE: Formerly used as an anthelmintic [R1], taken with honey or a tea.

COTO
NECTANDRA COTO L. AND OTHER SPECIES OF *NECTANDRA*
Fam. Lauraceae

SYNONYMS: Paracoto.

HABITAT: South America.

DESCRIPTION: Rarely found in commerce. The bark occurs as thick pieces 10–15 cm or more long, about 6 cm wide, and 1–1.5 cm thick, with a brown, corky outer surface with whitish patches, and a striated inner surface. Taste: pungent; odour: aromatic.

PART USED: Bark.

CONSTITUENTS: Largely unknown; alkaloids parastemine and cotoine, tannins, essential oil, resin etc. [R4].

MEDICINAL USE: Antiseptic and astringent; formerly used for catarrh, diarrhoea and dysentery [R1], as a decoction.

COTTON ROOT
GOSSYPIUM HERBACEUM L.
Fam. Malvaceae

HABITAT: Indigenous to India and the Arabian peninsula, but cultivated in China, southern Europe and North America.

DESCRIPTION: Flexible or quilled strips, light reddish-brown externally with faint, longitudinal ridges and small lenticels and occasionally attached rootlets. The cork is often exfoliating and easily separated. The inner surface is paler in colour with a silky sheen. Fracture: very fibrous. Taste: faintly acrid and astringent; odour: distinctive.

PART USED: Root bark, seeds.

CONSTITUENTS: (i) Oil, containing the sesquiterpene gossypol, with 6-methoxygossypol, 6,6'-dimethoxygossypol, and others, and in the seed, gossyfulvin, gossypurpurin [R16,1,2] (ii) Phenolic acids, betaine, resin, catechol and sterols [R2].

MEDICINAL USE: Emmenagogue, oxytocic, male contraceptive [R1]. The effects of gossypol were first discovered in China, when the oil used for cooking caused infertility in men. Since then it has been clinically tested there as a male contraceptive, and the effects found to be usually reversible [R20 and references therein]. It causes a marked decrease in sperm count, but also a degeneration of germ cells in the seminiferous tubules in male humans and animals [3]. Gossypol is reported to cause a transient weakness early in therapy, hypokalaemia, and changes in ECG among other side effects [4]. In female rats, it prevents ovum implantation, induces abortion and produces abnormalities in the surviving foetuses [5,6]. These results mean that gossypol is unlikely to be used clinically in other countries. It also has antiviral, anti-tumour and antibacterial activity both *in vitro* and *in vivo* [R16;1,2] and is an inhibitor of arachidonate 5- and 12-lipoxygenase [7], which supports the use of Cotton root bark in dysmenorrhoea. However, in view of the teratogenicity it cannot be recommended.

PREPARATIONS AND DOSE: Powdered root bark, dose: 2–4 g, or equivalent extract.

SPECIFIC REFERENCES: 1. Stipanovic R *et al* (1977) *Phytochem.* 14:1077. 2. Dorsett P *et al* (1975) *J. Pharm. Sci.* 64:1073. 3. Waller D *et al* (1981) *Contraception* 23:653. 4. Qian S *et al* (1980) *Chin. Med. J.* 93:477. 5. Lin Y *et al* (1985) *Life Sci.* 37:39. 6. Nath D *et al* (1997) *Fitoterapia* 68(2):1376. 7. Hamasaki Y *et al* (1985) *Biochim. Biophys. Acta* 843(1):37.

COUCHGRASS
AGROPYRON REPENS (L.) BEAUV.
Fam. Graminae

SYNONYMS: Twitch Grass, Quick Grass, Dog Grass (in North America), *Triticum repens* L.

HABITAT: Grows in most parts of the world. As Joseph Miller said, "...and is too frequent in gardens, whence it is hard to extirpate it".

DESCRIPTION: Rhizome slender, tubular, about 2 mm diameter, pale yellow, stiff, smooth with nodes at intervals of 2–3 cm. Taste: slightly sweet; odourless.

PART USED: Rhizome.

CONSTITUENTS: (i) Carbohydrates; triticin, a fructosan polysaccharide, about 8%, inositol, mannitol and mucilages (ii) Volatile oil, containing carvacrol, carvone and agropyrene (1-phenyl-2,4-hexadiyne) (iii) Hydroxycinnamic acid esters (iv) Silicic acid minerals including silica and iron [R2;1,2,3].

MEDICINAL USE: Diuretic, demulcent, aperient, anti-cholesteraemic [R1]. Used in urinary and bladder complaints, cystitis, nephritis etc., and for gout and rheumatism. Tests on the risks of calcium oxalate urolithiasis in rats did not show any particular effect [4]. However, a multi-centre post-marketing surveillance study of the fluid extract for the treatment of

143

urinary tract infections and irritable bladder indicated *Agripyron repens* drops to be safe and effective, and without adverse reactions [5].

PREPARATIONS AND DOSE: Powdered rhizome, dose: 4–8 g three times daily, or equivalent extract.

SPECIFIC REFERENCES: 1. Koetter U *et al* (1994) *Planta Med.* 60(5):488. 2. Schilcher H *et al* (1989) *Z. Phytother.* 10:77. 3. Boesel R *et al* (1989) *Planta Med.* 55:399. 4. Grases F *et al* (1995) *J. Ethnopharmacol.* 45(3):211. 5. Hautmann C *et al* (2000) *Z. Phytother.* 21(5):252.

COWHAGE
MUCUNA PRURIENS D.C.
Fam. Fabaceae

SYNONYMS: Cowage, Cowitch, *Dolichos pruriens* L.

HABITAT: India, Africa, South America.

DESCRIPTION: A tender, evergreen climber with downy leaves and clusters of purple or white pea-like flowers followed by flattened pods up to 9 cm long. These are covered with orange or brown bristles, about 2.5 mm long, barbed at the apex. They are extremely irritating to the skin and must be handled with caution.

PART USED: Whole plant.

CONSTITUENTS: (i) Alkaloids and indole amines, such as mucunadine, mucunine, prurienine, purieninine, mucuadine, mucuadinine, L-dopa, 5-hydroxytryptamine (serotonin), *N,N*-dimethyltryptamine, bufotenine and others [R12,R16;1,2] (ii) Sterols including beta-sitosterol, stigmasterol, ursolic and betulinic acids in the root [3] (iii) Mucuanain, a proteolytic enzyme [R12].

MEDICINAL USE: Traditionally used as an anti-Parkinsonian agent, anthelmintic, hypoglycaemic and aphrodisiac [R1]. L-dopa, one of the constituents, is well-known as a treatment for Parkinson's disease, but recent studies in rats have shown that *Mucuna pruriens* extract is superior to L-dopa alone [4] and a clinical study in humans has confirmed the use [R16]. The indole bases are reported to be spasmolytic and to depress respiration and blood pressure in animals [2]. The plant extract reduces blood sugar levels in rats [5,6] and the aphrodisiac activity has also been substantiated in animal tests [7]. The plant extract has antioxidant [8] and analgesic [9] activity. In West Africa, the plant is a traditional remedy for snakebite, an effect which has been supported to some extent since the extract reduces blood clotting time after treatment with *Echis cariatus* venom both *in vitro* [10] and *in vivo* in rats [11]. This has recently shown to be due to activation of prothrombin [12] and reduction of coagulation enzyme levels, which are normally increased by the venom [11].

SPECIFIC REFERENCES: 1. Bell E *et al* (1971) *Nature* 229:136. 2. Ghosal S *et al* (1971) *Planta Med.* 24:434. 3. Aruna V *et al* (1998) *Indian Drugs* 35(6):356. 4. Hussain G *et al* (1997) *Phytother. Res.*

11(6):419. 5. Rathi S *et al* (2003) *Phytother. Res.* 17 *In press.* 6. Grover J *et al* (2001) *J. Ethnopharmacol.* 76(3):233. 7. Amin K *et al* (1996) *Fitoterapia* 67(1):53. 8. Tripathi Y *et al* (2002) *Phytother. Res.* 16(6):534. 9. Jauk L *et al* (1993) *Int. J. Pharmacog.* 31(3):213. 10. Houghton P *et al* (1994) *J. Ethnopharmacol.* 44(2):99. 11. Aguiyi J *et al* (2001) *Phytother. Res.* 15(8):712. 12. Guerranti R *et al* (2001) *J. Ethnopharmacol.* 75(2–3):175.

COWSLIP

PRIMULA VERIS L.
Fam. Primulaceae

SYNONYMS: Paigles, Peagles, *P. officinalis.*

HABITAT: Common in Britain, Europe and temperate Asia.

DESCRIPTION: A short, hairy perennial, with oval, wrinkled leaves. The flowers are tubular, yellow, about 1 cm diameter, five-lobed and spotted with orange at the throat. Taste: sweetish; odour: apricot-like.

PART USED: Flowers, occasionally root.

CONSTITUENTS: (i) Saponin glycosides, especially in the root, based on the triterpene aglycones primulagenin A, dehydroprimulagenin A, primverogenins A and B, including primulic acid (about 5–10%), primulaveroside, primveroside etc. [1,2] (ii) Flavonoids, particularly in the flowers, consisting of quercetin, luteolin, kaempferol, isorhamnetin, and apigenin and their glycosides, and several methoxylated flavones [3,4,5] (iii) Tannins; epicatechin and epigallotannin [R7;3].

MEDICINAL USE: Sedative, antispasmodic, mild diuretic and aperient [R1]. The saponins are anti-inflammatory, antiviral [6] and anti-fungal [7]. The flowers are particularly high in flavonoids, which are anti-inflammatory and antispasmodic; they inhibit histamine release and act as free-radical scavengers [R7;8].

PREPARATIONS AND DOSE: Flowers, dose: 1–2 g, three times daily as an infusion.

SPECIFIC REFERENCES: 1. Calis I *et al* (1992) *J. Nat. Prod.* 55:1299. 2. Siems K *et al* (1998) *Planta Med.* 64(3):272. 3. Karl C *et al* (1981) *Planta Med.* 41:96. 4. Huck C *et al* (1999) *Planta Med.* 65(5):491. 5. Huck C *et al* (2000) *J. Chromatog.* 870(1–2):453. 6. Buechi S (1996) *Deutsche Apot. Ztg.* 136:89. 7. Sekizaki H (1995) *Natural Medicines* 49(1):97. 8. Middleton E *et al* (1984) *Biochem. Pharmacol.* 33:3333.

CRAMPBARK

VIBURNUM OPULUS L. AITON.
Fam. Caprifoliaceae

SYNONYMS: Guelder Rose, Snowball Tree.

HABITAT: Europe, Britain and America.

DESCRIPTION: A large bush, growing to a height of about 2.5 m. The bark is about 0.5–2 mm thick, in curved pieces, greyish-brown externally with scattered lenticels, and faintly cracked longitudinally.

Inner surface paler brown, laminate. Fracture: tough, with flat splinters. Taste: bitter, slightly astringent.

PART USED: Bark.

CONSTITUENTS: (i) Hydroquinones; arbutin, methylarbutin and traces of free hydroquinone (ii) Coumarins, such as scopoletin and esculetin (iii) Triterpenes including oleanolic and ursolic acid derivatives (iv) Iridoid glycoside esters (v) Polyphenolics; astragalin, paeonoside, catechins [R9;1 and refs therein, 2,3,4,5].

MEDICINAL USE: Antispasmodic, astringent, sedative, nervine [R1]. As its name suggests, it is used for cramp, particularly of menstruation, and other uterine dysfunctions. Scopoletin is antispasmodic [5] and uterine relaxant effects have been described [6]. Enzyme inhibiting and angioprotective effects have been described *in vivo* [2].

PREPARATIONS AND DOSE: Powdered bark, dose: 2–4 g, by decoction, or equivalent extract.

SPECIFIC REFERENCES: 1. Upton R (ed) *'Cramp Bark'. American Herbal Pharmacopoeia.* Pub: AHP, Sacramento, USA (2000). 2. Jonadet M *et al* (1989) *Pharm. Acta Helvetica* 64(3):94. 3. Ivanov V *et al* (1983) *Farmatsiya* 32(2):20. 32(4):113, and (1984) 33(4):26. 4. Bock *et al* (1978) *Phytochem.* 17:753. 5. Jarboe C *et al* (1967) *J. Med. Chem.* 10:488. 6. Jarboe C *et al* (1966) *Nature* 212(64):837.

CRANBERRY

VACCINIUM MACROCARPON AITON.
Fam. Ericaceae

SYNONYMS: *V. oxycoccus* L. is used as a substitute but is considered inferior.

HABITAT: North America, from the Carolinas to Canada.

DESCRIPTION: A small heath-like shrub with pink flowers, followed by shiny, red-black, edible berries, up to about 1 cm in diameter, in June and July.

PART USED: Berries, juice.

CONSTITUENTS: (i) Polyphenolics including flavonoids, anthocyanins (odain) and tannins such as catechin (ii) Plant acids; ascorbic, benzoic, citric, ellagic, quinic, beta-hydroxybutyric, malic and others (iii) Triterpenes [R7,R11;1].

MEDICINAL USE: Urinary antiseptic, used to treat cystitis. Numerous studies have suggested efficacy for cranberry juice, particularly in the treatment of acute urinary tract infection (UTI) and prevention of long-standing disease, although many of these are not rigorously controlled. It is usually well-tolerated although the taste is very sharp and has resulted in a high drop-out rate for some studies. Cranberry juice is thought to act by increasing levels of hippuric acid (a metabolite of benzoic acid), and therefore acidity of the urine, and also by preventing adhesion of bacteria to the bladder wall [R7,R11;1,2,3,4,5,6,7 and references therein].

PREPARATIONS AND DOSE: Juice: for treatment and prevention of UTI, dose up to 960 ml daily.

SPECIFIC REFERENCES: 1. Siciliano A (1995) *HerbalGram* 38:51. 2. Avorn J *et al* (1994) *JAMA* 271(10):751. 3. Ofek I *et al* (1991) *New Eng. J. Med.* 324(22):1599. 4. Kontiokari T *et al* (2001) *Brit. Med. J.* 322(7302):1571. 5. Howell A *et al* (1998) *New Eng. J. Med.* 339:1085. 6. Wilson T *et al.* (1998) *Life Sci.* 62:381. 7. Jepson R *et al* (2000) *Cochrane Library* 1, Oxford Press, UK.

CRANESBILL, AMERICAN
GERANIUM MACULATUM **L.**
Fam. Geraniaceae

SYNONYMS: Alumroot, Storksbill, Wild Geranium.

HABITAT: North America.

DESCRIPTION: Root about 3–5 cm long, 0.5–1 cm thick, dull brown, hard; knotty, with small protuberances. Fracture: short, cut surface pale or reddish-brown, with white dots. Taste: very astringent; odourless.

PART USED: Root, herb.

CONSTITUENTS: Gallotannins [R2]. Little information is available, although other species of *Geranium,* particularly G. *thunbergii* Sieb. et Zucc., and G. *sanguineum* L, have been investigated to a much greater extent. *G. thunbergii* contains tannins including geraniin, dehydrogeraniin, geraniic acids A and B, furosin, furosinin, phyllanthusiin F and others [1,2], and G. *sanguineum* contains gallocatechins, catechins and flavonoids [3,4].

CRANESBILL

MEDICINAL USE: Styptic, astringent, vulnerary, tonic [R1]. The root is even more astringent than the herb. An infusion or decoction is taken for diarrhoea, internal or external bleeding. It may be taken in the form of a douche for leucorrhoea and topically for ulcers and haemorrhoids. Tannins and polyphenols isolated from the other species have been shown to inhibit *Herpes* and influenza viruses [3,4,5] and geraniin prevents liver damage in experimental liver injury and nephrosis [6,7]. Tannin-containing crude drugs tend to have a uraemic toxin-decreasing action [8]. See also [9].

PREPARATIONS AND DOSE: Powdered herb or root, dose: 2–4 g, by infusion, or equivalent extract, three times daily.

SPECIFIC REFERENCES: 1. Okuda T *et al* (1982) *Chem. Pharm. Bull.* 30(1):1110. 2. Ito H *et al* (1999) *Chem. Pharm. Bull.* 47(8):1148. 3. Serkedjeva J (1995) *Fitoterapia* 63(2):111. 4. Serkedjeva J (1996) *Phytother. Res.* 10(5):441. 5. Serkedjeva J (1999) *J. Ethnopharmacol.* 64(1):59. 6. Nakanishi Y *et al* (1999) *Natural Medicines* 53(1):22. 7. Nakanishi Y *et al* (1999) *Natural Medicines* 53(2):94. 8. Yokozawa T *et al* (1995) *Phytother. Res.* 9(1):1. 9. *Geranium and Pelargonium.* Ed. Lis-Balchin M (2002). *Medicinal and Aromatic Plants – Industrial Profiles.* Pub: Taylor and Francis, London, UK.

CRATAEVA NURVALA

CRATAEVA NURVALA BUCH.
Fam. Capparidaceae

SYNONYMS: C. religiosa Hook f. and Thoms., *C. magna* (Lour.) D.C.
Three-leaved caper, Varuna.

HABITAT: Native to southern India.

DESCRIPTION: A small deciduous tree, with trifoliate, glabrous leaves.
The flowers are large and greenish-white; the fruits fleshy and ovoid.
The mature bark is greyish, wrinkled and rough with noticeable lenticels.

PART USED: Stem and root bark, leaves.

CONSTITUENTS: (i) Alkaloids, such as cadabicine and its diacetate,
in the stem bark [1] (ii) Triterpenes based on diosgenin; lupeol, varunol,
spinasterol, taraxasterol, lupenone and others [2] (iii) Tannins and
flavonoids [R16].

MEDICINAL USE: Used in Ayurvedic medicine for urinary calculi
and urinary tract infections, and as a digestive stimulant, tonic and
antimalarial. A beneficial effect on experimental urolithiasis has
been observed in rats [3,4], and supported by a clinical study [R16].
Anti-inflammatory activity has also been noted; these effects were
attributed to the lupeol content [R19].

SPECIFIC REFERENCES: 1. Ahmed V *et al* (1987) *J. Nat. Prod.*
50(6):1186. 2. Geetha T *et al* (1998) *Pharmacol. Res.* 37(3):191. 3.
Prabhakar Y *et al* (1990) *Fitoterapia* 61(2):99. 4. Varalakshmi P
et al (1991) *J. Ethnopharmacol.* 31(1):67.

CRAWLEY

CORALLORBIZA ODONTORHIZA NUTT.
Fam. Orchidaceae

SYNONYMS: Coral Root, Dragon's Claw, Chicken Toe.

HABITAT: North America.

DESCRIPTION: The rhizome appears in small, brown, coral-like,
branched pieces, about 2–3 cm long and 2 mm in thickness, with
minute warts and transverse scars. Fracture: short and horny.
Taste: sweetish then bitter; odour: strong and peculiar when fresh.

PART USED: Rhizome.

CONSTITUENTS: Unknown.

MEDICINAL USE: Reputed to be diaphoretic, antipyretic and sedative [R1].

CROSSWORT

GALIUM CRUCIATUM L.
Fam. Rubiaceae

SYNONYMS: Yellow Bedstraw.

HABITAT: A common wild plant in Britain and Europe, flowering in May.

DESCRIPTION: Stem slender, about 30–60 cm long, bearing whorls of four leaves, ellipsoidal, oblong, hairy. Flowers, yellow, in small clusters, about eight together in the axils of the upper leaves.

PART USED: Herb.

CONSTITUENTS: (i) Coumarins, including umbelliferone, scopoletin, and cruciatin, a monoglucoside (ii) Flavonoids such as hyperoside and rutin (iii) Tannins [1].

MEDICINAL USE: Formerly made into a salve, for wounds [R1].

SPECIFIC REFERENCES: 1. Borisov M (1974) *Khim. Prir. Soedin.* 10:82.

CROTON SEEDS
CROTON TIGLIUM L.
Fam. Euphorbiaceae

SYNONYMS: Tiglium, *Tiglium officinale* Klotsch., Badou (Chinese).

HABITAT: Widely distributed throughout Asia and China.

DESCRIPTION: The seeds have a brown, mottled appearance. The outer layer is easily removed, leaving a hard, black coat. The oil is yellowish- or reddish-brown and rather viscid, with an unpleasant odour. It is toxic and should be handled with extreme care.

PART USED: Oil expressed from seeds.

CONSTITUENTS: Diterpene esters of the tigliane type, at least 11 of which have been isolated. The most important of these is tetradecanoyl phorbol acetate (TPA; formerly known as phorbol myristate acetate or PMA). For full information see [1].

MEDICINAL USE: Irritant, rubifacient, cathartic [R1]. Should not be used medicinally. Strongly purgative, it causes hypotension, severe abdominal pain, rapid and weak pulse, and shock (1 ml is usually fatal). Croton oil is a co-carcinogen (tumour promoter). TPA has a wide range of pharmacological effects in addition to tumour promotion: it causes erythema, vesication and hyperplasia of the skin, platelet aggregation, interference with prostaglandin metabolism and many others. These properties are mostly mediated via activation of the enzyme protein kinase C. TPA is used widely as a biochemical probe to investigate carcinogenesis, inflammation and other cellular mechanisms [1].

PREPARATIONS AND DOSE: Croton oil: Use not recommended.

SPECIFIC REFERENCES: 1. Evans F (Ed.) 'Naturally Occurring Phorbol Esters', CRC Press (1986).

CUBEB
PIPER CUBEBA L.
Fam. Piperaceae

SYNONYMS: Tailed Pepper, *Cubeba officinalis* Miq.

HABITAT: Native to Indonesia, but cultivated elsewhere.

149

DESCRIPTION: The fruit resembles black pepper in size and colour, but tapers sharply into the stalk. The seed has a minute embryo in a small cavity at the apex. Taste: warm; aromatic and rather like turpentine.

PART USED: Unripe fruit.

CONSTITUENTS: (i) Volatile oil, 10–20%, consisting of mono- and sesquiterpenes including sabinene, alpha-thujene, alpha- and beta-pinene, alpha-terpinene and others [1,2] (ii) Lignans; mainly (–)-cubebine, with (–)-cubebinin and kinokinin; and (–)-dihydrocubebinin, (–)-clusin, and derivatives [3,4] (iii) Miscellaneous; cubebic acid, resins gums etc. [R19].

MEDICINAL USE: Aromatic, diuretic, expectorant, carminative [R1]. Used to treat bronchitis, coughs and urinary-tract infections. The fruits have been used for amoebic dysentery. The oil is reputedly antiviral *in vivo* and antibacterial *in vitro* [R19].

SPECIFIC REFERENCES: 1. Ohta T *et al* (1966) *Tet. Lett.* 52:6365. 2. Ikeda R *et al* (1962) *J. Food Sci.* 27:455. 3. Batterbee J *et al* (1969) *J. Chem. Soc.* (C). 2470. 4. Prabhu B *et al* (1985) *Phytochem.* 24(2):329.

CUCKOOPINT
ARUM MACULATUM L.
Fam. Araceae

SYNONYMS: Lords and Ladies, Wake Robin, Wild Arum, Starchwort, Ramp.

HABITAT: Europe and the British Isles.

DESCRIPTION: The plant consists of a one-leafed, erect and pointed spathe, enclosing the flower. Inside the spathe is the club-shaped, purplish or buff-coloured spadix. The root is ovoid and about the size of a hazel nut, showing annular scars left by the leaves and rootlets. Taste: acrid; odourless.

PART USED: Root.

CONSTITUENTS: (i) Polysaccharides, four of which are acetylated or glucomannans [1,2] (ii) An N-acetylgalactosamine-specific lectin [3] (iii) Miscellaneous; polyphenols, basic volatile substances and saponin glycosides of unknown structure [1].

MEDICINAL USE: Diaphoretic, expectorant [R1]. Has been used locally for sore throats. Large doses cause gastric inflammation, and fatal effects have been recorded. The glucomannan isolated from the root is thought to ameliorate stomach ulcers [2] and an extract is reported as having anti-fertility potential in female rats [4]. The plant has a long history of rather unusual uses; Dioscorides stated that the root has an effect against gout, "being laid on stamped with cow's dung"; and Gerard writes "Bears, after they have lain in their dens 40 days without any manner of sustenance but what they get from licking and sucking their own feet, do, as soon as they come forth eat the herb Cuckoo-pint; through the windy nature thereof, the hungry gut is opened and made fit enough to receive sustenance". The starch from the root was used to starch the ruffs worn in the days of Queen Elizabeth I, and Gerard also says that it was "the most pure white starch" but "it choppeth, blistereth and maketh the hands rough and rugged and withall smarting".

SPECIFIC REFERENCES: 1. Akhtardziev K T et al (1984) Farmatsiya 34(3):1. 2. Koleva M et al (1980) Pharmazie 35(11):712. 3. Allen A (1995) Biochim. Biophys. Acta 1244(1)129. 4. Elbctieha A et al (1996) Arch. STD/HIV Res. 10(3):181.

CUDWEED

GNAPHALIUM ULIGINOSUM L.
Fam. Asteraceae

SYNONYMS: Marsh Cudweed, Cottonweed, Cotton Dawes.

HABITAT: A native British plant.

DESCRIPTION: The plant is densely woolly, with small, narrow leaves, about 3 cm long and 0.5 cm wide; the flower-heads are composite, small, yellow corymbs.

PART USED: Herb.

CONSTITUENTS: Largely unknown. The herb contains volatile oil and tannins [R2].

MEDICINAL USE: Astringent, used for tonsillitis and laryngitis as a gargle [R1]. Reputed to be an antidepressant and aphrodisiac. In Russia it has been used clinically to treat hypertension, usually in combination with other herbs [1]. Other species of Gnaphalium, from Guatemala, have antibacterial activity [2,3].

SPECIFIC REFERENCES: 1. Scheptoin B T et al (1984) Vrach Delo 6:18. 2. Caceres A et al (1990) J. Ethnopharmacol. 30(1):55. 3. Caceres A et al (1991) J. Ethnopharmacol. 31(2):193.

CUMIN

CUMINUM CYMINUM L.
Fam. Apiaceae

SYNONYMS: Cummin, Jeera.

HABITAT: Cultivated widely along the Mediterranean and in India.

DESCRIPTION: Fruits about 6 mm long, 1 mm wide, longitudinally ribbed, often with pedicel attached, light brown in colour. Each mericarp has four dorsal and two commisural vittae. Odour and taste: characteristic, curry-like.

PART USED: Fruits.

CONSTITUENTS: (i) Volatile oil, about 2–5%, composed mainly of cuminaldehyde, 1,3- and 1,4-p-menthadien-7-al, 3 p-menthen-7-al, with alpha- and beta-pinene, alpha- and beta-phellandrene, limonene and many others [1] (ii) Flavonoids, including apigenin and luteolin glycosides [2] (iii) Petroselic and other acids [R19].

MEDICINAL USE: Antispasmodic, stimulant, carminative [R1]. The oil has anti-carcinogenic effects as measured by an increase in carcinogen detoxifying enzymes in mice [3] and dietary cumin seeds in rats reduced the incidence of tumours in experimental colon cancer [4]. The seeds also had an anti-diabetic effect in rats [5]. Cumin is widely used in cookery as a spice.

BIBLICAL REFERENCES: Isaiah 28:25–27; Matthew 23:23.

SPECIFIC REFERENCES: 1. Varo P *et al* (1970) *J. Agric. Food Chem.* 18:234 and 239. 2. Harborne J *et al* (1972) *Phytochem.* 11:1741. 3. Aruna K T *et al* (1996) *Phytother. Res.* 10(7):577. 4. Nalini N *et al* (1998) *Med. Sci. Res.* 26(11):781. 5. Willatgamuwa A *et al* (1997) *Nutr. Res.* 18(1):131.

CUPMOSS
CLADONIA PYXIDATA FRIES.
Fam. Cladoniaceae

SYNONYMS: Chin Cups.

HABITAT: British Isles and Europe on barren ground.

DESCRIPTION: It is a lichen, not a moss as the name suggests. The scyphi are greyish-white, about 2.5 cm long, wineglass shaped, with hollow stems and a terminal cup. Taste: mucilaginous and slightly sweet; odourless.

PART USED: Scyphi.

CONSTITUENTS: (i) Lichen acids such as fumaroprotocetraric, barbatic and psoromic acids (ii) An enzyme, emulsin [R4].

MEDICINAL USE: Expectorant and anti-tussive [R1]. Formerly used for whooping cough (or Chin-Cough, hence the synonym) as a decoction, sweetened with honey, but little information is available.

CUP-PLANT
SILPHIUM PERFOLIATUM L.
Fam. Asteraceae

SYNONYMS: Indian Cup Plant, Ragged Cup.

HABITAT: India.

DESCRIPTION: Rhizome cylindrical, crooked, elongated, pitted and rough, with small roots. The transverse section shows large resin canals.

PART USED: Rhizome.

CONSTITUENTS: Unknown. The aerial parts contain triterpene glycosides based on oleanolic acid [1].

MEDICINAL USE: Tonic, diaphoretic, alterative [R1]. No recent information is available.

SPECIFIC REFERENCES: 1. Davidyants E *et al* (1984) *Khim Prir. Soedin* 5:666.

D DAMIANA
TURNERA DIFFUSA WILL.
Fam. Turneraceae

HABITAT: Southern North America, Mexico and parts of sub-tropical America and Africa.

DESCRIPTION: Leaves wedge-shaped, about 1–2.5 cm long, up to 6 mm broad, shortly stalked, with a few serrate teeth and recurved margins. Taste: bitter; aromatic, with a fig-like flavour.

PART USED: Leaves.

CONSTITUENTS: (i) Volatile oil, about 0.5–1%, containing thymol, alpha-copaene, 8-cadinene and calamene,1,8-cineole, alpha- and beta-pinenes and calamenene (ii) Flavonoids such as 5-hydroxy-7,3', 4-trimethoxyflavone (iii) The hydroquinone, arbutin (iv) Miscellaneous; a cyanogenetic glycoside, tetraphylline B (= barterin), a bitter substance of undetermined structure called damianin, tannins etc. [R2,R19;1].

MEDICINAL USE: Aphrodisiac, tonic, stomachic [R1]. The aphrodisiac activity has not yet been properly demonstrated in humans, although a multi-herb preparation containing Damiana was reported to enhance sexual satisfaction in women [2]. An extract was shown to stimulate sexual activity in impotent (or sluggish) male rats, although it had no effect on normal, sexually potent, animals. It also had no effect on locomotor activity [3]. Damiana is sometimes incorporated into anti-obesity preparations with apparent benefits [4]. The leaves are reportedly antidepressant [5].

PREPARATIONS AND DOSE: Powdered leaf, dose: 2–4 g, or equivalent extract, three times daily.

SPECIFIC REFERENCES: 1. Dominguez X *et al* (1976) *Planta Med.* 30:68. 2. Ito T *et al* (2001) *J. Sex Marital Ther.* 27(5):541. 3. Arletti R *et al* (1999) *Psychopharmacology* 143(1):15. 4. Andersen T *et al* (2001) *J. Hum. Nutr. Diet* 14(3):243. 5. Jin J (1966) *Lloydia* 29(3):250.

DANDELION
TARAXACUM OFFICINALE WEBER.
Fam. Asteraceae

SYNONYMS: Taraxacum dens-leonis Desf., *Leontodon taraxacum* L.

HABITAT: Widely distributed throughout most of the world as a troublesome weed.

DESCRIPTION: Dandelion is so well-known it needs no description. Roots are collected in the autumn.

PART USED: Leaves, root.

CONSTITUENTS: (i) Sesquiterpene lactones; taraxacoside (an acylated gamma-butyrolactone glycoside), taraxinic acid, dihydrotaraxinic acid and taraxacolide glucosides, and others (ii) Polyphenolic caffeoyltartaric acids (iii) Coumarins (iv) Triterpenes; taraxol, taraxerol, taraxasterol,

153

beta-amyrin, stigmasterol and beta-sitosterol [R2,R19; 1,2,3]. The vitamin A content is reportedly higher than in carrots [R19].

MEDICINAL USE: Diuretic, tonic, anti-rheumatic and mild aperient [R1]. Used chiefly in kidney and liver disorders, for rheumatism and as a general tonic. The anti-inflammatory activity was confirmed in animal studies [4] and the polyphenols shown to have antioxidant activity [5]. The polysaccharides and aqueous extracts showed anti-tumour activity in animals [6]. The root, when roasted, is used as a coffee substitute or flavour additive, and the fresh young leaves may be used in salads. The flowers are used to make country-style wines.

PREPARATIONS AND DOSE: Powdered leaf, dose: 2–10 g, root, dose: 2–8 g, or equivalent extract, three time daily.

SPECIFIC REFERENCES: 1. Budzianowski J (1997) *Planta Med.* 63:288. 2. Rauwald H-W *et al* (1985) *Phytochem.* 24(7):1557. 3. Hansel R *et al* (1980) *Phytochem.* 19:857. 4. Mascolo N *et al* (1987) *Phytother. Res.* 1(1):28. 5. Hagymasi K *et al* (2000) *Phytother. Res.* 14:43. 6. Baba K *et al* (1981) *Yakugaku Zasshi* 10(6):538.

DEER'S TONGUE
TRILISIA ODORATISSIMA (J F GMEL) CASS.
Fam. Asteraceae

SYNONYMS: Vanilla Leaf, Wild Vanilla, Hound's Tongue, *Liatris odoratissima* Michx., *Carphephorus odoratissimus* (J F Gmel) Heb.

HABITAT: Eastern North America.

DESCRIPTION: Leaves obovate-lanceolate; those from the root are fleshy and taper at the base into a flattened stalk, stem leaves sessile. The dried leaves have a strong odour of new-mown hay.

PART USED: Leaves.

CONSTITUENTS: (i) Coumarin and dihydrocoumarin (ii) Sesquiterpenes; eudesmin and epieudesmin (iii) Triterpenes; lupeol, lupenone and beta-amyrin [1,2].

MEDICINAL USE: Diuretic, stimulant, tonic [R1]. No pharmacological information is available. The coumarin gives Deer's Tongue its vanilla-like flavour.

SPECIFIC REFERENCES: 1. Appleton R *et al* (1971) *Phytochem.* 10:440. 2. Karlsson K *et al* (1972) *Acta Chem. Scand.* 26:1383.

DEVIL'S BIT
SUCCISA PRATENSIS MOENCH.
Fam. Dipsacaceae

SYNONYMS: Devil's Bit Scabious, Ofbit.

HABITAT: Damp grassy places throughout Europe.

DESCRIPTION: Leaves opposite, stalked, lanceolate-ovate, with scattered glands. Flower-heads blue-purple, florets four lobed, receptacle hairy.

154

PART USED: Herb.

CONSTITUENTS: Iridoids, such as catalpol, verbenalin and loganin [1].

MEDICINAL USE: Diaphoretic, demulcent, febrifuge [R1]. It has been taken for coughs and fevers. Culpeper states, "The root was longer until the Devil bit it away, envying its usefulness to mankind," hence the common name.

SPECIFIC REFERENCES: 1. Suomi J *et al* (2001) *Electrophoresis* 22(12):2580.

DEVIL'S CLAW
HARPAGOPHYTUM PROCUMBENS D.C.
Fam. Pedaliaceae

HABITAT: Indigenous to southern and eastern Africa.

DESCRIPTION: The plant bears a large, hooked, claw-like fruit, which is dangerous to grazing cattle, and gives the plant its name. The tuber is up to about 6 cm in diameter, with a yellowish-brown longitudinally striated bark. In commerce it usually occurs cut, in circular orfan-shaped pieces. Fracture: short, showing a light grey-brown concentric and radiate xylem in transverse section, with occasional cavities. Taste: astringent; odourless.

PART USED: Tuber.

CONSTITUENTS: (i) Iridoid glycosides, including harpagide, harpagoside and procumbide (ii) Flavonoids, mainly kaempferol and luteolin glycosides (iii) Phenolic acids; chlorogenic and cinnamic acid (iv) A quinone, harpagoquinone (v) Triterpenes; oleanolic and ursolic acid derivatives [R7,R8,R17 and refs therein].

MEDICINAL USE: Anti-inflammatory, anti-rheumatic, analgesic, sedative. Numerous pharmacological tests have demonstrated *in vivo* anti-inflammatory activity, for instance in the rat paw oedema test, and analgesic effects comparable to that of phenylbutazone in rabbits. It exerts its activity via inhibition of eicosanoid biosynthesis and the whole extract is more potent than isolated harpagide [1]. More recently several clinical studies have shown the efficacy of standardized extracts in human patients with osteoarthritis, non-radicular back pain and other forms of chronic and acute pain. It is generally well-tolerated and appears to be a suitable alternative to non-steroidal anti-inflammatory agents, which often have gastrointestinal side effects [R7,R17;2,3,4 and refs therein].

PREPARATIONS AND DOSE: Powdered tuber, dose: 0.1–0.25 g, by decoction, or equivalent extract, three times daily.

SPECIFIC REFERENCES: 1. Loew D *et al* (2001) *Clin. Pharmacol. Ther.* 69:356. 2. Laudahn D *et al* (2001) *Phytother. Res.* 15(7):621. 3. Chubrasik S *et al* (1996) *Phytomed.* 3(1):1. 4. Chantre P *et al* (2000) *Phytomed.* 7(3):177.

DILL
ANETHUM GRAVEOLENS L.
Fam. Apicaeae

SYNONYMS: Peucedanum graveolens Benth.

HABITAT: Indigenous to the Mediterranean region and southern parts of Russia, cultivated widely elsewhere.

DESCRIPTION: Fruits normally separated into two mericarps; each ovoid, compressed, winged, about 2–3 mm wide with three longitudinal ridges on each side and four dorsal vittae. On the flat commisural surface there are two more vittae and the pale carpophore. Odour and taste: pleasant, aromatic and characteristic. Indian Dill is *A. sowa* Roxb., which has narrower and more convex fruits, with more pronounced ridges and narrower wings.

PART USED: Fruits; the herb is used in cookery.

CONSTITUENTS: (i) Volatile oil, consisting mainly of carvone (about 50%), with dihydrocarvone, limonene, dill apiole, alpha- and beta-phellandrene, eugenol, anethole, myristicin, carveole, alpha-pinene and others (ii) Flavonoids; kaempferol and its glucuronide, vicenin and others (iii) Coumarins such as scopoletin, esculetin, bergapten, umbelliferone etc. (iv) Xanthone derivatives such as dillanoside. (v) Phthalides such as butylphthalide, Z-ligustilide, neocnidilide and senkyunolide occur in the roots [R2;1,2].

MEDICINAL USE: Carminative, stomachic [R1]. Used frequently in gripe waters for wind and colic in infants. The seeds have been used as a diuretic, and the activity confirmed measured as an increase in urine flow in dogs [3].

PREPARATIONS AND DOSE: Dill Oil BP, dose: 0.05–2 ml; Concentrated Dill Water BPC 1973, dose: 0.3–1 ml.

SPECIFIC REFERENCES: 1. Kosawa M *et al* (1976) *Chem. Pharm. Bull.* 24:220. 2. Gijbels M *et al* (1983) *Sci. Pharm.* 51:414. 3. Mahran G *et al* (1991) *Phytother. Res.* 5(4):169.

DODDER
CUSCUTA EPITHYMUM MURR.
Fam. Convolvulaceae

SYNONYMS: Lesser Dodder, Dodder of Thyme, Hell-weed, Devil's Guts.

HABITAT: A parasite growing in most parts of the world.

DESCRIPTION: Stem thread-like, curled and twisted, without leaves but with small, globular clusters of flowers. Taste: saline and slightly acrid; odourless.

PART USED: Herb.

CONSTITUENTS: Largely unknown. Flavonoids including kaempferol, quercetin and its 3-glucoside and substituted *p*-hydroxycinnamic acids have been reported [1]. Other species of *Cuscuta* have been investigated more thoroughly; in general they contain glycoproteins, and also polyphenols, saponins and alkaloids depending on the host plant [2,3,4].

MEDICINAL USE: Hepatic, laxative [R1]. Has been used in urinary, spleen and liver disorders. The related species C. *reflexa* decreased heart rate and blood pressure in anaesthetized rats [5] and *C. campestris* had a tranquillizing and anti-inflammatory effect in rats [6].

SPECIFIC REFERENCES: 1. Pagnani F *et al* (2001) *Boll. Chim. Pharm.* 113(1):30. 2. Stanilova S *et al* (2000) *Int. J. Immunopharmacol.* 22(1):15. 3. Istudor V *et al* (1984) *Farmacia* 32(3):173. 4. Baumel P *et al* (1993) *Planta Med.* 59(7S):A643. 5. Gilani A *et al* (1992) *Int. J. Pharmacog.* 30(4):296. 6. Agha A *et al* (1996) *Phytother. Res.* 10(2):117.

DOG ROSE
ROSA CANINA L. AND OTHER SPP.
Fam. Rosaceae

SYNONYMS: Wild Briar, Rosehips, Cynosbatos.

HABITAT: Europe, North Africa and parts of Asia. Extensively cultivated.

DESCRIPTION: The fruits, or hips, are oval, fleshy, scarlet when fresh and blackish when dried, with the remains of the calyx teeth at the apex. Seeds angular, whitish, densely covered with hairs, taste, sweetish and acidulous.

PART USED: The ripe or nearly ripe fruit.

CONSTITUENTS: (i) Vitamins; vitamins A, C and K, thiamine, riboflavine and niacin (ii) Flavonoids such as rutin (iii) Tannins 2–3% (iv) Miscellaneous; sugars, pectin, plant acids, carotenoids, traces of essential oil and vanillin [R2,R19].

MEDICINAL USE: Astringent, anti-diarrhoeal [R1]. Syrup made from the fruits is given to infants as a source of vitamin C.

DRAGON'S BLOOD
DAEMONOROPS DRACO BLUME
D. PROPINQUUS BECC.
Fam. Palmae

SYNONYMS: Dracorubin, Sanguis Dranconis.

HABITAT: Malaysia, Indonesia.

DESCRIPTION: A red resin produced by the fruits, softened with water and pressed and dried. Occurs as lumps, tears or sticks.

PART USED: Resin.

CONSTITUENTS: Red tannin derivatives called dracoresinotannols, with benzoic acid and its esters [R4].

MEDICINAL USE: Astringent in diarrhoea [R1], colouring agent.

DWARF ELDER
SAMBUCUS EBULUS L.
Fam. Caprifoliaceae

SYNONYMS: Ground Elder, Danewort, Wallwort.

HABITAT: Europe, including the British Isles, where it is a troublesome weed in gardens.

DESCRIPTION: Leaves pinnate, leaflets longer than those of the common Elder (q.v.), often with stipules at the base. Flowers white with pink anthers. In North America the name 'Dwarf Elder' is given to a completely different plant, *Aralia bispida* Vent. (Araliaceae).

PART USED: Leaves.

CONSTITUENTS: (i) Flavonoids, sterols, tannins (unspecified) [1] (ii) Ribosome-inactivating proteins known as ebulins and ebulitins have also been described [2]. Little information is available.

MEDICINAL USE: Expectorant, diuretic, anti-ulcer agent [R1]. An extract demonstrated anti-nociceptive and anti-inflammatory effects in rats, using the tail flick and formalin experimental methods, and was suggested as having a centrally-acting effect [1]. An extract showed anti-ulcer activity *in vivo* in rats [3]. The ribosome inactivating proteins are considered to be non-toxic [2].

SPECIFIC REFERENCES: 1. Ahmadiani A *et al* (1998) *J. Ethnopharmacol.* 61(3):229. 2. De Benito F *et al* (1995) *FEBS Lett.* 360(3):299. 3. Yesilada E *et al* (1993) *Phytother. Res.* 7(3):263.

DYER'S GREENWEED
GENISTA TINCTORIA L.
Fam. Fabaceae

SYNONYMS: Greenweed, Dyer's Weed, Dyer's Broom.

HABITAT: Indigenous to Europe, cultivated elsewhere.

DESCRIPTION: Stems almost unbranched, about 15–20 cm long, angular, with erect lanceolate sessile, hairless leaves, about 2 cm long and 4 mm broad. Flowers: yellow, typically papilionaceaous, in terminal spikes. Taste: bitter; odourless.

PART USED: Twigs, leaves.

CONSTITUENTS: (i) Isoflavone glycosides including genistein, its 7-O-glucoside and daidzein (ii) Flavonoids, mainly luteolin glycosides (iii) Alkaloids such as anagyrine, ammodendrine, cytisine, *N*-methyl-cytisine, isosparteine, lupanine and tinctorine [R2;1,2,3,4].

MEDICINAL USE: Diuretic, cathartic, emetic [R1]. It has been used in the past for gout. The isoflavones are phytoestrogens and genistein is a tyrosine kinase inhibitor. However because of the toxic alkaloids, the use of *Genista* for these purposes cannot be recommended (see Broom). It was formerly used as a dye, but this is rare nowadays.

SPECIFIC REFERENCES: 1. Harborne J (1969) *Phytochem.* 8:1449. 2. Ulubelen A *et al* (1971) *Lloydia* 34(2):258. 3. Lewis J *et al* (1971) *J. Chem. Soc* (C) 4:629. 4. Swiatek L *et al* (1984) *Farm. Pol.* 40:729. 5. Inoue H *et al* (1970) *Chem. Pharm. Bull.* 1856.

ECHINACEA

ECHINACEA ANGUSTIFOLIA (D.C.) HELLER
E. PALLIDA (NUTT.) BRITT.
E. PURPUREA MOENSCH.
Fam. Asteraceae

SYNONYMS: Coneflower, Purple Coneflower (*E. purpurea*), Black Sampson, *Brauneria angustifolia, B. pallida.*

HABITAT: Native to the northern North America, cultivated widely in Europe and elsewhere.

DESCRIPTION: The dried rhizome is greyish-brown, often twisted, longitudinally furrowed, up to about 1 cm in diameter. The transverse section shows a thin bark, and a yellowish porous wood flecked with black. Taste: slightly sweet then bitter, leaving a tingling sensation on the tongue; odour: faintly aromatic.

PART USED: Roots and rhizome; aerial parts and juice.

CONSTITUENTS: (i) Caffeic acid conjugates, such as cichoric acid, echinacoside, 6-caffeoyl echinacoside, cynarine, verbascoside, chlorogenic and rosmarinic acids, and others (ii) Unsaturated isobutyl amides, including echinacin and others, such as undeca-, dodeca-, trideca- and pentadeca-dien-diynoic acid isobutylamides. These are fairly unstable (iii) Polysaccharides; mainly heteroxylans and arabinorhamnogalactans (iv) Essential oil, containing humulene, caryophyllene and its epoxide, germacrene D, and methyl-*p*-hydroxy-cinnamate (v) Miscellaneous; vanillin, linolenic acid derivatives, a labdane derivative, and the flavonoid rutin. The alkaloids tussilagine and isotussilagine have been reported, in very small quantities. The constituents vary between species in both quality and quantity; for example, echinacoside is absent from *E. angustifolia* and *E. purpurea,* and cichoric acid is found in *E. purpurea* and *E. pallida* but not *E. angustifolia.* For full details see references [R7,R8;1,2,3,4,5,6,7].

MEDICINAL USE: Antibacterial, antiviral, vulnerary, alterative [R1]. It is used especially for skin diseases, boils, carbuncles, septicaemia and to aid wound healing generally, and for upper respiratory-tract infections such as tonsillitis and pharyngitis, as a preventative as well as a treatment. It is usually taken internally in the form of drops or tablets. Antibacterial, antiviral and antioxidant effects have been documented, but the most important action of Echinacea is probably its ability to stimulate the immune system, a property demonstrated by total extracts and by the polysaccharide fraction in a number of *in vivo* and *in vitro* tests. These include the stimulation of phagocytosis, and effects have been observed clinically. The polysaccharide fraction activates macrophages, causing an increase in secretion of free radicals and interleukin I, possibly explaining its activity against infections and in some anti-tumour systems. Echinacin has been shown to inhibit the formation of hyaluronidase by bacteria; this would help to localize the infection and stop it spreading. The results of clinical trials of Echinacea are becoming increasingly available and support the use,

159

and although not all are of good quality, the overall evidence is fairly good. Taking Echinacea during pregnancy was not associated with an increased rate of birth defects. See [R7,R8,R11,R17;2,8,9,10 and refs therein].

PREPARATIONS AND DOSE: Powdered root, dose: 1–2 g, by decoction, or equivalent extract, three times daily.

SPECIFIC REFERENCES: 1. Perry N *et al* (2001) *J. Agric. Food Chem.* 49(4):1702. 2. Duff Sloley B *et al* (2001) *J. Pharm. Pharmacol.* 53:849. 3. Bauer R *et al* (1989) *Phytochem.* 28:505. 4. Bauer R *et al* (1988) *Phytochem.* 27:2339. 5. Von Roder E *et al* (1984) *Deutsch Apot. Ztg.* 124(45):2316. 6. Bohlmann F *et al* (1983) *Phytochem.* 22:1173. 7. Lindenmuth G *et al* (2000) *J. Alt. Complement. Med.* 6(4):327. 8. Facino R *et al* (1995) *Planta Med.* 61:510. 9. Gallo M *et al* (2000) *Arch. Int. Med.* 160:3141.

ECLIPTA

ECLIPTA ALBA (L.) HASSAK.

Fam. Asteraceae

SYNONYMS: Trailing eclipta *E. prostrata* (L.).

HABITAT: India and many other parts of Asia, growing as a common weed.

DESCRIPTION: An erect or prostrate, highly branched annual herb, with a daisy-like flower and hairy leaves.

PART USED: Whole plant.

CONSTITUENTS: (i) Triterpene oleanane saponins known as eclalbasaponins I-VI, and other sterols (ii) Flavonoids and isoflavonoids including wedelolactone, desmethylwedelolactone and their glucosides (iii) Columbin, a sesquiterpene lactone, coumarins and terthienyl derivatives [R16;1].

MEDICINAL USE: Liver protectant, and treatment for jaundice, hepatitis and liver and spleen enlargement. It has also been used as a hair dye and for alopecia and ringworm. It is an important herb in Ayurvedic medicine as a general tonic and for a number of other conditions [R16]. The hepatoprotective activity has been confirmed in experimental liver damage in rodents [2,3,4] and anti-inflammatory and analgesic activity has also been reported [5]. The leaves are eaten as food in Java.

PREPARATIONS AND DOSE: Powdered herb, dose: 3–6 g, by decoction, or equivalent extract.

SPECIFIC REFERENCES: 1. Yahara S *et al* (1994) *Chem. Pharm. Bull.* 42(6):1336. 2. Saxena A *et al* (1993) *J. Ethnopharmacol.* 40(3):155. 3. Singh B *et al* (1993) *Phytother. Res.* 7(2):154. 4. Lin S-C *et al* (1996) *Phytother. Res.* 10(4):483. 5. Leal L *et al* (2000) *J. Ethnopharmacol.* 70(2):151.

ELDER
SAMBUCUS NIGRA L.
Fam. Caprifoliaceae

SYNONYMS: Black Elder, European Elder.

HABITAT: Europe, and the British Isles, commonly growing in hedges and on waste ground.

DESCRIPTION: The flowers, appearing in May, are small, creamy-white with yellow anthers, four-petalled, in flat-topped umbel-like clusters, with a mucilaginous taste and a characteristic odour. The flowers are followed in September by small, shiny, purplish-black berries, also in hanging clusters. Leaves pinnate, leaflets broad with serrate margins. Bark light grey, with wide fissures revealing the smooth white inner surface. Taste: sweetish, then nauseous.

PART USED: Flowers, berries, leaves, bark.

CONSTITUENTS: Flowers: (i) Triterpenes including ursolic acid, 30-beta-hydroxyursolic acid, oleanolic acid, alpha- and beta-amyrin and free and esterified sterols (ii) Fixed oil, containing free fatty acids; mainly linoleic, linolenic and palmitic acids, and alkanes (iii) Flavonoids, including rutin, quercetin, nicotoflorin, hyperoside, kaempferol etc. (iv) Miscellaneous; phenolic acids, e.g. chlorogenic acid, pectin, sugars etc. [R2,R7,R8,R9;1,2,3,4]. Leaves: (i) Triterpenes similar to those found in the flowers (ii) Cyanogenetic glycosides, e.g. sambunigrin, holocalin and prunasin and others; cyanohydrins (iii) Flavonoids including rutin and quercetin [4,5].

MEDICINAL USE: Alterative, diuretic, anti-inflammatory [R1]. The flowers are used most frequently, as an infusion or herbal tea. Their anti-inflammatory action was demonstrated in rats and it was suggested that it was due to the ursolic acid content [6]. A decoction of the flowers or berries enhanced phenobarbitone induced sleep in rats, and the berry extract decreased the analgesic effect of morphine [7]. Other documented effects include an anti-diabetic action, by stimulation of insulin secretion, *in vitro* [8]. The flowers and berries are often used to make wine, for their flavour rather than medicinal effect; however the wine taken hot, or a mixture of elder flowers and peppermint, are a traditional remedy for colds and influenza. Recent studies show an *in vitro* activity against several strains of influenza virus, and a clinical study in human patients demonstrated a reduction in the duration of flu symptoms. The effect was thought to be due to increasing inflammatory cytokine production as well as a direct antiviral action [9].

PREPARATIONS AND DOSE: Powdered flowers, dose: 2–4 g, by infusion, or equivalent extract, three times daily.

SPECIFIC REFERENCES: 1. Richter W *et al* (1977) *Pharm. Ztg.* 122:1567. 2. Inoue T *et al* (1975) *Phytochem.* 14:1871. 3. Petitjean-Freytet C *et al* (1991) *J. Pharm. Belg.* 46(4):241. 4. Della Greca M *et al* (2000) *Tet. Lett.* 41(33):6507. 5. Della Greca M *et al* (2000) *Nat.*

161

Prod. Lett. 14(3):175. 6. Mascolo N *et al* (1987) *Phytother. Res.* 1(1):28. 7. Jakovljevic V *et al* (2001) *Pharm. Biol.* 39(2):142. 8. Gray A *et al* (2000) *J. Nutr.* 130(1):15. 9. Barak V *et al* (2001) *Eur. Cytokine Network* 12(2):290.

ELECAMPANE
INULA HELENIUM L.
Fam. Asteraceae

SYNONYMS: Scabwort, Yellow Starwort, *Helenium grandiflorum* Gilib., *Aster officinalis* All., *A. helenium* (L.) Scop.

HABITAT: Indigenous to Europe and temperate Asia, naturalized in North America, and cultivated widely.

DESCRIPTION: Roots light grey, hard, horny, in cylindrical pieces of varying length, usually 1–2 cm thick and often attached to large pieces of the crown of root. Fracture: short, the transverse section showing a radiate structure with numerous dark oil glands. Taste: bitter, acrid; odour: aromatic, sweet, and faintly camphoraceous.

PART USED: Root.

CONSTITUENTS: (i) Volatile oil, about 1–4%, containing sesquiterpene lactones, mainly alantolactone (= helenalin or elecampane camphor), isoalantolactone and their dihydro derivatives, alantic acid and azulene (ii) Inulin; up to 44% (iii) Miscellaneous; sterols, resin etc. [R7;1,2].

MEDICINAL USE: Diaphoretic, diuretic, expectorant, alterative, tonic [R1]. Used principally in combination with other herbs for coughs, bronchitis and other pulmonary disorders, and for nausea, diarrhoea and as an anthelmintic. The essential oil is anti-fungal and antibacterial [1,2], and a smooth muscle relaxant. Alantolactone is anti-inflammatory in animals and has been shown to stimulate the immune system; it is also anthelmintic and hypotensive in animals and antibacterial and anti-fungal *in vitro* [R7].

PREPARATIONS AND DOSE: Dried root, dose: 1.5–4 g, or equivalent extract, three times daily.

SPECIFIC REFERENCES: 1. Boatto G *et al* (1994) *Fitoterapia* 65(3):279. 2. Cantrell C *et al* (1999) *Planta Med.* 65(4):351.

ELM
ULMUS MINOR (MILL.) RICH.
Fam. Ulmaceae

SYNONYMS: Common Elm, English Elm, European Elm, Field Elm, *U. carpinifolia* Ruppius ex Suckow, *U. campestris* L.

HABITAT: A common tree throughout Europe.

DESCRIPTION: The inner bark only is used; it occurs in thin strips 2–3 mm thick, externally rusty-brown colour but paler on the inner surface. Fracture: laminate and fibrous. Taste: mucilaginous, astringent and faintly bitter; odourless.

PART USED: Bark.

CONSTITUENTS: (i) Sterols, including campesterol, beta-sitosterol and cholesterol (ii) Mucilages; a complex mixture of pentoses, methylpentoses and hexoses (iii) Tannins and proanthocyanins [R2].

MEDICINAL USE: Astringent, demulcent, diuretic [R1]. The related 'Slippery Elm' (q.v.) is more commonly used.

BIBLICAL REFERENCES: Hosea 4:13, probably the terebinth *Pistachia terebinthus.*

EMBELIA
EMBELIA RIBES BURM.
Fam. Myrsinaceae

HABITAT: India.

DESCRIPTION: A large, climbing shrub, with simple, lanceolate, coreaceous leaves. The flowers are small and white or greenish, followed by the small globular, reddish-brown berries which have a wrinkled or warty surface when dried, with a small projection at the apex. Each contains a single red seed. Taste: pungent and astringent; odour: faintly aromatic.

PART USED: Fruit.

CONSTITUENTS: (i) Naphthaquinones; embelin (= embelic acid), rapanone and vilangin (ii) Chrisembine, an alkaloid (iii) Fatty acids, in the seed [R16;1].

MEDICINAL USE: Contraceptive. The berries are important in Ayurvedic medicine and are also used as an anthelmintic, carminative and diuretic. Embelin is being investigated as a contraceptive, it has anti-fertility effects in animals and appears to act both by preventing implantation in the female and inhibiting spermatogenesis in the male, without being blastotoxic. It was found to be oestrogenic and weakly progestogenic at the minimum effective dose [1,2,3,4]. Anthelmintic, insecticidal, antimicrobial and anti-tumour activities have been described, which are common properties of quinones, and analgesic activity has been reported [5].

PREPARATIONS AND DOSE: Powdered fruit, dose: 2–4 g, or equivalent extract.

SPECIFIC REFERENCES: 1. Bhargava S (1988) *Fitoterapia* 59(3):163. 2. Prakash O (1981) *Planta Med.* 41:258. 3. Dixit V *et al* (1983) *Andrologia* 15(5):486. 4. Gupta S *et al* (1989) *Contraception* 39(3):307. 5. Atal C *et al* (1984) *J. Ethnopharmacol.* 11(3):309.

EPHEDRA
EPHEDRA SINICA STAPF.
E. EQUISETINA BUNGE
E. GERARDIANA WALL. AND OTHER SPECIES
Fam. Ephedraceae

SYNONYMS: Ma Huang.

163

HABITAT: China, *E. gerardiana* is Indian.

DESCRIPTION: Slender green stems jointed in branches of about 20 tufts about 15 cm long. Leaves reduced to sheaths surrounding the stems, which terminate in a sharp, recurved point.

PART USED: Stems.

CONSTITUENTS: (i) Alkaloids, up to about 3%, but widely varying. *E. sinica* usually has higher concentrations than the other species. The major alkaloid is (–)-ephedrine, together with many others including (+)-pseudoephedrine, norephedrine, norpseudoephedrine, N-methyle-phedrine, ephedroxane, maokonine, transtorine, the ephedradines A-D, feruloylhistamine and benzylmethylamine (ii) Volatile oil, containing alpha-terpineol, tetramethylpyrazine, terpinen-4-ol, linalool and others (iii) Tannins, particularly catechin derivatives (iv) Diterpenes including ephedrannin A and mahuannin A have been isolated from other species of *Ephedra* [R7;1,2,3,4,5,6,7,8].

MEDICINAL USE: Anti-asthmatic, bronchodilator, sympathomimetic, CNS and cardiac stimulant [R1]. Ephedra has been used since ancient times in China for asthma and hay fever. Herbalists use it to treat enuresis, allergies, narcolepsy and other disorders, and anti-inflammatory activity has been observed in extracts [2]. The use as an anti-allergic agent has been supported by evidence that it induced production of immunoglobulin A in Peyer's patches cells [9] and blocked complement activation by the classical and alternative pathways [10]. The tannins inhibit the influenza A virus *in vitro* [4]. Recently the water extract of Ephedra has been shown to have anti-tumour, anti-angiogenic and anti-invasive effects using *in vitro* cell culture methods [11]. The herb has been used with some success as a slimming aid [12], but this can be dangerous if high doses are used for long periods, for example hypertension and other cardiovascular events, and a case of exacerbation of hepatitis have been noted [13,14]. Both ephedrine and pseudoephedrine are widely used in the form of nasal drops, tablets and elixirs as decongestants [R7,R8,R14]. Absorption of ephedrine and pseudoephedrine was found to be much slower after ingestion of the herb than for isolated alkaloid preparations [15], and these should be avoided by hypertensive patients. The herb is not considered to have these side effects since it contains other components, such as the ephedradins, mahuanins, maokonine and feruloylhistamine, which are actually hypotensive [5,6,7,8]. Ephedroxane is anti-inflammatory [16]. For evaluation of possible toxicity see [17].

PREPARATIONS AND DOSE: Powdered herb, dose: 1–4 g, or equivalent extract. Ephedrine, dose: 15–60 mg orally three times daily; nasal drops 0.5–1%.

SPECIFIC REFERENCES: 1. Liu Y-M *et al* (1993) *Planta Med.* 59(4):376. 2. Hikino H *et al* (1980) *Chem. Pharm. Bull.* 28(10):2900. 3. Miyazawa M *et al* (1997) *Flav. Fragr. J.* 12(1):15. 4. Mantani N *et al* (2001) *Planta Med.* 67(3):240. 5. Hikino H *et al* (1982) *Heterocycles* 17:155 and 19:1381. 6. Hikino H *et al* (1983) *Planta Med.* 48:108. 7. Kasahara Y *et al* (1983) *Heterocycles* 20:1953 and 1741. 8.

Konno C *et al* (1980) *Heterocycles* 14:295. 9. Bae E-A *et al* (2000) *Korean J. Pharmacog.* 31(3):259. 10. Ling M *et al* (1995) *Clin. Exp. Immunol.* 102(3):582. 11. Nam N-H *et al* (2003) *Phytother. Res.* 17 *in press.* 12. Boozer C *et al* (2002) *Int. J. Obesity* 26(5):593. 13. Haller C *et al* (2000) *New Eng. J. Med.* 343(25):1833. 14. Borum M. (2001) *Am. J. Gasteroenterol.* 96(5):1654. 15. White L *et al* (1997) *J. Clin. Pharmacol.* 37(2):116. 16. Konno C *et al* (1979) *Phytochem.* 18:697. 17. Hathcock J (2001) *HerbalGram* 53:21.

ERGOT

CLAVICEPS PURPUREA TUL.

Fam. Clavicipitaceae

SYNONYMS: Ergot of Rye, Smut of Rye, Spurred Rye, *Secale cornutum* Nees.

HABITAT: Grows on rye.

DESCRIPTION: The hard mycelium of the fungus is formed from the grains of rye; it is purplish, up to about 3 cm long, 0.5 cm diameter, cylindrical, compressed, with a longitudinal furrow down each side and tapering to rounded ends. Fracture: short and horny; interior whitish with a purplish tinge. Odour: disagreeable.

PART USED: Fungus.

CONSTITUENTS: (i) Indole alkaloids; including the ergometrine (ergonovine) group which includes ergometrine and ergometrinine, the ergotamine group which includes ergotamine and ergotaminine, the ergotoxine group which includes ergocristine, ergocristinine, ergocryptine, ergocryptinine, ergocornine and ergocorninine, agroclavine, elymoclavine and the more recently isolated ergobine and ergobinine [R3;1,2] (ii) Triacyl glycerols based on C16 and C18 fatty acids including ricinoleic acid [3] (iii) Miscellaneous; histamine, tyramine and other amines, sterols and acetylcholine [R3].

MEDICINAL USE: Oxytocic, vasoconstrictor, alpha-adrenergic receptor blocker [R1]. The alkaloids ergotamine and ergometrine are normally used individually because of their potency and slightly different effects. Ergotamine is used to relieve migraine headaches, because it is a vasoconstrictor and has anti-serotonin activity. It can also prevent the hyperalgesia induced by morphine withdrawal in mice [4]. Ergometrine has been used after childbirth, in the third stage of labour and for post-partum haemorrhage; it is a powerful uterine stimulant but rather unpredictable. Both should be used only under careful medical supervision. The ergot alkaloids have also been used as templates for the development of new compounds (e.g. bromocriptine) for use in Parkinson's disease and other conditions. The European plagues of the Middle Ages, referred to as St Anthony's Fire, were due to contamination of flour with ergot; the toxic symptoms included hallucinations and gangrene and are known as 'Ergotism' [R3;5]. Small amounts of Ergot alkaloids may be found in foodstuffs and sub-acute toxicity testing in rats suggests effects are not serious [6]. For a recent full review, see [7]. Ergot is the starting material for the illicit

165

manufacture of the hallucinogen LSD and its supply is monitored.

SPECIFIC REFERENCES: 1. Perellino N *et al* (1993) *J. Nat. Prod.* 56(4):489. 2. Fiserova A *et al* (1997) *Physiol. Res.* 46(2):119. 3. Batrakov S *et al* (1997) *Chem. Phys. Lipids* 86(1):1. 4. Ghelardini C *et al* (1998) *Phytother. Res.* 12:S10. 5. Van Dongen P *et al* (1995) *Eur. J. Obs. Gyn. Rep. Biol.* 60(2):109. 6. Peters-Volleberg G *et al* (1996) *Food Chem. Toxicol.* 34(10):951. 7. Ergot. Ed. Kren V (1999) *Medicinal and Aromatic Plants – Industrial Profiles.* Pub: Harcourt Academic, Amsterdam, The Netherlands.

ERYNGO
ERYNGIUM MARITIMUM L.
Fam. Apiaceae

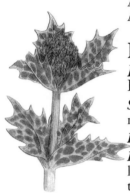

ERYNGO

SYNONYMS: Eringo, Sea Holly. Field Eryngo is *E. campestre* L. and may be substituted.

HABITAT: Sandy soils near the sea in Britain and Europe.

DESCRIPTION: A hairless perennial with leathery blue-green spiny leaves showing whitish veins and margins. The flowers are blue, in tight umbels with spiny bracts. The root is up to about 8 cm long, transversely wrinkled, dark brown and crowned with the remains of the leaf stalks. Fracture: spongy, coarsely fibrous, with a small, radiate, yellow centre. Taste: sweetish, mucilaginous; odour: faint.

PART USED: Root.

CONSTITUENTS: (i) Saponins; these are haemolytic, based on the barrigenols esterified with angelic and tiglic acids and containing arabinose, glucose and xylose (ii) Coumarins, including egelinol and its benzoate, agasyllin and grandivetin (iii) Polyphenolic acids such as rosmarinic and chlorogenic acids [R2;1,2]. *P. campestre* contains flavonol acyl glycosides [3].

MEDICINAL USE: Diuretic, anti-inflammatory, expectorant [R1]. Mostly used for urinary tract conditions such as cystitis, urethritis, polyuria and renal colic, and for prostate disorders. Anti-inflammatory activity by a hydrophilic extract has been demonstrated in an animal model [4].

PREPARATIONS AND DOSE: Powdered root, dose: 2–4 g, or equivalent extract.

SPECIFIC REFERENCES: 1. Erdelmeier C *et al* (1985) *Planta Med.* 51(5):407. 2. Gracza L *et al* (1985) *Arch. Pharm.* 312:1090. 3. Hohmann J *et al* (1997) *Planta Med.* 63(1):96. 4. Lisciani R *et al* (1984) *J. Ethnopharmacol.* 12(3):263.

ETERNAL FLOWER
HELICHRYSUM STOECHAS D.C.
Fam. Asteraceae

SYNONYMS: Goldilocks, *Gnaphalium stoechas* L., *G. citrinum* Lam., *Stoechas citrina.*

HABITAT: A garden plant in Britain and Europe.

DESCRIPTION: Flower-heads ovate, compositous, arranged in a crowded corymb; the outer florets are yellow and shiny. Taste: bitter, pungent; odour: faint.

PART USED: Tops.

CONSTITUENTS: (i) Flavonoids including the helichrysins, helipyron, gnaphaliin, and luteolin, quercetin, isoquercetin, apigenin and kaempferol glycosides (ii) Triterpenes such as ursolic acid (iii) Polyphenolic acids; caffeoyl quinic, chlorogenic, neochlorogenic and others [1,2,3,4] (iv) Volatile oil, the major components of which are nerol and neryl acetate [R19].

MEDICINAL USE: Expectorant, liver protectant, choleretic, detoxicant [R1]. The antioxidant properties have been demonstrated against enzymatically induced lipid peroxidation in microsomal fractions of rat liver [3] and anti-inflammatory effects confirmed in mice [4]. The extract was also reported to be antimicrobial [5].

SPECIFIC REFERENCES: 1. Mericli A *et al* (1992) *Fitoterapia* 63(5):475. 2. Carini M *et al* (2001) *J. Pharm. Biomed. Anal.* 24(3):517. 3. Czinner E *et al* (2001) *J. Ethnopharmacol.* 77(1):31. 4. Recio M *et al* (1991) *Planta Med.* 57(Suppl.2)A56. 5. Rios J *et al* (1990) *Planta Med.* 56(6):646.

EUCALYPTUS
EUCALYPTUS GLOBULUS LABILL.
Fam. Myrtaceae

SYNONYMS: Blue Gum, Gum Tree. Other species used for oil production include *E. polybracteata* R T Baker, and *E. smithii* R T Baker. A lemon scented Eucalyptus is obtained from *E. citriodora*, which grows in Queensland.

HABITAT: Victoria and Tasmania in Australia, cultivated in southern Europe, the Nilgiri Hills of India, and elsewhere.

DESCRIPTION: The leaves are scimitar-shaped, 10–15 cm long and about 3 cm wide, shortly stalked and rounded at the base, with numerous transparent oil glands. Taste and odour: characteristic.

PART USED: Leaves and the oil distilled from them.

CONSTITUENTS: (i) Volatile oil, the major component of which is 1, 8-cineole (= eucalyptol), with terpineol, alpha-pinene, *p*-cymene and small amounts of ledol, aromadendrene and viridoflorol; aldehydes, ketones and alcohols (ii) Tannins and polyphenols; catechin, macrocarpals H, I and J, euglobals I-VIII, tellimagrandin I, eucalalbin C; and ellagic, caffeic, ferulic, gallic and protocatechuic acids (iii) Flavonoids: eucalyptin, hyperoside, sakainol, rutin and many others [R16,R13;1,2,3,4].

MEDICINAL USE: Antiseptic, antispasmodic, expectorant, stimulant, febrifuge, insect repellent [R1]. Eucalyptus is a traditional Aboriginal remedy for coughs, colds and bronchitis. The oil is taken internally in small doses, as an ingredient of cough mixtures, sweets and pastilles, and as an inhalation; and externally in the form of a liniment, ointment or 'vapour rub' as a rubifacient, decongestant and antiseptic. The leaf extract and oil have well-defined antiseptic effects against a variety of bacteria and yeasts [6,7] and antioxidant activity has been noted [8]. The euglobals inhibit Epstein-Barr virus activation [9]. Other potential uses, including anti-diabetic and diuretic effects have been reported [R16]. The oil is insect repellent and larvicidal, and is used in pharmaceuticals for these properties, as well as an antiseptic and flavouring for dentifrices and other cosmetics. For full recent review, see [10].

PREPARATIONS AND DOSE: Eucalyptus Oil BP, dose: 0.05–0.2 ml; Menthol and Eucalyptus Inhalation BPC.

SPECIFIC REFERENCES: 1. Dethier M *et al* (1994) *J. Ess. Oil Res.* 6(5):469. 2. Manguro L *et al* (1995) *Nat. Prod. Lett.* 7(3):16. 3. Conde E *et al* (1997) *Phytochem. Anal.* 8:186. 4. Osawa K *et al* (1996) *J. Nat. Prod.* 59(9):823. 5. Santos G (1997) *Phytochem.* 44(7):1309. 6. Navarro V *et al* (1996) *J. Ethnopharmacol.* 53:143. 7. Osawa K *et al* (1998) *Natural Medicines* 52(1):33. 8. Dessi M *et al* (2001) *Phytother. Res.* 15(6):511. 9. Takasaki M *et al* (1990) *Chem. Pharm. Bull.* 38(10):2737. 10. '*Eucalyptus*'. Ed: Coppen J. (2002) *Medicinal and Aromatic Plants – Industrial Profiles.* Pub: Taylor and Francis, London, UK.

EUCALYPTUS KINO

EUCALYPTUS ROSTRATA SCHLECHT
E. CAMADULENSIS AND OTHER SPP.
Fam. Myrtaceae

SYNONYMS: Red Gum.

HABITAT: Madras and Sri Lanka.

DESCRIPTION: Dark reddish-brown, irregularly shaped pieces of gum. Taste: astringent; adheres to the teeth and colours the saliva red.

PART USED: Dried juice of the tree.

CONSTITUENTS: (i) Volatile oil, reported to contain about 70% citronellal (ii) Tannins; kinotannic acid, catechol, pyrocatechol and 'kino red' [R4].

MEDICINAL USE: Astringent and tonic [R1]. Formerly used for inflamed mucous membranes and for diarrhoea, and as a gargle or lozenge for sore throats.

EUPHORBIA

EUPHORBIA HIRTA L.
Fam. Euphorbiaceae

SYNONYMS: Snake Weed, Pill-Bearing Spurge, Asthma-Weed, *E. pilulifera* Jaquin, *E. capitata* Lam.

HABITAT: A widespread pan-tropical weed.

DESCRIPTION: Stem: slender, cylindrical, with bristly hairs and opposite leaves, which are lanceolate, about 2 cm long and 1 cm wide, toothed at the margin. Flowers: very small, in dense, round clusters in the axils of the leaves. Taste: bitter; odourless.

PART USED: Herb.

CONSTITUENTS: (i) Flavonoids; euphorbianin, leucocyanidanol, myricitrin, quercetin and others (ii) Tannins and polyphenols including the euphorbins A-E, gallic acid and derivatives (iii) Sterols including alpha amyrin, methylene cycloartenol [R16,1,2,3,4]. Toxic diterpene esters, similar to those found in Euphorbium (q.v.) were reported to be present but this work was discredited and they have been shown conclusively to be absent [4].

MEDICINAL USE: Anti-asthmatic, anti-inflammatory, anti-fungal and amoebicidal [R1]. Anti-inflammatory activity has been observed for both the triterpene fraction and the aqueous extract, which is also analgesic, antipyretic and sedative [5]. The extract is anti-diarrhoeal in mice [3] and also has anti-amoebic and spasmolytic effects [6]. Other properties including anti-mycotic, anti-fertility and galactogenic effects have been described [R16].

SPECIFIC REFERENCES: 1. Blanc P *et al* (1972) *Plantes Med. Phytother.* 6(2):106. 2. Yoshida T *et al* (1988) *Chem. Pharm. Bull.* 36(8):2940. 3. Galvez J *et al* (1993) *Planta Med.* 59(4):333. 4. Martinez V *et al* (1999) *Rev. Soc. Quim. Mex.* 43(3-4):103. 4. Evans F (1986) *Naturally Occurring Phorbol Esters.* Pub: CRC Press, USA. 5. Lanhers M *et al* (1991)) *Planta Med.* 57(3):225. 6. Tona L *et al* (2000) *Phytomed.* 7(1):31.

EUPHORBIUM

EUPHORBIA RESINIFERA BERG.
Fam. Euphorbiaceae

HABITAT: Native to North Africa.

DESCRIPTION: The plant has fleshy quadrangular stems, covered with spines and resembling a cactus. The latex is collected by incision. The milky juice exudes and hardens on exposure to the air. Tasting and inhaling inadvisable, it is acrid and highly sternutatory.

PART USED: Dried latex.

CONSTITUENTS: Diterpene esters; mainly derivatives of 12-deoxyphorbol [1].

MEDICINAL USE: Euphorbium was formerly used as a drastic purgative [R1], but it is irritant, vesicant and toxic and should not be taken in any form. The 12-deoxyphorbol esters are tumour promoting, pro-inflammatory and cause platelet aggregation [1,2]; they activate protein kinase C, and are being used to investigate various biochemical processes. For review see [3].

SPECIFIC REFERENCES: 1. Williamson E *et al* (1981) *Biochem. Pharmacol.* 30(18):2691. 2. Williamson E *et al* (1981) *Acta. Pharmacol. et Toxicol.* 4847. 3. Evans F (Ed.) In: *Naturally Occurring Phorbol Esters.* Pub: CRC Press, USA (1986).

EVENING PRIMROSE

OENOTHERA BIENNIS L.
AND OTHER OENOTHERA SPP.
Fam. Onagraceae

SYNONYMS: Tree Primrose, Sun Drop.

HABITAT: North America, especially sandy soil, and cultivated as a garden plant elsewhere.

DESCRIPTION: The plants are medium or tall hairy perennials with alternate, lanceolate leaves and large, yellow, four-petalled flowers, followed by long elongated capsules.

PART USED: Oil from the seed. The roots and leaves have also been used, much less frequently.

CONSTITUENTS: (i) The seed oil contains about 70% cis-linoleic acid and about 9% *cis*-gamma-linolenic acid (GLA).

MEDICINAL USE: The leaves were formerly used as a poultice and for a variety of 'female' disorders, but the oil is now much more important, and has been extensively investigated. The therapeutic benefits are ascribed mainly to the GLA content. The main indications for which clinical evidence exists are: atopic eczema, especially in infants, mastalgia, rheumatoid arthritis and premenstrual syndrome. Many other claims have been made, but are unsubstantiated. GLA appears to lower blood pressure and has been shown to correct some defects, including restoring the motility of red cells, in the blood of patients with multiple sclerosis. The oil is usually taken in conjunction with Vitamin E to prevent oxidation, in a similar way to Borage (q.v.). See [R7 and refs therein].

PREPARATIONS AND DOSE: Evening Primrose Oil, dose: very variable. For eczema, up to 6 g per day has been recommended; for mastalgia and premenstrual syndrome, usually 2–4 g daily.

EYEBRIGHT

EUPHRASIA OFFICINALIS L.
AND OTHER SPP.
Fam. Scrophulariaceae

HABITAT: Meadows and grassy places throughout Europe and temperate Asia.

DESCRIPTION: Up to 15 cm in height; leaves opposite near the base and alternate above, about 1 cm long and 0.5 cm broad, lanceolate, dentate. Flowers small, white, often tinged with purple or with a yellow spot, axillary, two-lipped, with four yellow stamens. Taste: saline, bitter; odourless.

PART USED: Herb.

Constituents: (i) Iridoid glycosides; aucubin, geniposide, catalpol, luproside, adoxoside, eurostoside, euphroside, ixoroside veronicoside, verproside and others (ii) Lignans including coniferyl glucosides and eukovoside (iii) Tannins and polyphenolic acids, including gallic, caffeic and ferulic acids, and flavonoids [R7,R17;1,2,3]

MEDICINAL USE: Astringent, tonic, anti-catarrhal. Used principally as a remedy in disorders of the eye such as conjunctivitis, as an eye lotion [R1]. Eye drops containing *Euphrasia* were evaluated recently in a clinical prospective cohort trial for conjunctivitis, and efficacy and tolerability deemed "good to very good" by both patients and physicians [4]. Aucubigenin is active against some bacteria, fungi and viruses [5], and has anti-tumour activity [6]; it also increases growth of neurites in cultured cell lines [7]. It is thought to be responsible for much of the activity of aucubin, to which it is hydrolysed by gut bacteria [8]. Aucubin also protects against liver damage in animals, induced by alpha-amanitin and carbon tetrachloride [9] and is anti-inflammatory in mice [10]. Anti-hyperglycaemic effects for the leaves have also been shown in experimentally diabetic rats [11].

PREPARATIONS AND DOSE: Powdered herb, dose: 2–4 g, by infusion for catarrh, or as an eye lotion.

SPECIFIC REFERENCES: 1. Luczak S *et al* (1990) *Plantes Med. Phytother.* 24:66. 2. Sticher O *et al* (1980) *Planta Med.* 39:269 and (1981) 42:122. 3. Salama O *et al* (1983) *Planta Med.* 47:90. 4. Stoss M *et al* (2000) *J. Alt. Comp. Med.* 6(6):499. 5. Chang I *et al* (1997) *Phytother. Res.* 11:189. 6. Ishiguro K *et al* (1986) *Chem. Pharm. Bull.* 34(6):2375. 7. Matsumi Y *et al* (1996) *Biol. Pharm. Bull.* 19(6):791. 8. Hattori M *et al* (1990) *Phytother. Res.* 4(2):66. 9. Chang I *et al* (1993) *Phytother. Res.* 7:53. 10. Recio M *et al* (1994) *Planta Med.* 60:232. 11. Porchezhian E *et al* (2000) *Fitoterapia* 71(5):522.

EYE BRIGHT

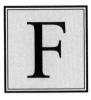

FENNEL
FOENICULUM VULGARE MILL.
Fam. Apiaceae

SYNONYMS: Sweet Fennel is the variety generally used; it is sometimes referred to as *Foeniculum vulgare* var *dulce* and Bitter Fennel as *F. vulgare* var *vulgare*.

HABITAT: Indigenous to the Mediterranean region but widely cultivated elsewhere.

DESCRIPTION: The fruit is about 1 cm long and 0.25 cm broad, oblong, cylindrical and slightly curved. Each half-fruit has four longitudinal ridges, the two lateral thicker than the two dorsal. The colour varies from greenish to brown. Taste: sweet, aromatic; odour: characteristic.

PART USED: Fruit. The herb and fresh bulb are used in cooking.

CONSTITUENTS: (i) Volatile oil, up to about 8%, consisting mainly of anethole; approximately 80% in sweet fennel and 60% in bitter fennel. Some varieties are anethole-free with up to 80% estragole, these are not suitable for normal use. The other major component of the oil is fenchone, higher in bitter than sweet fennel. Minor ingredients include limonene, anisaldehyde, alpha- and beta-pinene, alpha-phellandrene, myrcene, ocimene, alpha- and beta-terpinene and apiole, and the polymers of anethole, dianethole and photoanethole [1,2] (ii) Terpene and hemiterpene glycosides, such as the foeniculo-sides I-IX, which are hydroxycineole glucosides; zizybeoside, icavisideisopentenyl glycosides, and erythroanethole glucosides, [3,4,5,] (iii) Sugar alcohols, nucleosides and glucides [6] (iv) Flavonoids; mainly rutin, quercetin and kaempferol glycosides (v) Coumarins; bergapten, imperatorin, xanthotoxin, sessalin and marmesin [7]. The essential oil from the root contains a substantial amount of apiole and that from the aerial parts is similar in composition to the oil from the fruit.

MEDICINAL USE: Stomachic, carminative, anti-inflammatory, orexigenic [R1]. Fennel is used particularly to treat flatulence and colic in infants. The volatile oil is spasmolytic and carminative [8] and has been shown to increase liver regeneration in partially hepatectomized rats [9]. It also has useful antimicrobial and anti-fungal properties. The root has diuretic activity [10]. Fennel is anti-inflammatory in rats and also reportedly slightly oestrogenic [2]. Anethole is anti-inflammatory, acting by inhibiting TNF-mediated signalling [11]. It is a popular flavouring in drinks and foods.

PREPARATIONS AND DOSE: Dried fruits, dose: 0.3–0.6g, or equivalent extract.

SPECIFIC REFERENCES: 1. Miraldi E *et al* (1999) *Flav. Frag. J.* 14(6):379. 2. Albert-Puleo M (1980) *J. Ethnopharmacol.* 2(4):337. 3. Ono M *et al* (1996) *Chem. Pharm. Bull.* 42(2):337. 4. Kitajima J *et al* (1998) *Chem. Pharm. Bull.* 46(10):1587, 1591 and 1643. 5. Ishikawa

T *et al* (1998) *Chem. Pharm. Bull.* 46(10):1599, 160 and 346; and (1999)(11):1738 and 1748. 6. Kitajima J *et al* (1999) *Chem. Pharm. Bull.* 47(7):988. 7. El Khrisy E *et al* (1980) *Fitoterapia* 51:273. 8. Forster H *et al* (1980) *Planta Med.* 40(4):309. 9. Gershbein L *et al* (1977) *Food Cosmet. Toxicol.* 15(3):173. 10. Susplugas P *et al* (1991) *Plantes Med. Phytother.* 25(4):163. 11. Chainy G *et al* (2000) *Oncogene* 19(25):2943.

FENUGREEK

TRIGONELLA FOENUM-GRAECUM L.
Fam. Fabaceae

SYNONYMS: Foenugreek, Bird's Foot, Methi.

HABITAT: Mediterranean Europe, North Africa, India, cultivated worldwide.

DESCRIPTION: An annual aromatic herb reaching about 60 cm, with compound leaves up to 5 cm long. Seeds: brownish-yellow, 4–7 mm long, oblong or rhomboid, with a deep longitudinal furrow, encased in a pod with a narrow 'beak'. Taste and odour: savoury, aromatic and characteristic.

PART USED: Seeds, leaves.

CONSTITUENTS: (i) Volatile oil, in small quantities, containing 3-hydroxy-4,5-dimethyl-2-furanone, dihydrobenzofuran, dihydroactinidi-olide, beta-elemene, beta-selinene (ii) Alkaloids, including trigonelline, gentianine and carpaine (iii) Saponins, the trigoneosides I-VIII, trigo-foenosides A,B,C and D, fenugrin B, based on diosgenin, yuccagenin, sarsapogenin, yamogenin, gitogenin, tigogenin and others (iv) Coumarins; trigocoumarin, methyl- and thrimethyl coumarin (v) Flavonoids, including vitexin and its glycosides and esters, isovitexin, orientin, vicenins 1 and 2, quercetin and luteolin (vi) Mucilage; mostly a galactomannan [1,2,3,4,5 and refs therein].

MEDICINAL USE: Demulcent, nutritive, laxative, digestive, antipyretic and expectorant [R1]. Saponin-rich extracts of Fenugreek are anti-diabetic in animal models and reduce blood levels of cholesterol and blood lipids. Clinical studies in human diabetic patients have confirmed these findings [5,6], and fenugreek is well-tolerated. It is already widely used in cooking as an ingredient of curry powders. The aqueous extract promotes healing of gastric ulcers produced experimentally in rats, and exhibits a mild smooth muscle relaxant effect in rabbits without affecting either the heart or blood pressure, which substantiates its claim as an aid to digestion. Fenugreek extracts are anti-inflammatory in rats, and have antioxidant and antimicrobial activities [7,8,9,10].

SPECIFIC REFERENCES: 1. Girardon P *et al* (1985) *Planta Med.* 51(6):533. 2. Yoshikawa M *et al* (1998) *Heterocycles* 47(1):397. 3. Gupta R *et al* (1986) *J. Nat. Prod.* 49(6):1153. 4. Khurana S *et al* (1982) *Phytochem.* 21(8):2154. 5. Al-Habbori M *et al* (1998) *Phytother. Res.* 12(4):233. 6. Shapiro K *et al* (2002) *J. Am. Pharm. Ass.* 42(2):217.

173

7. Zia T *et al* (2001) *J. Ethnopharmacol.* 75(2–3):191. 8. Ravikumar P *et al* (1999) *Phytother. Res.* 13(3):197. 9. Sharma R *et al* (1996) *Phytother. Res.* 10:519. 10. 'Fenugreek'. Ed. Petropoulos G (2002) *Medicinal and Aromatic Plants – Industrial Profiles.* Taylor and Francis, London, UK.

FEVERBUSH

GARRYA FREMONTII TORR.
Fam. Garryaceae

SYNONYMS: Skunkbush, California Feverbush.

HABITAT: California, North and Middle America.

DESCRIPTION: Elliptical leaves up to 8 cm long, with an entire margin and apex pointed. Taste: bitter; odour: slight.

PART USED: Leaves.

CONSTITUENTS: Diterpene and norditerpene alkaloids [1].

MEDICINAL USE: Tonic, bitter, febrifuge [R1].

SPECIFIC REFERENCES: 1. Pelletier S (1992) *J. Nat. Prod.* 55(1):1.

FEVERFEW

TANACETUM PARTHENIUM (L.) SCHULTZ BIP.
Fam. Asteraceae

SYNONYMS: Featherfew, Featherfoil, Midsummer Daisy, *Chrysanthemum parthenium* (L.) Bernh., *Leucanthemum parthenium* (L.) Gren and Godron, *Pyrethrum parthenium* (L.) Sm.

HABITAT: Grows wild in many parts of Europe and the British Isles.

DESCRIPTION: A perennial herb reaching up to 60 cm, with a downy erect stem. The leaves are yellowish-green, alternate, stalked, ovate and pinnately divided with an entire or crenate margin. The flowers, which appear in June to August, are up to about 2 cm in diameter and arranged in corymbs of up to 30 heads, with white ray florets and yellow disc florets and downy involucral bracts. Taste: bitter and nauseous; odour: strongly aromatic, characteristic.

PART USED: Herb.

CONSTITUENTS: (i) Volatile oil, containing alpha-pinene and derivatives, bornyl acetate and angelate, costic acid, beta-farnesine, camphor and several spiroketal ethers (ii) Sesquiterpene lactones; the major one being parthenolide, with santamarine (= balchanin), esters of parthenolide, reynosin, artemorin and its epoxide, 3-beta-hydroxyparthenolide, 3-beta-hydroxycostunolide, 8-alpha-hydroxyestafiatin, artecanin and others, partholide and chrysantholide cranolide, chrysanthemonin, and others (iii) Acetylene derivatives, mainly in the root (iv) Melatonin has been reported in some samples [R7;1,2, and refs therein].

MEDICINAL USE: Febrifuge, analgesic, anti-rheumatic, stomachic, anthelmintic [R1]. Used formerly to treat rheumatism and menstrual

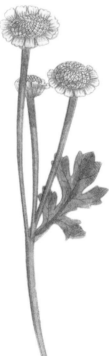

FEVERFEW

problems, however the main use now is as a prophylactic and treatment for migraine, where clinical trials have shown it to be effective. The fresh leaves may be eaten, usually with other foods to disguise the nauseous taste, to prevent migraine attacks. The active components are thought to be the sesquiterpene lactones, which inhibit prostaglandin production and arachidonic acid release, which explains the anti-platelet and anti-febrile actions to some extent. Extracts also inhibit secretion of serotonin from platelet granules and proteins from poly-morphonuclear leucocytes (PMNs). Since serotonin is implicated in the aetiology of migraine and PMN secretion is increased in rheumatoid arthritis, these findings substantiate the use of Feverfew in these conditions. The digestive effect may be due to the spiroketal ethers, which are known to be spasmolytic. Recent studies have focused on parthenolide, which is anti-inflammatory and known to inhibit the production of interleukin 12 and NF-Kappa-B [3]. It also prevents intercellular adhesion molecule-1 expression in human synovial fibroblasts [4] and inhibits phorbol ester-induced transcriptional activation of inducible nitric oxide synthase gene in a human monocyte cell line [5]. The essential oil is antimicrobial against numerous species of bacteria and fungi. Feverfew may have side effects in a few individuals; these are usually dermatitis and soreness or ulceration of the mouth, and more pleasantly, a mild tranquillizing effect. For more information see [R2,R7,R8;1,2,6,7,10,11,12 and refs therein].

PREPARATIONS AND DOSE: For migraine prophylaxis, dose: fresh leaf, 2–3 leaves per day; freeze-dried leaf, dose: 50 mg daily.

SPECIFIC REFERENCES: 1. Knight D (1995) *Nat. Prod. Rep.* 12:271. 2. Williams C *et al* (1999) *Phytochem.* 51(3):417. 3. Kang B *et al* (2001) *Immunol. Lett.* 77:159. 4. Piela-Smith T *et al* (2001) *Cell Immunol.* 209:89. 5. Fukuda K *et al* (2000) *Biochem. Pharmacol.* 60:595. 6. Deweerdt C *et al* (1996) *Phytomed.* 3:225. 7. Adad M *et al* (1995) *Phytother. Res.* 9:79. 8. Johnson E *et al* (1985) *Br. Med. J.* 291:569. 9. Heptinstall S *et al* (1986) *Lancet* i:1071. 10. Palevitch D *et al* (1997) *Phytother. Res.* 11(7):508. 11. Kalodera Z *et al* (1997) *Pharmazie* 52(11):885. 12. Pittler M *et al* (2001) Cochrane Review, *Cochrane Library* Issue 3.

FIG

FICUS CARICA L.
Fam. Moraceae

HABITAT: Cultivated in most Mediterranean countries, especially Greece, Turkey and Spain.

DESCRIPTION: The fig is a fleshy inflorescence containing the minute ovaries of the female flowers. The male flowers occupy the small orifice at the apex.

PART USED: Fleshy inflorescence or 'fruit', leaves.

CONSTITUENTS: Fruit: (i) Flavonoids; schaftoside and isoschaftoside, which are isomeric C-glycosides of apigenin [1] (ii) Miscellaneous;

175

sugars, mainly glucose, vitamins A and C with minor amounts of B and D, plant acids and enzymes including ficin. Leaf: (i) Triterpenes based on oleanolic acid and lupeol [2].

MEDICINAL USE: Nutritive, emollient, demulcent, mild laxative [R1]. The fresh and dried fruits are used in mild constipation and as food. The leaf is a traditional remedy for diabetes and hypoglycaemic effects have been confirmed in streptozocin-diabetic rats [3,4]. A clinical study of the leaf extract in patients with type I diabetes mellitus found that it helped to control post-prandial glycaemia, when taken along with a normal diabetes diet and insulin injections [5]. The leaf extract reduces triglyceride and cholesterol levels in experimentally diabetic and hyperlipidemic rats [6,7], and contains angiotensin I-converting enzyme inhibitors [8].

PREPARATIONS AND DOSE: Compound Fig Elixir BPC, dose: 2.5–10 ml.

BIBLICAL REFERENCES: Numbers 13:23 and 20:5; II Kings 20:7; Nehemiah 13:15; Song of Solomon 2:13; Isaiah 38:21; Jeremiah 24: 1–8 and 29:17; Matthew 7:16; Mark 11:13; Luke 6:44; James 3:12; Revelation 6:13. Also, at least 39 references to the tree.

SPECIFIC REFERENCES: 1. Siewek F *et al* (1980) *Z. Naturforsch.* 40(1–2):8. 2. Ahmed W *et al* (1990) *Fitoterapia* 61(4):373. 3. Perez C *et al* (1996) *Phytother. Res.* 10(1):82. 4. Perez C *et al* (2000) *Pharm. Biol.* 38(3):181. 5. Serraclara A *et al* (1998) *Diabetes Res. Clin. Prac.* 39(1):19. 6. Dominguez E *et al* (1996) *Phytother. Res.* 10(6):526. 7. Perez C *et al* (1999) *Phytother. Res.* 13(3):188. 8. Maruyama S *et al* (1989) *Agr. Biol. Chem.* 53(10):2763.

FIG, SACRED
FICUS RELIGIOSA L.
Fam. Moraceae

SYNONYMS: Peepul, Bo-tree.

HABITAT: Indigenous to India and Southeast Asia, cultivated widely, especially in the vicinity of temples.

DESCRIPTION: A large tree with a characteristic, milky, latex. The bark is greyish and covered with epiphytes, and peels off in patches. The leaves are large and ovate. The figs are small and fleshy and purplish when ripe. The tree lives to a great age.

PART USED: Fruits, bark, leaves and latex.

CONSTITUENTS: (i) Sterols, including lanosterol, campesterol, lupeol, isofucosterol and their glucosides, in the bark (ii) Coumarins; bergapten and bergaptol, in the bark (iii) Miscellaneous; tannins in the leaf, vitamin K in the bark and others [R16].

MEDICINAL USE: Used for many different purposes, the tree is of great religious significance to Buddhists and Hindus. Siddhartha is reputed to have been sitting under the tree when he received enlightenment to become the Buddha, and Hindus offer prayers beneath it whilst facing east. It forms a component of many Ayurvedic formulations.

Medicinally the main use is for diarrhoea and dysentery, and for diabetes, and these activities are supported to a limited extent by experimental results. Most of the research has been carried out in India [R16;1, and refs therein].

SPECIFIC REFERENCES: 1. Mousa O *et al* (1994) *J. Ethnopharmacol.* 41(1–2):71.

FIGWORT
SCROPHULARIA NODOSA L.
Fam. Scrophulariaceae

SYNONYMS: Rosenoble, Throatwort, Carpenter's Square, Scrofula Plant.

HABITAT: A European and British wild plant.

DESCRIPTION: The stem is quadrangular, bearing opposite, stalked leaves which are 10–12 cm long and 3–5 cm broad, rounded but unequal at the base and tapering to a point at the apex. The margin is sharply serrate and the veins depressed above and prominent beneath. Taste: bitter; odour: characteristic.

PART USED: Herb.

CONSTITUENTS: (i) Iridoids, including aucubin, harpagide, scrophuloside A4, scopolioside, scrovalentinoside, acetyl harpagide and 6-alpha-rhamnopyranosylcatalpol [1,2] (ii) Flavonoids; diosmin and hesperidin (iii) Phenolic acids; ferulic, isoferulic, p-coumaric, caffeic, vanillic and chlorogenic acids [R7].

FIGWORT

MEDICINAL USE: Vulnerary, anti-inflammatory and diuretic [R1]. Aucubin is a mild laxative and has been shown to stimulate the excretion of uric acid from the kidneys in animals. Figwort is taken as an infusion or applied as a poultice to aid wound-healing. This use which has been supported by evidence that the iridoid glycosides stimulate the growth of human dermal fibroblasts *in vitro* [2]. The iridoids of other species of *Scrophularia* have been shown to be immunostimulant and anti-hepatotoxic [3].

PREPARATIONS AND DOSE: Dried herb, dose: 2–8 g, or equivalent extract.

SPECIFIC REFERENCES: 1. Miyase T *et al* (1999) *J. Nat. Prod.* 62(8):1079. 2. Stevenson P *et al* (2002) *Phytother. Res.* 16(1):33. 3. Garg H *et al* (1994) *Phytother. Res.* 8:224.

FIRE-FLAME BUSH
WOODFORDIA FRUTICOSA KURTZ.
Fam. Lythraceae

SYNONYMS: *W. floribunda* Salisb. Shiranji Tea.

HABITAT: A common Asian shrub, widely cultivated as an ornamental.

DESCRIPTION: A leafy shrub or small tree, with fluted stems and long spreading branches. The flowers are numerous, and bright red, hence the name 'fire-flame', in dense terminal panicles.

PART USED: Flowers.

CONSTITUENTS: (i) Tannins; oenothein A and B, woodfordins A-I and others (ii) Flavones; cyanidin, pelargonidin and myricetin glucosides (iii) Chrysophanol glucopyranoside, an anthraquinone [R16;1,2,3,4].

MEDICINAL USE: The flowers are used in the form of a herbal tea, and in Ayurvedic medicine an infusion is often fermented before use. The plant is astringent and stimulant, and used particularly to treat dysentery, diarrhoea and haemorrhage. The woodfordins have anti-tumour activity *in vivo* and *in vitro,* and woodfordin C appears to be the most potent. It is an inhibitor of the enzyme topoisomerase II and inhibits intracellular DNA (but not RNA) synthesis [3,4]. Antiviral activity has been observed without cytotoxicity [5] and anti-inflammatory and antipyretic activity in rats [R16]. Immunomodulatory effects were shown in human polymorphonuclear leucocytes by a fermented preparation of the flowers [6].

SPECIFIC REFERENCES: 1. Yoshida T *et al* (1992) *Chem. Pharm. Bull.* 40(8):2023. 2. Yoshida T *et al* (1991) *Chem. Pharm. Bull.* 39(5):1157. 3. Yoshida T *et al* (1990) *Chem. Pharm. Bull.* 38(5):1211. 4. Kuramochi-Motegi A *et al* (1992) *Biochem. Pharmacol.* 44(10):1961. 5. Kusumoto I *et al* (1992) *Phytother. Res.* 6:241. 6. Kroes B *et al* (1993) *J. Ethnopharmacol.* 40(2):117.

FIVE-LEAF-GRASS
POTENTILLA REPTANS L.
Fam. Rosaceae

SYNONYMS: Cinquefoil, Fivefinger.

HABITAT: A common British wild plant.

DESCRIPTION: Slender creeping stems with five leaflets, bluntly serrate, about 3 cm long, with scattered hairs on the veins and margins. Flowers small, bright yellow, five-petalled with numerous stamens. Taste: astringent; odourless.

PART USED: Herb, root.

CONSTITUENTS: Tannins and flavonoids based on quercetin [R2].

MEDICINAL USE: Astringent, febrifuge [R1]. The herb has been taken as an infusion for diarrhoea and externally as an astringent lotion. Other species of *Potentilla* such as 'Silverweed' and 'Tormentil' (q.v.) are used more frequently.

FLAX
LINUM USITATISSIMUM L.
AND OTHER SPECIES.
Fam. Linaceae

SYNONYMS: Linseed.

HABITAT: Cultivated in many temperate and tropical countries.

DESCRIPTION: The seeds are brown, oval, pointed at one end, polished and about 0.5 cm long although this varies. Taste: mucilaginous, slightly unpleasant; odour: faint.

PART USED: Seeds and the oil expressed from the seed. The pericyclic fibres from the stem are used to prepare flax fibre (linen), and the oil to produce resins and other chemicals.

CONSTITUENTS: (i) Fixed oil, consisting mainly of glycerides of linoleic and linolenic acids (ii) Lignans, the most important being secoisolariciresinol and its diglucoside (SECO and SDG) (iii) Mucilage, about 6% (iv) Linamarin and lotaustralin, cyanogenetic glucosides [1,2,3,4 and refs therein].

MEDICINAL USE: Demulcent, emollient, laxative, pectoral [R1]. It has been used in bronchitis and coughs, and for internal laxative and demulcent use. Externally it may be used as poultice for burns, scalds and boils etc. The lignans are being investigated for anti-cancer effects, as a result of the metabolic conversion of SECO and SDG to the mammalian lignans enterolactone and enterodiol. These compounds are thought to affect the human female hormone cycle and are present in much lower amounts than usual in patients with breast cancer. Experimental results in animals support the hypothesis. Exposure of female rats during early life to SDG improves bone density of the femur; this only occurs when endogenous oestrogen levels are low and does not persist into adulthood. No negative effects on bone strength were observed [5]. A recent double blind, placebo-controlled, randomized study in post-menopausal women given three months' supplementation with 40 g/day flaxseed resulted in lower serum cholesterol levels, but had no effect of markers of bone metabolism [6]. Flaxseed in men has been suggested as having beneficial effects on the progression of prostate cancer following a pilot study in 25 men [7]. For further details, see review references [1,2,3,4 and refs therein].

SPECIFIC REFERENCES: 1. Haggerty W (1999) *HerbalGram* 45:51. 2. Boik J In: *Natural Compounds in Cancer Therapy.* Oregon Medical Press, pp. 282–284 (2001). 3. Ayres D *et al* In: *Lignans: Chemical, Biological and Clinical Properties.* Cambridge University Press, UK, (1990). 4. MacRae W *et al* (1984) *Phytochem.* 23:1207. 5. Eard W *et al* (2001) *Br. J. Nutr.* 86(4):499. 6. Lucas E *et al* (2002) *Clin. Endocrinol. Metab.* 87(4):1527. 7. Demark-Wahnefried W *et al* (2001) *Urology* 58:47.

FLEABANE

ERIGERON CANADENSE L.
Fam. Asteraceae

SYNONYMS: Canada Fleabane, Coltstail, Prideweed.

HABITAT: Europe and North America.

179

DESCRIPTION: Stem unbranched, lower leaves oblanceolate and short stalked, with five teeth, the upper leaves becoming linear with an entire margin, 2.5–5 cm long. Flower-heads numerous, bell-shaped, about 0.5 cm long and broad, whitish. Taste: astringent, aromatic and bitter; odour: slight.

PART USED: Herb, seeds.

CONSTITUENTS: (i) Volatile oil, containing *d*-limonene, terpineol, linalool, germacrene D, nerolidol, beta-caryophyllene, alpha-humulene and dipentene (ii) Flavonoids, including apigenin, luteolin and quercetin (iii) Terpenes such as spinasterol and beta-sitosterol (iv) Plant acids; vanillic, caffeic, succinic [1,2].

MEDICINAL USE: Astringent, diuretic, tonic [R1]. Formerly used for diarrhoea and kidney disorders, often as an infusion. An aqueous extract has a transient hypotensive effect in rats [3].

SPECIFIC REFERENCES: 1. Jirovetz L *et al* (1999) *Scientia Pharmaceutica* 67(1):89. 2. Grancia D *et al* (1985) *Cesk. Pharm.* 34(6):209. 3. Lassere B *et al* (1983) *Naturwissensch.* 70:95.

FLUELLEN
KICKXIA ELATINE (L.) DUM.
K. SPURIA (L.) DUM.
Fam. Scrophulariaceae

SYNONYMS: Fluellin. Sharp-leaved Fluellen is *K. elatine* (= *Linaria elatine* L.) Mill., Round-leaved Fluellen is *K. spuria* (= *Linaria spuria* L.) Mill.

HABITAT: A British and European wild plant.

DESCRIPTION: A partly recumbent, much branched annual. Leaves greyish-green, round or oval and, in *K. elatine*, somewhat pointed. Flowers yellow, two-lipped, the lower lip is three-lobed and the upper two-lobed.

PART USED: Herb.

CONSTITUENTS: *K. spuria* contains the flavonoids salvigenin and sinensetin [1].

MEDICINAL USE: Astringent [R1]. Taken as a tea, or applied externally, for nasal and other bleeding.

SPECIFIC REFERENCES: 1. Toth L *et al* (1980) *Pharmazie* 35:334.

FOOL'S PARSLEY
AETHUSA CYNAPIUM L.
Fam. Apiaceae

SYNONYMS: Dog Parsley, Dog Poison.

HABITAT: A British and European wild plant.

DESCRIPTION: Resembles parsley somewhat, may be distinguished by the three long slender bracts hanging from the base of the flowers.

PART USED: Herb.

CONSTITUENTS: (i) Polyines; aethusin, aethusanol A and B and cicutoxin [1] (ii) Alkaloids such as cynapine, with traces of coniine (iii) Volatile oil [R4;1].

MEDICINAL USE: Formerly used as a sedative and stomachic (in small doses) [R1]. Its use is not advisable as it is very poisonous and has been mistaken for parsley, with unfortunate results.

SPECIFIC REFERENCES: 1. Tuescher E *et al* (1990) *Pharmazie* 45(7):537.

FOXGLOVE
DIGITALIS PURPUREA L.
Fam. Scrophulariaceae

SYNONYMS: Purple Foxglove. The Woolly Foxglove, *D. lanata* L., and other species are also used.

HABITAT: British Isles and Europe.

DESCRIPTION: Leaves ovate, about 10–30 cm long and up to 10 cm wide, with a sub-acute apex and a crenate margin; petiolate with a decurrent base. The veins are prominent on the undersurface and depressed on the upper surface, anastomozing near the margin. Taste: very bitter; odour: faint.

PART USED: Leaves.

CONSTITUENTS: (i) Cardenolides; glycosides based on digitoxigenin, gitoxigenin and gitaloxigenin. There are many, but the most important ones are digitoxin and gitoxin. *D. lanata* contains related glycosides, including digoxin and lanatosides. It is the main source of digoxin for the pharmaceutical industry (ii) Anthraquinones such as alizarin derivatives and others, in both species (iii) Miscellaneous; flavonoids and saponins [R3,R14].

MEDICINAL USE: Cardiac tonic [R1]. Digitalis glycosides increase the force of contraction of the heart without increasing the oxygen consumption, and slow the heart rate when auricular fibrillation is present. They are used to treat congestive heart failure. Digitalis leaf, even in the standardized form, is rarely used due to the potency and different onset of action of the individual glycosides. These are only used under close medical supervision. Digoxin is usually the glycoside of choice since it is the least cumulative and most rapidly excreted, and it is very widely prescribed. Due to their cumulative effect the glycosides can easily give rise to toxic symptoms; these include nausea, vomiting and anorexia [R3,R14].

FOXGLOVE

PREPARATIONS AND DOSE: Digoxin BP, dose: 0.0625–0.25 mg daily.

FRANGULA
FRANGULA ALNUS MILL.
Fam. Rhamnaceae

SYNONYMS: Alder Buckthorn, *Rhamnus catharticus* L.

HABITAT: Europe and North America.

DESCRIPTION: A small, thornless tree, with broadly elliptical, smooth leaves. The bark occurs as thin, quilled pieces, greenish-black externally with numerous elongated white lenticels. There is a crimson layer just beneath the surface, which is visible when abraded. Fracture: fibrous; taste: sweetish at first, then bitter; odourless.

PART USED: Bark.

CONSTITUENTS: (i) Anthraquinone derivatives, including frangulosides (= frangulins) A and C, glucofrangulinanthrones A and B, glucofranguloside A and its diacetate, glucofranguloside B, palmidin C and others (ii) Naphthoquinones (iii) Traces of peptide alkaloids including frangularine [R2,R3,R7,R8,R9;1,2,3,4].

MEDICINAL USE: Stimulant laxative [R1], often incorporated in preparations with a bulk laxative such as Sterculia or Ispaghula (q.v.). The bark is dried and seasoned for two years before use to avoid the violent griping pains, sickness and nausea induced by the fresh bark [R3].

PREPARATIONS AND DOSE: Dried bark, dose: 0.5–2.5g, or equivalent extract.

SPECIFIC REFERENCES: 1.Wagner H *et al* (1978) *Planta Med.* 33:244. 2. Van Os F (1976) *Pharmacol.* 14(S1):18. 3. Helmholz H *et al* (1993) *Pharm. Zeit.* 138:3478. 4. Rauwald H *et al* (1990) *Planta Med.* 56(6):563.

FRINGETREE
CHIONANTHUS VIRGINICUS L.
Fam. Oleaceae

SYNONYMS: Old Man's Beard, Snowdrop Tree.

HABITAT: Southern parts of North America.

DESCRIPTION: The root bark occurs in irregular, quilled pieces up to about 8 cm long and about 3 mm thick, externally dull brown with concave scars. The inner surface is quite smooth and buff-coloured. Fracture short, dense, showing projecting bundles of stone cells.

PART USED: Rootbark.

CONSTITUENTS: Largely unknown. Chionanthin, and phillyrin, which are reputed to be haemolytic saponin glycosides, have been reported [R2].

MEDICINAL USE: Alterative, hepatic, cholagogue, diuretic, tonic [R1]. Fringetree is thought to be of particular use in liver disorders, jaundice and for gallstones.

FROSTWORT
HELIANTHEMUM CANADENSE MICHX.
Fam. Cistaceae

SYNONYMS: Rock Rose, Frostweed, *Cistus canadense* L.

HABITAT: Europe and North America.

DESCRIPTION: Twigs slender, purplish-green, with opposite leaf scars. Leaves linear, up to 1.5 cm long, greyish-green, downy. Flowers apetalous in small clusters. Taste: astringent and bitter; odourless.

PART USED: Herb.

CONSTITUENTS: (i) Tannins, about 10% (ii) Helianthinin, a glycoside [R4].

MEDICINAL USE: Astringent, alterative, tonic. It may be taken internally as an infusion or applied externally as a wash for ulcers etc.

FUMITORY
FUMARIA OFFICINALIS L.
Fam. Fumariaceae

SYNONYMS: Common Fumitory, Earthsmoke. Indian Fumitory is *F. indica* Pugsley (= *F. parviflora* Lank.)

HABITAT: Common in Europe and the British Isles, especially in cultivated fields, flowering throughout the summer. Indian fumitory is found widely in Asia and also in Europe.

DESCRIPTION: Leaves pinnate, glabrous. Flowers slender, tubular, two-lipped, pink with darker tips, in short spikes. Fruit, globular, containing one seed. Taste: bitter and saline; odour: faint. Indian fumitory is much larger, with paler flowers.

PART USED: Herb.

CONSTITUENTS: (i) Isoquinoline alkaloids, including bulbocapnine, canadine, coptisine, corydaline, dicentrine, cryptopine, fumaricine, fumariline, fumaritine, N-methylhydrastine, protopine, sanguinarine, sinactine and others (ii) Hydroxycinnamic acid derivatives [R2,R7,R9;1,2,3,4]. *F. indica* contains similar alkaloids, as well as fumariflorine, bicuculline, hydrastine, aldumine, parfumidine, parfumine and others [R16 and refs therein].

FUMITORY

MEDICINAL USE: Tonic, mild diuretic and laxative, anti-inflammatory [R1]. Used mainly in stomach disorders, liver complaints and skin infections. Culpeper wrote, "The juice of the Fumitory and Docks mingled with vinegar and the places gently washed therewith, cures all sorts of scabs, pimples, blotches, wheals and pushes which arise on the face or hands and any other part of the body." The herb is spasmolytic to the bile duct and gastrointestinal tract [1,5], and at least some of these actions are due to the presence of sanguinarine, which is antiseptic. Fumariline is anticonvulsant [6] and analgesic, and extracts of *F. indica* have been shown to be hepatoprotective [7]. For further details see [R2,R7,R9, R16 and refs therein].

PREPARATIONS AND DOSE: Dried herb, dose: 2–4 g, or equivalent extract, three times daily.

SPECIFIC REFERENCES: 1. Duke J (1985) *Ztg. Allg. Med.* 34:1819. 2. Hahn R *et al* (1993) *Planta Med.* 3. Mardirossian Z *et al* (1983) *Phytochem.* 22:759. 4. Sousek J *et al* (1999) *Phytochem. Anal.* 10(1):6. 5. Hentschel C *et al* (1995) *Fortschr. Med.* 113(19):291. 6. Rao K *et al* (1998) *J. Ethnopharmacol.* 60(3):207. 7. Kumar A *et al* (1986) *Planta Med.* 4:324.

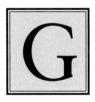

GALANGAL
ALPINIA OFFICINARUM HANCE
Fam. Zingiberaceae

SYNONYMS: Galanga, East India Root, Lesser Galangal. Greater Galangal is A. *galanga* Willd.

HABITAT: Southeast Asia, cultivated in India.

DESCRIPTION: The rhizome is dark reddish-brown, cylindrical, about 1–2 cm diameter and 3–6 cm long, marked at short intervals with raised rings, which are the scars of the leaf bases. Fracture hard and tough, showing a paler inside with a darker central column. Taste: pungent and spicy; odour: aromatic, rather like ginger. Greater Galangal is larger and paler, and less pungent.

PART USED: Rhizome.

CONSTITUENTS: (i) Volatile oil, containing a number of diaryl heptanoids including galangol, gingerols, and alpha-pinene, cineole, linalool and other mono- and sesquiterpenes (ii) Flavonoids including galangin and its 3-methyl ether (iii) Curcuminoids such as hexahydrocurcumin [R2;1,2]. Greater galangal, A. *galanga*, contains (i) Volatile oil, with hydroxychavicol, 1'-acetoxychavicol, cinnamyl alcohol, 1'-acetoxyeugenol and their acetates (ii) Diterpenes of the labdane type (iii) Flavonoids including galangin [R2;3,4].

MEDICINAL USE: Carminative, stimulant, anti-inflammatory [R1]. It is used mainly for dyspepsia and in the Middle East for rheumatism and arthritis. Extracts are anti-inflammatory in animals, and inhibit prostaglandin synthesis [2]. Antioxidant activity has been described [5] and larvicidal activity against *Toxocara canis* reported [6]. A. *galanga* has anti-ulcer activity in animals [7] and anti-fungal effects have been observed for the diterpenes and acetoxychavicol acetate [4]. Anti-tumour effects have been seen *in vitro* [3]. Antibacterial effects have been ascribed to the flavonoids [8]. No toxic effects were observed in mice although, over a 90-day period, A. *galangal* caused an increase in sperm counts and motility, and an increased red-blood-cell count [9].

PREPARATIONS AND DOSE: Powdered rhizome (root), dose: 1–2 g.

SPECIFIC REFERENCES: 1. Itokawa H *et al* (1985) *Chem. Pharm. Bull.* 33(11):4889. 2. Kiuchi F *et al* (1982) *Chem. Pharm. Bull.* 30(6):2279. 3. Itokawa H *et al* (1987) *Planta Med.* 53(1):32. 4. Haraguchi H *et al* (1996) *Planta Med.* 62(4):308. 5. Kim B *et al* (1997) *Int. J. Cosmet. Sci.* 19(6):299. 6. Kiuchi F *et al* (1989) *Jap. J. Pharmacog.* 43(4):353. 7. Al-Yahya M *et al* (1990) *Phytother. Res.* 4(3):112. 8. Chit K *et al* (2001) *Pharm. Biol.* 39(3):181. 9. Qureshi S *et al* (1992) *Planta Medica* 58(2):124.

GALBANUM

FERULA GUMMOSA BOISS.
AND OTHER SPECIES.
Fam. Apiaceae

SYNONYMS: F. galbaniflua Boiss. et Buhse.

HABITAT: Middle East and the Levant.

DESCRIPTION: The gum-resin occurs in translucent, yellowish- or bluish-green masses of tears. Soft Galbanum (Levant) is more viscous and may contain small pieces of root; Hard Galbanum (Persian) is friable and may contain pieces of stem. Odour: rather like musk or turpentine.

PART USED: Gum-resin.

CONSTITUENTS: (i) Volatile oil, up to 30%, the highest being in the soft variety, containing mono- and sequiterpenes, alcohols and acetates including alpha- and beta-pinene, carene, limonene, terpinolene, linalool, terpineol, borneol, myrcene, cadinene, guaiol, galbanol, 10-epijunenol and others; azulenes such as guiazulene (ii) Thiol esters such as *S*-isopropyl-3-methylbutanethioate and *S*-sec-butyl-3-methylbutanethioate (iii) Undecatrienes including *n*-1,3,5-undecatriene (iv) The coumarin umbelliferone (v) Resinic acids, 30–40% [1,2,3,4].

MEDICINAL USE: Carminative, stimulant, expectorant, vulnerary [R1]. It may be taken internally or applied as an ointment or ingredient of plasters. Recently it has been shown to alleviate morphine withdrawal syndrome, induced by naloxone, in mice [5] and exhibit spamolytic effects on isolated rat ileum [6].

BIBLICAL REFERENCES: Exodus 30:34, an ingredient of incense.

SPECIFIC REFERENCES: 1. Wichtl M (1974) *Planta Med.* 11:53. 2. Thomas A *et al* (1976) *Tetrahedron* 32:2261. 3. Burrell J *et al* (1976) *Tet. Lett.* 30:2837. 4. Jessenne M *et al* (1974) *Plantes Med. Phytother.* 8:241. 5. Ramezani M *et al* (2001) *J. Ethnopharmacol.* 77(1):71. 6. Sadraei H *et al* (2001) *Phytomed.* 8(5):370.

GALE, SWEET

MYRICA GALE L.
Fam. Myricaceae

SYNONYMS: Bog Myrtle, Dutch Myrtle.

HABITAT: Native to Britain, Scandinavia, France, Portugal, North America and parts of Russia.

DESCRIPTION: Leaves leathery, lanceolate-obovate, about 2–3 cm long and 1 cm wide, with small resinous glands. Taste: astringent; odour: aromatic, recalling that of bay leaves.

PART USED: Shrub.

CONSTITUENTS: (i) Essential oil, containing cineole, germacrone,

185

myrcene, nerolidol, cineole, limonene, dipentene and others (ii) Dihydrochalcones; 2'-hydroxy-4,6'-dimethoxy-3'-methyldihydrochalcone, myrigalone A and B, and others (iii) Myricitrin and other flavonoids (iv) Esters of fatty acids [R2,R4;1,2].

MEDICINAL USE: Aromatic, astringent [R1]. The methylated dihydrochalcones are bacteriostatic and fungistatic *in vitro* [1] and are free radical scavengers and antioxidants in various *in vitro* systems [2,3]. Myrigalone B inhibits low-density lipoprotein oxidation in cholesterol-fed rabbits [4].

SPECIFIC REFERENCES: 1. Malterud K *et al* (1982) *Acta Pharm. Sueca* 19:43. 2. Malterud K *et al* (1996) *Pharmacol. Toxicol.* 78(2):111. 3. Mathieson L *et al* (1995) *Planta Med.* (61(6):515. 4. Mathieson L *et al* (1996) *Pharmacol. Toxicol.* 78(3):143.

GALLS
QUERCUS INFECTORIA OLIVIER.
Fam. Fagaceae

SYNONYMS: Nutgalls, Blue Galls, Oak Galls, *Gallae ceruleae.*

HABITAT: Mediterranean countries, the Middle and Far East.

DESCRIPTION: Galls are formed as a result of the bark being punctured by an insect for laying eggs, after which an excrescence grows. The plant itself is of the oak family but rarely grows to more than a shrub. Taste: very astringent and slightly acid, then sweetish; odourless.

PART USED: Gall.

CONSTITUENTS: 'Tannic acid', or gallotannic acid (60–70%), which a complex mixture of glycosides of phenolic acids, mainly gallic acid polymers. Varies widely in composition but is generally regarded as a pentadigalloylglucose polymer [R19].

MEDICINAL USE: Astringent [R1]. Formerly used for diarrhoea and dysentery but may have cytotoxic effects as well as its antiviral, antimicrobial and other properties. These are probably due to the ability of tannins to precipitate proteins. Antibacterial activity has been described for the ethanol extract [1]. A more recent use of tannic acid is for the removal of tattoos, although it is caustic and may cause burning [2,3].

BIBLICAL REFERENCES: The biblical word refers to a bitter herb, Matthew 27:34; Acts 8:23.

SPECIFIC REFERENCES: 1. Nimri L *et al* (1999) *Pharm. Biol.* 37(3):196. 2. Mercer N *et al* (1991) *Br. Med. J.* 303:380. 3. Scott M *et al* (1991) *Br. Med. J.* 303:720.

GAMBOGE

GARCINIA HANBURYI HOOK, F.
G. CAMBOGIA (GAERTN) DESR.
AND OTHER SPECIES
Fam. Guttiferae

SYNONYMS: Camboge, Gutta Cambodia, Gutta Gamba.

HABITAT: Southeast Asia.

DESCRIPTION: Usually in the form of cylindrical sticks, deep orange brown and opaque. The transverse fracture should be smooth and conchoidal. Taste: very acrid; the powder is strongly sternutatory.

PART USED: Gum-resin.

CONSTITUENTS: (i) Resins, 70–75%, consisting mainly of alpha- and beta-garcinolic acids, with gambogic and neo-gambogic acids [1] (ii) Flavonoids, catechins, benzophenones and hydroxycitric acid have been reported in *G. cambogia* [2,3].

MEDICINAL USE: Laxative, usually in combination with other agents [R1]. More research has been carried out on *G. cambogia*, which is thought to be less purgative and is normally used as an anti-obesity agent and to lower blood cholesterol and lipid levels. These effects have been confirmed in rats fed with a flavonoid extract of *G. cambogia* and a high-fat diet [4]. The fruit extract prevents undesirable changes in lipid profiles in rabbits induced by dexamethasone [5], and reduces peroxidative damage by ethanol in the rat [6]. It is thought to act by inhibiting lipid droplet accumulation in fat cells, without affecting adipose conversion, since glycerophosphate dehydrogenase enzyme was not inhibited by the extract [7]. It has also been suggested as an aid to weight loss because of the content of hydroxycitric acid, which inhibits lipogenesis in the liver [3], and a small clinical study of 20 patients has supported this use [8]. Anti-ulcer activity has recently been reported for *G. cambogia* [9].

SPECIFIC REFERENCES: 1. Liu G *et al* (1984) *Yao Hsueh Pao* 19(8):636. 2. Waterman P *et al* (1983) *Biochem. System. Ecol.* 11:21. 3. Vasselli J *et al* (1998) *FASEB J.* 12:A505. 4. Koshy A *et al* (2001) *Phytother. Res.* 15(5):395. 5. Mahendran P *et al* (2001) *Indian J. Physiol. Pharmacol.* 45(3):345. 6. Mahendran P *et al* (2001) *Indian J. Pharmacol.* 33(2):87. 7. Hasegawa N (2001) *Phytother. Res.* 15(2):172. 8. Ramos R *et al* (1996) *Investigacion Medica Internacional* 22(3):97. 9. Mahendran P *et al* (2002) *Phytother. Res.* 16(1):81.

GARLIC

ALLIUM SATIVUM L.
Fam. Alliaceae

HABITAT: Cultivated worldwide.

DESCRIPTION: The bulb is well-known, creamy-white, composed of a number of small bulbs or 'cloves' covered with membranous bracts.

187

PART USED: Bulb.

CONSTITUENTS: (i) Sulphur compounds, including allicin (= S-allyl-2-propenthiosulphinate), allylmethyltrisulphide, diallyldisulphide, diallyl-trisulphide, diallyltetrasulphide, allylpropyldisulphide, ajoene (= 4,5,9-trithiododeca-1,6,11-triene 9-oxide), 2-vinyl-4*H*-1,3-dithiin, mercaptan, alliin (which breaks down enzymatically to allicin) and others (ii) Glycosides including sativoside B1 (iii) Monoterpenoids; citral, geraniol, linalool and alpha- and beta-phellandrene (iv) Sulphur-containing peptides such as glutamyl S-methyl cysteine, glutamyl S-methyl cysteine sulphoxide and many more (v) Miscellaneous; enzymes including allinase, vitamins of the B group, minerals, flavonoids based on kaempferol and quercetin etc. [R7,R8,R16, R17;1,2,3].

MEDICINAL USE: Antibiotic, expectorant, hypotensive, antithrombotic, anti-diabetic [R1]. Used most frequently at present for respiratory infections such as colds, flu and bronchitis, for nasal and throat catarrh, and for its cardiovascular protection from blood-clotting, atherosclerosis and related conditions. It is very often taken as a prophylactic. Different types of garlic preparations are available, such as standardized allicin-rich powders, aged garlic extracts (AGE) and capsules containing the oil. All have different individual compositions but it is generally recognized that the sulphur-containing compounds must be present for any type of therapeutic effect. The allyl sulphides have antibacterial, antiviral and even more potent anti-fungal activity, which has also been demonstrated *in vitro* to be synergistic with amphotericin B. Hypolipidaemic activity has been observed in animals treated with cool-dried garlic powder, and S-allyl cysteine (SAC) is regarded as important in this activity. SAC inhibits NF-kappa-B synthesis and low-density lipoprotein (LDL) oxidation, which are implicated in atherosclerosis. Allicin is also antioxidant and garlic extracts protect endothelial cells from oxidized-LDL damage. Cardiovascular benefits are supported by the antithrombotic activity, which has been shown in several studies, and an anti-platelet effect demonstrated by AGE in humans. It is known that ajoene is a potent antithrombotic agent, as well as 2-vinyl-4*H*-1,3-dithiin to a lesser extent. Immunomodulatory activity has been described and also chemopreventative activity against carcinogenesis in various experimental models. Diallyl sulphide is thought to inhibit carcinogen activation via cytochrome-P450 (CYP) mediated oxidative metabolism. Epidemiological evidence suggests that a diet rich in garlic reduces the incidence of cancer, and laboratory studies point to a general mechanism of action involving CYP enzymes and antimutagenesis by enhancing glutathione transferase and related enzymes. Hepatoprotection against paracetamol (acetaminophen)-induced liver damage has been described and attributed to similar mechanisms. Allicin and allylpropyldisulphide are hypoglycaemic in humans and animals; however garlic also contains hyperglycaemic compounds, which may account for the discrepancies in some early publications. Other properties of garlic described include antihypertensive, diuretic and anti-aging (*in vitro*, in human fibroblast cells), and even enhancement of spermatogenesis in mice. There is a huge amount of information available, of highly variable scientific quality, but overall the evidence for the health benefits of taking garlic is extremely good. For more information see [R7,R8,R11,R16,R17; 4,5,6,7,8,9,10,11 and refs therein].

PREPARATIONS AND DOSE: Dried bulb, dose: 2–4 g, or equivalent extract; oil, dose: up to 12 mg.

BIBLICAL REFERENCES: Numbers 11:5.

SPECIFIC REFERENCES: 1. Sendi A (1995) *Phytomed.* 4:323. 2. Block E *et al* (1992) *Angew. Chem.* 31:1135. 3. Matsura H *et al* (1989) *Chem. Pharm. Bull.* 37(10):2741. 4. Avato P *et al* (2000) *Phytomed.* 7(3):239. 5. Hughes B *et al* (1991) *Phytother. Res.* 5:154. 6. Shen J *et al* (1996) *Planta Med.* 62:415. 7. Ho S P *et al* (2001) *Phytomed.* 8(3):39. 8. Steiner M *et al* (2001) *J. Nutr.* 131:980S. 9. Kyo E *et al* (2001) *J. Nutr.* 131:1075S. 10. Jeong H *et al* (1998) *Cancer Lett.* 134(1):73. 11. Balasenthil S *et al* (2001) *Fitoterapia* 72(5):524. 12. Guyonnet D *et al* (2001) *Mutat. Res.* 495(1-2):135.

GELSEMIUM

GELSEMIUM SEMPERVIRENS (L.) JAUME ST. HIL.
Fam. Loganiaceae

SYNONYMS: Yellow Jasmine, Wild Jasmine, Yellow Jessamine, Wild Jessamine, Wild Woodbine, *Bignonia sempervirens* L., *Gelsemium nitidum* Michx.

HABITAT: Southern North America, cultivated elsewhere as an ornamental.

DESCRIPTION: The root is twisted, brown and smooth, with a thin bark and woody centre showing broad medullary rays. The rhizome is less tortuous and is distinguished by the distinct pith and purplish longitudinal lines on the bark. The fracture is short and woody, showing a few silky fibres in the bark. Taste: slightly bitter; odour: faintly aromatic. The plant should not be confused with the yellow flowering jasmine.

PART USED: Root, rhizome.

CONSTITUENTS: (i) Indole alkaloids, consisting mainly of gelsemine, with gelsedine, gelsemicine, gelsemidine, gelsevirine and others (ii) Iridoids; gelsemide and its 7-glucoside, gelsemiol and its 1- and 3-glucosides, 9-hydroxy-semperoside, semperoside and brasoside (iii) Coumarins such as fabiatin and scopoletin (= 'gelsemic acid') [1,2].

MEDICINAL USE: Sedative, diaphoretic, antispasmodic and febrifuge [R1]. It was formerly used in small doses for neuralgia, nervous excitement, insomnia, inflammation of the bowels and diarrhoea. The alkaloids are CNS depressants and Gelsemium must be used with caution. Toxic effects include respiratory depression, giddiness, double vision and even convulsions, and it has been known to be fatal. Low doses of the extract have been shown to have neurotropic and protective effects against experimentally induced stress in mice [3].

189

SPECIFIC REFERENCES: 1. Wenkert E *et al* (1971) *Experientia* 28:377. 2. Jensen S *et al* (1987) *Phytochem.* 26(6):1725. 3. Bousta D *et al* (2001) *J. Ethnopharmacol* 74(3):205.

GENTIAN
GENTIANA LUTEA L.
Fam. Gentianaceae

SYNONYMS: Yellow Gentian.

HABITAT: Mountainous parts of Europe.

DESCRIPTION: Occurs in commerce as cylindrical pieces, 2–4 cm in diameter, yellowish-brown or brown externally. The upper part, or rhizome, often bears encircling leaf scars and the lower part is longitudinally wrinkled. Fracture: short and hard, showing a transverse surface, which is orange-brown with a dark ring of cambium. Taste: initially sweet and then bitter; odour: characteristic.

PART USED: Root and Rhizome.

CONSTITUENTS: (i) Iridoids, including amarogentin, gentiopicroside (= gentiopicrin) and swertiamarin (ii) Xanthones such as gentisein, gentisin (gentianin), isogentisin, 1,3,7-trimethoxyxanthone and others (iii) Alkaloids; mainly gentianine and gentialutine (iv) Phenolic acids including gentisic, caffeic, protocatechuic, syringic and sinapic acids [R7,R8;1,2].

MEDICINAL USE: Bitter, tonic. The most popular of the herbal gastric stimulants and widely used to improve the digestion, stimulate the appetite and treat all types of gastrointestinal disorders including dyspepsia, gastritis, heartburn, nausea and diarrhoea [R1]. Extracts stimulate gastric secretion in cultured rat gastric mucosal cells [3]. Gentiopicroside has been shown to suppress chemically and immunologically-induced liver damage in mice [4]. Gentisin and isogentisin are mutagenic in the Ames test [5] and have anti-tubercular activity against *Mycobacterium bovis* [6]. Gentian extracts are choleretic in rats [7] and preliminary studies have shown that Gentian extracts have adaptogenic and mild analgesic activity in mice [8].

PREPARATIONS AND DOSE: Powdered root, dose: 0.5–2 g; Alkaline Gentian Mixture BPC, dose: 10–20 ml; Acid Gentian Mixture BPC, dose: 10–20 ml.

SPECIFIC REFERENCES: 1. Verotta L (1985) *Fitoterapia* 56:25. 2. Menkovic N *et al* (2000) *Planta Med.* 66(2):178. 3. Gebhardt R (1997) *Pharm. Pharmacol. Lett.* 7(2–3):106. 4. Kondo Y *et al* (1994) *Planta Med.* 60(5):414. 5. Morimoto I *et al* (1983) *Mutat. Res.* 116:103. 6. Menkovic N *et al* (1999) *Pharm. Pharmacol. Lett.* 9(2):74. 7. Ozturk N *et al* (1998) *Phytomed.* 5:283. 8. Ozturk N *et al* (2002) *Phytother. Res.* 16 (7):627.

GERMANDER
TEUCRIUM CHAMAEDRYS L.
Fam. Lamiaceae

SYNONYMS: Wall Germander.

HABITAT: A common European wild plant, rare in Britain.

DESCRIPTION: Leaves dark green, shiny, rather leathery, up to 3 cm long and 1 cm broad, oval, pointed, with rounded teeth. Flowers purplish-red, two-lipped, with the upper lip deeply bifid, and projecting stamens. Taste: bitter; odourless.

PART USED: Herb.

CONSTITUENTS: (i) Iridoid glycosides, including harpagide and acetyl harpagide (ii) Clerodane and neoclerodane diterpenes; the teucrins A-G, teucvin, teucvidin, teuflin, teugin and acetylteugin, teuflidin, isoteuflidin and marrubiin (iii) Phenylpropanoids such as teucroside [602] (iv) Volatile oil, containing mainly beta-caryophyllene with humulene [R2,R7;1,2,3].

MEDICINAL USE: Gastric stimulant, tonic, diuretic, diaphoretic and anti-rheumatic [R1]. It is used to stimulate bile secretion and to treat gout, and also used topically as an antiseptic and vulnerary. Recent studies have shown that high doses are hepatotoxic and attributed to the teucrin A at least in part [4,5,6].

PREPARATIONS AND DOSE: Dried herb, dose: 2–4 g, or equivalent extract, three times daily.

SPECIFIC REFERENCES: 1. Rodriguez M *et al* (1984) *Phytochem.* 23:1467 and 2960. 2. Sticher O *et al* (1982) *Planta Med.* 30:124. 3. Savona M *et al* (1982) *Phytochem.* 21:721. 4. Kouzi A *et al* (1994) *Chem. Res. Toxicol.* 7(6):850. 5. De Smet P (1992) *Pharm. Weekblad* 127(26):646. 6. Perez A *et al* (2001) *Gastroenterologia y Hepatologia* 24(5):240.

GINGER
ZINGIBER OFFICINALE ROSE.
Fam. Zingiberaceae

HABITAT: Native to Southeast Asia but cultivated in India, China, the West Indies, Nigeria and elsewhere in the tropics.

DESCRIPTION: The appearance is well-known. The rhizome is freed from rootlets and may be peeled before drying. Some types are sun-bleached to improve appearance. African dried ginger is usually unpeeled, and the fresh rhizome is widely available and always unpeeled. Fracture: short and fibrous; odour and taste: characteristic, aromatic and pungent.

PART USED: Rhizome.

CONSTITUENTS: (i) Volatile oil, containing zingiberene and bisabolene, with zingerone, zingiberol, zingiberenol, curcumene, camphene, citral, cineole, borneol, linalool, methylheptenone and many other minor components (ii) Pungent principles; a mixture of phenolic compounds with carbon side chains consisting of seven or more carbon atoms,

191

referred to as gingerols, gingerdiols, gingerdiones, dihydrogingerdiones and shogaols. The shogaols are produced by dehydration and degradation of the gingerols and are formed during drying and extraction. The shogaols are twice as pungent as the gingerols, which accounts for the fact that dried ginger is more pungent than fresh (iii) A series of monoacyldigalactosylglycerols, known as gingerglycolipids A, B and C (iv) 6-gingesulphonic acid [R7,R16;1,2,3 and refs therein].

MEDICINAL USE: Carminative, anti-emetic, spasmolytic, anti-flatulent, antitussive, heptoprotective, anti-platelet and hypolipidaemic agent [R1]. 6-Gingerol and 6-shogaol have been shown to suppress gastric contractions, and ginger capsules containing the dried rhizome were found to be superior to dimenhydrinate in preventing the gastrointestinal symptoms of motion sickness, morning sickness of pregnancy and vertigo [4,5,6,7]. Both the fresh and dried rhizome suppress gastric acid secretion and reduce vomiting. Anti-ulcer activity has been described in animals and attributed to the volatile oil constituents, especially the 6-gingesulfonic acid [1,2]. Hepatoprotective effects have been noted in cultured hepatocytes by the gingerols, which are more active than the homologous shogaols, and both are also antioxidants and free radical scavengers [3,8]. The gingerols and shogaols inhibit the synthesis of PGF_{2alpha} in the bowel, which is thought to reduce bowel activity. Ginger inhibits cholesterol biosynthesis and has been shown to lower blood cholesterol in animal tests [9]; it also exhibits other types of cardiovascular activity such as producing a positive inotropic effect on the heart and inducing transient hypotension [10]. Antipyretic, anti-platelet, analgesic and anti-inflammatory effects have been observed and ginger has been suggested as of potential use in the treatment of migraine [11]. It has shown immunomodulatory [12], and also antiviral activity, which was ascribed to the sesquiterpenes [13]. Ginger is known to produce a warming effect when ingested, and the pungent principles stimulate thermogenic receptors. In addition, zingerone induces catecholamine secretion from the adrenal medulla. In Oriental medicine ginger is so highly regarded that it forms an ingredient of about half of all multi-item prescriptions. A distinction is made between the indications for the fresh rhizome (vomiting, coughs, abdominal distension and pyrexia) and the dried or processed rhizome (abdominal pain, lumbago and diarrhoea). This is probably justifiable since the constituents are present in different proportions. There are numerous recent papers on ginger; for further details on these as well as of the less frequent uses of ginger, such as insect repellent and molluscicidal effects, see reviews [R7,R8,R17,R18]. Ginger is of course a very important culinary spice, both fresh and dried.

PREPARATIONS AND DOSE: Dried rhizome, dose: 0.25–1 g, or equivalent extract, three times daily.

SPECIFIC REFERENCES: 1. Yamahara J et al (1992) Chem. Pharm. Bull. 40(8):2239. 2. Yoshikawa M et al (1994) Chem. Pharm. Bull. 42(6):1226. 3. Aeschbach R et al (1994) Food Chem. Toxicol. 32(1):31. 4. Kawai T et al (1994) Planta Med. 60:17. 5. Grontved A et al (1986)

J. Oto-Rhino-Laryngology 48(5):282. 6. Vutyavanich T *et al* (2001) *Obstet. Gynecol.* 97:577. 7. Niebyl J *et al* (2002) *Am. J. Obstet. Gynecol.* 86(5c):S253. 8. Hikino H *et al* (1985) *J. Ethnopharmacol.* 14:31. 9. Tanabe M *et al* (1993) *Chem. Pharm. Bull.* 41(4):710. 10. Shoji N *et al* (1982) *J. Pharm. Sci.* 71(10):1174. 11. Mustafa T *et al* (1990) *J. Ethnopharmacol.* 29:267. 12. Sohni Y *et al* (1996) *J. Ethnopharmacol.* 54(2–3):119. 13. Denyer C *et al* (1994) *J. Nat. Prod.* 57(5):658.

GINGER, WILD

ASARUM CANADENSE L.
Fam. Aristolochiaceae

SYNONYMS: Indian Ginger, Canadian Snakeroot.

HABITAT: North America, Canada.

DESCRIPTION: Rhizome slender, hardly branched, about 10 cm long and 3 mm thick, wrinkled, greyish- or purplish-brown. Rootlets whitish, occurring on the nodes. Fracture: short; taste: bitter and pungent; odour: aromatic.

PART USED: Rhizome.

CONSTITUENTS: (i) Volatile oil, 3.5–4.5%, containing methyleugenol (ii) Aristolochic acid [R4;1].

MEDICINAL USE: Expectorant, carminative, stimulant [R1]. It has been used for amenorrhoea. Aristolochic acid is carcinogenic (see Birthwort) so use is not recommended. It is certainly not a substitute for Ginger (q.v.).

SPECIFIC REFERENCES: 1. Doskotch R *et al* (1967) *Lloydia* 30:141.

GINKGO

GINKGO BILOBA L.
Fam. Ginkgoaceae

SYNONYMS: Maidenhair-Tree.

HABITAT: A dioeceous fossil tree, indigenous to China and Japan and cultivated elsewhere as an ornamental. It is a hardy tree, and reputed to be the only species to ever have survived a nuclear explosion.

DESCRIPTION: Leaves petiolate, glabrous, bilobed; each lobe triangular, up to about 6 cm long and 4 cm wide, with fan-like, fine, prominent, radiate veins and an entire margin.

PART USED: Leaves. The fruits are eaten in China.

CONSTITUENTS: (i) Terpene lactones, the ginkgolides A, B and C, with bilobalide and other minor components (ii) Flavonoids, the most important being the biflavone glycosides such as ginkgetin, isoginkgetin, bilobetin, 5-methoxybilobetin, with some quercetin and kaempferol derivatives (iii) Miscellaneous; terpenes such as bilobanone, traces of essential oil, tannins, nonacosane and

193

nonacosanol (= ginnol) (iv) Ginkgolic acids are present in the fruit but normally only in very minor amounts in the leaf [R2,R7,R8;1].

MEDICINAL USE: At present the most important use of Ginkgo is an aid to memory deterioration, due to aging and milder forms of dementia. It enhances cognitive processes, possibly by improving blood circulation to the brain and having anti-inflammatory and antioxidant affects [2,3]. Among the many clinical studies carried out, the extract was shown to improve the mental performance in healthy volunteers [2] and geriatric patients where this was impaired [4,5,6], and recently, an improvement in cognitive abilities was seen in a pilot study of 23 patients with multiple sclerosis [7]. Ginkgo alleviates some of the symptoms of tinnitus, intermittent claudication [8] and altitude sickness [9]. It is often used for circulatory disorders in general. Ginkgo extracts have complex vasoactive effects on isolated blood vessels. Ginkgo is also an anti-asthmatic agent and bronchodilator, due to the presence of the ginkgolides. These, and particularly ginkgolide B (= BN 52021), are specific platelet activating factor (PAF) antagonists, which has useful and far-reaching effects, since PAF is involved in allergic inflammation, anaphylactic shock and asthma. A small study found it to be effective in treating asthma in children (although it is not in clinical use for this purpose), and anecdotal evidence suggests that asthmatic patients taking Ginkgo for other reasons find their asthma attacks and use of bronchodilators is reduced. The ginkgolides also inhibit other pharmacological effects produced by PAF, such as platelet aggregation and the wheal-and-flare response in skin. The effects on the central nervous system are complex and include effects on neurotransmitter uptake, neurotransmitter receptors during ageing, cerebral ischaemia, and neuronal injury [10]. It has been suggested that inhibition of nitric oxide plays a part in this [11]. A recent report also demonstrates that Ginkgo extract ameliorates gentamicin-induced nephrotoxicity in rats [12]. A review of trials of Ginkgo for dementia (including Alzheimer's) concludes that it is at least as effective as anticholinesterase therapy, with a more acceptable side effect profile than tacrine [13]. A recent study, in patients with Alzheimer's disease, suggests that Ginkgo extract is more effective in mild to moderate cases, but in severe dementia it appears to slow down deterioration [14]. The effects on the central nervous system are complex, due to the combined effects of the various components of the extract, and have been well reviewed [15]. Ginkgo has been reported to cause dermatitis and gastrointestinal disturbances, though these symptoms are rare and are more likely to be a result of ingestion of the fruits, due to the alkyl phenols [13] or from overdosage. Many studies have been conducted, of variable quality, and the evidence to support the use of Ginkgo is generally good. See [R7,R8,R17;2,6,8,10,11,12,15,16,17,18 and refs therein].

PREPARATIONS AND DOSE: Dried leaf, dose: 120–600 mg; dried leaf extract, standardized to terpene lactone content (2–6%) and biflavone content (24%), dose: 120–240 mg daily.

SPECIFIC REFERENCES: 1. Braquet P *et al* (1986) *Trends Pharm, Sci.*

7:397. 2. Rigney U *et al* (1999) *Phytother. Res.* 13(5):408 . 3. Bridi R *et al* (2001) *Phytother. Res.* 15(5):449. 4. Le Bars P *et al* (1997) *JAMA* 278(16):1327. 5. Kanowski S *et al* (1997) *Phytomedicine* 4(1):3. 6. Ernst E *et al* (1999) *Clin. Drug Invest.* 17(4):301. 7. Kenny C *et al* (2002) *Am. Acad. Neurol. 54th Meeting, Denver, Colorado,* USA: P06.081. 8. Peters H *et al* (1998) *Vasa* 27:106. 9. Roncin J *et al* (1996) *Aviation Space Environ. Med.* 67(5):445. 10. Di Renzo G (2000) *Fitoterapia* 71:S43. 11. Calapai G *et al* (2000) *Life Sci.* 67(22):2673. 12. Naidu M *et al* (2000) *Phytomed.* 7(3):191. 13. Wettstein A (1999) *Phytomed.* 6(6):393. 14. Le Bars P *et al* (2002) *Neuropsychobiol.* 45(1):19. 15. DeFeudis F *et al* (2000) *Curr. Drug Targets* 1(1):25. 16. Baron-Ruppert G *et al* (2001) *Phytomed.* 8(2):133. 17. Mix J *et al* (2002) *Hum. Psychopharmacol. Clin. Exp.* (17(2):267. 18. Ginkgo biloba. Ed. Teris A (2000) *Medicinal and Aromatic Plants – Industrial Profiles.* Pub: Taylor and Francis, London, UK.

GINSENG

PANAX GINSENG C. A. MEYER
Fam. Araliaceae

SYNONYMS: Chinese Ginseng, Korean Ginseng, *P. schinseng* Nees. American Ginseng is *P. quinquefolius* L. Japanese Ginseng is *P. japonicas* C A Meyer (= *P. pseudo-ginseng* Wall.) var *japonica* C A Meyer. Himalayan Ginseng is *P. pseudo-ginseng* Wall. San-chi Ginseng is *P. notoginseng* Burk. Siberian Ginseng is *Eleutherococcus senticosus* Maxim (= *Acanthopanax senticosus*). Many other species and varieties are used.

HABITAT: *P. ginseng* is native to China and cultivated in China, Korea, Japan and Russia.

DESCRIPTION: *P. ginseng*: The root is spindle-shaped, pale brownish-yellow, about 1–2 cm in diameter, ringed above and divided into two or three equal branches which are longitudinally wrinkled. Fracture: short, mealy, showing a thin bark containing numerous reddish resin glands; wood wedges narrow, yellowish, with broad medullary rays.
Taste: sweetish; odour: faintly aromatic.

PART USED: Root.

CONSTITUENTS: (i) Saponin glycosides. These are the ginsenosides (or referred to less frequently as panaxosides). There is also series of notogensenoside saponins, and methyl ginsenosides. The ginsenosides are designated ginsenosides Ra, Rb... Rg1, Rg2... Rs etc. (The panaxoside nomenclature uses the suffixes A–F, it does not correspond to that of the ginsenosides.) In *Eleutherococcus* the saponins are chemically different, they are the eleutherosides A–F (ii) Glycans; the panaxans A–E, in *P. ginseng* (iii) Miscellaneous; volatile oil, containing beta-elemene; panaxynol, acetylenic compounds, panaxydol, panaxytriol, falcarinol, falcarintriol and others [R7;1]. The actual composition depends upon the species and method of preparation of the root.

MEDICINAL USE: Tonic, stimulant and adaptogen. Ginseng is taken

195

to improve stamina and concentration, for debility, ageing, sexual inadequacy, diabetes, insomnia, stress and many other real (or imaginary) ailments. Extensive research is still ongoing into the effects of Ginseng. The two main indications are sometimes divided into the tonic and adaptogenic properties. The tonic effect is a general enhancement of mental and physical performance, including improvements in memory and learning, thought to be the result of changes in cholinergic activity [2] and protection of hippocampal neurones [3]. Most of the activity is due to the ginsenosides, although nicotinic effects have been observed in a non-ginsenoside extract [4]. Clinical studies support these effects to some extent [5] and recently it has been demonstrated that in healthy volunteers Ginseng extract improves cognitive performance and mood [6]. The adaptogenic effect is the ability to enhance non-specific resistance to stress in the body, attributed to elevation of serum levels of corticosteroids and reduction of catecholamines, resulting in homoeostasis [2,7]. Ginsenoside R_{b-1} acts as a CNS sedative and R_{g-1} has anti-fatigue and stimulant properties. In animals, an extract increases the capacity of skeletal muscle to oxidize free fatty acids (in preference to glucose) to produce cellular energy, which would help to explain the anti-fatigue activity seen in conventional exhaustion tests. Ginseng has a traditional use in diabetes and a small study has supported this [8]. Panaxans A–E are known to be hypoglycaemic in mice and are probably responsible for at least some of the effects of Ginseng on carbohydrate metabolism. Other documented effects include immunomodulatory activity [9], potentiation of analgesic activity [10], and anti-cancer effects by ginsenosides Rs3 and Rs4 [11]. A recent trial of Ginseng involving thirty volunteers for improving 'quality of life' measures, including mental health issues, showed that it produced beneficial effects, which stopped after eight weeks of treatment. Adverse effects were reported by about one third of those taking it [12]. Ginseng is taken widely, and fatalities are unknown, but even so, side effects are well-documented and include oestrogenic effects, irritability and related symptoms. Hypertension is usually described as a side effect of Ginseng use, but recently a study found that supplementation with Ginseng (200 mg/day for 28 days) reduced diastolic blood pressure in a randomized, double blind, placebo controlled study of 30 patients [13]. A 'Ginseng abuse' syndrome has been described but does not appear to be a major problem. For clinical and other details of *Eleutherococcus*, see [R7;15]; for further information on Ginseng, see [R2,R7,R20;1,7,12,14,16 and refs therein].

PREPARATIONS AND DOSE: Dried root: short-term (up to 20 days), dose: 0.5–1g daily; long-term, dose: 0.4–0.8g.

BIBLICAL REFERENCES: Ezekiel 27:17.

SPECIFIC REFERENCES: 1. Attele S *et al* (1999) *Biochem. Pharmacol.* 58:1685 2. 7:397. 2. Tachikawa E *et al* (1995) *J. Pharmacol. Exp. Ther.* 273:629. 3. Lim J *et al* (1997) *Neurosci. Res.* 28:191. 4. Lewis R *et al* (1999) *Phytother. Res.* 13(1):59. 5. Sorensen H *et al* (1996) *Curr, Ther. Res.* 57:959. 6. Kennedy D *et al* (2001) *Nutr. Neurosci.* 4(4):295. 7. Nocerino E *et al* (2000) *Fitoterapia* 71:S1. 8. Sotaniemi E *et al* (1995)

Diabetes Care 18(10):1373. 9. Singh V *et al* (1984) *Planta Med.* 50:462. 10. Kumar S *et al* (2000) *Pharm. Pharmacol. Commun.* 6:527. 11. Kim S *et al* (1999) *Eur. J. Cancer.* 35(3):507. 12. Ellis J *et al* (2002) *Ann. Pharmacother.* 36:375. 13. Caron M *et al* (2002) *Ann. Pharmacother.* 36(5):758-763. 14. Dharmananda S (2002) *HerbalGram* 54:34. 15. Szolomicki S *et al* (2000) *Phytother. Res.* 14(1):30. 16. Ginseng. Ed. Court W (2000) *Medicinal and Aromatic Plants – Industrial Profiles.* Pub: Taylor and Francis, London, UK.

GLADWIN
IRIS FOEDIDISSIMA L.
Fam. Iridaceae

SYNONYMS: Stinking Iris, Gladwine, Stinking Gladdon, Roastbeef Plant.

HABITAT: Woods and shady places in Britain and parts of Europe.

DESCRIPTION: Long narrow leaves; flowers bluish-purple, shaped like the common Iris but smaller; bright orange seeds. Odour when bruised: sickly, unpleasant.

PART USED: Rhizome.

CONSTITUENTS: Unknown.

MEDICINAL USE: Antispasmodic, cathartic, anodyne [R1].

GOA
ANDIRA ARAROBA AG.
Fam. Leguminosae

SYNONYMS: Araroba, Bahia Powder, Brazil Powder, Chrysarobin.

HABITAT: South America, mainly Brazil.

DESCRIPTION: The yellowish powder is scraped out of longitudinal fissures in the tree after felling, and purified by sifting and solvent extraction. It is very irritating to eyes and mucous membranes.

CONSTITUENTS: A complex mixture of anthraquinone derivatives known as 'chrysarobin' [R3].

MEDICINAL USE: Taenifuge, anti-parasitic [R1]. It has been used externally as an ointment for ringworm and other parasitic infections. It is highly irritant, and should not be used internally.

GOAT'S RUE
GALEGA OFFICINALIS L.
Fam. Fabaceae

SYNONYMS: French Lilac.

HABITAT: Grows wild in Europe, naturalized in Britain.

DESCRIPTION: An erect, branched plant reaching 1.5 m. The leaves have 6–8 pairs of elongated leaflets and the tip terminates in a small

197

point. Flowers pale bluish-purple, or more rarely pink or white, borne on short stalks in an erect spike. Pods almost cylindrical.

PART USED: Herb.

CONSTITUENTS: (i) Galegine (= isoamylene guanidine), its 4-hydroxy derivative and peganine (ii) Flavonoids including galuteolin (iii) Saponins and lectins [R2;1,2].

MEDICINAL USE: Galactagogue, diuretic, vermifuge, anti-diabetic. Goat's Rue is a traditional herb used to treat diabetes and hypoglycemic effects in animals have been observed for extracts [3,4]. It has also been advocated as an aid to weight reduction, and both these effects are ascribed to the presence of galegine. Mice fed with galegine showed reduced food intake and consequent weight loss, with no overt toxicity [4].

PREPARATIONS AND DOSE: Powdered herb, dose: 0.3–1.2 g, or equivalent extract.

SPECIFIC REFERENCES: 1. Palit P *et al* (1998) *J. Pharm. Pharmacol.* 50S:80. 2. Petricic J *et al* (1982) *Acta Pharm. Yugoslav.* 32:219. 3. Lemus I *et al* (1999) *Phytother. Res.* 13(1):91. 4. Palit P *et al* (1999) *J. Pharm. Pharmacol.* 51S:97.

GOLDEN ROD
SOLIDAGO VIRGAUREA L.
Fam. Asteraceae

HABITAT: A common garden and wild plant in Europe and Asia.

DESCRIPTION: A tall upright perennial herb, with oblong-lanceolate leaves, pointed and finely serrate. The flowers, which appear in July to September, are golden yellow, composite, shortly rayed and on branching spikes. Taste: acrid and bitter; odour: when dry, agreeable and slightly aromatic.

PART USED: Leaves.

CONSTITUENTS: (i) Saponins. In the European form, these are the acyl virgaurea saponins 1,2 and 3, based on polygalic acid; in the Asian form, the solidago saponins I-XXIX, acyl virgaurea saponins 1 and 2, and bellis saponin BA2 (ii) Clerodane diterpenes, at least 12 of which have been isolated; these include solidagolactones I–VII and elonga-tolides C and E, isolated from Asian varieties (iii) Phenolic acids and glucosides, including salicylic, vanillic, caffeic virgaureoside A and leicarposide (iv) Volatile oil, in the European samples composed of alpha- and beta-pinene, limonene, elemene, myrcene and others; in Asian samples mainly limonene, germacrene-B and D and betacaryophyllene (v) Flavonoids such as rutin, astragalin, hyperoside, quercitrin and many others [R2;1,2,3,4,5].

MEDICINAL USE: Diaphoretic, anti-inflammatory, antiseptic, carminative, diuretic [R1]. Golden Rod is used mainly for inflammatory diseases of the urinary tract, and for bladder and kidney stones. An extract of the plant exhibited anti-inflammatory activity in the rat paw oedema test [6] and isolated leicarposide has been shown to have this effect [4]. The saponins are anti-fungal against *Candida* species [1]. An extract of the leaves and flowers shows a transient hypotensive effect in rats [7].

SPECIFIC REFERENCES: 1. Bader G *et al* (1987) *Pharmazie* 42(2):140. 2. Bader G (1999) *Z. Phytother.* 20:196. 3. Goswami G *et al* (1984) *Phytochem.* 23(4):837. 4. Metzer J *et al* (1984) *Pharmazie* 39(12):869. 5. Inose Y *et al* (1991) *Chem. Pharm. Bull.* 39:2037. 6. El-Ghazaly M *et al* (1992) *Arzneim. Forsch.* 42(3):333. 7. Lassere B *et al* (1983) *Naturwissenschaft.* 70:95.

GOLDEN SEAL

HYDRASTIS CANADENSIS L.
Fam. Ranunculaceae

SYNONYMS: Orange Root, Yellow Root.

HABITAT: Native to North America; mostly cultivated.

DESCRIPTION: The rhizome is yellowish-brown, about 5 cm long and 1 cm thick, knotty and twisted, wrinkled longitudinally and encircled by leaf scars. Rootlets frequently present in abundance. Fracture: short, showing a dark yellow cut surface, thick bark, large pith and broad medullary rays. Taste: very bitter; odour: strong, characteristic and disagreeable.

PART USED: Rhizome, gathered in the autumn.

CONSTITUENTS: (i) Isoquinoline alkaloids, mainly beta-hydrastine, berberine and canadine (= tetrahydroberberine), with lesser amounts of canadaline, hydrastidine and isohydrastidine etc. [1,2,3] (ii) Miscellaneous; fatty acids, resin, polyphenolic acids and a small amount of volatile oil [R19].

MEDICINAL USE: Tonic, hepatoprotective, anti-dysenteric, haemostatic, anti-inflammatory [R1]. Used internally for dyspepsia, dysentery, gastritis, peptic ulceration, colitis, menorrhagia and other menstrual disorders; and topically for conjunctivitis, eczema and inflammation of the ear. The alkaloid berberine has antimicrobial, anti-diarrhoeal, enterotoxin-inhibiting, cytotoxic and anti-carcinogenic activity, as well as being anti-inflammatory, choleretic and anticholinesterase. Hydrastine is reportedly sedative, choleretic and antibacterial. Synergistic activity between the alkaloids has been observed in antimicrobial and isolated organ studies [4]. An extract has relaxant effects on rabbit bladder detrusor muscle, as well as rat uterus and guinea pig trachea; many of these effects are not elicited by the isolated alkaloids [5,6]. A large number of clinical studies have been carried out and support these uses; for full details see [R11,R17]. Golden Seal is used in a similar way to Barberry (q.v.).

PREPARATIONS AND DOSE: Powdered herb, dose: 0.5–1 g. For extracts standardized to 5% hydrastine, the usual dose is 250–500 mg three times daily.

SPECIFIC REFERENCES: 1. Gleye J *et al* (1974) *Phytochem.*13:674. 2. Galeffi C *et al* (1997) *Planta Med* 63:194. 3. Messana I *et al* (1980) *Gazz. Chim. Ital.* 10:539. 4. Palmery M *et al* (1996) *Phytother. Res.* 10(1):47. 4. Simeon S *et al* (1989) *Plantes Med. Phytother.* 23(3):202. 5. Bolle P *et al* (1998) *Phytother. Res.* 12:S86. 6. Cometa M *et al* (1998) *Phytother. Res.*12:S83.

GOLD THREAD

COPTIS TRIFOLIA L. (SALIS.)
C. GROENLANDICA (OED.) FERN.
Fam. Ranunculaceae

SYNONYMS: Mouth Root, Vegetable Gold.

HABITAT: *C. trifolia* is Indian in origin and *C. groenlandica* is from North America and Canada. In Chinese medicine the rhizomes of *C. chinensis* Franch, *C. deltoidiea* C Y Cheng et Hasio, and *C. teetoides* C Y Cheng are widely used and referred to as Huanglian.

DESCRIPTION: Rhizomes thread-like, golden yellow, matted, with very small roots. Taste: very bitter; odour: slight.

PART USED: Rhizome.

CONSTITUENTS: (i) Isoquinoline alkaloids; mainly berberine and coptisine [R2]. The Chinese species are better investigated and berberine, palmitine, coptisine, jatrorrhizine and many others have been isolated [R5].

MEDICINAL USE: Bitter tonic [R1]. Used to promote digestion and for similar indications as Barberry and Golden Seal (q.v.).

PREPARATIONS: Powdered rhizome, dose: 0.5–1.2 g.

GOUTWORT

AEGOPODIUM PODAGRARIA L.
Fam. Apiaceae

SYNONYMS: Ground Elder, Goutweed, Gout Herb, Ashweed, Ground Ash, Herb Gerarde.

HABITAT: A troublesome weed throughout Britain and Europe. Gerard, in the 16th century, remarked that "it groweth of it selfe in gardens without setting or sowing and is so fruitful in his increase, that where it hath once taken root, it will hardly be gotten out againe, spoiling and getting every year more ground, to the annoying of better herbs". This sentiment still applies for most gardeners.

DESCRIPTION: A creeping perennial with white or pink, typically umbelliferous flowers and 1–2 trefoil leaves, sometimes variegated or reddish coloured.

PART USED: Herb.

CONSTITUENTS: (i) Flavonoids including hyperoside, isoquercitrin and kaempferol rhamnoglucoside (ii) Furanocoumarins such as umbelliferone, peucedanin and xanthotoxin (iii) Polyynes, in the fresh herb (iii) Volatile oil (iv) Caffeic acid derivatives such as chlorogenic acid [R2;1,2].

MEDICINAL USE: Diuretic, sedative [R1]. Formerly used externally as a poultice and internally for gout. Culpeper is quoted as saying "the very carrying of it about in the pocket will defend the bearer from any attack of the aforesaid complaint". The fresh foliage has been eaten as a vegetable. The coumarins are phototoxic, and as would be expected, an extract of the leaf is lethal to brine shrimp [2].

SPECIFIC REFERENCES: 1. Harborne J *et al* (1972) *Phytochem.* 11:1741. 2. Ojala T *et al* (1999) *Planta Med.* 65(8):715.

GRAINS OF PARADISE

AFRAMOMUM MELEGUETA (ROSCOE) K. SCHUM.
Fam. Zingiberaceae

SYNONYMS: Guinea Grains, Melegueta Pepper, Alligator Pepper.

HABITAT: Tropical West Africa.

DESCRIPTION: The seeds are red-brown, small, hard, shiny and oyster-shaped. Taste and odour: aromatic and pungent.

PART USED: Seeds.

CONSTITUENTS: (i) Volatile oil, containing mainly humulene and caryophyllene, with a small amount of their oxides (ii) Pungent principles such as the paradols (hydroxyphenyl alkanones), gingerols (hydroxyphenyl alkanols), 6-shogaol and gingerone [1,2] (iii) Miscellaneous; tannin, starch [R2].

MEDICINAL USE: Formerly used as a stimulant [R1]. Antibacterial and anti-fungal activity has been reported for extracts [3], and 6-paradol shown to inhibit the growth of various species of *Mycobacterium* and also *Candida* [2]. Anti-ulcer, inhibition of gastric secretion, and other cytoprotective effects have been noted in experimental ulcers and gastric damage induced by various methods [4,5] as would be anticipated from its constituents, which are similar to those found in Ginger (q.v.).

SPECIFIC REFERENCES: 1. Ajaiyeoba E *et al* (1999) *Flav. Frag. J.* 14(2):109. 2. Galal A (1996) *Int. J. Pharmacog.* 34(1):64. 3. Oloke J *et al* (1988) *Fitoterapia* 59(5):384. 4. Rafatullah S *et al* (1995) *Int. J. Pharmacog.* 33(4):311. 5. Enyikwola O (1994) *Int. J. Pharmacog.* 32(1):37.

GRAVEL ROOT

EUPATORIUM PURPUREA L.
Fam. Asteraceae

SYNONYMS: Gravelweed, Joe-Pye Weed, Queen of the Meadow Root.

HABITAT: North America.

DESCRIPTION: Rhizome up to 3 cm diameter, very hard and tough, with a thin, greyish-brown bark and thick, whitish wood, often hollow in the centre and with wide medullary rays. The short lateral branches usually

201

have crowded, tough, slender, woody roots attached. Taste: bitter, astringent and slightly acrid.

PART USED: Rhizome and root.

CONSTITUENTS: (i) Benzofuran derivatives, including cistifolin, euparin, euparone, 6-hydroxy-3-beta-methoxytrematone and others (ii) Volatile oil, of unknown composition (iii) Flavonoids, including eupatorin [R7;1,2].

MEDICINAL USE: Diuretic, stimulant, tonic, anti-inflammatory [R1]. Used principally in the treatment of rheumatoid arthritis, and for stones (or 'gravel') in the kidney and bladder, as well as other kidney and urinary disorders including cystitis and urethritis. Cistifolin and other benzofurans from the extract have been shown to inhibit cell adhesion mediated by leukocyte integrins, which supports the anti-inflammatory use, since the integrins play a crucial role in the development of many inflammatory diseases [1,2,3].

PREPARATIONS AND DOSE: Powdered root, dose: 2–4 g, or equivalent extract, three times daily.

SPECIFIC REFERENCES: 1. Habtemariam S (2001) *Phytother. Res.* 15(8):687. 2. Habtemariam S (1998) *Planta Med.* 64(8):683. 3. Habtemariam S (1998) *Phytother. Res.* 12(6):422.

GRINDELIA
GRINDELIA CAMPORUM GREEN
G. SQUARROSA NUTT.
Fam. Asteraceae

SYNONYMS: Gum Plant, Gum Weed, Tar Weed, *G. robusta* (= *G. camporum*).

HABITAT: North and South America.

DESCRIPTION: Leaves lanceolate, glabrous, those of *G. camporum* being broader at the base, leathery, brittle, serrated at the margins, about 610 cm long and 1–3 cm broad. Flower-heads globular, about 2 cm in diameter, with yellow florets and reflexed, linear, pointed involucral scales. Taste: bitter; odour: faint, aromatic, balsamic.

PART USED: Herb.

CONSTITUENTS: (i) Diterpenes of the grindelane type, including grindelic acid and its 17-hydroxy derivative, 13-isogrindelic acid, and many others (ii) Flavonoids; including acacetin, kumatakenin, quercetin and its 3,3'-dimethyl ether derivative [1] (iii) Essential oil, containing bornyl acetate, borneol and alpha-pinene [2] (iv) Polyphenolic acids including caffeic, gallic, protocatechuic and vanillic acids [3] (v) Polyynes such as matricarianol and its acetate [R2] (vi) Saponins based on grindeliasapogenins, bayogenin and oleanolic acid [4].

MEDICINAL USE: Antispasmodic, expectorant, anti-asthmatic [R1]. Used mainly for asthma and bronchitis, and infections of the upper respiratory tract, for cystitis and in the form of a lotion for dermatitis. Antibacterial effects have been demonstrated and ascribed to the polyphenolic acid fraction [3], and an aqueous extract has anti-inflammatory activity in the rat paw oedema test [5].

PREPARATIONS AND DOSE: Powdered herb, dose: 2–4 g, or equivalent extract, three times daily.

SPECIFIC REFERENCES: 1. Timmermann B *et al* (1985) *Phytochem.* 24(5):1031. 2. Kaltenbach G *et al* (1993) *J. Ess. Oil Res.* 5:107. 3. Didry N *et al* (1982) *Plantes Med. Phytother.* 16(1):7. 4. Kreutzer S *et al* (1990) *Planta Med.* 56(4):392. 5. Mascolo N *et al* (1987) *Phytother. Res.* 1(1):28.

GROUND IVY
GLECHOMA HEDERACEA L.
Fam. Lamiaceae

SYNONYMS: Nepeta hederacea (L.) Trev., *N. glechoma* Benth.

HABITAT: A common wild plant in Europe and the British Isles.

DESCRIPTION: Stems quadrangular, unbranched, often purplish, hairy, bearing opposite leaves, which are kidney-shaped, hairy, bluntly serrate and long-stalked. Flowers blue, two-lipped, in groups of two or three in the axils of the leaves. Taste: bitter; odour: aromatic.

PART USED: Herb.

CONSTITUENTS: (i) Essential oil, containing sesquiterpenes including glechomafuran, with linalool, limonene, pulegone, menthone, terpineol and others (ii) Flavonoids; isoquercitin, hyperoside, and apigenin and luteolin glycosides (iii) Triterpenes including alpha- and beta-ursolic acids and oleanolic acid (iv) Hydroxy octadecadienoic acid derivatives (v) Marrubiin, a diterpene (vi) Polyphenolic acids including rosmarinic [R7,1,2,3,4,5,6].

MEDICINAL USE: Astringent, tonic, diuretic, expectorant [R1]. Used mainly for bronchitis and catarrh, but also for haemorrhoids. Externally it may be used to soothe inflammation. Several instances of anti-inflammatory activity have been described: ursolic and oleanolic acid inhibit Epstein-Barr activation induced by the inflammatory tumour promoter tetradecanoyl phorbol acetate in Raji cells [6]. One of the hydroxyoctadecadienoic acid derivatives was found to be a partial agonist at prostaglandin E1 and D2 receptors [4]. Anti-inflammatory activity for the whole herb extract has also been demonstrated using the rat paw oedema test [7].

PREPARATIONS AND DOSE: Powdered herb, dose: 2–4 g, or equivalent extract, three times daily.

SPECIFIC REFERENCES: 1. Barberan F *et al* (1986) *Fitoterapia* 57(2):67. 2. Okuyama E *et al* (1983) *Shoyakugaku Zasshi* 106:1108. 3. Stahl E *et al* (1972) *Justus Leibigs Ann. Chem.* 757:23. 4. Henry D *et al* (1988) *Eur. J. Biochem.* 170(1–2):389. 5. Kuhn H *et al* (1989) *Eur. J. Biochem.* 186(1–2):155. 6. Ohigashi H *et al* (1986) *Cancer Lett.* 30(2):143. 7. Mascolo N *et al* (1987) *Phytother. Res.* 1(1):28.

GROUND PINE, AMERICAN

LYCOPODIUM COMPLANATUM L.
Fam. Lycopodiaceae

HABITAT: North America, Europe, Russia.

DESCRIPTION: Stem long, creeping, yellowish-green, scaly, about 2 mm in diameter, giving off at intervals erect, fan-shaped, forked branches with minute, scale-like leaves, and bearing stalked tufts of four to five cylindrical spikes of spore cases in the axils of minute bracts. Taste and odour: aromatic, slightly terebinthinate.

CONSTITUENTS: (i) Piperidine alkaloids, including lycopodine, complanatine, complanadine A and nicotine (ii) Triterpenes including alpha-onocerin, lycoclavatol, serratendiol, campesterol stigmasterol and others (iii) Flavonoids; chrysoeriol, luteolin and apigenin glycosides [R2;1,2].

MEDICINAL USE: Little used here apart from in homoeopathic medicine. In Chinese medicine it is highly regarded as a tonic and for skin disorders. Lycopodine produces uterine contractions and increases peristalsis in the small intestine of animals. Lycopodium alkaloids are toxic [1, and refs therein].

SPECIFIC REFERENCES: 1. Ayer W (1991) *Nat. Prod. Rep.* 8:455. 2. Kobayashi J *et al* (2000) *Tet. Lett.* 41(47):9069.

GROUND PINE, EUROPEAN

AJUGA CHAMAEPITYS (L.) SCHREB.
Fam. Lamiaceae

HABITAT: Grows in bare, sparse, stony places in Britain and parts of Europe.

DESCRIPTION: A low greyish annual, with narrow, erect, deeply trifid leaves with single yellow two-lipped flowers in the axils. Taste and odour: terebinthinate.

PART USED: Leaves.

CONSTITUENTS: (i) Iridoid glycosides, including acetyl harpagide (ii) Phyto-ecdysterols; ajugalactone, cyasterone, makisterone and beta-ecdysone (iii) Caffeic acid derivatives [R2;1,2,3].

MEDICINAL USE: Stimulant, diuretic, emmenagogue [R1]. Used for gout and rheumatism and female disorders, combined with other herbs, often as an infusion. Medicinal activity is probably due to the iridoids, but the ecdysterols are insect anti-feedants. See also Bugle and Devil's Claw.

SPECIFIC REFERENCES: 1. Camps F *et al* (1985) *Ann. Quim.* 81C(1):74. 2. Kooiman P *et al* (1972) *Acta Bot. Nederl.* 21(4)417. 3. Lamaison C *et al* (1991) *Fitoterapia* 62(2):166.

GROUNDSEL
SENECIO VULGARIS L.
Fam. Asteraceae

SYNONYMS: Grounsel.

HABITAT: A common weed worldwide.

DESCRIPTION: A low annual, with pinnately lobed leaves and ray-less, brush-like yellow flower heads, about 6 mm long and 3 mm broad, in loose clusters, with black-tipped sepal-like bracts. Taste: salty; odour: imperceptible.

PART USED: Herb.

CONSTITUENTS: (i) Pyrrolizidine alkaloids; seneciphylline, senecionine, reddelline, retrorsine and others, mainly as the N-oxides [1,2] (ii) Volatile oil, the main component of which is beta-caryophyllene, with myrcene, alpha-copaene, beta-farnesine and germacrene D [3] (iii) Flavonoids; glucuronides of quercetin and isorhamnetin [4].

MEDICINAL USE: Formerly used as a diuretic and diaphoretic and to relieve bilious pains [R1]. Internal use is not recommended as the alkaloids are hepatotoxic, and veno-occlusive disease has been reported clinically for a patient taking the herb [5]. Senecionine and its N-oxide have anti-fertility effects in rats [6].

SPECIFIC REFERENCES: 1. Ingolfsdottir H *et al* (1990) *Acta Pharm. Nord.* 2(5):343. 2. Toppel G *et al* (1986) *Planta Med.* 52:25P. 3. Van Dooren-Bos R *et al* (1981) *Planta Med.* 42:385. 4. Mansour R *et al* (1981) *Phytochem.* 20:1180. 5. Vilar II (2000) *Gastroenterologia y Hepatologia* 23(6):285. 6. Tu Z-B *et al* (1988) *J. Pharm. Sci.* 77(5):461.

GUAIACUM
GUAIACUM OFFICINALE L.
G. SANCTUM L.

Fam. Zygophyllaceae

SYNONYMS: Guaiac, *Lignum vitae, Lignum sanctum.*

HABITAT: West Indies, Florida and South America.

DESCRIPTION: The wood is normally sold as shavings. The heartwood is greenish brown, heavier than water and with an aromatic and irritating taste. The resin, which accounts for about 20%, is produced by firing the logs, and collected when melted.

PART USED: Wood, resin.

CONSTITUENTS: (i) Lignans; furoguaiacidin, guaiacin, furoguaiacin, tetrahydrofuroguaiacin A and B, furoguaiaoxidin and others (ii) Resin acids: (–)-guaiaretic, (–)-hydroguaiaretic, guaiacic and alpha- and beta-guaiaconic acids (iii) Terpenoids based on oleanolic acid, including guaiagutin, guaiasaponin etc. (iv) Volatile oil, containing guaiol, which rearranges to guaiazulene on steam distillation [R2,R7;1,2,3,4,5,6].

MEDICINAL USE: Anti-rheumatic, anti-inflammatory, diuretic, diaphoretic, mild laxative [R1]. Used mainly for rheumatic pain and gout. An extract of the rhizome showed calcium antagonism using inhibition of contraction of aortic strips [7]. The chemistry of *Guaiacum* wood is well-characterized, but little pharmacological or clinical work has been carried out, apart from confirming the anti-inflammatory activity [8].

PREPARATIONS AND DOSE: Powdered wood, dose: 1–2 g, by decoction, or equivalent extract, three times daily.

SPECIFIC REFERENCES: 1. Ahmad V *et al* (1984) *Phytochem.* 23:2612. 2. Ahmad V *et al* (1986) *Phytochem.* 25:951. 3. Ahmad V *et al* (1984) *J. Nat. Prod.* 47:977. 4. Ahmad V *et al* (1986) *J. Nat. Prod.* 49:784. 5. Majumder P *et al* (1975) *J. Chem. Soc. Chem. Commun.* 702. 6. Kratochvil J *et al* (1975) *Phytochem.* 10:2529. 7. Rauwald H *et al* (1994) *Phytotherapy Res.* 8(3):135. 8. Duwiejua M *et al* (1994) *J. Pharm. Pharmacol.* 46(4):286.

GUAR GUM
CYAMOPSIS TETRAGONOLOBUS (L.) TAUBERT.
Fam. Fabaceae

SYNONYMS: Cluster Bean.

HABITAT: Africa, parts of Asia.

DESCRIPTION: The gum obtained from the ground endosperms of the seeds is a yellowish-white powder.

PART USED: Seeds.

CONSTITUENTS: (i) Polysaccharides, composed of straight and branched chains of D-galactose and D-mannose polymers [R2,R14].

MEDICINAL USE: Used as a source of fibre and adjunct to the treatment of diabetes. It reduces pre- and post-prandial glucose levels and is usually given with meals. It may also be of use in lowering blood lipid levels [R14;1,2]. Other clinical effects such as alleviation of diarrhoea have been described [3], but the use of guar as a slimming aid does not appear to be justified [4]. It is also used as a thickening and suspending agent in foods, and as a tablet binder.

PREPARATIONS AND DOSE: Powdered gum, dose: 5 g with meals.

SPECIFIC REFERENCES: 1. Todd P (1990) *Drugs* 39:917. 2. Salenius J-P *et al* (1995) *Br. Med. J.* 310:95. 3. Sapen H *et al* (2001) *Clin. Nutr.* 20(4):301. 4. Pittler M *et al* (2001) *Am. J. Med.* 110(9):724.

GUARANA
PAULLINIA CUPANA KUNTH EX H.B.K.
Fam. Sapindaceae

SYNONYMS: Brazilian Cocoa *Paullinia sorbilis* Mart.

HABITAT: Brazil and Venezuela.

DESCRIPTION: The paste is formed from the pulverized and roasted seeds, formed into rolls or bars and dried. These have an astringent, bitter then sweet taste; and an odour recalling that of chocolate.

PART USED: Seeds.

CONSTITUENTS: (i) Caffeine, (= guaranine) up to 7%, with theobromine, theophylline, xanthine and other xanthine derivatives (ii) Oligomeric proanthocyanidins, including d-catechin (iii) Miscellaneous; saponins, starch, fats, choline, pigments (iii) Essential oil, containing estragole, anethole and others [R2;1,2].

MEDICINAL USE: Stimulant, astringent [R1]. The pharmacological effects are mainly due to the caffeine content. Guarana acts as an antioxidant and inhibits lipid peroxidation in rats and mice [3]. It also has antithrombotic effects in rabbit platelets [4]. Guarana is widely used as a tonic or food supplement to alleviate tiredness and promote alertness. This is supported by the fact that it contains caffeine, and a water extract has been shown to increase blood glucose levels and deplete glycogen levels in rats given maltose, both before and after exercising [5]. It does not appear to have any toxic effects (beyond those to be expected by caffeine overdose) [2].

PREPARATIONS AND DOSE: Powdered Guarana, dose: 0.5–4 g, or equivalent extract.

SPECIFIC REFERENCES: 1. Frohne D (1993) *Deutsch Apot. Ztg.* 133:218. 2. Benoni H *et al* (1996) *Z. Lebensmitt. Untersuch. Forsch.* 203(1):95. 3. Mattei R *et al* (1998) *J. Ethnopharmacol.* 60(2):111. 4. Bydlowski S *et al* (1991) *Brazil. J. Med. Biol. Res.* 24(4):421. 5. Miura T *et al* (1998) *Biol. Pharm. Bull.* 21(6):646.

GYMNEMA

GYMNEMA SYLVESTRIS R. BR.
Fam. Asclepidaceae

SYNONYMS: Periploca of the Wood.

HABITAT: India, Sri Lanka and tropical Africa.

DESCRIPTION: A large woody climber with opposite leaves, which are ovate and hairy on both surfaces, and small yellow flowers. Taste: slightly bitter, followed by a temporary loss of sensitivity to the taste of sugar and other sweeteners.

PART USED: Leaves, root.

CONSTITUENTS: (i) Saponin glycosides known collectively as 'gymnemic acid', consisting of a mixture of glycosides, the gymnemic acids A-D and V-Z. There are many others, e.g. the gymnemasins A-D, gymnasides I-VII, gymnemosides A-F and their aglycones (ii) Gurmarin, a polypeptide (iii) Miscellaneous; amino acids, including gamma-aminobutyric acid, and an alkaloid 'gymnamine' [R16;1,2,3,4].

MEDICINAL USE: Anti-diabetic. The herb is a traditional treatment for diabetes in India. It also has the remarkable property of inhibiting the palatal response to all sweet tastes for a short time after chewing the

207

leaves, although other taste perceptions are unaffected. The anti-hyperglycaemic property is due to the gymnemic acids and other saponins and was shown in animal studies to affect only diabetic mice. Increased circulating levels of insulin were observed [5] and insulin release was stimulated via increased membrane permeability [6]. It has also been suggested that regeneration of the Islets of Langerhans may occur [7]. The loss of sensation to sweet tastes is mainly due to the polypeptide gurmarin [8]. The leaf extract has hypolipidemic activity in human patients [9], and animals fed a high fat diet [10]. Other activities of the leaf include smooth muscle relaxant, hepatoprotective, antiviral, antibacterial, and antioxidant activity [R16].

SPECIFIC REFERENCES: 1. Yoshikawa K *et al* (1991) *Phytochem.* 31(1):237. 2. Yoshikawa M *et al* (1997) *Chem. Pharm. Bull.* 45(10):1671. 3. Yoshikawa M *et al* (1997) *Chem. Pharm. Bull.* 45(12):2034. 4. Ota M *et al* (1998) *Biopolymers* 45(3):231. 5. Sugihara Y *et al* (2000) *J. Asian Nat. Prod. Res.* 2(4):321. 6. Persaud S *et al* (1999) *J. Endocrinol.* 163(2):207. 7. Shanmugasundaram E *et al* (1990) *J. Ethnopharmacol.* 30(3):265. 8. Miyasaka A *et al* (1995) *Brain Res.* 676(1):63. 9. Shanmugasundaram E *et al* (1990) *J. Ethnopharmacol.* 30(3): 281. 10. Bishayee A *et al* (1994) *Phytother. Res.* 8:118.

HAIR CAP MOSS
POLYTRICHUM JUNIPERUM WILLD.
Fam. Polytrichaceae

SYNONYMS: Ground Moss, Bear's Bed.

HABITAT: A common European moss found in dry places, the margins of woods and poor sandy soil.

DESCRIPTION: Stems slender, unbranched, 5–8 cm long, with small, short, awl-shaped, red-tipped 'leaves', overlapping and crowded in the upper part of the stem. Fruit stalks terminate in a quadrangular capsule containing the spores.

PART USED: Whole plant.

CONSTITUENTS: Very little information available: tannins have been reported [R4].

MEDICINAL USE: Diuretic, styptic [R1]. Formerly used in dropsy (congestive heart failure) and urinary calculi. Extracts have been shown to have weak anti-tumour effects in mice [1]. It is said that this moss is found growing on human skulls, which gives it the name.

SPECIFIC REFERENCES: 1. Belkin M *et al* (1952) *J. Nat. Cancer Inst.* 13:742.

HARTSTONGUE
SCOLOPENDRIUM VULGARE SM.
Fam. Polypodiaceae

SYNONYMS: Asplenium scolopendrium L., *Phyllitis scolopendrium* Green.

HABITAT: It grows in gardens and woodlands in parts of Europe, North America, South-western and eastern Asia.

DESCRIPTION: Fronds stalked, up to about 60 cm long and 5 cm wide, with transverse simple veins and on the reverse side, lines of spore cases in transverse series. Taste: unpleasant; odourless.

PART USED: Herb.

CONSTITUENTS: (i) Flavonoids including leucodelphidin and kaempferol glucosides (ii) Thiaminase (in the fresh plant) (iii) Miscellaneous tannins, mucilage etc. [R2,R4].

MEDICINAL USE: Diuretic, laxative, pectoral [R1]. It has been taken as a decoction.

HAWTHORN
CRATAEGUS OXYCANTHOIDES THUILL.
C. MONOGYNA JACQ.
Fam. Rosaceae

SYNONYMS: Haw, May, Whitethorn.

HABITAT: A common British and European hedge plant.

DESCRIPTION: A hairless, thorny, deciduous shrub with 3–5 lobed leaves, bearing white or pink dense clusters of flowers, followed by deep red false

209

fruits containing one seed (in *C. monogyna*), or two seeds (in *C. oxycanthoides*). The flowers appear in early summer and the berries or 'haws' in September.

PART USED: Berries, leaves, flowers.

CONSTITUENTS: (i) Flavonoids; vitexin, vitexin-4-rhamnoside, quercetin and quercetin-3-galactoside, hyperoside, rutin, vicentin, orientin and others (ii) Procyanidins, catechins and epicatechin dimers (iii) Phenolic acids including chlorogenic and caffeic acids (iv) 2-phenylchromone derivatives in the flowers, leaves and buds (v) Amines; phenethylamine, methoxyphenethylamine, dopamine, acetylcholine and tyramine (vi) Triterpenes based on ursolic and oleanolic acid [R2,R7,R9;1,2,3,4].

MEDICINAL USE: Cardiac tonic, hypotensive, coronary and peripheral vasodilator, antiarrhythmic, anti-sclerotic [R1]. Animal studies have shown beneficial effects on coronary blood flow, blood pressure and heart rate, as well as improve circulation to the extremities. Hawthorn inhibits myocardial sodium and potassium ATP-ase and exerts a positive inotropic effect and relaxes the coronary artery, and the procyanidins inhibit angiotensin-converting enzyme (ACE). Hawthorn extracts block repolarising potassium current in ventricular muscle and so prolongs the refractory period, exerting an antiarrhythmic effect [1,5,6,7,8,9]. Clinical trials have supported some of these pharmacological effects, although a recent study showed that tolerance to exercise was not improved in 20 patients with class II congestive heart failure [10]. However, in combination with diuretic treatment, in a trial in 209 patients with class III heart failure, Hawthorn did show an increased level of tolerance to exercise [11]. A new double blind pilot study has also indicated a promising role for Hawthorn extract in mild, essential hypertension [12]. A recent review summarises these effects [13].

PREPARATIONS AND DOSE: Powdered leaf and flower, dose: 200–500 mg twice daily; dry extract, dose: 160–900 mg corresponding to 3.5–20 mg total flavonoids; powdered berry, dose: 0.3–1 g three times daily.

SPECIFIC REFERENCES: 1. Upton, R (Ed.) (1999) '*Hawthorn Leaf and Flower*' and '*Hawthorn Berry*' *American Herbal Pharmacopoeia*, Pub: AHP, Sacramento, USA. 2. Wagner H *et al* (1982) *Planta Med.* 45:98. 3. Rehwald A *et al* (1993) *Planta Med.* 59:A628. 4. Ammon H *et al* (1981) *Planta Med.* 43:105. 5. Bahorun T *et al* (1994) *Planta Med.* 60:323. 6. Mueller A *et al* (1999) *Planta Med.* 65:333. 7. Lacaille-Dubois M *et al* (2001) *Phytomedicine* 8(1):47. 8. Schussler M *et al* (1995) *Arneim. Forsch.* 45:842. 9. Schmidt U *et al* (1994) *Phytomedicine* 1(1):17. 10. Zapfe G (2001) *Phytomedicine* 8(4):62. 11. Tauchert M (2002) *Am. Heart J.* 143(5):910. 12. Walker A *et al* (2002) *Phytother. Res.* 16(1):48. 13. Chang Q *et al* (2002) *J. Clin. Pharmacol.* 42(6):605.

HEARTSEASE
VIOLA TRICOLOR L.
Fam. Violaceae

SYNONYMS: Wild Pansy.

HABITAT: A common British wild and garden plant.

DESCRIPTION: Leaves oval to broad lanceolate; stipules leafy, pinnately lobed. Flowers 1–2.5 cm in diameter, blue to violet, or yellow, with a spurred calyx. The herb has little taste or odour.

PART USED: Herb.

CONSTITUENTS: (i) Flavonoids, including violanthin (which is a di-glucoside of apigenin), vitexin, vicinine-2, saponarine, scoparin, violanthin, rutin (violaquercitrin) (ii) Methylsalicylate, traces [R2,R9;1,2].

MEDICINAL USE: Expectorant, diuretic, anti-inflammatory [R1]. Used for bronchitis, rheumatism, skin eruptions and eczema, and urinary disorders, often taken as an infusion or applied as a lotion.

SPECIFIC REFERENCES: 1. Molnar P *et al* (1986) *Phytochemistry* 25:195. 2. Komorowski T *et al* (1983) *Herba Pol.* 29:5.

HEATHER
CALLUNA VULGARIS (L.) HULL.
Fam. Ericaceae

SYNONYMS: Common or Scottish Heather; Ling.

HABITAT: A common European and North American wild and ornamental plant found particularly on moors, bogs and open woods.

DESCRIPTION: A carpeting, evergreen undershrub, with small, undivided, linear leaves arranged alternately. The flowers are pale purple, bell-shaped, borne on leafy spikes from July to September.

PART USED: Flowers.

CONSTITUENTS: (i) Hydroquinone and its glycosides; mainly arbutin (ii) Flavonoids, such as quercitrin and myricitrin (iii) Triterpenes including ursolic acid and uvaol (iii) Coumarins; scopoletin [R2;1,2,3,4].

MEDICINAL USE: Diuretic, urinary antimicrobial, anti-inflammatory and cholagogue. Heather flowers are used mainly to treat cystitis, gout and rheumatism. Aqueous extracts of heather have antimicrobial properties against *Staphylococcus aureus* and *S. epidermidis, Candida albicans* and *Cryptococcus neoformans* which were attributed to the hydroquinone (the aglycone of arbutin) and ursolic acid content [5]. Ursolic acid and uvaol are anti-inflammatory and inhibit both lipoxygenase and cyclo-oxygenase enzymes, as well as being anti-proliferative *in vitro* in a number of tumour cell lines [2,5,6,7]. Heather is often used in a similar way to Uva Ursi (q.v.) which also contains arbutin. The plant is prized as a source of pollen for honey (a constituent of the liqueur Drambuie) as well as forming a habitat for grouse and other game birds.

SPECIFIC REFERENCES: 1. Es-Saady D *et al* (1995) *Fitoterapia* 66(4):366.   211

2. Najid A *et al* (1992) *FEBS Lett.* 299(3):213. 3. Waksmundzka-Hajnos M *et al* (1997) *Acta Pol. Pharm.* 54(3):237. 4. Simon A *et al* (1994) *Phytochem.* 36:1043. 5. Braghirolli L *et al* (1996) *Phytother. Res.* 10(Suppl. 1):S86. 5. Es-Saady D *et al* (1994) *Mediators Inflam.* 3(3):181. 6. Tunon H *et al* (1995) *J. Ethnopharmacol.* 48(2):61

HEDGE HYSSOP

GRATIOLA OFFICINALIS L.
Fam. Scrophulariaceae

SYNONYMS: Gratiola.

HABITAT: A British and European wild plant found in damp places.

DESCRIPTION: A medium hairless perennial, with opposite, lanceolate, sessile leaves about 3 cm long and 0.5 cm broad, with a toothed margin near the tip. Flowers white or pale pink, tubular, with five stamens. Taste: acrid and bitter; odourless.

PART USED: Herb, root.

CONSTITUENTS: (i) Cucurbitacin glycosides, including gratiotoxin, and gratioside, elatineride and desacetyl elatineride (ii) Triterpene saponins including gratiolone (iii) Flavonoids [R2,R4;1].

MEDICINAL USE: Diuretic, emetic, cathartic [R1]. The cucurbitacins are cathartic and cytotoxic (see Bryony, White). The internal use of this plant is therefore not recommended.

SPECIFIC REFERENCES: 1. Muller A *et al* (1979) *Pharm. Ztg.* 124:1761.

HEDGE MUSTARD

SISYMBRIUM OFFICINALE L.
Fam. Brassicaceae

HABITAT: Common throughout Europe.

DESCRIPTION: The flowers are about 3 mm diameter, with pale yellow petals in the shape of a cross, followed by the pods which are 6–20 mm long and pressed to the stem. The stems long and spreading and the rosette leaves deeply pinnately lobed. Odour and taste: mustard-like.

PART USED: Herb.

CONSTITUENTS: (i) Glucosinolates; sinigrin, glucoputranjivin, gluconapin, glucocochlearin, glucocheirolin, glucobrassicin and neoglucobrassicin (ii) Cardioactive glycosides including corchoroside and helveticoside [R2;1,2,3].

MEDICINAL USE: Formerly used for hoarseness, weak lungs and to help the voice [R1]. The glucosinolates decompose to release volatile mustard oils.

SPECIFIC REFERENCES: 1. Bachelard H *et al* (1963) *Austral. J. Biol. Sci.* 16:147. 2. Ockendon J G *et al* (1979) *Trans. Br. Mycol. Soc.* 72:156. 3. Carnat A *et al* (1998) *Ann. Pharm. Francais.* 56(1):39.

HELLEBORE, AMERICAN

VERATRUM VIRIDE AIT.
Fam. Melanthiaceae

SYNONYMS: Green Hellebore, American Veratrum, Indian Poke.
White Hellebore is *V. album.*

HABITAT: North America and Canada. *V. album* is from
Central Europe.

DESCRIPTION: The rhizome is blackish, obconical, 5–8 cm long
and 1–3 cm diameter, with tufts of stem leaf remains at the top and
numerous shrivelled yellowish-brown rootlets. Internally it is whitish
with a ring of air spaces in the cortex and the endodermis and
vascular bundles visible in the centre. It closely resembles that of
White Hellebore. Taste: bitter and acrid; odourless but sternutatory.

PART USED: Rhizome.

CONSTITUENTS: (i) Steroidal alkaloids, classified into the jerveratrum
type, which are present as glycosides or free alkamines and include
pseudojervine and veratrosine; and the ceveratrum type which are
usually found as esters and include protoverine and veracevine esters.
V. album contains similar alkaloids (ii) Cardioactive glycosides;
hellebrin and glucohellebrin [R2,R3;1,2].

MEDICINAL USE: Hypotensive, cardiac depressant [R1]. Occasionally
used for high blood pressure, and formerly for toxaemia of pregnancy,
although not recommended for this purpose, as many of these
alkaloids are teratogenic. For example, the lambs of ewes fed on
White Hellebore are born with a single central eye, possibly the
inspiration for Homer's cyclops, Polyphemus. The ceveratrum-type
alkaloids are hypotensive; they cause peripheral vasodilatation, probably
by inhibition of the vasomotor centre and stimulation of the vagus
nerve. When taken by mouth overdose causes immediate vomiting,
so poisoning in this way is rare despite the toxicity of the plant. The
extract is insecticidal (see also Cevadilla). Veratrum is used more often
in homoeopathic medicine.

SPECIFIC REFERENCES: 1. Kupchan S *et al* (1961) *Lloydia* 24(1):17.
2. El-Sayed K *et al* (1996) *Int. J. Pharmacog.* 34:111.

HELLEBORE, BLACK

HELLEBORUS NIGER L.
Fam. Ranunculaceae

SYNONYMS: Christmas Rose, Melampodium.

HABITAT: Native to sub-alpine woods in southern and eastern
Europe, cultivated in Britain as an ornamental. The plant flowers in
mid-winter, hence the synonym.

DESCRIPTION: The rhizome is blackish, occurring as a tangled mass
of short branches, bearing straight, slender, rather brittle black rootlets
with a central cord. Taste: bitter and acrid; odour: faint, fatty.

PART USED: Rhizome.

CONSTITUENTS: Cardiac glycosides; helleborin, helleborein, hellebrin and others based on helleborigenin [R3;1,2].

MEDICINAL USE: Cardiac tonic, purgative, abortifacient [R1]. The glycosides have digitalis-like action (see Foxglove). They are dangerous and should be used only under medical supervision. The plant was formerly used to treat lice; however it has caused abortion in a pregnant woman using it for this purpose.

SPECIFIC REFERENCES: 1. Krenn K et al (1998) Phytochem. 48(1):1. 2. Steyn P et al (1998) Nat. Prod. Rep. 15(4):397.

HELLEBORE, FALSE
ADONIS VERNALIS L.
Fam. Ranunculaceae

SYNONYMS: Yellow Pheasant's Eye.

HABITAT: Northern Europe and Asia.

DESCRIPTION: Stem about 15–25 cm long, bearing feathery 2–3 pinnate leaves and a single large yellow flower, 40–80 mm across with ten or more petals and numerous stamens. Taste: slight; odourless.

PART USED: Herb.

CONSTITUENTS: (i) Cardiac glycosides, including adonitoxin, k-strophanthoside, cymarin, vernadigin and 16-hydroxystrophanthidin and others, based on the aglycones adonitoxigenin and adonitogenin (ii) 2,6-dimethoxybenzoquinone [R2;1,2].

MEDICINAL USE: Cardiac tonic, diuretic [R1]. The glycosides have digitalis-like action (see Foxglove). They stimulate the vagus nerve and increase the contractility and work output of the heart. This plant should be used only under medical supervision.

SPECIFIC REFERENCES: 1. Winkler C et al (1985) Pharm. Acta Helv. 60:234. 2. Kopp B et al (1992) Phytochem. 31:3195.

HEMLOCK
CONIUM MACULATUM L.
Fam. Apiaceae

HABITAT: Great Britain and Europe.

DESCRIPTION: Typically umbelliferous in appearance. The leaves are hairless, repeatedly pinnate, and the stem hollow, with distinctive and characteristic purplish blotches. Fruits ovate, plano-convex, indented on the flat surface with five ridges. Taste and odour: unpleasant, foetid. Hemlock has long been used as a poison, and was used by Socrates as a means of suicide.

PART USED: Leaves, unripe fruits.

CONSTITUENTS: (i) Alkaloids; mainly coniine, with gamma-coniceine, methylconiine, conhydrin, pseudoconhydrin and N-methylpseudoconhydrin (ii) Volatile oil (usually very low), the major component of which is myrcene [R3;1,2].

MEDICINAL USE: Sedative, anodyne. Formerly used for neuralgia. The alkaloids are very toxic and it should be used only under medical supervision, if at all.

BIBLICAL REFERENCES: Hosea 10:4; Amos 6:12 where Wormwood is meant (q.v.).

SPECIFIC REFERENCES: 1. Roberts M (1975) *Phytochem.* 14:2395. 2. Roberts M (1980) *Planta Med.* 39:216.

HEMP AGRIMONY
EUPATORIUM CANNABINUM L.
Fam. Asteraceae

SYNONYMS: Water Hemp.

HABITAT: A common European and British wild plant found in damp places.

DESCRIPTION: Stem angular, often reddish, striated, rough; leaves palmate, with 3–5 lobes, the segments lanceolate, irregularly serrate. Flower-heads: slender, tubular, pinkish, with all the florets rayless. Taste: sweetish, then bitter; odour: faintly aromatic.

PART USED: Herb.

CONSTITUENTS: (i) Volatile oil, containing alpha-terpinene, *p*-cymene, thymol, azulenes, neryl acetate, germacrene D and many others (ii) Sesquiterpene lactones, the major one being eupatoriopicrin, with eupatolide, eucannabolide, hydroxy eupatoriopicrin, peroxycannabinolide, sachalinin and others (iii) Pyrrolizidine alkaloids; supinine, intermedine, lycopsamine, trachelanthamine and amabiline (iv) Polysaccharides (v) Phenolics such as chlorogenic acid and luteolin [R2;1,2,3,4].

MEDICINAL USE: Diuretic, alterative [R1]. The polysaccharides have immunostimulatory activity; they enhance phagocytosis in a number of immunological test systems. However, eupatoriopicrin is considered to be the main active principle, and has been shown to be cytostatic as well as cytotoxic. It delayed transplanted tumour growth in mice in a dose-dependent manner and has shown a number of other anti-cancer activities [5,6]. Extracts of the herb have hepatoprotective effects in mice [7] despite the fact that the alkaloids are known hepatotoxins, probably because this is an effect shown after chronic administration. The sesquiterpene lactones can be allergenic [3]. The herb should not be taken internally unless the alkaloids are shown to be absent from the sample.

SPECIFIC REFERENCES: 1. Katochvil J *et al* (1971) *Phytochem.* 10:2529. 2. Zdero C *et al* (1986) *Planta Med.* 53(2):169. 3. Rucker G *et al* (1997) *Natural Toxins* 5(6):223. 4. Hendriks H *et al* (1987) *Planta Med.* 53(5):456. 5. Woerdenbag H *et al* (1987) *Phytother. Res.* 1(2):76 and (1988)2(3):109. 6. Woerdenbag H *et al* (1989) *Br. J. Cancer* 59(1):68. 7. Lexa A *et al* (1990) *Phytother. Res.* 4(4):148.

HENBANE

HYOSCYAMUS NIGER L.
Fam. Solanaceae

HABITAT: Grows in waste places in Britain and Europe.

DESCRIPTION: A slightly sticky, hairy, annual or biennial, with alternate leaves. In the annual plant these are smaller and usually sessile. In the biennial they are larger in the first year, up to 30 cm long, ovate or lanceolate, petiolate; and in the second year, 10–20 cm long with a deeply dentate margin and much more hairy. The flowers are five-lobed, tubular, creamy yellow with purplish veins. Taste and odour: unpleasant, characteristic.

PART USED: Leaves and flowering tops.

CONSTITUENTS: Tropane alkaloids, 0.045–0.14%, the principal ones being hyoscyamine and hyoscine (= scopolamine). Egyptian Henbane, *H. muticus*, contains higher concentrations of the alkaloids; this and other species of *Hyoscyamus* are used as a source of hyoscine [R3].

MEDICINAL USE: Antispasmodic, anodyne, sedative, mydriatic [R1]. The alkaloids are parasympatholytic, with similar actions to Belladonna (q.v.); although with less cerebral excitement. Henbane is used mainly for its antispasmodic effect on the digestive and urinary tracts, and to counteract griping due to purgatives. It is an ingredient of some anti-asthmatic smoking mixtures and herbal cigarettes. The alkaloid hyoscine is used very widely, as a pre-operative medication, to prevent travel sickness in the form of tablets and trans-dermal patches, and for many other purposes. The N-butyl bromide derivative is used to treat irritable bowel syndrome [R3,R14].

PREPARATIONS AND DOSE: Hyoscyamus Dry Extract BPC 2002, dose: 15–60 mg.

REGULATORY STATUS: POM or P, with restrictions.

HENNA

LAWSONIA INERMIS L.
Fam. Lythraceae

SYNONYMS: Henne, *L. alba* Lam.

HABITAT: Egypt, the Middle East, India.

DESCRIPTION: Leaves shortly stalked, smooth, lanceolate, up to 5 cm long, with revolute, entire margins and a mucronate apex. Taste: astringent; odour: tea-like.

PART USED: Leaves.

CONSTITUENTS: (i) Naphthaquinones, such as lawsone, isoplumbagin, lawsaritol and hennoside (ii) Coumarins; laxanthone I, II, and III (iii) Flavonoids; luteolin and its 7-O-glucoside, acacetin-7-O-glucoside (iv) Miscellaneous; beta-sitosterol-3-O-glucoside and other sterols, tannins etc. [1,2,3,4,5].

MEDICINAL USE: Astringent, anti-haemorrhagic, anti-inflammatory [R1]. It has been used to treat skin infections such as *Tinea*, and lawsone is known to be antibacterial, anti-fungal, cytotoxic and tuberculostatic *in vitro* and in rodents [1,6,7,8]. Extracts of the leaf have anti-inflammatory, analgesic and antipyretic effects [5,7] and show some liver protecting activity [9]. A fraction isolated from the leaf showed nootropic activity in various memory tests in mice [10]. Care should be taken if given internally due to suspected anti-fertility activity and other cytotoxic effects [11]. It is non-toxic when applied externally, although the practice by Bedouin people of covering baby boys with the dye has led to reports of haemolysis in G6PD deficient newborn babies [12]. Henna is used more often as a dye for the hair and in some eastern countries to stain the hands and feet orange-red, and to produce temporary 'tattoos', a practice which is now leading to an increasing number of allergic reactions [13].

BIBLICAL REFERENCES: In Song of Solomon 1:4 & 4:13 as 'camphire'.

SPECIFIC REFERENCES: 1. Karawya M *et al* (1969) *Lloydia* 32:76. 2. Mahmood Z *et al* (1983) *Fitoterapia* 4:153. 3. Gupta S *et al* (1994) *Nat. Prod. Lett.* 4(3):195. 4. Gupta S *et al* (1993) *Fitoterapia* 64(4):365. 5. Bardwaj D *et al* (1978) *Phytochem.* 17:1440. 6. Ali N *et al* (2001) *J. Ethnopharmacol.* 74(2):173. 7. Ali B *et al* (1995) *Pharmacol.* 52(6):356. 8. Sharma V (1990) *Tubercle* 71(4):293. 9. Anand K *et al* (1992) *Planta Med.* 58(1):22. 10. Iyer M *et al* (1998) *Indian J. Pharmacol.* 30(3):181. 11. Munshi S *et al* (1977) *Planta Med.* 31(1):73. 12. Kandil H *et al* (1996) *Ann. Trop. Paediatrics* 16(4):287. 13. Chung W *et al.* (2002). *Arch Dermatol* 1389(1):88.

HIMALAYAN CEDAR

CEDRUS DEODARA (D. DON) G. DON F.
Fam. Pinaceae

SYNONYMS: Deodar.

HABITAT: The western Himalayas and cultivated elsewhere.

DESCRIPTION: A majestic large evergreen reaching up to 85 m, with ascending spreading branches. The leaves are needle-like, dark green with a silver sheen, and arranged in whorls. The male cones are cylindrical and the female cones ovoid, with overlapping scales, both up to 12 cm long.

PART USED: Leaves, bark, heartwood.

CONSTITUENTS: (i) Essential oil, containing sesquiterpene hydrocarbons, beta-himachalene being the major component, up to around 90%, with alpha-himachalene and other isomers, himachol, atlantone, *p*-methylacetophenone and others (ii) Flavonoids, in the stem bark, including deodarin, taxifolin and quercetin [R16;1].

MEDICINAL USE: The oil is used in skin disorders, such as sores and ulcers, and to treat parasites. Veterinary studies have found it to be useful in treating mite infestations and mange. It is anti-fungal, in

217

secticidal, larvicidal and molluscicidal. Himachol is spasmolytic, and in general the plant exhibits low toxicity [R16 and refs therein; 2,3,4].

PREPARATIONS AND DOSE: Powdered wood, dose: 3–6 g; oil, dose: 0.5–3 ml.

SPECIFIC REFERENCES: 1. Nigam M (1990) *Indian Perfumer.* 34(4):278. 2. Kar K *et al* (1975) *J. Pharm. Sci.* 64(2):258. 3. Mall H *et al* (1985) *Indian Drugs* 22(6):296. 4. Singh D *et al* (1984) *Naturwissenschaften* 71(5):265.

HOLLY
ILEX AQUIFOLIUM L.
Fam. Aquifoliaceae

SYNONYMS: Holm, Hulm.

HABITAT: Grows freely in Britain and Europe.

DESCRIPTION: The bush is well-known; the leaves are shiny, leathery and with a spiny margin; the berries appear in early winter and are globular and bright red.

PART USED: Leaves, berries.

CONSTITUENTS: (i) Glycosides such as menidaurin (a nitrile, but not cyanogenetic) (ii) Flavonoids; mainly kaempferol and quercetin glycosides, including rutin (iii) Triterpenes including alpha- and beta-amyrin, ursolic acid, stigmasterol and campesterol (iv) Theobromine (in the leaf, unconfirmed) (v) Caffeic acid derivatives; chlorogenic acid [R2;1].

MEDICINAL USE: Diuretic, febrifuge, cathartic [R1]. Rarely used medicinally. An ethanolic extract has been shown to inhibit leukotriene B4 synthesis and have a free radical scavenging effect [2] and high doses cause a fatal drop in blood pressure in rats [3].

SPECIFIC REFERENCES: 1. Catalano S *et al* (1978) *Planta Med.* 33:416. 2. Muller K *et al* (1998) *Planta Med.* 64(6):536. 3. Lasser B *et al* (1983) *Naturwissenschaften* 70:95.

HOLLYHOCK
ALTHAEA ROSEA (L.) CAV.
Fam. Malvaceae

HABITAT: A well-known garden plant.

DESCRIPTION: The dried flowers are deep purplish black, about 6 cm in diameter. The corolla is united with the stamens, which form a tube; although the anthers, which are reniform, are free.

PART USED: Flowers.

CONSTITUENTS: (i) Flavonoids and anthocyanidins, based on malvidin (ii) mucilages (unspecified) [R4;1].

MEDICINAL USE: Emollient, demulcent, diuretic [R1]. Used in a similar way to Marshmallow (q.v.). An aqueous extract given to rats produced a significant elevation in androgens together with a decrease in estrogens, indicating a weak anti-oestrogenic effect and general effect on steroid metabolism [2].

SPECIFIC REFERENCES: 1. Takeda K et al (1988) Phytochem. 28(2):499. 2. Papiez M (2001) Fol. Histochem. Cytobiol. 39(2):219.

HOLY THISTLE
CNICUS BENEDICTUS L.
Fam. Asteraceae

SYNONYMS: Blessed Thistle, Carbenia benedicta Berul. Carduus benedictus Steud.

HABITAT: Coastal regions of the Mediterranean.

DESCRIPTION: Leaves greyish-green, thin and brittle, with prominent, pale veins and irregularly toothed margins, each tooth ending in a spine. Flower-heads are about 2 cm long and 4 cm broad, with bristly involucral scales. Taste: very bitter; odourless.

PART USED: Herb.

CONSTITUENTS: (i) Lignans; arctigenin, trachelogenin, nortracheloside, 2-acetylnortracheloside, and in the fruit, arctiin (ii) Sesquiterpene lactones; cnicin, salonitenolide (iii) Volatile oil, containing cinnamaldehyde, cuminaldehyde, citronellol, fenchone and paraffins (iv) Polyacetylenes (v) Miscellaneous; lithospermic acid, tannins and mucilages, potassium and manganese salts [R7;1,2,3,4,5,6,7].

MEDICINAL USE: Stomachic, bitter, anti-haemorrhagic, expectorant, antiseptic, vulnerary [R1]. It is used internally for anorexia, dyspepsia and catarrh; and externally for wounds and ulcers. Cnicin is anti-inflammatory [8] and has some antibiotic activity, and the essential oil and polyacetylenes are bacteriostatic [2,4]. The lignans are similar to those found in Burdock (q.v.) and have anti-tumour activity in human hepatoma and mouse sarcoma cell lines [6], as well as anti-HIV and PAF activity [7]. The bitter substances such as cnicin, are considered to have choleretic and hypolipidemic activities [8].

PREPARATIONS AND DOSE: Powdered herb, dose: 1.5–3 g or equivalent extract.

SPECIFIC REFERENCES: 1. Vanhaelen M et al (1975) Phytochem. 14:2709. 2. Vanhaelen-Fastre R (1974) Planta Med. 25:47. 3. Vanhaelen-Fastre R et al (1975) Planta Med. 26:375. 4. Vanhaelen-Fastre R et al (1973) Planta Med. 24:165. 5. Ulubelen A et al (1977) Planta Med. 31:375. 6. Moritani et al (1996) Biol. Pharm. Bull. 19:1515. 7. Tamayo C et al (2000) Phytother. Res. 14(1):1. 8. Schneider G et al (1987) Planta Med. 53:247.

HONEYSUCKLE
LONICERA CAPRIFOLIUM L.
Fam. Caprifoliaceae

SYNONYMS: Dutch Honeysuckle. Chinese or Japanese Honeysuckle is *L. japonica* Thunb.

HABITAT: Widespread in many parts of the world.

DESCRIPTION: The dried flowers are yellowish-brown, mostly tubular flower-buds mixed with the stalked heads of young fruits. Leaves, thin, up to 5 cm long and about 2–3 cm broad, oval and shortly stalked. Taste: sweet and mucilaginous; odour: imperceptible when dried.

PART USED: Flowers, leaves.

CONSTITUENTS: Unknown. Saponins and loganic acid have been reported [R2]. *L. japonica* contains: (i) Iridoids including loganin, secologanin, vogeloside and epivogeloside (ii) Saponins based on oleanolic acid or hederagenin (iii) Essential oil containing linalool, 2,6,6-trimethyl-2-vinyl-5-hydroxytetrahydropyran, geraniol, eugenol, carvacrol, hex-1-ene, hex-3-en-1-ol and others (iv) Flavones; lonicerin and loniceraflavone (v) Chlorogenic acid [R5:1].

MEDICINAL USE: Expectorant, laxative [R1]. Rarely used. However, *L. japonica* is widely used in traditional Chinese medicine for fever, inflammation, dysentery and abscess. The extract is bacteriostatic [R5].

SPECIFIC REFERENCES: 1. Kawai H *et al* (1988) *Chem. Pharm. Bull.* 36:3664 and 4769.

HOPS
HUMULUS LUPULUS L.
Fam. Cannabinaceae

HABITAT: Native to Europe, parts of Asia and North America, and extensively cultivated.

DESCRIPTION: The female flower (or strobile) is yellowish-green, cone-like, about 2.5–3 cm long and 2–2.5 cm broad, formed from two membranous scales, one of which bears the small seed-like fruit at the base. It is scattered with shining yellow glands; these can be separated by sifting and are then known as lupulin. Taste: bitter; odour: aromatic and characteristic.

PART USED: Strobiles.

CONSTITUENTS: (i) Volatile oil, composed mainly of humulene (= alpha-caryophyllene, about 90%), with beta-caryophyllene, myrcene, farnesene, 2-methylbut-3-ene-2-ol, 3-methylbut-2-ene-1-al, 2,3,5-trithiahexane and similar compounds (ii) Chalcones and other flavonoids; xanthohumol and isoxanthohumol, and a series of prenylated flavonoids and chalcones including 6-prenylnaringenin, 6-geranyl-naringenin, 6,8-diprenylnarigenin, and also glycosides of kaempferol and quercetin (iii) Oleo-resin, composed of alpha-bitter acids such as humulone, cohumulone, adhumulone, posthumulone and others; and beta-bitter acids such as lupulene, colupulone, adlupulone etc. and traces of 2-methylpropanoic and 3-methylbutanoic acids (v) Miscellaneous; tannins, lipids, and phenolic acids [R2,R7;1,2,3,4,5].

MEDICINAL USE: Sedative, tranquillizer, hypnotic, tonic, diuretic, anodyne and aromatic bitter [R1]. The sedative and tranquillizing activity is well-established in a variety of animal tests; it is due at least in part to the 2-methylbut-3-ene-2-ol. This substance, which is present in fresh extract, has been found to be absent from many commercial preparations; however these preparations are still efficacious and it is thought that the compound may be formed in the body from the alpha-bitter acids [3,4]. Hop pillows are a popular remedy for sleeplessness. Other pharmacological actions of hops include spasmolytic and antimicrobial activity; the bitter acids are antimicrobial [6] and anti-fungal [5] and an extract of hops is spasmolytic on isolated smooth muscle preparations. The presence of oestrogenic substances has been disputed [R7], but recently 6-prenylnaringenin and related compounds have been identified as phytoestrogens. The content is not high enough in hops (or beer) to be thought a problem with normal doses [7]. These compounds also have anti-proliferative and cytotoxic effects on certain human cancer cell lines *in vitro* [1] and inhibit those human cytochrome P450 enzymes responsible for the activation of some carcinogens [7]. Hop polyphenols also inhibit calcium flux in clonal rat pituitary cells [8]. Together these effects may account for the chemopreventive effect of hops, and the phytoestrogens may protect against breast and ovarian cancer to some extent. Most of the hops grown are used to produce beer, but whether all of the useful pharmacological effects of hops survive the brewing process is arguable.

PREPARATIONS AND DOSE: Powder, dose: 0.5–1 g or equivalent extract.

SPECIFIC REFERENCES: 1. Miranda C *et al* (1999) *Food Chem. Toxicol.* 37(4):271. 2. Song-San S *et al* (1989) *Phytochem.* 28:1776. 3. Wohlfart R *et al* (1982) *Arch. Pharm.* 315:132. 4. Hansel R *et al* (1982) *Planta Med.* 45:224. 5. Mizobuchi S *et al* (1985) *Agric. Biol. Chem.* 49:399. 6. Schmalreck A *et al* (1975) *Can. J. Microbiol.* 21:205. 7. Milligan S *et al* (2000) *J. Clin. Endocrinol. Metab.* 85(12): 4912. 8. Henderson M *et al* (2000) *Xenobiotica* 30(3):235.

HOREHOUND, BLACK

BALLOTA NIGRA L.
Fam. Lamiaceae

SYNONYMS: Marrubium nigrum Crantz.

HABITAT: Similar to White Horehound.

DESCRIPTION: Lower leaves cordate, upper leaves ovate; downy, with a crenate margin. Flowers purplish, labiate; calyx with five spreading, broadly ovate teeth. Taste and odour: unpleasant.

PART USED: Herb.

BLACK HOREHOUND

CONSTITUENTS: (i) Diterpenoids, including marrubiin, ballonigrin, ballotinone (= 7-oxomarrubiin), ballotenol, 7-alpha-acetoxymarrubiin,

221

13-hydroxyballonigrinolide and preleosibirin (ii) Phenylpropanoids such as verbascoside, forsythoside B, arenaioside, ballotetroside, allysonoside-5, lavandulifolioside-6, and angoroside A7. Iridoids have been shown to be absent [1,2,3,4,5].

MEDICINAL USE: Stimulant, antiemetic, antispasmodic [R1]. Also used for similar indications to Horehound (q.v.) although not so widely because of the unpleasant taste. The phenylpropanoids are antibacterial [3] and inhibit *in vitro* low-density lipoprotein (LDL) peroxidation. This activity is independent of any capacity to chelate copper induced LDL oxidation [6]. They act as antioxidants and are also sedative [7].

PREPARATIONS AND DOSE: Powdered herb, dose: 2–4 g or equivalent extract, three times daily.

SPECIFIC REFERENCES: 1. Savarona G *et al* (1976) *J. Chem. Soc. Perkin Trans.* I 1607 and (1977):497. 2. Bruno M *et al* (1986) *Phytochem.* 25:538. 3. Didry N *et al* (1999) *J. Ethnopharmacol.* 67(2):197. 4. Seidel V *et al* (1998) *Ann. Pharm. Francais* 55(1):31. 5. Seidel V *et al* (1998) *J. Pharm. Belgique* 51(2):72. 6. Seidel V *et al* (2000) *Phytother. Res.* 14(2):93. 7. Daels-Rakotoarison D *et al* (2000) *Arzneim. Forsch.* 50(1):16.

HOREHOUND, WHITE
MARRUBIUM VULGARE L.
Fam. Lamiaceae

SYNONYMS: White Horehound, Hoarhound.

HABITAT: Found growing wild throughout Europe, cultivated in Britain.

DESCRIPTION: A downy perennial. Leaves cordate-ovate, bluntly serrate, wrinkled and stalked; flowers small, white, in dense whorls, the calyx having 10 hooked teeth. Taste: bitter, aromatic; odour: characteristic.

PART USED: Herb.

CONSTITUENTS: (i) Labdane diterpenes, the major component being marrubiin, a lactone, together with premarrubiin and the alcohols marrubiol, marrubenol, sclareol, peregrinin, vulgarol and dihydroperegrinin (ii) Volatile oil, containing alpha-pinene, sabinene, limonene, camphene, bisabolol, p-cymol, fenchoene and alpha-terpinolene (iii) Alkaloids; traces of betonicine and its isomer turicine (iv) Miscellaneous; choline, alkanes, phytosterols, tannins etc [1,2,3,4].

MEDICINAL USE: Expectorant, bitter tonic, antiseptic [R1]. Horehound is used particularly for bronchitis and asthma. Marrubiin is considered to be responsible for the expectorant activity, as well as most of the other therapeutic effects of Horehound. It has been shown to normalize extrasystolic arrhythmias, and when the lactone ring is open the corresponding acid is strongly choleretic. Marrubiin is antinociceptive, but the analgesic activity is not due to any interaction with the opioid system [5]. It is also hypotensive and the activity is attributed to vascular relaxation [6]. The essential oil, although present only in traces, has antimicrobial properties and is also reported to be vasodilatory and hypotensive. Extracts of horehound are anti-inflammatory in the rat paw oedema test [7] and also have anti-serotonin activity [5]. Horehound is an ingredient of some tonics, candies and ales.

PREPARATIONS AND DOSE: Powdered herb, dose: 1–2 g, or equivalent extract, three times daily.

SPECIFIC REFERENCES: 1. Knoss W *et al* (1999) *Planta Med.* 64(4):357. 2. Kowalewski Z *et al* (1978) *Herba Pol.* 183. 3. Saleh M *et al* (1989) *Planta Med.* 55:105. 4. Popa D *et al* (1974) *Rastit. Resur.* 9(3):384, and (1975) 10(3):365. 5. De Jesus R *et al* (2000) *Phytomedicine* 7(2):1116. 6. El Bardai S *et al* (2001) *Clin. Exp. Hypertension* 23(4):329. 7. Mascolo N *et al* (1987) *Phytother. Res.* 1(1):28.

HORSE CHESTNUT

AESCULUS HIPPOCASTANUM L.
Fam. Hippocastanaceae

SYNONYMS: Hippocastanum vulgare Gaertn.

HABITAT: Native to western Asia but widely cultivated and naturalized in most temperate regions.

DESCRIPTION: A large tree reaching 30 m high, bearing large sticky buds, which open in early spring to produce leaves composed of 5–7 large, oval, sessile leaflets. The flowers are erect, candle-like, dense panicles, white or pink in colour. The tree bark in commerce is thick, greyish-brown externally, with elongated warts; pinkish-brown and finely striated internally; fracture finely fibrous and laminate. Taste: bitter and astringent; odourless. The fruits are characteristic spiny capsules, each with two to four compartments containing the large shiny brown seeds or 'conkers'.

PART USED: Seeds, occasionally bark.

CONSTITUENTS: (i) Saponins, a complex mixture known as 'aescin' or 'escin', composed of acylated glycosides of protoescigenin and barring-togenol-C. There are at least 30 of these, the most important being alpha and beta escin, and the escins Ia, Ib, IIa, IIb, IIIa etc. The acyl groups are often tiglic or angelic acids (ii) Sterols and triterpenes such friedelin, taraxerol and spinasterol (iii) Coumarins such as esculin (aesculin) and fraxin, and their aglycones (iv) Flavonoids based on quercetin and kaempferol (v) Procyanidins and anthocyanins, catechins and tannins [R7;1, and refs therein, 2,3].

MEDICINAL USE: Anti-inflammatory, venotonic and astringent [R1]. Extracts of Horse Chestnut, or more usually preparations of escin, are used particularly for chronic venous insufficiency (CVI), haemorrhoids and varicose veins, or feelings of 'heaviness' in the legs [7]. It can be used to decrease the likelihood of deep-vein thrombosis (DVT) after surgery and applied topically to bruises and sports injuries. Escin has been shown to reduce oedema and exudation, decreasing capillary permeability, increasing venous tone and reducing hypoxia. It antagonizes some of the effects of bradykinin and produces an increase in plasma levels of ACTH, corticosterone and glucose in rats. A number of clinical studies have shown benefits in CVI, DVT, varicose veins (including those of pregnancy), and for the prevention of oedema in the ankle and foot during an aeroplane flight (of 15 hours). It has been found to be effective in the treatment of cerebral oedema and a rise in intra-cranial pressure following road accidents. Venotonic effects, and an improvement in capillary resistance, have also been noted in healthy volunteers [R17;2,3,4,5,6,7,8,9,10]. Escin is also widely used in cosmetics [10]. For further information on the numerous clinical trials and pharmacological activities, see [R17,:11 and refs therein].

PREPARATIONS AND DOSE: Standardized extract, dose: usually 300 mg daily, equivalent to 100 g aescin.

SPECIFIC REFERENCES: 1. Bombardelli E *et al* (1996) *Fitoterapia* 67(6): 483. 2. Matsuda H *et al* (1994) *Biol. Pharm. Bull.* 20(10):1092. 3. Yoshikawa M *et al* (1994) *Chem. Pharm. Bull.* 42(6):1357. 4. Diehm C *et al* (1996) *Lancet* 347:292. 5. Marshall M *et al* (1987) *Phlebology* 2:123. 6. Wienert V (1997) *Int. J. Angiol.* 6(2):115. 7 . Diehm C *et al* (1996) *Phlebology* 11(1):23. 8. Leskow P (1996) *Therapie Woch.* 46:874. 9. Pittler M *et al* (1998) *Arch. Dermatol.* 134:1356. 10. Wilkinson J *et al* (1999) *Int. J. Cosmet. Sci.* 21:437. 11. Sirtori C *et al* (2001) *Pharm. Res.* 44(3):183.

HORSEMINT, AMERICAN
MONARDA PUNCTATA L.
Fam. Lamiaceae

SYNONYMS: American Horsemint.

HABITAT: North America.

DESCRIPTION: Leaves opposite, lanceolate, smooth. The flowers occur in axillary tufts, the corolla is yellow with purple spots and two stamens and the sessile bracts yellow and purple. Taste: pungent and bitter; odour: rather like thyme.

PART USED: Leaves, tops.

CONSTITUENTS: Volatile oil, the major component of which is thymol [R4]. The related species, *M. fistulosa* contains thymol and thymoquinone [1].

MEDICINAL USE: Stimulant, carminative, emmenagogue. Experiments on the related *M. fistulosa* showed that thymoquinone has cytotoxic effects against various human tumour cells lines, particularly for CNS, prostate, breast, melanoma and ovarian tumours [1].

SPECIFIC REFERENCES: 1. Johnson H *et al* (1998) *Nat. Prod. Lett.* 11(4):241.

HORSEMINT, ENGLISH

MENTHA LONGIFOLIA (L.) HUDS.
Fam. Lamiaceae

SYNONYMS: Mentha sylvestris L.

HABITAT: Throughout Britain and Europe.

DESCRIPTION: Leaves opposite, nearly sessile, ovate- lanccolate, serrate and downy on the undersurface. Flowers lilac, typically labiate, in axillary clusters or a terminal spike. Taste and odour recalling that of garden mint.

PART USED: Herb.

CONSTITUENTS: (i) Volatile oil, the major components of which vary widely, but include diosphenol, rotundifolone, piperitone oxide, beta-caryophyllene, germacrene-D, menthol, menthofuran, menthone, epoxypulegone, carvone and others [R2;1] (ii) Flavone glycosides such as isoorientin, vicenin-2, lucenin-1, hypolaetin, and apigenin-, tricetin- and luteolin glycosides (iii) Phenolic acids [2,3].

MEDICINAL USE: Carminative, stimulant [R1]. The essential oil exhibits CNS-depressant activity [1] and the crude ethanol extract, which is rich in polyphenols, has been found to be a CNS stimulant, with hepatoprotective and choleretic effects [3,4].

SPECIFIC REFERENCES: 1. Perez-Raya M *et al* (1990) *Phytother. Res.* 4(6):232. 2. Sharaf M *et al* (1999) *Fitoterapia* 70(5):478. 3. Mimica-Dukic N *et al* (1996) *Int. J. Pharmacog.* 34(5):359. 4. Mimica-Dukic N *et al* (1999) *Pharm. Biol.* 37(3):221.

HORSENETTLE

SOLANUM CAROLINENSE L.
Fam. Solanaceae

SYNONYMS: Bullnettle, Sandbrier.

HABITAT: Eastern North America, growing on sandy soil

DESCRIPTION: Root cylindrical, smooth with a few slender rootlets, with a thin pale brown bark which is easily abraded, showing white underneath. Fracture, tough, woody. Taste: bitter then sweetish; odourless.

PART USED: Root, berries.

CONSTITUENTS: Alkaloids; anabasine, cuscohygrine, solanine, solasodine, solamine and solaurethine [1].

MEDICINAL USE: Antispasmodic, sedative [R1]. An aqueous extract is antibacterial [1].

SPECIFIC REFERENCES: 1. Evans W *et al* (1977) *Phytochem.* 16:1859.

HORSERADISH
RADICULA ARMORACIA (L.) ROBINSON.
Fam. Brassicaceae

SYNONYMS: *Armoracia rusticana* (Gaertn) Mey. and Scherb. *A. lapathifolia* Gilib., *Cochlearia armoracia* L. *Nasturtium armoracia* Fries., *Roripa armoracia* Hitch.

HABITAT: Eastern Europe, but cultivated in Britain and North America.

DESCRIPTION: Root yellowish-white, cylindrical, about 2 cm thick, with a fleshy consistency. Usually sold fresh. Taste and odour when crushed or scraped, pungent, mustard-like.

PART USED: Root.

CONSTITUENTS: (i) Glucosinolates, mainly sinigrin, gluconasturtiin, glucoberteroin, glucocapparin, glucocheirolin, glucocochlearin and glucobrassicin, which releases volatile isothiocyanates on contact with the enzyme myrosin during crushing (ii) Coumarins including scopoletin and aesuletin (iii) Caffeic and hydroxycinnamic acid derivatives (higher in the leaf than the root) (iv) Peroxidase enzymes, in large amounts (v) Miscellaneous; vitamins, asparagine, resin, sugars [R4,R7,1,2,3].

MEDICINAL USE: Stimulant, diaphoretic, diuretic, antiseptic [R1]. Formerly used for respiratory and urinary infections, kidney stones and externally as a poultice in inflammatory conditions. The oil is highly irritant and isothiocyanates are known to be goitrogenic, so large doses of horseradish should be avoided. The peroxidase enzymes caused hypotension in the cat, when injected intravenously, thought to be due to stimulation of arachidonic acid metabolites [3]. However this is unlikely to be relevant to oral ingestion of Horseradish. Now used more often as a condiment or relish.

SPECIFIC REFERENCES: 1. J Harborne and H Baxter (Eds) *Phytochemical Dictionary.* Pub: Taylor and Francis London, UK (1993). 2. Stoehr H *et al* (1975) *Z. Lebens. Unters Forsch.* 159:219. 3. Sjaastad O *et al* (1984) *J. Histochem. Cytochem.* 32:1328.

HORSETAIL
EQUISETUM ARVENSE L.
Fam. Equisetaceae

HABITAT: Common on wet ground and waste places throughout Europe, Asia, China, Japan and North America.

DESCRIPTION: A perennial herb reaching up to 80 cm but usually less. Stems hollow, grooved, green, bearing whorls of branches at the nodes, leaves reduced to sheaths above the nodes. Taste and odour: slight.

PART USED: Herb.

CONSTITUENTS: (i) Alkaloids, including nicotine, palustrine and palustrinine (ii) Flavonoids, mainly apigenin, genkwanin, kaempferol, luteolin and quercetin glycosides (iii) Sterols including cholesterol, isofucosterol, campesterol and others (iv) Silicic acid, up to 8% (v) Caffeic acid derivatives (vi) Miscellaneous; loliolide, equisetumpyrone, equisitonin, dimethylsulphone, thiaminase and aconitic acid [R2;1,2,3,4,5,6,7].

MEDICINAL USE: Haemostatic, astringent [R1]. Horsetail is taken for genito-urinary complaints such as cystitis, prostatitis, urethritis and enuresis. It may be used internally as an anti-haemorrhagic and externally as a styptic and vulnerary. Diuretic and spasmolytic effects have been observed in animals, and silicic acid from Horsetail protected against experimental liver injury in rats [8]. Uptake of silicon and calcium was determined over two years in 122 post menopausal women with osteoporosis, using a Horsetail extract with a calcium supplement, and an increase in bone density demonstrated [9]. A feeding study in rats suggested that Horsetail should not be taken by individuals who consume a cholesterol-rich diet [10]. Extracts can cause dermatitis. The related species *E. myriochaetum* reduced blood glucose levels in a small placebo controlled crossover study of 11 patients with recently diagnosed type 2 diabetes [11].

PREPARATIONS AND DOSE: Powdered herb, dose:1–4 g or equivalent extract.

SPECIFIC REFERENCES: 1. Veit M *et al* (1990) *Phytochem.* 30:527. 2. Carnat A *et al* (1991) *Plantes Med. Phytother.* 25(1):32. 3. Veit M *et al* (1992) *Phytochem.* 31:3483. 4. Veit M *et al* (1993) *Phytochem.* 32:1029. 5. Fabre B *et al* (1993) *Plantes Med. Phytother.* 26(3):1904. 6. Veit M *et al* (1995) *Phytochem.* 39:915. 7. Hiraga Y *et al* (1997) *Nat. Prod. Lett.* 10(3):181. 8. Li S-Y *et al* (1992) *Chin. J. Pharmacol. Toxicol.* 6(1):67. 9. Corletto F (1999) *Minerva Ortoped. Traumatol.* 50(5):201. 10. Maeda H *et al* (1997) *J. Nutr. Sci. Vitaminol.* 43(5):553. 11. Revilla M *et al* (2002) *J. Ethnopharmacol.* 81(1):117.

HOUNDSTONGUE
CYNOGLOSSUM OFFICINALE L.
Fam. Boraginaceae

SYNONYMS: Dog's Tongue.

HABITAT: Grows in dry grassy places and dunes.

DESCRIPTION: A greyish biennial, softly downy, with alternate, long, lanceolate leaves and dark red, funnel-shaped flowers. Odour: like mice.

PART USED: Herb.

CONSTITUENTS: (i) Pyrrolizidine alkaloids; cynoglossine, consolidine, heliosupine, echinatine [1] (ii) Allantoin (iii) Miscellaneous; tannin 8–9%, choline, mucilage, resin [R4].

MEDICINAL USE: Anodyne, demulcent, astringent [R1]. Due to the toxic alkaloids its use is not recommended.

SPECIFIC REFERENCES: 1. Van Dam N *et al* (1993) *Planta Med.* 59(7S):A646.

HOUSELEEK

SEMPERVIVUM TECTORUM L.
Fam. Crassulaceae

HABITAT: A common garden plant in Britain and Europe.

DESCRIPTION: Leaves forming a rosette 5–8 cm in diameter, fleshy, sessile, oblong-ovate, incurved, pointed and hairy at the margin. Taste: saline, astringent and acid; odourless.

PART USED: Fresh leaves.

CONSTITUENTS: (i) Polyphenolic compounds including phenolcarboxylic acids and anthocyanidins (ii) Flavone and flavanol mono- and di-glycosides (unspecified) [1].

MEDICINAL USE: Refrigerant, astringent [R1]. The fresh leaves have been bruised and applied as a poultice for burns and stings etc. The juice has potent antioxidant, free-radical scavenging and membrane-stabilizing abilities, reducing ascorbic acid and ferric-chloride-induced lipid peroxidation in microsomal suspensions of rat liver [1]. A freeze-dried extract lowered HDL-cholesterol levels and protected against experimental liver damage [1,3], and also improved various parameters of liver function, such as normalizing cytochrome P450 enzymes and restoring reactivity of spleen cells in rats fed an atherogenic diet [2,3].

SPECIFIC REFERENCES: 1. Blazovics A *et al* (1993) *Phytother. Res.* 7(1):95 and 98. 2. Blazovics A *et al* (1994) *Phytother. Res.* 8(1):33. 3. Blazovics A *et al* (2000) *J. Ethnopharmacol.* 73(3):479.

HYDRANGEA

HYDRANGEA ARBORESCENS L.
Fam. Saxifragaceae

SYNONYMS: Wild Hydrangea, Seven Barks.

HABITAT: North America. Hydrangea species are widely cultivated as ornamentals.

DESCRIPTION: Root pale fawn-coloured, smooth with tapering branches; bark very thin. Fracture hard and woody, showing a radiate structure and in larger pieces, a distinct pith. Taste: sweetish then pungent; odourless.

PART USED: Root.

CONSTITUENTS: Largely unknown (i) Flavonoids; kaempferol and quercetin (ii) Other reported constituents include umbelliferone (= hydrangin), saponin, volatile oil etc. Tannins are reportedly absent [R7;1,2]. Other species of *Hydrangea*, notably *H. macrophylla* Ser. *var thunbergii* Makino, have been more extensively investigated. This species contains (i) Stilbene derivatives, such as hydrangenol and hydrangeic acid [3] (ii) Secoiridoid glucoside complexes, the hydramacrosides A and B [4] (iii) Isocoumarins including phyllodulein, phyllodulcin, thunberginol and hydrangenol glucosides (iv) Umbelliferone [5].

MEDICINAL USE: Diuretic, nephritic [R1]. Used traditionally to treat, and prevent urinary complaints, including kidney and bladder stones. The extract has been shown to be non-toxic in animals [2]. Other species are used for their anti-allergic effects and the hydramacrosides A and B inhibit histamine release from mast cells induced by antigen-antibody reaction [4]. Hydrangenol also exhibits anti-allergic properties and inhibits activation of hyaluronidase [6].

PREPARATIONS AND DOSE: Powdered root and rhizome, dose: 2–4 g or equivalent extract.

SPECIFIC REFERENCES: 1. Bate-Smith E (1978) *Phytochem.* 17:267. 2. Der Mardirossian A *et al* (1976) *J. Toxicol. Environ. Health* 1:939. 3. J Harborne and H Baxter (Eds) *Phytochemical Dictionary.* Pub: Taylor and Francis London, UK (1993). 4. Yohikawa M *et al* (1994) *Chem. Pharm. Bull.* 42(8):1691. 5.Yohikawa M *et al* (1999) *Chem. Pharm. Bull.* 47(3):383. 6. Kakegawa H *et al* (1988) *Planta Med.* 54:385.

HYDROCOTYLE

CENTELLA ASIATICA (L.) URBAN.
Fam. Apiaceae

SYNONYMS: Indian Pennywort, Gotu Kola, *Hydrocotyle asiatica* L.

HABITAT: Indian and Pakistan, China, Madagascar, South Africa and most countries in Southeast Asia

DESCRIPTION: A small, herbaceous, slender, creeping perennial. The leaves are glabrous, kidney-shaped, up to 2.5 cm in diameter, with a crenate margin and rounded apex. The flowers are pale violet and the umbels each bear 2–5 fruits with a hard pericarp. Taste and odour: faint, tobacco-like.

PART USED: Herb.

CONSTITUENTS: (i) Saponins; asiaticoside, oxyasiaticoside, brahminoside, brahmoside, centelloside, madecassoside, isothankuniside, thankuniside and others; and free asiatic, brahmic, centellinic, isobrahmic, madecassic and betulinic acids (ii) Volatile oil, containing trans-farnesene, germacrene-D, beta-caryophyllene, beta-elemene, bicycloelemene and other minor components (iii) Flavonoids based on quercetin and kaempferol (iv) Phytosterols; stigmasterol and beta-sitosterol [R2,R7,R16;1,2,3].

MEDICINAL USE: Vulnerary, dermatic, anti-leprotic, anti-inflammatory [R1]. The main uses are for the treatment of certain skin conditions, particularly ulcers, wounds and for keloid and hypertrophic scars, and as an immunomodulator. The wound-healing effects have been demonstrated in a number of studies in animals, and included radiation burns. The activity was shown to be due to the saponin content. Tensile strength and collagen content were increased, and antioxidant activity was considered to play an important part in the effect [4,5,6]. It was shown to improve subjective and objective clinical findings in a small trial of patients with venous disorders of the lower limbs [7] and to

229

prevent and treat scarring both after burns and post-operatively [8]. The extract inhibited the growth of human fibroblasts *in vitro* and stimulated phagocytosis in mice. A recent clinical trial has demonstrated the healing properties of a tincture on wounds [9]. It may be taken orally, often as an infusion, and applied topically. The immunomodulating effects of the herb have been shown *in vitro* and *in vivo* in mice, and other reported effects include anti-ulcer activity [10], and psychoneurological, anti-tubercular and spasmolytic effects. For further information see [R7,R11,R16 and refs therein].

PREPARATIONS AND DOSE: Powdered leaf, dose: 0.5–1 g daily, or equivalent extract.

SPECIFIC REFERENCES: 1. Asakawa Y *et al* (1982) *Phytochem.* 21(10):2590. 2. Singh B *et al* (1969) *Phytochem.* 8:917. 3. Wong K *et al* (1994) *J. Ess. Oil Res.* 6(3):307. 4. Shukla A *et al* (1999) *J. Ethnopharmacol.* 65(1):1. 5. Maquart F *et al* (1999) *Eur. J. Dermatol.* 9(4):289. 6. Shukla A *et al* (1999) *Phytother. Res.* 13(1):50. 7. Allegra G *et al* (1981) *Clin. Ther.* 99:507. 8. Bosse J-P *et al* (1979) *Ann. Plastic Surg.* 3(1):13. 9. Morisset (1987) *Phyther. Res.*1(3):117. 10. Cheng C *et al* (2000) *Life Sci.* 67(21):2647.

HYSSOP
HYSSOPUS OFFICINALIS L.
Fam. Lamiaceae

HABITAT: Indigenous to southern Europe but cultivated elsewhere.

DESCRIPTION: Leaves linear-lanceolate, nearly sessile, about 2 cm long and 23 mm broad, hairy on the margin. Flowers small, blue, labiate, in axillary tufts arranged on one side, with a calyx of five uneven teeth. Taste: bitter; odour: aromatic and camphoraceous.

PART USED: Herb.

CONSTITUENTS: (i) Volatile oil, composed mainly of camphor, pinocamphone, pinocarvone, thujone and isopinocamphone, with alpha- and beta-pinene, alpha-terpinene, linalool, bornyl acetate and many others (ii) Flavonoids, including diosmin and hesperidin (iii) Diterpenes including marrubiin (iv) Triterpenes; oleanolic and ursolic acids (v) Caffeic acid derivatives including rosmarinic acid (vi) A polysaccharide referred to as MAR-10 [R2;1,2,3].

MEDICINAL USE: Stimulant, carminative, pectoral, sedative [R1]. Hyssop is used for bronchitis, coughs and colds. It contains marrubiin, which is an expectorant (see Horehound) and ursolic acid, which has anti-inflammatory activity. The plant extract shows anti-HIV (human immunodeficiency virus) activity *in vitro* [4], and the polysaccharide MAR-10 strongly inhibits replication of HIV-Type 1 [3] in cultured peripheral blood mononucleocytes. The essential oil of Hyssop is antispasmodic [1] and bacteriostatic [6].

PREPARATIONS AND DOSE: Powdered herb, dose: 2–4g or equivalent extract, three times daily.

BIBLICAL REFERENCES: Exodus 12:22; Leviticus 14:4, 6, 49, 51, 52; Numbers 19:6, 18; Psalm 51:7 probably Syrian marjoram (*Origanum syriacum*), also John 19:29 and Hebrews 9:19.

SPECIFIC REFERENCES: 1. Mazzanti G *et al* (1998) *Phytother. Res.* 12:S92. 2. Varga E *et al* (1998) *Acta Pharm. Hungarica* 68(3):183. 3. Gollspufi S *et al* (1995) *Biochem. Biophys. Res. Commun.* 210(1):145. 4. Kreis W *et al* (1990) *Antiviral Res.* 14(6):323. 5. Bedoya L *et al* (2002) *Phytother. Res.* 16(6):550. 6. Marino M *et al* (2001) *Int. J. Food Microbiol.* 67(3):187.

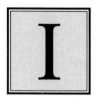

IBOGA
TABERNANTHE IBOGA STAPF.
Fam. Apocynaceae

SYNONYMS: Ibogo.

HABITAT: Central and West Africa, especially the Congo and Cameroon.

DESCRIPTION: A shrub with simple, entire leaves and an extensive network of laticifers, which yield a milky sap.

PART USED: Root bark.

CONSTITUENTS: Terpenic indole alkaloids, mainly ibogaine, ibogamine, ibogaline, voacangine and derivatives, and 18-methylcoronaridine [1,2].

MEDICINAL USE: Narcotic, stimulant, hallucinogenic. Extracts of the root bark have been used by indigenous peoples to ameliorate thirst, hunger and fatigue, as an aphrodisiac, and in many rituals. Ibogaine is hallucinogenic, and a CNS stimulant; in large doses can cause paralysis and respiratory arrest. More recently it has been advocated as a method of reducing the craving of heroin addiction and has been used clinically for this purpose. Experiments with rats demonstrate that ibogaine interferes with naloxone-induced morphine withdrawal [3] and numerous mechanisms of action have been postulated. Ibogaine is metabolised to noribogaine *in vivo* and both compounds increase corticosterone levels in the body [4]. Noribogaine is more potent as a serotonin agonist than ibogaine, with fewer side effects than the parent compound [5]. Ibogaine is a non-competitive NMDA receptor antagonist [6]. Both ibogaine and 18-methyl coronaridine are antagonists at the alpha-3beta-4 nicotinic receptor [7] and inhibit cholinergic contraction of guinea pig ileum, which was not affected by naloxone; both enhance purinergic contractions of rat isolated vas deferens [8]. Iboga alkaloids have been suggested as an aid to alcohol withdrawal [9]. However, ibogaine is not only hallucinogenic but also neurotoxic, thought to be by inhibiting glutamate uptake [10], so it should only be used under medical supervision.

SPECIFIC REFERENCES: 1. Popik P *et al* (1999) *The Alkaloids* 52:197. 2. Popik P *et al* (1995) *Pharmacol. Rev.* 47:235. 3. Parker L *et al* (2002) *Prog. Neuropsychopharmacol. Biol. Psychiatry* 26(2):293. 4. Szumlinski K *et al* (2001) *Pharmacol. Biochem. Behav.* 69(3–4):485. 5. Baumann M *et al* (2001) *J. Pharmacol. Exp. Ther.* 297(2):531. 6. Leal M *et al* (2000) *Neurochem. Res.* 25(8):1083. 7. Glicks *et al* (2002) *Eur. J. Pharmacol.* 438(1–2):99. 8. Mundey M *et al* (2000) *Br. J. Pharmacol.* 129(8):1561. 9. Rezvani A *et al* (1995) *Pharmacol. Biochem. Behav.* 52:615. 10. Leal M al (2001) *NeuroReport.* 12(12):263.

ICELAND MOSS
CETRARIA ISLANDICA (L.) ACH.
Fam. Parmeliaceae

SYNONYMS: Iceland Lichen.

Habitat: Grows in most northern countries.

Description: Thallus smooth, greyish- or olive-brown, about 6 cm long, curled or channelled, terminating in spreading, flattened lobes which are fringed with small papillae. The undersurface is paler with minute, depressed, white spots. Taste: bitter; odour: when wet, recalls that of seaweed.

Part Used: Lichen.

Constituents: (i) Lichenic acids (depsidones); mainly fumarprotocetraric, protocetraric, cetraric, protolichesteric, lichesteric, lichesterenic, protolichesterinic, and usnic acids (ii) Polysaccharides, mainly glucans such as lichenan and isolichenan (iii) Miscellaneous; furan derivatives, fatty acid lactones and terpenes [1,2,3].

Medicinal Use: Demulcent, expectorant, antiemetic, nutritive [R1]. Extracts of Iceland Moss are an ingredient of some cough lozenges and have been used to treat inflammation and dryness of the pharyngeal mucosa. A clinical trial of patients who had undergone surgery of the nasal septum supported this type of use, and no side effects were observed [4]. The emollient properties are due mainly to the polysaccharides; however the other constituents also have useful biological activities. Usnic acid and related compounds inhibit tumour promoter-induced Epstein-Barr activation [5]. Protolichesterinic acid inhibits arachidonic acid lipoxygenase activity and shows anti-proliferative effects in malignant cell lines [6], and inhibits HIV-1 reverse transcriptase *in vitro* [7]. It also shows antimicrobial activity against *Mycobacterium aurum* (a non-pathogenic organism with a similar sensitivity profile to *M. tuberculosis*) [8] and against *Helicobacter pyloris*, one of the causes of peptic ulcer [9]. Iceland Moss is generally non-toxic but can concentrate heavy metals, and the lichenic acids are bitter and potentially toxic in large doses [10].

Preparations and Dose: Dried lichen, dose: 1–2 g or equivalent extract.

Specific References: 1. Kramer P *et al* (1995) *Arzneim. Forsch.* 45(6):726. 2. Gudjonsdottir G *et al* (1997) *J. Chromatog.* 757(1–2):303. 3. Ingolfsdottir K *et al* (1994) *Planta Med.* 60(6):527. 4. Kempe C *et al* (1997) *Laryngo-Rhino-Otologie* 76(3):186. 5. Yamamoto Y *et al* (1995) *Chem. Pharm. Bull.* 43(8):1388. 6. Ogmundsdottir H *et al* (1998) *J. Pharm. Pharmacol.* 50(1):107. 7. Pengsuparp T *et al* (1995) *J. Nat. Prod.* 58(7):1024. 8. Ingolfsdottir K *et al* (1998) *Eur. J. Pharm. Sci.* 6(2):141. 9. Ingolfsdottir K *et al* (1997) *Antimicrob. Agents Chemother.* 41(1):215. 10. Airaksinen M *et al* (1986) *Arch. Toxicol.* 59(Suppl.9):406.

IGNATIUS BEANS

Strychnos ignatii Berg.
Fam. Loganiaceae

Synonyms: S. *cuspida* A. W. Hill, S. *lanceolaris* Miq., S. *ovalifolia* Wall ex G. Don.

HABITAT: The Philippines and other parts of Southeast Asia.

DESCRIPTION: Seeds ovoid, irregularly angular, about 2.5 cm long and 2 cm across, with a distinct hilum at one end. Externally dull grey, with occasional fragments of brown epidermis still adhering. Fracture: hard, horny. Taste: intensely bitter; odourless.

PART USED: Seeds.

CONSTITUENTS: Indole alkaloids; brucine and its *N*-oxide, alpha- and beta-colubrine, diaboline, icajine, novacine, strychnine and its *N*-oxide, 10-hydroxystrychnine, isostrychnine, pseudostrychnine, protostrychnine, macusine B and its *O*-methyl derivative, normelinonine B, vomicine and others [1].

MEDICINAL USE: Stimulant, tonic [R1]. The alkaloids and their properties are similar to those of Nux Vomica (q.v.), including their extremely poisonous nature.

REGULATORY STATUS: Schedule 1 Poison.

SPECIFIC REFERENCES: 1. Datta B *et al* (1990) *Planta Med.* 56(1):133.

INDIAN PHYSIC
GILLENIA TRIFOLIATA MOENSCH.
G. STIPULACEA PURSH.
Fam. Rosaceae

SYNONYMS: Indian Hippo, *Spiraea trifoliata* L., *S. stipulata* Muhl.

HABITAT: North America.

DESCRIPTION: The roots are cylindrical, usually fissured transversely, 2–4 mm in diameter and up to 15 cm long. The external surface is blackish, and the transverse section shows a thick reddish bark which easily separates from the white woody centre. Taste: pleasantly bitter; odourless.

PART USED: Root bark.

CONSTITUENTS: No information available. A substance known as 'gillein' has been reported [R2].

MEDICINAL USE: Expectorant, cathartic, emetic [R1]. The American Indians are thought to have used it in a similar way to Ipecacuanha (q.v.).

IPECACUANHA
CEPHAELIS IPECACUANHA (BROTERO) A. RICH.
C. ACUMINATA KARSTEN
Fam. Rubiaceae

SYNONYMS: Ipecac. Rio, Matto Grosso or Brazilian Ipecac, *Psychotria ipecacuanha* Stokes apply to *C. ipecacuanha*; Cartagena, Nicaragua or Panama Ipecac to *C. acuminata.*

HABITAT: *C. ipecacuanba* is native to tropical South America, including Brazil, and cultivated in southern Asia; *C. acuminata* is from Central America.

DESCRIPTION: C. ipecacuanha root is slender, tortuous, reddish-brown, up to about 4 mm in diameter, with a characteristic annular appearance. *C. acuminata* has fewer annulations and is larger, up to 7 mm diameter, and externally greyish-brown. Taste: bitter; odour: slight. The powder is sternutatory.

PART USED: Root, rhizome.

CONSTITUENTS: (i) Isoquinoline alkaloids; usually about 2–3%, consisting mainly of emetine and cephaeline, with psychotrine, O-methylpsychotrine, emetamine and protoemetine (ii) Monoterpene isoquinoline glucosides such as ipecoside and alangiside (iii) Iridoids including sweroside and 7-dehydrologanin (iv) Tannins; ipecacuanhin and ipecacuanhic acid [R3;1,2,3,4].

MEDICINAL USE: Expectorant, emetic, stimulant, diaphoretic, amoebicide. Ipecac extract is an ingredient of many cough preparations because of its expectorant activity. It is well-known as an emetic [5] and is routinely employed to induce vomiting in cases of drug overdose, particularly in children, although this usage has been questioned recently [6]. The alkaloids are clinically useful in the treatment of amoebiasis and although active in a number of anti-tumour systems *in vitro*, have not proved effective in treating leukaemia. Emetine and cephaeline are metabolized by cytochrome P450 enzymes, but a study has shown that they are unlikely to affect plasma levels of any other drugs which may be co-administered with them [7].

PREPARATIONS AND DOSE: Ipecacuanha Liquid Extract (LE) BP, dose: 0.25–1 ml; tincture BP 1973 0.25–1 ml. Ipecacuanha Emetic Mixture BP (contains 0.7 ml Ipecac LE in 10 ml), dose: 10 ml (infants) to 30 ml (adults).

SPECIFIC REFERENCES: 1. Fujii T *et al* (1998) *The Alkaloids* 51:271. 2. Itoh A *et al* (1989) *Chem. Pharm. Bull.* 37:1137. 3. Itoh A *et al* (1991) *Phytochem.* 30:3117. 4. Itoh A *et al* (1993) *Phytochem.* 32:761. 5. Rudd J *et al* (1998) *Eur. J. Pharmacol.* 352(22–3):143. 6. Quang L *et al* (2000) *Curr. Opinion Pediatrics* 12(2):153. 7. Asano T *et al* (2001) *Biol. Pharm. Bull.* 24(6):678.

IRISH MOSS
CHONDRUS CRISPUS (L.) STACKH.
Fam. Gigartinaceae

SYNONYMS: Carrageenan, Carragheen. Other related spp. of the order Gigartinales (red algae), including *Mastocarpus stellatus* and species of *Euchema* and *Gigartina* may be used.

HABITAT: The Atlantic coast of Europe and North America.

DESCRIPTION: The seaweed has a cylindrical base and a flat, forked frond with a fan-shaped outline, reaching up to 25 cm long, 0.3–1.25 cm wide and 1–2 mm thick. Taste: mucilaginous and saline.

PART USED: Whole seaweed.

CONSTITUENTS: (i) Polysaccharides. The extract, also known as

235

'carrageenin', consists of sulphated, straight chain galactans (called carrageenins or carrageenans). There are several different types, a gelling fraction known as kappa-carrageenin and a non-gelling fraction known as lambda-carrageenin, together with iota- and nu- and mixed carrageenins. They are composed of *O*-galactose and 3,6-anhydrogalactose residues with a high proportion of sulphate esters, but are differentiated by the relative proportions and the number, type and position of the sulphate esters [1] (ii) Hordenine, an amine, in *M. stellatus* [2] (iii) Fatty acids such as palmitic, oleic, arachidonic and eicosapentaenoic acids [3].

MEDICINAL USE: Demulcent, antitussive, nutritive [R1]. Used for coughs, bronchitis and for irritations of the kidney and bladder. The carrageenins of low molecular weight (around 20,000), including the degraded forms, have been reported to have toxic effects in animals when injected and ingested but no toxicity has been observed in humans when taken orally. Food grades of high molecular weight are not normally absorbed through the gut and are considered to be non-toxic. Injected carrageenin is used to produce experimental inflammation for testing the effects of drugs, where it produces a type of adjuvant-induced arthritis, the mechanisms of which are complex [4,5,6]. The carrageenins also inhibit herpes simplex virus types 1 and 2 and human immunodeficiency virus [1,7,8], and have anti-ulcer effects [9]. Irish Moss extracts are used extensively in the preparation of manufactured foods.

PREPARATIONS AND DOSE: Dried thallus, dose: 5–10 g, as an infusion.

SPECIFIC REFERENCES: 1. Carlucci M *et al* (1999) *Chemotherapy* 45(6):429. 2. Barwell C *et al* (1989) *Phytother. Res.* 3(2):67. 3. Pettitt T *et al* (1988) *Phytochem.* 28(2):399. 4. Silvan A *et al* (1996) *Gen. Pharmacol.* 27(4):639. 5. Suganuma T *et al* (1998) *Biol. Pharm. Bull.* 21(7):756. 6. Gao X *et al* (2000) *Eur. J. Pharmacol.* 406(1):53. 7. Carlucci M *et al* (1999) *Antiviral Res.* 43(2):93. 8. Schaeffer D *et al* (2000) *Ecotoxicol. Environ. Safety* 45(3):208. 9. Nagaoka M *et al* (2000) *Biofactors* 12(1–4):267.

ISPAGHULA

PLANTAGO OVATA FORSK.
Fam. Plantaginaceae

SYNONYMS: Blond Psyllium, Spogel, Indian Plantago, *P. decumbens* Forsk., *P. ispaghula* Roxb.

HABITAT: Native to the Mediterranean region, cultivated widely throughout the world, including Russia and China. *P. ovata* is cultivated in India and Pakistan.

DESCRIPTION: The seeds are pinkish- or greyish-brown, boat-shaped, 1.8–3.3 mm long.

PART USED: Seeds, seed husk.

CONSTITUENTS: (i) Mucilage, 10–30%, consisting of a mixture of polysaccharides composed of mainly of D-xylose units, with smaller amounts of L-arabinose and aldobiouronic acid (ii) Monoterpene alkaloids; (+)-boschniakine (= indicaine) and (+)-boschniakinic acid (= plantagonine) (iii) Iridoids such as aucubin (iv) Triterpenes including the sterols stigmasterol, beta-sitosterol, campesterol, and alpha- and beta-amyrin (v) Fixed oil rich in polyunsaturated fatty acids etc. (vi) Sugars [R2,R7].

MEDICINAL USE: Bulk laxative; anti-dysenteric [R1]. The seeds swell when moistened into a gelatinous mass, promoting peristalsis and hydrating the faeces. The bulk thus formed also has a beneficial effect in diarrhoea. *P. ovata* seed has also been shown in rats to absorb a mixture of food additives including cyclamate, thus preventing harmful effects [1]. Ispaghula is thought to have a stimulant laxative effect in addition to the effect of the fibre [2]. More recently, it has been found clinically that supplementation of orlistat (the anti-obesity drug) with ispaghula husk reduced adverse gastrointestinal side effects [3]. In another study, a randomized, placebo, crossover trial, it also reduced plasma LDL-cholesterol concentrations when given at a dose of 15 g/day for 30 days to various groups of people. In these cohorts, it was also found that supplementation reduced plasma triglyceride levels in men, increased triglyceride levels in post-menopausal women, and had no effect on pre-menopausal women [4]. The seed is more effective than the husk in reducing serum cholesterol levels [5] and the mucilage appears to exert its effect without fermentation or decomposition in the gut [6]. The mucilage also suppressed the humoral immune response in animals, possibly indicating a useful additional effect in inflammatory bowel disease [7]. Extracts of the husk showed anti-amoebic effects against three species of *Entamoeba, in vitro* [8], supporting the traditional use of Isphagula in diarrhoea and dysentery.

PREPARATIONS AND DOSE: For constipation: dried seed husk, dose: 3.5–7 g; dried seeds, dose: 5–10 g taken after soaking in warm water for several hours.

SPECIFIC REFERENCES: 1. Ershoff B *et al* (1976) *J. Food Sci.* 41:949. 2. Gilani A *et al* (1998) *Phytother. Res.* 12:S63. 3. Cavaliere H *et al* (2001) *Int. J. Obesity* 25(7):1095. 4. Vega-Lopez S *et al* (2001) *Am. J. Clin. Nutr.* 74(4):435. 5. Gelissen I *et al* (1994) *Am. J. Clin. Nutr.* 59(2):385. 6. Marteau P *et al* (1994) *Gut* 35(12):1747. 7. Rezaeipoor R *et al* (2000) *J. Ethnopharmacol.* 72(1–2):283. 8. Zaman V *et al* (2002) *Phytother. Res.* 16(1):78.

IVY

HEDERA HELIX L.
Fam. Araliaceae

HABITAT: A common European plant, found also in northern and eastern Asia and introduced into America.

DESCRIPTION: Leaves dark green, paler beneath, leathery, shiny, long-stalked, about 5–10 cm wide, radiate veined with three to four triangular lobes. The upper leaves may be ovate. The berries are purplish-black, globular, 48 mm in diameter, with the calyx ring visible at the apex. Taste: bitter and nauseous; odour: aromatic and slightly resinous when rubbed.

PART USED: Leaves, berries.

CONSTITUENTS: (i) Saponins; based on oleanolic acid, bayogenin and hederagenin, including hederosaponins (hederacosides) B, C and D, alpha- and beta-hederin, hederacolchiside and others (ii) Sterols such as campesterol and beta-sitosterol (iii) Polyacetylenes such as falcarinol and derivatives (iv) Essential oil containing methyl ethyl ketone and methyl isobutyl ketone (v) Flavonoids including rutin, quercetin, astragalin and others (vi) Caffeic acid derivatives including chlorogenic, neochlorogenic, protocatechuic and rosmarinic acids [R2;1,2,3,4,5].

MEDICINAL USE: Cathartic, febrifuge, diaphoretic, anthelmintic [R1]. It is widely used in preparations for bronchitis and catarrh, as an expectorant [5,6]. A recent post-marketing, multi-centre surveillance study in 1350 patients confirmed the efficacy of Ivy leaf extract (97.5 or 130 mg/day) for chronic bronchitis. Improved expectoration and pain in respiration were observed after four weeks of treatment [6]. The saponins and sapogenins are the main active ingredients; they are expectorant, amoebicidal, anti-fungal and molluscicidal and kill liver flukes both *in vitro* and *in vivo* [1,5,7]. Hederagenin, hederocolchiside A1, alpha- and beta-hederins and hederosaponins B,C and D are anti-leishmanial *in vitro* [8,9]. The saponins are antimutagenic and anticlastogenic [10,11], and inhibit hyaluronidase activity [12]. Both the saponin and the flavonoid fractions are spasmolytic [2]. Extracts have been shown to have antithrombin effects *in vitro* [13]. Occasionally allergic reactions may be seen; these are due at least in part to the falcarinol content [14]. Ivy extracts are often used in cosmetic preparations to treat cellulite, with some success [15]; however in general, few clinical studies have been carried out.

PREPARATIONS AND DOSE: Dried leaf, dose: 300 mg or equivalent extract.

SPECIFIC REFERENCES: 1. Balansard G *et al* (1980) *Planta Med.* 39:234. 2. Trute A *et al* (1997) *Planta Med.* 63(2):125 and 177. 3. Elias R *et al* (1991) *J. Nat. Prod.* 54(1):98. 4. Hansen L *et al* (1985) *Phytochem.* 25:285. 5. Landgrebe H *et al* (1999) *Pharm. Ztg.* 144(35):11. 6. Hecker M *et al* (2002) *Forsch. Komplement. Klass Naturheil.* 9(2):77. 7. Julien J *et al* (1985) *Planta Med.* 51(3):205. 8. Majester-Savornin B *et al* (1991) *Planta Med.* 57(3):260. 9. Ridoux O *et al* (2001) *Phytother. Res.* 15(4):298. 10. Elias R *et al* (1990) *Mutagenesis* 5(4):327. 11. Amara-Mokrane Y *et al* (1996) *Mutagenesis* 11(2):161. 12. Facino R *et al* (1995) *Arch. Pharm.* 328(10):720. 13. De Medeiros J *et al* (2000) *J. Ethnopharmacol.* 72(1–2):157. 14. Gafner F *et al* (1988) *Contact Dermatitis* 19(2):125. 15. Maffei F *et al* (1990) *Acta Therapeutica* 16(4):337.

IVY, AMERICAN

PARTHENOCISSUS QUINQUEFOLIA K. PLANCH.
Fam. Vitaceae

SYNONYMS: Virginian Creeper, Woodvine, *Cissus hederacea* Ross, *C. quinquefolia* Desf., *Vitis quinquefolia* Lam.

HABITAT: North America, but cultivated as an ornamental in Europe and elsewhere.

DESCRIPTION: The bark occurs in quilled pieces, externally brown, with enlarged, transverse lenticels. The fracture shows a whitish bark with coarse, flattened fibres in the inner portion. Taste: insipid; odour: faintly aromatic.

PART USED: Bark, twigs.

CONSTITUENTS: Anthocyanins [R4]. The berries contain oxalic acid, but the main active constituents are unknown [R2].

MEDICINAL USE: Tonic, expectorant, astringent [R1]; as a decoction.

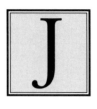

JABORANDI
PILOCARPUS MICROPHYLLUS STAPF.
AND OTHER SPP. OF *PILOCARPUS*
Fam. Rutaceae

SYNONYMS: Maranham Jaborandi. Pernambuco Jaborandi is from *P. jaborandi* Holmes, and Paraguay Jaborandi from *P. pinnatifolius* Lemaire.

HABITAT: Brazil.

DESCRIPTION: Leaflets dull green, up to 5 cm long and 3 cm wide, with entire, slightly recurved margins and an unequal base. The veins are prominent on the upper surface and oil cells are visible. The other species are larger, with only minor differences. Taste: bitter, odour: slightly aromatic.

PART USED: Leaves.

CONSTITUENTS: (i) Imidazole alkaloids; pilocarpine, isopilocarpine, pilosine, isopilosine, epiisopilosine (ii) Volatile oil, containing limonene, sabinene, alpha-pinene and caryophyllene [R3;1,2,3]. The other two species have a lower alkaloid content than *P. microphyllus.*

MEDICINAL USE: Stimulant, expectorant, diaphoretic, miotic [R1]. Jaborandi has also been used in hair tonics to stimulate hair growth. Pilocarpine is a sympathomimetic agent, causing salivation and has been licensed in North America for use in dryness of the mouth following radiation treatment for cancer of the head and neck [R3]. It also produces tachycardia and other effects. Its main use is in ophthalmic preparations as a miotic, in open-angle glaucoma and to contract the pupil after the use of atropine.

PREPARATIONS AND DOSE: Pilocarpine Eye Drops BP, 1%, 2% and 4%.

SPECIFIC REFERENCES: 1. Pinheiro C (1997) *Econ. Bot.* 51:49. 2. Hill, K In: *The Alkaloids* Pub: Wiley, UK (1983). 3. Craveiro A *et al* (1979) *J. Nat. Prod.* 42:169.

JACOB'S LADDER
POLEMONIUM COERULEUM L.
Fam. Polemoniaceae

SYNONYMS: Greek Valerian, English Greek Valerian.

HABITAT: Northern Europe, rare in Britain.

DESCRIPTION: Leaves pinnate, alternate; flowers in a cluster, purplish-blue, open, with five petal-lobes. Taste: slightly bitter; odourless.

PART USED: Herb.

CONSTITUENTS: (i) Triterpene saponins, polemonium saponins 1-3, based on camelliagenin (ii) Miscellaneous; volatile oil, resins and organic acids [R2,1,2,3].

MEDICINAL USE: Diaphoretic, astringent [R1]. Thought to be similar in effect to Abscess Root (q.v.). The saponins are anti-fungal [4] and the ethanol extract of the plant is both cytostatic and cytotoxic to human lymphoma Raji cells and others [5].

SPECIFIC REFERENCES: 1. Reznicek G *et al* (1993) *Planta Med.* 59:A612. 2. Reznicek G *et al* (1994) *Pharmazie* 49(1):58 and (4):300. 3. Aurada E *et al* (1982) *Sci. Pharm.* 50(4):331. 4. Hiller K *et al* (1981) *Pharmazie* 36(2):133. 5. Narimov A *et al* (1996) *Eksper. Onkol.* 18(3):287.

JALAP
IPOMOEA PURGA HAYNE
Fam. Convolvulaceae

SYNONYMS: Mexican Jalap, Vera Cruz Jalap, *I. jalapa* Scheide and Deppe, *Convolvulus jalapa* L., *C. purga* Wend., *Exogonium purga* Benth. Brazilian Jalap is *I. operculata.*

HABITAT: Mexico.

DESCRIPTION: Roots usually ovoid, up to about 15 cm long, very hard and heavy. Externally dark brown, wrinkled, with paler, transverse lenticels. Fracture: hard, horny, showing a greyish interior.

PART USED: Tuberous root.

CONSTITUENTS: Resin, containing glycoretins such as jalapin, convolvin, convulvin. The resins are composed of short chain fatty acids, e.g. valeric, tiglic and exegonic acid, and sugars such as quinovosides [R2,R3;1,2]. Brazilian Jalap contains similar compounds called operculins [3].

MEDICINAL USE: Cathartic, purgative [R1]. Usually used with carminatives and other laxatives to prevent griping. Brazilian Jalap is sometimes substituted; it has similar effects.

SPECIFIC REFERENCES: 1. Singh S *et al* (1973) *Phytochem.* 12:1701. 2. Linajes A *et al* (1994) *Econ. Bot.* 48:84. 3. Ono T *et al* (1992) *Chem. Pharm. Bull.* 40:1400.

JAMAICA DOGWOOD
PISCIDIA PISCIPULA (L.) SARG.
Fam. Fabaceae

SYNONYMS: Fish Poison Tree, *P. erythrina* L.

HABITAT: West Indies, South America.

DESCRIPTION: The bark occurs in quilled pieces, up to about 15 cm long and 3–6 mm thick, dark grey-brown externally with thin, longitudinal and transverse ridges, roughish and wrinkled, and somewhat fissured. Fracture: tough, fibrous, showing blue-green or brownish-green patches. Taste: bitter and acrid; odour: characteristic.

PART USED: Bark.

CONSTITUENTS: (i) Isoflavones; lisetin, jamaicin, ichthyone,

241

piscerythrone, piscidone and the rotenoids rotenone, milletone, isomilletone, sumatrol, and others (ii) Organic acids, including piscidic acid (*p*-hydroxybenzyltartaric acid), its mono- and diethyl esters, fukiic acid and its 3'-O-methyl ester (iii) Miscellaneous; beta-sitosterol, tannins etc [R3;1,2,3,4,5].

MEDICINAL USE: Analgesic, sedative, antispasmodic [R1]. Used particularly for neuralgia, migraine, insomnia, female complaints, whooping cough and asthma. An extract has been demonstrated to have antispasmodic, antitussive, antipyretic, anti-inflammatory and sedative actions in animals, with very low toxicity [6]. The spasmolytic principles were shown to be the isoflavones [4]. Rotenones are insecticidal and piscicidal and Jamaica Dogwood has been used for this purpose; they are irritant but relatively harmless to mammals.

PREPARATIONS AND DOSE: Dried root bark 1–2g as a decoction, or equivalent extract, three times daily.

SPECIFIC REFERENCES: 1. Pietta P *et al* (1983) *J. Chromatog.* 260:267. 2. Redaelli C *et al* (1984) *Phytochem.* 23:2976. 3. Delle Monache F *et al* (1984) *Phytochem.* 23:2945. 4. Della Loggia R *et al* (1988) *Prog. Clin. Biol. Res.* 280:365. 5. Heller W A *et al* (1975) *Helv. Chim. Acta* 58:974. 6. Aurousseau M *et al* (1965) *Ann. Pharm. Fr.* 23:251.

JAMBUL
SYZYGIUM CUMINI (L.) SKEELS.
Fam. Myrtaceae

SYNONYMS: Java Plum, Jamun, *S. jambolanum* D.C., *S. jambos* Alston, *Eugenia jambolana* Lam., *E. cumini* Druce, *Myrtus cumini* L.

HABITAT: Native to India, Indonesia and Australasia, but cultivated and naturalized widely throughout Asia, tropical America, the Caribbean and Africa.

DESCRIPTION: The tree is an evergreen reaching up to 50 m, with lanceolate, coriaceous leaves dotted with visible oil glands. The bark is smooth, greyish and exfoliating; the seeds sub-cylindrical, about 6 mm long and rather less in diameter; one end truncated and with a central depression. Externally hard and tough, blackish-brown; internally pinkish-brown. Taste: faintly astringent and aromatic; odour: slight.

PART USED: Bark, fruits, leaves.

CONSTITUENTS: (i) Triterpenes, such as Eugenia triterpenes A and B in the fruit; and betulinic acid, friedelin, daucosterol and others in the bark (ii) Phenolics, including methylxanthoxylin and 2,6-dihydroxy-4-methoxyacetophenone; ellagic, gallic and caffeic acids in the bark and fruit (iii) Flavonoids such as quercetin in the fruit pulp and bark, and astragalin, myricetin and others in the bark (iv) Essential oil containing eugenol, beta-phellandrene, terpinolene and others (v) Miscellaneous sugars, vitamins (in the pulp) and fatty acids (in the seeds) [R12,R16 and refs therein].

MEDICINAL USE: Anti-diabetic, astringent, diuretic [R1]. The bark and seeds are commonly used as anti-diabetic agents. A number of studies have demonstrated hypoglycaemic activity in animals [1,2,3], together with a reduction in hyperlipidemia, and also in human volunteers [4] and diabetic patients [R12]. The leaf extract is anti-inflammatory and antipyretic [5], and the seeds and bark are also anti-inflammatory as shown in the rat paw oedema test [6,7]. Anti-diarrhoeal effects have also been observed in rats [8]. Extracts of the seeds have some central nervous system depressant effects, including anticonvulsant and sedative properties [9]. For further detail see [R12 and R16].

PREPARATIONS AND DOSE: Bark, dose: 3–6 g daily; seed, dose: 2 g daily; leaf, dose: 15–20 g; or equivalent extract.

SPECIFIC REFERENCES: 1. Grover J *et al* (2000) *J. Ethnopharmacol.* 73(3):461. 2. Grover J *et al* (2001) *J. Ethnopharmacol.* 76(3):233. 3. Vikrant V *et al* (2001) *J. Ethnopharmacol.* 76(2):139. 4. Bhatt H *et al* (1983) *Asian Med. J.* 26(7):489. 5. Slowing K *et al* (1994) *J. Ethnopharmacol.* 43(1):9. 6. Mahapatra P *et al* (1986) *Planta Med.* 6:540. 7. Muruganandan S *et al* (2001) *Fitoterapia* 72:369. 8. Mukherjee P *et al* (1989) *J. Ethnopharmacol.* 60(1):85. 9. De Lima M *et al* (1998) *Phytother. Res.* 12(7):488.

JAVA TEA
ORTHIOSIPHON STAMINEUS BENTH.
Fam. Lamiaceae

SYNONYMS: O. aristatus Miq., *O. spicatus* Bak.

HABITAT: Native to Indonesia, cultivated elsewhere.

DESCRIPTION: The leaf is lanceolate-ovate, up to 7.5cm in length, with an acute apex, cuneate base and a short petiole. The upper surface is pale greyish-green, and the lower surface dark green or brownish. The margin is irregularly dentate. Flowers, if present, are bluish-white or purplish. Taste and odour: astringent and aromatic.

PART USED: Leaves.

CONSTITUENTS: (i) Flavonoids including sinensetin, eupatorin, slavigenin, cirsimaritin, pilloin, rhamnazin, tetramethylscutellarein and others (ii) Diterpenes of the isopimarane type, such as orthosiphonones A and B, orthosiphols A, B, F, G H, and the pimaranes neoorthosiphols A and B, and staminol (iii) Essential oil containing beta-elemene, alpha-humulene, beta-caryophyllene oxide and others (iv) Benzochromones including orthochromene A, methylripariochromene and acetovanillochromene (v) Phenolic acids such as caffeic and rosmarinic acids [R7;1,2,3,4,5,6,7,8,9].

MEDICINAL USE: Traditionally used in Java as an anti-diabetic, diuretic and antihypertensive. It is also used for kidney and bladder disorders, gallstones and gout. Diuretic properties have been recorded for the extracts [10,11,12] and attributed to the methylripari-ochromene content [8] and the flavonoids [5]. Hypoglycaemic effects observed in experimentally diabetic rats [13]. The neoorthosiphols

243

suppressed the contractile effect on isolated rat thoracic aorta [14]. The flavonoids inhibit lipoxygenase, which supports the anti-inflammatory usage [7]. Other reported effects of Java tea include antibacterial, anti-fungal and cytostatic effects *in vitro,* activity against a melanoma cell line, and antioxidant properties. Clinical studies are sparse and so far inconclusive for most indications. For further information, see [R7 and refs therein].

PREPARATIONS AND DOSE: Powdered leaf, dose: 6–12 g daily, or equivalent extract.

SPECIFIC REFERENCES: 1. Shibuya H *et al* (1999) *Chem. Pharm. Bull.* 47:695 and 911. 2. Guerin J-C *et al* (1989) *J. Nat. Prod.* 52:171. 3. Matsuda T *et al* (1992) *Tetrahedron* 48:6787. 4. Stampoulis P *et al* (1999) *Tet. Lett.* 40:4239. 5. Schut G *et al* (1986) *Planta Med.* 52:240. 6. Malterud K *et al* (1989) *Planta Med.* 55:569. 7. Lyckander I *et al* (1992) *Acta Pharm. Nord.* 4:159. 8. Matsubara T *et al* (1999) *Biol. Pharm. Bull.* 22:1083. 9. Sumaryono W *et al* (1991) *Planta Med.* 57:176. 10. Englert J *et al* (1992) *Planta Med.* 58:237. 11. Schut G *et al* (1993) *Fitoterapia* 64:99. 12. Beaux D *et al* (1998) *Phytother. Res.* 12:498. 13. Mariam A *et al* (1996) *Fitoterapia* 67:465. 14. Ohashi K *et al* (2000) *Chem. Pharm. Bull.* 48:433.

JEWEL WEED
IMPATIENS AURENS MUHL.
I. BIFLORA WALT.
Fam. Balsaminaceae

SYNONYMS: Balsam Weed, Pale Touch-Me-Not, *I. pallida* Nutt., (*I. aurea*); Spotted Touch-Me-Not, Speckled Jewels, *I. fulva* (*I. biflora*).

HABITAT: Indonesia, North America.

DESCRIPTION: Leaves grey-green, thin, ovate, more or less dentate; stem jointed. Flowers axillary, solitary, slipper-shaped with a long, recurved spur. Those of *I. aurea* are pale yellow and those of *I. biflora* are orange-yellow and spotted. The valves of the fruit curl up when dehisced.

PART USED: Herb.

Constituents: Naphthalene derivatives; mainly 2-hydroxy-2,4-naphthoquinone (lawsone) [R2]. For details of the effects of lawsone, see Henna. The related plant *I. balsamina* L. has been investigated to a greater extent; it contains (i) Naphthoquinones including lawsone, di-(2-hydroxy-1,4-naphthoquinone)-3-methane and 2-methoxy-1,4-naphthoquinone (ii) Flavonoids such as rutin, astragalin, quercetin and nicotiflorin [1].

MEDICINAL USE: Aperient, diuretic [R1]. The fresh plant has been made into an ointment for the treatment of haemorrhoids, and the juice is reputed to remove warts and corns, and to cure ringworm. A clinical study, using a topically applied extract against poison ivy-induced dermatitis, did not show any beneficial effect [2].

I. balsamina is used topically for all types of itching and insect bites; it has anti-allergic and anti-anaphylactic properties which have been demonstrated in a number of pharmacological models, including atopic dermatitis and chronic pruritis. These effects appear to involve platelet activating factor (PAF) as well as histamine [1,3,4,5,6].

SPECIFIC REFERENCES: 1. Fukumoto H *et al* (1996) *Phytother. Res.* 10:202. 2. Long D *et al* (1997) *Am. J. Contact Dermatitis* 8(93):150. 3. Fukumoto H *et al* (1995) *Phytother. Res.* 9(4):567. 4. Ishiguro K *et al* (1997) *Phytother. Res.* 11:48 and 343. 5. Ishiguro K *et al* (1999) *Phytother. Res.* 13:521. 6. Oku H *et al* (2001) *Phytother. Res.* 15:506.

JUJUBE
ZYZYPHUS JUJUBE MILL.
Fam. Rhamnaceae

SYNONYMS: The closely related *Z. vulgaris* Lamk. is also used.

HABITAT: Africa, Middle East, Far East.

DESCRIPTION: Fruits of variable size, depending on origin, usually up to 3 cm long and 1.5 cm in diameter, red, smooth and shiny when fresh, brownish-red and wrinkled when dried; fleshy and containing one or two seeds. Taste: sweet and mucilaginous.

PART USED: Berries.

CONSTITUENTS: (i) Saponins of the dammarane type, known as the jujubasaponins I-III, the zyzyphus saponins I, II and III, jujubosides A and B, zizybeosides I and II, and zizyvyosides I and II, proto-jujubosides A, B etc. together with at least 11 pentacyclic triterpenoids including betulinic, oleanolic and ursolic acids [1,2,3,4,5,6] (ii) Cyclopeptide alkaloids such as jubanine-C, scutianine-C, and zizyphine A [7].

MEDICINAL USE: Emollient, sedative, antitussive, anti-allergic and nutrient [R1]. In the Far East it is taken to improve muscular strength, increase body weight, protect the liver and kidney, lower blood pressure and prevent stress ulcer formation. Recent work there has shown that extracts of the fruit increase levels of cyclic AMP in leucocytes, and that the fruit itself contains very high levels of both cyclic AMP and cyclic GMP [4]. It stimulates release of nitric oxide from cultured endothelial cells and kidney tissues, which may help to explain the traditional use for kidney diseases and hypertension [8]. The triterpenes are cytotoxic *in vitro* and have anti-hepatitis B virus activity [2], and the protojujubo-sides show potent immunological adjuvant activity [6]. Leaf extracts are hypoglycaemic in rats [9].

SPECIFIC REFERENCES: 1. Okamura N *et al* (1981) *Chem. Pharm. Bull.* 29:676 and 3507. 2. Huang R *et al* (2001) *Chin. Pharm. J.* 53:179. 3. Yagi A *et al* (1978) *Chem. Pharm. Bull.* 26:3075. 4. Cyong J *et al* (1982) *Chem. Pharm. Bull.* 30:1081. 5. Yoshikawa K *et al* (1991) *Chem. Pharm. Bull.* 32(48):7059. 6. Matsuda H *et al* (1999) *Chem. Pharm. Bull.* 47(12):1744. 7. Tripathi M *et al* (2001) *Fitoterapia* 72(5):507. 8. Kim H *et al* (1996) *Asia Pacific J. Pharmacol.* 11(3–4):121. 9. Erenmemisoglu A *et al* (1995) *J. Pharm. Pharmacol.* 47(1):72.

JUNIPER

JUNIPERUS COMMUNIS L.
Fam. Cupressaceae

HABITAT: Widely distributed throughout the world, particularly Europe.

DESCRIPTION: The fruit, usually called a 'berry' which it resembles, is about 0.5–1 cm in diameter, globular, purplish-black with a grey bloom, and three lines or furrows joined at the apex, indicating the junction of the three seeds. Taste and odour: characteristic.

PART USED: Fruit.

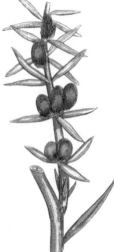

JUNIPER

CONSTITUENTS: (i) Volatile oil, up to 2%, containing mainly myrcene, sabinene and alpha-pinene, with 1,4-cineole, p-cymene, camphene, limonene, beta-pinene, terpinen-4-ol, gamma-terpinene, alpha-thujene and others (ii) Condensed tannins; (+)-afzelechin, (–)-epiafzelechin, (+)-catechin, (–)-epicatechin, (+)-gallocatechin and (+)-epigallocatechin (iii) Diterpene acids; myrceocommunic, communic, sandaracopimaric, isopimaric, torulosic acids and other diterpenes such as geijerone (iv) Flavonoids: armentoflavone, apigenin and others (v) Miscellaneous: desoxypodophyllotoxin, 1,4-dimethyl-3-cyclohexen-1-yl methyl ketone sugars, resin, vitamin C [R2,R7;1,2,3,4,5].

MEDICINAL USE: Diuretic, antiseptic, carminative, anti-inflammatory [R1]. Juniper is used mainly for acute and chronic cystitis and rheumatism, and the anti-inflammatory effects have been demonstrated *in vivo* [6]. The diuretic activity of an extract has been confirmed in rats and shown to be due to various constituents including the essential oil [7]. Hypoglycaemic and hypotensive effects have also been observed [R7;8]. The anti-fertility effects are well-known, and have been confirmed in animals [9,10]. It should be avoided during pregnancy, and accounts for the notorious reputation of gin, of which Juniper is the main flavour ingredient.

PREPARATIONS AND DOSE: Dried fruits, dose: 1–2 g three times daily; Juniper Berry Oil BPC 1949, dose: 0.03–0.2 ml three times daily; Juniper Liquid Extract 1:1, dose: 2–4 ml three times daily.

BIBLICAL REFERENCES: 1 Kings 19:4–5; Job 30:4; Psalm 120:4.

SPECIFIC REFERENCES: 1. Chandler R (1986) *Rev. Parm. Canada* 563. 2. Freidrich H *et al* (1978) *Planta Med.* 33:251. 3. Koukos P *et al* (1997) *J. Ess. Oil Res.* 9:35. 4. Ochoka J *et al* (1997) *Phytochem.* 44:869. 5. Hiermann A *et al* (1996) *Sci. Pharm.* 64:437. 6. Mascolo N *et al* (1987) *Phytother. Res.* 1(1):28. 7. Stanic G *et al* (1998) *Phytother. Res.* 12(7):494. 8. Sanchez de Medina F *et al* (1994) *Planta Med.* 60:197. 9. Agrawal O *et al* (1980) *Planta Med.* 40:S98. 10. Schlicher H *et al* (1994) *Z. Phytother.* 15:205.

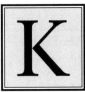

KAMALA
MALLOTUS PHILIPPINENSIS MULL. ARG.
Fam. Euphorbiaceae

SYNONYMS: Kameela, *Rottlera unctoria* Roxb.

HABITAT: Eastern Africa, India, Saudi Arabia.

DESCRIPTION: The hairs and glands covering the fruit are obtained by sifting; they form a red mobile powder, which floats on water. Tasteless, and nearly odourless.

PART USED: Capsule hairs and glands.

CONSTITUENTS: (i) Phloroglucinol derivatives; rottlerin, isorottlerin, isoallorottlerin, and methylene-bis-methylphloroacetophenone (ii) Kamalins I and II [1,2].

MEDICINAL USE: Taenifuge, purgative [R1]. Formerly used to treat leprosy and skin diseases, and still used in India and elsewhere for the treatment of tapeworm infestation.

SPECIFIC REFERENCES: 1. Widen C-J *et al* (1980) *Planta Med.* 40:3284. 2. Lounasmaa M *et al* (1975) *Planta Med.* 28:16.

KARELA
MOMORDICA CHARANTIA L.
Fam. Cucurbitaceae

SYNONYMS: Bitter Gourd, Bitter Melon, Cerassie.

HABITAT: Grown as a vegetable throughout India, China, Africa and parts of America.

DESCRIPTION: A slender, branched, climbing shrub with kidney-shaped, lobed leaves. The flowers are monoecious and yellow; the male flowers solitary and the female flowers bracteate. The fruit resembles a cucumber with numerous ridges or warts and soft spines, up to 7 cm long with tapering ends. Taste: intensely bitter.

PART USED: Leaf, fruit.

CONSTITUENTS: (i) Triterpene (cucurbitane-type) glycosides called the momordicosides A-L and the goyaglycosides A-H, charine, vicine, momordicin, momordicinin, and cucurbitanes I, II and III, and in the leaf, the goyasaponins I, II, and III (ii) Proteins; alpha-, beta-, and gamma-momorcharins, momordins a and b, and other lectins (iii) Sterols (campesterol, beta-sitosterol etc.) and fatty acids (mainly palmitic and oleic acids) (iv) Volatile oil, containing pentenyl, hexenyl and other aldehydes, menthol, nerolidol, myrtenol, sabinol and others [R12,R16;1,2,3,4,5,6,7,8].

MEDICINAL USE: The plant is widely used in the treatment of diabetes, and the fruit is eaten as a vegetable. The leaf may be made into a tea called 'cerassie'; both have hypoglycaemic effects. It has also been used to treat asthma, skin infections and hypertension. The extract causes hypoglycaemia in animals and human diabetic patients

[9,10]. Cytotoxicity and anti-tumour effects have been described in a wide range of systems; the crude extract, lectin fraction, and proteins have these properties and it is thought that they may have clinical applications [R12,R16;11,12 and refs therein]. Contraceptive and teratogenic effects have also been described in animals [13,14], so care should be taken in pregnant women; although cooking the vegetable may well destroy many of the toxins. Other effects such as antimicrobial and antiviral properties [15,16], lipolytic activity and hepatoprotection have been described: see reviews [R12,R16 and refs therein for more detail].

SPECIFIC REFERENCES: 1. Murakami T *et al* (2001) *Chem. Pharm. Bull.* 49(1):54. 2. Begum S *et al* (1997) *Phytochem.* 44:1313. 3. Fatope M *et al* (1990) *J. Nat. Prod.* 53(6):1491. 4. El-Gengaihi *et al* (1995) *Pharmazie* 50(5):361. 5. Okabe H *et al* (1982) *Chem. Pharm. Bull.* 30:3977 and 4334. 6. Okabe H *et al* (1980) *Chem. Pharm. Bull.* 28:2753. 7. Miyahara Y *et al* (1981) *Chem. Pharm. Bull.* 29:1561. 8. Pu Z *et al* (1998) *Biochem. Biophys. Res. Commun.* 253(1):143. 9. Binder F *et al* (1989) *J. Agric. Food Chem.* 37(2):418. 10. Srivastava Y *et al* (1993) *Phytother. Res.* 7(4):285. 11. Raza H *et al* (2000) *Biochem. Mol. Toxicol.* 14(3):131. 12. Ng T *et al* (1994) *Gen. Pharmacol.* 25(1):75. 13. Singh A *et al* (1998) *Toxicol. Lett.* 94(1):37. 14. Chan W *et al* (1986) *Contraception* 34(5):537. 15. Lee-Huang S *et al* (1995) *Proc. Natl. Acad. Sci.* 92(19):8818. 16. Bourinbaiar A *et al* (1996) *Biochem. Biophys. Res. Commun.* 219(3):923.

KAVA

PIPER METHYSTICUM FORST.
Fam. Piperaceae

SYNONYMS: Kava Kava, Kawa.

HABITAT: South Sea Islands.

DESCRIPTION: Root large, externally blackish-grey, internally whitish. Fracture mealy and somewhat splintery, central portion porous, with irregularly twisted thin woody bundles, separated by broad medullary rays, which form a mesh. Taste: pungent, numbing; odour: reminiscent of lilac.

PART USED: Root.

CONSTITUENTS: (i) Pyrone derivatives (kava lactones); kawain, dihydrokawain, methysticin, 5,6-dehydromethysticin, dihydromethysticin, yangonin, 11-methoxy-nor-yangonin and desmethoxyyangonin (ii) Flavonoids, chalcones known as flavokavins A and B (iii) Alkaloids; pipermethysticine, a piperidine alkaloid [R2,R17;1 and refs therein].

MEDICINAL USE: Stimulant, relaxant, tonic, diuretic [R1]. Kava was traditionally used in bronchitis, rheumatism and gout, and as a diuretic, but more recently for its relaxing and anti-fatigue effects. The plant is very highly regarded in the South Pacific islands, where it is cultivated for preparation as a ceremonial and psychoactive recreational drink. The active constituents are the kavalactones which have anxiolytic, anticonvulsant and muscle relaxant effects. In general the traditional uses have been substantiated in both clinical and animal tests [1,2]. Kava extract causes reversible inhibition of monoamine oxidase B and inhibits noradrenaline uptake from synaptosomes [3,4] and appears to affect the GABA-A binding site [5]; all of which may contribute to the anxiolytic activity. It produces changes in brain waves similar to those of other anxiolytics, but without apparent dependency, and sedation is rarely a problem with Kava use [6]. Other properties of kava include antimicrobial, fungistatic, neuroprotective and antithrombotic effects [R17]. A Kava abuse syndrome, manifested as a form of dermatitis, has been identified in drinkers of the intoxicating drink, and ascribed to niacin deficiency [7]. Kava is also taken in combination with other sedative herbs, particularly Valerian (q.v.), and beneficial properties have been observed for this combination as well as the individual herbs, as measured by a reduction in mental stress during laboratory tests [8,9] and the alleviation of stress-induced insomnia [10]. It also reduced withdrawal symptoms of benzodiazepines in anxious patients [11]. For further detail, see [R2,R8,R17,1,2,13 and refs therein]. Kava is usually well tolerated, with few side effects in most patients, although liver toxicity has been reported in a few susceptible individuals [12] and products containing the herb have now been withdrawn for sale in many countries.

PREPARATIONS AND DOSE: Extract, dose: usually 120 mg, when required.

SPECIFIC REFERENCES: 1. Singh Y *et al* (1997) *HerbalGram* 39:33. 2. Pittler M *et al* (2000) *J. Clin. Psychopharmacol.* 20:84. 3. Uebelhack R *et al* (1998) *Pharmacopsychiatry* 31:187. 4. Gleitz J *et al* (1996) *Eur. J. Pharmacol.* 315:89. 5. Boonen G *et al* (1998) *Planta Med.* 64:504. 6. Gleitz J *et al* (1997) *Planta Med.* 63:27. 7. Ruze P (1990) *Lancet* 335:1442. 8. Cropley M *et al* (2002) *Phytother. Res.* 16(1):23. 9. Wheatley D (2001) *Phytother. Res.* 15:549. 10. Wheatley D (2001) *Hum. Psychopharmacol. Clin. Exp.* 16:353. 11. Malsch U *et al* (2001) *Psychopharmacology* 157(3):277. 12. Escher M *et al* (2001) *Br. Med. J.* 322:139. 13. Cairney S *et al* (2002) *Aust. NZ. J. Psychiatry* 36(5):657.

KHAT

CATHA EDULIS FORSK.
Fam. Celastraceae

SYNONYMS: Abyssinian tea, African tea, Chat, Kat, Qat, Mirra.

HABITAT: Indigenous to Ethiopia but found throughout Yemen, Somalia, Saudi Arabia, Kenya and other parts of East Africa, the Arabian peninsula and Afghanistan.

DESCRIPTION: A small tree, when occurring naturally, but can reach 25 m when cultivated. It is polymorphic, and the leaves, which are lanceolate with a serrated margin, can be either opposite or alternate, and ranging from dark to pale green. Taste and odour: aromatic, astringent, very bitter.

PART USED: Fresh young leaves and shoots.

CONSTITUENTS: (i) Proto-alkaloids, known as khatamines, the most important being cathinone, which is only found in the fresh plant, cathine (norpseudoephedrine) and norephedrine (ii) Cathedulines (sesquiterpene alkaloids) known as K1, K2, K3 (from Kenya) or Y1, Y2 etc. (from Yemen) (iii) Phenylpentenylamines such as merucathine, merucathinone and pseudomerocathinone (iv) Tannins (v) Miscellaneous essential oil, triterpenes [1,2,3,4,].

MEDICINAL USE: Stimulant. The leaves are chewed to increase alertness and wakefulness. Originally chewed by religious practitioners as a means of keeping awake for all night prayer and for soldiers to reduce fatigue, Khat is still widely used socially, particularly by men in Somalia and Yemen. Khat parties are occasionally held where current affairs are discussed and music listened to, and are a means of welcoming strangers into the community. It has mildly amphetamine-like effects and is becoming increasingly abused in the West [1]. Khat has constipating and spasmolytic properties and delays gastric emptying. The main stimulatory properties arise from the cathinone content, which can induce psychosis and dependence with excessive use. Other documented toxic effects include acute autonomic responses such as elevated blood pressure and tachycardia, insomnia and anorexia, hyperthermia, mydriasis and endocrine disruption [1,4,5,6]. The high incidence of oesophageal carcinoma in the Yemen is attributed to the high tannin content of Khat [1,6] and an increased susceptibility to acute myocardial infarction has been reported [1,7]. Abnormalities in the male reproductive system in animals have been observed, although were not noted with moderate doses [8,9]; however an increase in plasma liver enzymes, and histopathological lesions in the liver and kidney, have been described [10]. The pharmacological, medical and social aspects of Khat have been well reviewed recently [1].

SPECIFIC REFERENCES: 1. Al-Motarreb *et al* (2002) *Phytother. Res.* 16(5):401. 2. Brenneisen R *et al* (1987) *J. Nat. Prod.* 50:1188. 3. Crombie L *et al* (1979) *J. Chem. Soc. Perk. Trans.*1:2976. 4. Kalix P *et al* (1996) *Pharm. World. Sci.* 18(2):69. 5. Makonnen E (2000) *Phytomed.* 7(4):309. 6. Heymann T *et al* (1995) *Aliment. Pharmacol. Ther.* 9(1):81. 7. Al-Motarreb *et al* (2001) *Heart* 87:279. 8. Islam M *et al* (1990) *Toxicol.* 60:223. 9. El-Shoura S *et al* (1995) *Hum. Reprod.* 10:2295. 10. Al-Mamary M *et al* (2002) *Phytother. Res.* 16(2):127.

KHELLA

AMMI VISNAGA (L.) LAM.
Fam. Apiaceae

SYNONYMS: Toothpick Plant, Visnaga.

HABITAT: Indigenous to the Mediterranean region and Egypt.

DESCRIPTION: A herbaceous annual reaching 1.5 m, with divided filiform leaves and typically umbelliferous flowers. The fruits are very small, broadly ovoid, and usually found as separate greyish-brown, merocarps. Taste and odour: very bitter, slightly aromatic. The dried, stout pedicels have been used as toothpicks in the Middle East, hence the name.

PART USED: Fruits (seeds).

CONSTITUENTS: (i) Furanocoumarins, the most important being khellin, together with visnagin, visnadin and khellol glucoside (ii) Essential oil, in very small amounts [R3;1,2].

MEDICINAL USE: The drug has a long history of use in the Middle East, especially Egypt, as an antispasmodic in renal colic, anti-asthmatic and coronary vasodilator for the treatment of angina pectoris. Khellin, visnadin and visnagin are vasodilators, with calcium channel blocking activity, and also have spasmolytic effects [2,3,4,5]. Khellin reduced serum LDL and total cholesterol levels in rats fed a high fat diet [2]. Khellin was the starting material for the development of several important semi-synthetic derivatives such as nifedipine (a calcium channel antagonist and vasodilator) used in heart disease, and amiodarone, a cardiac antiarrhythmic. Sodium cromoglycate was also developed from khellin and is widely used as a prophylactic treatment for asthma, hay fever and other allergic conditions [R3,R11].

SPECIFIC REFERENCES: 1. Elgamal M *et al* (1998) *Fitoterapia* 69(9):549. 2. Duarte J *et al* (1995) *Eur. J. Pharmacol.* 286(2):115. 3. Rauwald H *et al* (1994) *Planta Med.* 60(2):101. 4. Rauwald H *et al* (1994) *Phytother. Res.* 8(3):135. 5. Duarte J *et al* (1997) *Planta Med.* 63(3):233. 6. Naser H *et al* (1992) *Arzeim. Forsch.* 742(2):140.

KINO
PTEROCARPUS MARSUPIUM ROXB.
Fam. Fabaceae

HABITAT: India and Sri Lanka.

DESCRIPTION: The gum appears in commerce as small, blackish, shining fragments or as a coarse powder. Taste: very astringent. It adheres to the teeth when chewed.

PART USED: Juice.

CONSTITUENTS: Polyphenolic compounds which are diverse but structurally related: (i) Tannins, such as (–)-epicatechin (ii) Stilbenes; such as pterostilbene (iii) Flavonoids; liquiritigenin, pterosupin, isoliquiritigenin, 7-hydroxyflavanone, 7,4-dihydroxyflavanone and 5-deoxykaempferol (iv) Miscellaneous; marsupsin, a benzofuranone, and *p*-hydroxybenzaldehyde etc. [1,2,3].

MEDICINAL USE: Astringent [R1]. Used mainly for diarrhoea and dysentery and as a local application for sore throats and leucorrhoea. In India it is also used for diabetes; pterostilbene and marsupsin have been shown to reverse hyperglycaemia in alloxan-diabetic rats in a manner comparable to that of metformin [4]. A recent study showed that Kino extract inhibited glucose uptake by brush border membrane vesicles *in vitro*; insulin secretion was not affected [5].

PREPARATIONS AND DOSE: Powdered gum, dose: 0.3–1 g.

SPECIFIC REFERENCES: 1. Maurya R *et al* (1984) *J. Nat. Prod.* 47:179. 2. Maurya R *et al* (1985) *J. Nat. Prod.* 48:313. 3. Seshadri T (1972) *Phytochem.* 11:881. 4. Manickam M *et al* (1997) *J. Nat. Prod.* 60(6):609. 5. Srijayanta S *et al* (1998) *J. Pharm. Pharmacol.* 50:S219.

KNAPWEED
CENTAUREA NIGRA L.
Fam. Asteraceae

SYNONYMS: Black Knapweed, Star Thistle, Black Ray Thistle, Ironweed.

HABITAT: A native European wild plant.

DESCRIPTION: Globular flower-heads, about 5 cm long, the outer scales of which have blackish appendages at the apex with comb-like teeth. Florets are purplish, tubular. Taste: bitter, slightly saline.

PART USED: Herb.

CONSTITUENTS: Flavonoids including cantaurein and jacein [1].

MEDICINAL USE: Diuretic, diaphoretic, tonic [R1]. The flavones are antiviral *in vitro* [1].

SPECIFIC REFERENCES: 1. Kay-Kamb A *et al* (1991) *J. Pharm. Belg.* 46(5):325.

KNOTGRASS
POLYGONUM AVICULARE L.
Fam. Polygonaceae

SYNONYMS: Knotweed, Wireweed.

HABITAT: Europe, Russia, and parts of Asia.

DESCRIPTION: Stem slender, cylindrical, striated. Leaves narrowly lanceolate, about 1 cm long; stipules lanceolate. Taste: astringent; odourless.

PART USED: Herb.

CONSTITUENTS: (i) Polyphenolics, including gallic, caffeic and chlorogenic acids, catechin, oxymethyl anthraquinone, polygonic acid, fuglanin and others (ii) Flavonoids and anthocyanins; delphinidin, avicularin and glycosides based on quercetin (iii) Miscellaneous; lignans, silicic acid, sugars, mucilage etc. [R4,R16,1].

MEDICINAL USE: Astringent, as an infusion, for diarrhoea, dysentery and jaundice [R1]. The methanolic extract has anti-fibrotic activity in rat liver induced by bile tube ligation and other liver protective effects [2]. It is anti-inflammatory, and inhibits prostaglandin synthesis and platelet activating factor [3]. Antimicrobial effects against various dermatophyte fungi have been reported [R16]. A recent clinical trial in gingivitis showed a reduction in inflammation of the gums after two weeks treatment with a mouthwash containing the extract [4]. For further detail, see [R16].

SPECIFIC REFERENCES: 1. Kim H *et al* (1994) *J. Nat. Prod.* 57(5):581.
2. Nan J *et al* (2000) *Biol. Pharm. Bull.* 23(2):240. 3. Tunon H *et al*
(1995) *J. Ethnopharmacol.* 48(2):61. 4. Gonzalez Begne M *et al* (2001)
J. Ethnopharmacol. 74(1):45.

KOUSSO
HAGENIA ABYSSINICA J. F. GMEL.
Fam. Rosaceae

SYNONYMS: Kooso, Cusso, *Brayera anthelmintica* Kunth.

HABITAT: Northeast Africa.

DESCRIPTION: Flowers about 1 cm across, petals minute, linear;
10-veined leaf-like sepals in two rows. The female inflorescence is
normally used and occurs in commerce in the form of a cylindrical roll.

PART USED: Dried flowers.

CONSTITUENTS: (i) Acylphloroglucinols; known as kosins (or 'cosins'),
such as alpha-kosin, kosin K6, and kosin K8 (which are monomeric
phloroglucinol compounds); kosotoxin ('cussotoxin', a dimer) and
protokosin (a trimer) [1,2,3,4] (ii) Phenolic acids including
protocatechuic, vanillic and *p*-hydroxybenzoic acid [1].

MEDICINAL USE: Anthelmintic [R1]. Used as an infusion and
powder, in conjunction with purgatives such as Castor Oil (q.v.). The
kosins are cytotoxic and have anti-tumour activity against murine
adenocarcinoma cells [3] and kosotoxin is spasmolytic in guinea pig
ileum and rabbit jejunum against a range of spasmogens [5]. Excessive
doses are dangerous, causing irritation of the gastrointestinal tract,
salivation, vision disorders and collapse.

SPECIFIC REFERENCES: 1. Woldemariam T *et al* (1990) *J. Pharm.
Biomed. Anal.* 8:859. 2. Schiemenz G *et al* (1985) *Z. Naturforsch.*
40B:669. 3. Woldemariam T *et al* (1992) *J. Pharm. Biomed. Anal.*
10:555. 4. Metzner J *et al* (1983) *Planta Med.* 47:240. 5. Bogale M
et al (1996) *Phytother. Res.* 10 (Suppl):S112.

KUMARHOU
POMADERRIS ELLIPTICA L.
Fam. Rhamnaceae

SYNONYMS: Papapa, Gumdiggers Soap, Poverty Weed.

HABITAT: New Zealand.

DESCRIPTION: It is a branching shrub, up to 3 m in height, leaves 5–8
cm long, shiny above and downy on the undersurface. The inflorescence
is a multi-flowered cyme; the petals and sepals are yellowish-white.

PART USED: Herb.

CONSTITUENTS: Unknown.

MEDICINAL USE: Used by Maoris for asthma, bronchitis, kidney
troubles and as a blood purifier.

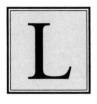

LABRADOR TEA
LEDUM LATIFOLIUM L.
Fam. Ericaceae

SYNONYMS: St James's Tea. *L. palustre* L. is also referred to as Labrador Tea, but more frequently as Marsh Tea or Wild Rosemary.

HABITAT: North America and Canada. *L. palustre* grows in northern Europe, Asia and America.

DESCRIPTION: Leaves linear-lanceolate, with a revolute margin, alternate, almost sessile, up to 5 cm long and 0.5 cm broad. The upper surface is dark green and smooth, the undersurface coated with red-brown hairs. Taste: bitter and camphoraceous; odour: aromatic.

PART USED: Leaves.

CONSTITUENTS: (i) Essential oil, containing sesquiterpenes including ledol (= ledum camphor), palustrol, aromadendrene, myrcene and in some samples, ascaridole [R2;1] (ii) Coumarins such as scopoletin and palustroside [2] (iii) Flavonoids; e.g. hyperoside [R2]. These are mainly specified for *Ledum palustre*, which has been investigated to a greater extent.

MEDICINAL USE: Pectoral, expectorant, diuretic [R1].

SPECIFIC REFERENCES: 1. Ylipahkala T *et al* (1992) *Chromatographia* 34(3–4):159. 2. Dubois M-A *et al* (1990) *Planta Med.* 56(6):664.

LACHNANTHES
LACHNANTHES TINCTORIA ELL.
Fam. Haemodoraceae

SYNONYMS: Spiritweed, Red Root, Paint Root, Wool Flower.

HABITAT: West Indies.

DESCRIPTION: Rhizome about 3 cm long, surrounded by long, slender, deep red roots. Leaves scythe-shaped, somewhat succulent, in a basal rosette, reddish-brown when dried. Flowers arranged in a woolly cyme. Taste: acrid; odourless.

PART USED: Root, herb.

CONSTITUENTS: A dimeric 9-phenylphenalenone has been isolated [1].

MEDICINAL USE: Tonic, narcotic [R1]. Has been used for coughs, pneumonia etc., but large doses produce vertigo, headache and other unpleasant symptoms.

SPECIFIC REFERENCES: 1. Edwards J *et al* (1979) *J. Nat. Prod.* 42(6):681.

LADY'S BEDSTRAW
GALIUM VERUM L.
Fam. Rubiaceae

SYNONYMS: Yellow Bedstraw, Cheese Rennet.

HABITAT: A common herb growing in dry grassy places in Britain, throughout Europe and parts of North America.

DESCRIPTION: Stems are slender, angular, bearing whorls of linear leaves with downy undersurfaces and revolute margins. Flowers very small, bright yellow, in terminal panicles. Taste: astringent, slightly bitter and acid; odourless.

PART USED: Herb.

CONSTITUENTS: (i) Iridoids, including asperuloside and galioside (ii) Flavonoid glycosides; quercetin-3-glucoside, quercetin-7-glucoside, quercitin-3-rutinoside, luteolin-7-glucoside and others (iii) Anthraquinone derivatives, such as alizarin, in the root (iv) *n*-Alkanes, mainly C_{31} and C_{29} [1,2].

MEDICINAL USE: Diuretic, alterative [R1]. Contains similar compounds to Clivers (q.v.) and used for similar purposes. The flowers have been used to make cheese instead of rennet, hence the synonym.

SPECIFIC REFERENCES: 1. Mathe I *et al* (1982) *Planta Med.* 45(3):P25. 2. Corrigan D *et al* (1973) *Phytochem.* 17:1131.

LADY'S MANTLE
ALCHEMILLA VULGARIS L.
Fam. Rosaceae

SYNONYMS: Lion's Foot.

HABITAT: A common British and European wild plant.

DESCRIPTION: A variable group of similar microspecies, usually hairy but sometimes glabrous. Leaves up to about 5 cm in diameter, having 7–11, rounded, serrate, palmate lobes. Flowers green, apetalous, in small clusters, borne on a forked stem which has small three-lobed leaves and broad stipules at the base of each fork. Taste: slightly astringent; odourless.

PART USED: Herb.

CONSTITUENTS: (i) Flavonoids, mainly glycosides of quercetin and kaempferol (ii) Tannins, consisting mainly of ellagitannins, including the dimer agrimoniin and laevigatiin [R2;1,2,3,4].

MEDICINAL USE: Astringent, styptic [R1]. Used for excessive menstruation and diarrhoea, with some success [5], and topically for leucorrhoea and pruritis. The flavonoids inhibit elastase and trypsin *in vitro* and confer angio-protective effects [2].

PREPARATIONS AND DOSE: Dried herb, dose: 2–4g as an infusion, or equivalent extract, three times daily.

SPECIFIC REFERENCES: 1. D'Agostino M *et al* (1998) *Phytother. Res.* 12(Suppl.1):S162. 2. Jonadet M *et al* (1986) *J. de Pharmacologie* 17(1):21. 3. Dorne A *et al* (1986) *Phytochem.* 25:65. 4. Geiger C *et al* (1990) *Planta Med.* 56:585. 5. Petcu P *et al* (1979) *Clujul Medical* 52(3):266.

LADY'S SLIPPER

CYPRIPEDIUM CALCEOLUS VAR *PUBESCENS* R BR.
Fam. Orchidaceae

SYNONYMS: Nerve Root, American Valerian, *C. pubescens* Willd.,
C. hirsutum Mill., *C. parviflorum* Salisb.

HABITAT: Indigenous to Canada and North America, cultivated in Europe.

DESCRIPTION: Rhizome up to 8 cm long, 0.5 cm in diameter, reddish-brown, with numerous cup-shaped bud scars and a few buds on the upper surface, and many slender, matted roots on the lower surface. Fracture: short; taste: bitter and pungent; odour: characteristic, slightly valerianic.

PART USED: Rhizome.

CONSTITUENTS: (i) Quinones, including cypripedone (2,8-dimethoxy 7-hydroxy-1,4-phenanthrene) (ii) Essential oil, tannins [R2;1].

MEDICINAL USE: Antispasmodic, nervine, sedative, mild hypnotic [R1]. Used for anxiety states, headache, neuralgia and emotional tension.

PREPARATIONS AND DOSE: Dried herb, dose: 2–4 g as an infusion, or equivalent extract, three times daily.

SPECIFIC REFERENCES: 1. Schmalle H *et al* (1979) *Naturwissensch.* 66(10):527.

LANTANA

LANTANA CAMARA L.
Fam. Verbenaceae

SYNONYMS: Sweet, Wild, White, or Yellow Sage; Common, Large-leaved or Prickly Lantana.

HABITAT: A native of tropical America, now found as a pan-tropical weed, especially in coconut plantations, fields and on waste ground; widely cultivated as an ornamental.

DESCRIPTION: An erect, branching shrub, reaching up to 2 m. The stems are quadrangular, with hooked prickles. Leaves are ovate, with a serrate margin, up to 10 cm long. The flowers vary in colour from pink, through red and orange, to yellow; occurring in dense, flat-topped clusters.

PART USED: Leaves.

CONSTITUENTS: (i) Triterpenes including lantadenes A, B, C and D, linaroside, lantanoside, and lantanone; lantic, lantanilic, camarilic, camaracinic, betulinic, ursolic and oleanolic acids, and a series of translactone containing euphane derivatives [R12;1,2,3,4,5,6] (ii) Essential oil containing limonene, alpha-phellandrene, germacrene-D, bicyclogermacrene, 1,8-cineole, alpha-humulene, beta-caryophyllene, sabinene and others [7,8,9] (iii) Flavonoid and phenylpropanoid glycosides including camaraside, lantanaside, verbascoside, geniposide, theveside and theveridoside [10,11,12].

MEDICINAL USE: Anti-inflammatory, antiseptic, vermifuge, emmenagogue. An infusion of the fresh leaves is taken for coughs and colds, rheumatism, digestive and many other disorders. A paste of the leaves is applied externally to skin infections such as leprosy and scabies. The plant is toxic to grazing animals and causes photosensitization, and liver and kidney damage. Several of the translactone triterpenes have thrombin inhibiting properties [2], and also inhibit Epstein-Barr virus activation [12]. Lantic acid is strongly antibacterial [4], and lantanoside, linaroside and camarinic acids are nematocidal [6]. The essential oil also shows a wide spectrum of antibacterial and anti-fungal activity [14] and the phenylpropanoids are weakly cardioactive [10]. Verbascoside is an inhibitor of protein kinase C, which is thought to confer anti-tumour activity to some extent [15]. Analgesic and antipyretic effects have been demonstrated for the extract [16]; however the toxic effects give cause for concern about the general medicinal use of this plant.

SPECIFIC REFERENCES: 1. Ghisalberti E (2000) Fitoterapia 71(5):467. 2. O'Neill M et al (1998) J. Nat. Prod. 61(11):1328. 3. Begum S et al (1995) J. Nat. Prod. 58(10):1570. 4. Saleh M et al (1999) Pharm. Biol. 37(1):63. 5. Sharma O et al (2000) Fitoterapia 71(5):487. 6. Begum S et al (2000) J. Nat. Prod. 63(6):765. 7. Sefidkon F (2002) Flav. Frag. J. 17(1):78. 8. Khan M et al (2002) Flav. Frag. J. 17(1):75. 9. Da Silva M et al (1999) Flav. Frag. J. 14(4):208. 10. Syah Y et al (1998) Fitoterapia 69(3):285. 11. Taoubi K et al (1997) Planta Med. 63(2):192. 12. Mahato S et al (1994) Tetrahedron 50(31):9439. 13. Inada A et al (1995) Planta Med. 61(6):558. 14. Deena M et al (2000) Fitoterapia 71(4):453. 15. Herbert J et al (1991) J. Nat. Prod. 54(6):1595. 16. Forestieri A et al (1996) Phytother. Res. 10(2):100.

LAPACHO

TABEBUIA AVELLANEDAE LORENTZ EX GRISEB
T. ROSEA BERTOL.
T. SERRATIFOLIA (VAHL) NICHOLSON
AND OTHERS
Fam. Bignoniaceae

SYNONYMS: Taheebo, Pau D'arco. *T. impetiginosa* (= *T. avellanedae*), *T. pentaphylla* (= *T. rosea*).

HABITAT: South America.

DESCRIPTION: A large tropical tree reaching 38 m in height. The leaves are compound, with long petioles, and the flowers large, red or purple, in terminal spikes or panicles. The seeds are winged.

PART USED: Inner bark.

CONSTITUENTS: (i) Naphthoquinones, the most important being lapachol, with deoxylapachol, xyloidone, alpha- and beta-lapachone, dehydro-alpha-lapachone and others (ii) Anthraquinones (iii) Benzoic acid and benzaldehyde derivatives (iv) Miscellaneous coumarins, flavonoids and carnesol [R17;1,2].

257

MEDICINAL USE: Used traditionally for infectious diseases, including bacterial, fungal and viral infections, to enhance immune function and for treatment of various cancers. The antimicrobial effects are documented for *Candida albicans, Brucella* and *Staphylococcus* species [3,4,5] and for several viruses [6]. These effects are usually attributed to lapachol, which is also anti-protozoal against *Leishmania, Trypanosoma* and *Schistosoma* species [7]. Lapachol is also anti-inflammatory [8]. Lapacho is becoming popular throughout the world, often as an anti-cancer treatment, after being used in hospitals in Brazil for treating terminal-cancer patients [R17]. Anti-tumour activity has been shown *in vitro* and *in vivo* [9,10] but this use is not yet supported by good clinical data, although a few uncontrolled trials have been carried out. Lapachol is usually regarded as the most active component, and semi-synthetic derivatives are being prepared in order to increase activity. Lapachol is an anticoagulant [6]; it has anti-inflammatory and analgesic properties [8] and is anti-ulcerogenic [11]. Although lapachol is known to be toxic in large doses, and inhibits pregnancy in mice [12] there is little evidence of toxicity for the herb when used in normal doses. For further details and more data on Lapacho, see [R17 and refs therein].

PREPARATIONS AND DOSE: (Example): extract equivalent to 250 mg lapachol, three times daily.

SPECIFIC REFERENCES: 1. Girard M *et al* (1988) *J. Nat. Prod.* 51(5):1023. 2. Fujimoto Y *et al* (1991) *J. Chem. Soc. Perkin Trans.* 1:2323. 3. Perez C *et al* (1994) *Fitoterapia* 65(2):169. 4. Giraud P *et al* (1994) *Planta Med.* 60(4):373. 5. Anesini C *et al* (1993) *J. Ethnopharmacol.* 39(2):119. 6. Preusch P *et al* (1989) *Arch. Biochem. Biophys.* 269(1):18. 7. Teixeira M *et al* (2001) *Phytother. Res.* 15(1):44. 8. De Almeida E *et al* (1990) *J. Ethnopharmacol.* 29(2):239. 9. Ueda S *et al* (1990) *Planta Med.* 56:669. 10. Houghton P *et al* (1994) *Planta Med.* 60(5):430. 11. Goel R *et al* (1987) *J. Pharm. Pharmacol.* 39(2):138. 12. Sareen V *et al* (1995) *Phytother. Res.* 9(2):139.

LARCH
LARIX DECIDUA MIQ.
Fam. Pinaceae

SYNONYMS: European Larch, *L. europea* D.C., *Pinus larix* L. *L. laricina* is Tamarac (q.v.), or American Larch.

HABITAT: Europe, including the British Isles.

DESCRIPTION: The inner bark of the tree, deprived of the grey outer inert bark, is preferred for medicinal use. The external surface is reddish-brown, the inner surface with a pinkish or yellowish tint. Fracture: short, slightly fibrous; Taste: astringent, bitter; odour: reminiscent of turpentine.

PART USED: Bark.

CONSTITUENTS: (i) Lignans; lariciresinol, liovil, and secoisolariciresinol (ii) Resins, consisting of the resin acids larinolic and laricinolic acids and others [2] (iii) Essential oil, containing alpha- and beta-pinene, limonene, phellandrene, borneol etc. (iv) Polysaccharides and gums; mainly arabinogalactans [R4;1,2]. *L. kaempferi* contains at least eight abietane diterpenes [3].

MEDICINAL USE: Astringent, balsamic, diuretic [R1]. Larch has been used as a tincture to treat bronchitis and urinary inflammation. The abietane diterpenes from *L. kaempferi* inhibit Epstein-Barr virus activation [3].

SPECIFIC REFERENCES: 1. Freudenberg K *et al* (1959) *Tet. Lett.* 17:19. 2. Holm Y *et al* (1997) *Flav. Frag. J.* 12(5):335. 3. Ohtsu H *et al* (2001) *Planta Med.* 67(1):55.

LARKSPUR
DELPHINIUM CONSOLIDA L.
and related species
Fam. Ranunculaceae

SYNONYMS: Lark's Claw, Knight's Spur.

HABITAT: A common garden plant.

DESCRIPTION: Seeds black, tetrahedral, flattened, up to about 2 mm in diameter, with acute edges and pitted surface. Taste: bitter and acrid; odourless.

PART USED: Seeds.

CONSTITUENTS: Diterpene alkaloids, of the aconitine type (see Aconite) including anthranoyllycoctonine, lycoctonine, delcosine and delsoline [R2;1,2,3,4].

MEDICINAL USE: Parasiticide, insecticide, antispasmodic [R1]. A tincture has been used to destroy nits and lice in the hair; the alkaloids also have insect-repellant activity [2]. These products should be used with great care as the alkaloids are cardiotoxic and neurotoxic and are being investigated for clinical usage as analgesics and antiarrhythmic agents [3,4].

SPECIFIC REFERENCES: 1. Pelletier S *et al* (1984) In: *The Alkaloids* Vol. Wiley, UK. 2. Ulubelen A *et al* (2001) *Phytother. Res.* 15(2):170. 3. Heubach J *et al* (1998) *Planta Med.* 64(1):22. 4. Manners G *et al* (1995) *J. Nat. Prod.* 58(6):863.

LAUREL
LAURUS NOBILIS L.
Fam. Lauraceae

SYNONYMS: Bay, Sweet Bay, Bay Laurel.

HABITAT: Native to the Mediterranean region, cultivated widely.

DESCRIPTION: The leaves are leathery, dark green with a paler undersurface, up to about 7 cm long and 2.5 cm across, elliptic-lanceolate, with an entire or slightly wavy margin. Taste and odour: characteristic, aromatic.

259

PART USED: Leaves, essential oil.

CONSTITUENTS: (i) Volatile oil, up to about 3%, containing cineole as the major component, with linalool, alpha-pinene and alpha-terpineol acetate; and in minor concentrations sabinene, limonene, methyleugenol, *p*-cymene, thuj-2-en-4-ol (ii) Sesquiterpenes including costunolide, eremanthine, zaluzanin C and D, reynosin, santamarine, magolialide and laurenolide (iii) Lignan glycosides based on isolariciresinol, including shizandraside [1,2,3,4,5,6,7].

MEDICINAL USE: Stomachic, cholagogue, diaphoretic and stimulant [R1]. The oil has been used as an external application for rheumatism and in hair-dressing for dandruff. Bay leaves are an important culinary spice. This plant should not be confused with West Indian Bay, from *Pimenta racemosa* (q.v.), which is an ingredient of Bay Rum. The sesquiterpenes inhibit alcohol absorption in rats and retard gastric emptying [4,8] and also inhibit nitric oxide production in activated mouse peritoneal macrophages, thought to be due to induction of heat shock protein 72 and prevention of NFkappaB activation [5]. An extract of Laurel seeds has anti-ulcerogenic effects in rats [9].

SPECIFIC REFERENCES: 1. Tada H *et al* (1976) *Chem. Pharm. Bull.* 24:667. 2. Novak M *et al* (1982) *Phytochem.* 24(4):585. 3. Hokwerda H *et al* (1982) *Planta Med.* 44(2):116. 4. Yoshikawa M *et al* (2000) *Bioorg. Med. Chem.* 8(8):2071. 5. Matsuda H *et al* (2000) *Life Sci.* 66(2):2151. 6. Yohara S *et al* (1992) *Jpn. J. Pharmacog.* 46(2):184. 7. Garg S *et al* (1992) *J. Nat. Prod.* 55(9):1315. 8. Matsuda H *et al* (1999) *Bioorg. Med. Chem. Lett.* 9(18):2647. 9. Afifi F *et al* (1997) *J. Ethnopharmacol.* 58(1):9.

LAVENDER

LAVANDULA ANGUSTIFOLIA MILL.
Fam. Lamiaceae

SYNONYMS: Garden Lavender, *L. officinalis*, Chaix., *L. vera* D. C. Spike Lavender is *L. latifolia* Medic., (= *L. spica* D.C.). 'Lavandin' is a hybrid of these.

HABITAT: Native to the Mediterranean region.

DESCRIPTION: The calyx is tubular, veined, purplish-grey, and five-toothed, one tooth being larger than the others. The corolla is also tubular, blue or mauve, two-lipped, the upper lip having two lobes and the lower having three. Taste and odour: pleasant, characteristic.

PART USED: Flowers.

CONSTITUENTS: (i) Volatile oil, containing linalyl acetate (up to 40%), with linalool, lavandulyl acetate, borneol, camphor, limonene, caryophyllene, 4-butanolide, and similar compounds (ii) Coumarins; umbelliferone, herniarin, coumarin, dihydrocoumarin (iii) Triterpenes such as ursolic acid (iv) Flavonoids such as luteolin (v) Caffeic acid derivatives including rosmarinic acid. Spike Lavender oil contains mainly 1,8-cineole and camphor, with little linalyl acetate [R8,R19;1,2].

MEDICINAL USE: Carminative, sedative, spasmolytic, anticonvulsant, antidepressant [R1]. Many of these uses have been supported by experimental and clinical results. The oil has central nervous system depressant activity in mice [3,4] and clinical studies have demonstrated the sedative effect of inhaled Lavender oil, including in patients who had been taking benzodiazepines and neuroleptics [R8;5]. The oil is spasmolytic in a number of isolated smooth muscle preparations [6], and has local anaesthetic properties [7]. A recent review on the physiological and psychological parameters of Lavender oil suggests that clinical and scientific data substantiates the traditional use of the oil, but methodological and identification problems (for example, the species from which is obtained) makes conclusive proof difficult to obtain at present [8]. The phenolic constituents are antioxidants [9]. Lavender oil kills mites, the activity due mainly to linalool [10]. For reviews, see [8,11]. Lavender is used extensively in perfumery, and Spike Lavender is used as an insect repellent.

SPECIFIC REFERENCES: 1. Timiner R et al 1975) J. Agric. Food. Chem. 23:53. 2. Kaiser R et al (1977) Tet. Lett. 7:665. 3. Guillemain J et al (1989) Ann. Pharm. Francais 47(6):337. 4. Buchbauer G et al (1991) Z. Naturforsch. 46C:1067. 5. Hardy M et al (1995) Lancet 346:701. 6. Lis-Balchin M et al (1999) Phytother. Res. 13(6):540. 7. Ghelardini C et al (1999) Planta Med. 65(8):700. 8. Cavanagh H et al (2002) Phytother. Res. 16(4):301. 9. Hohmann J et al (1999) Planta Med. 65(6):576. 10. Perrucci S et al (1996) Phytother. Res. 10(1):5. 11. Lavender. Ed. Lis-Balchin M (2002) Medicinal and Aromatic Plants – Industrial Profiles. Pub: Taylor and Francis, London, UK.

LAVENDER COTTON
SANTOLINA CHAMAECYPARISSUS L.
Fam. Asteraceae

HABITAT: Mediterranean countries.

DESCRIPTION: Leaves linear, about 2.5 cm long and 6 mm broad, with short obtuse teeth. Flowers sub-globular, on long, leafless stalks, yellow with lanceolate, pointed outer bracts and membranous inner bracts. Stems white, with cottony hairs. Taste: bitter; odour: reminiscent of chamomile.

PART USED: Herb.

CONSTITUENTS: (i) Essential oil, containing artemisia ketone as the major constituent, with myrcene and alpha-pinene (ii) Flavonoids, particularly 6-methoxy flavones; pectolinarigenin, hispidulin, nepetin and others (iii) Sterols, including beta-sitosterol glucoside [R2;1,2,3].

MEDICINAL USE: Anti-inflammatory, stomachic, emmenagogue, anthelmintic [R1]. The anti-inflammatory effects of various extracts were demonstrated in a number of assays, with no ulcerogenic or other signs of toxicity, and attributed to the beta-sitosterol content [1]. It inhibited mouse paw oedema induced by arachidonic acid and phorbol ester and was active against phospholipase A2 *in vitro* [4]. Spasmolytic

261

effects on isolated rat duodenum and uterus were also observed [1,5]. The oil is anti-candidal *in vivo* and *in vitro*, and was shown to be synergistic with clotrimazole [6].

SPECIFIC REFERENCES: 1. Giner R *et al* (1988) *Phytother. Res.* 2(1):37. 2. Becchi M R *et al* (1980) *Planta Med.* 38(3):267. 3. Rios J *et al* (1989) *Phytother. Res.* 3(5):212. 4. Sala A *et al* (2000) *Life Sci.* 66(2):PL35. 5. Giner R *et al* (1989) *J. Ethnopharmacol.* 27(1–2):1. 6. Suresh B *et al* (1997) *J. Ethnopharmacol.* 55(2):151.

LEMON
CITRUS LIMON (L.) BURM.
Fam. Rutaceae

SYNONYMS: Limon.

HABITAT: Native to Asia, cultivated widely throughout the world.

DESCRIPTION: The fruit is too well known to require description.

PART USED: Fruit, juice, peel and essential oil.

CONSTITUENTS: (i) Essential oil, in the peel, consisting of limonene, the major component (ca. 70%), with citral, alpha-terpinene, alpha- and beta-pinene, myrcene and sabinene; and sesquiterpenes such as bisabolene and caryophyllene (ii) Coumarins including limettin, bergamottin, imperatorin, sinensetin, nobiletin and 8-geranyloxypsoralen (iii) Flavonoids, often referred to as citrus bioflavonoids; mainly hesperidin, neohesperidin, naringin and eryocitrin and rutin (iv) Vitamin C, mucilage, calcium oxalate [R2,R5,R19 and refs therein].

MEDICINAL USE: The citrus bioflavonoids are frequently used in vascular disorders where venous insufficiency results in haemorrhoids and varicose veins, since they affect vascular permeability to liquids and proteins by decreasing porosity [R1]. They are also antihistaminic, diuretic, induce apoptosis in HL-60 cells, and inhibit bacterial mutagenesis [1,2,3]. The coumarins inhibit *in vitro* tumour promotion and superoxide and nitric oxide generation [4]. The fruit extract was shown to neutralize the haemorrhagic effect *in vitro* of snake venom (from *Bothrops atrox*) [5]. Lemons are a well-known source of vitamin C and are more usually used as a food and flavouring. For a full recent review of the genus *Citrus*, see [6].

SPECIFIC REFERENCES: 1. Paris R *et al* (1977) *Plantes Med. Phytother.* 11(Suppl):129 and 198. 2. Ogata S *et al* (2000) *Biosci. Biotech. Biochem.* 64(5):1075. 3. Calomme M *et al* (1996) *Planta Med.* 62:222. 4. Miyake Y *et al* (1999) *J. Agric. Food Chem.* 47(8):3151. 5. Otero R *et al* (2000) *J. Ethnopharmacol.* 73(1–2):233. 6. Citrus. Ed. Dugo G (2002) *Medicinal and Aromatic Plants – Industrial Profiles.* Pub: Taylor and Francis, London, UK.

LEMONGRASS

CYMBOPOGON CITRATUS (DC) STAPF.
C. FLEXOSUS (STEUDEL) J WATSON
Fam. Poaceae

SYNONYMS: West Indian Lemongrass is *C. citratus* (= *Andropogon citratus*) and East Indian Lemongrass is *C. flexosus* (= *A. flexosus*). These species are also known as Citronella in North America and India, but should not be confused with *C. nardus* or *C. winterana*, which are more commonly known as Citronella (q.v.).

HABITAT: Thought to be indigenous to tropical Asia, but now found widely in throughout the tropics.

DESCRIPTION: A densely tufted grass with tapering leaves up to 1 m long, and 5–10 mm wide, with the inflorence (which is 30–60 cm long) rarely formed. Odour and taste: lemony.

PART USED: Leaves, oil.

CONSTITUENTS: (i) Volatile oil, composed of citral (up to 75%), with myrcene, limonene, dipentene, linalool, nerol and geraniol, eugenol, furfural, citronellol, citronellal, nerolidol, menthol, humulene, cymbopogone and others (ii) Flavonoids including luteolin glycosides [R12,R18,R19;1].

MEDICINAL USE: Antimicrobial, sedative, antipyretic, analgesic. The antibacterial effects have been demonstrated in a number of studies, and it was found to inhibit *Staphyloccus aureus, Bacillus subtilis, Escherichia coli* [2], *Enterococcus faecalis, Klebsiella pneumoniae, Serratia marcescens* and others [3,4]. The oil is also anti-fungal against *Candida albicans* [3], and various *Trichophyton* species [5,6], and a cream containing a minimum of 2.5% was considered suitable for further clinical study [7]. The sedative and anxiolytic properties have also been assessed, but toxicity remains a concern [R18;8] and the analgesic effects confirmed; these are thought to be due at least in part to the myrcene content [9]. Lemongrass oil can cause sensitivity and oral use should be avoided, although when used as flavouring in cookery the herb is considered safe.

SPECIFIC REFERENCES: 1. Ayoub S *et al* (1984) *Fitoterapia* 55(6):368. 2. Alam K *et al* (1994) *Int. J. Pharmacog.* 32(4):396. 3. Hammer K *et al* (1999) *J. Appl. Microbiol.* 86(6):985. 4. Inouye S *et al* (2001) *Mycoses* 44(3–4):99. 5. Inouye S *et al* (2001) *J. Infect. Chemother.* 7(4):251. 6. Onawunmi G (1989) *Int. J. Crude Drug Res.* 27(2):121. 7. Wannisorn B *et al* (1996) *Phytother. Res.* 10(7):551. 8. Leite J *et al* (1986) *J. Ethnopharmacol.* 17(1):75. 9. Lorenzetti B *et al* (1991) *J. Ethnopharmacol.* 43(1):43.

LEMON VERBENA

ALOYSIA TRIPHYLLA (L'HER) BRITT.
Fam. Verbenaceae

SYNONYMS: Lemon Verbena, Herb Louisa, *Lippia citriodora* (Lam.)

263

HBK, *L. triphylla* L'Her, *Verbena citriodora* Cav. It is also known as Cedron in Mexico (not to be confused with *Simaba cedron*, q.v.).

HABITAT: Native to Argentina and Chile, cultivated in Europe and North Africa and elsewhere.

DESCRIPTION: The leaves occur in whorls of three or four on the stem, lanceolate, up to 10 cm long with the lateral veins almost at right angles to the midrib. Odour and taste: lemony.

PART USED: Leaves.

CONSTITUENTS: (i) Volatile oil, composed of citral, with cineole, limonene, dipentene, linalool, borneol, nerol and geraniol, and a C9-aldehyde (ii) Flavonoids including apigenin, diosmetin and luteolin glycosides, eupatorin and eupafolin (iii) Iridoids including verbascoside (acteoside) and geniposidic acid [1,2,3,4,5,6].

MEDICINAL USE: Antispasmodic, sedative, antipyretic. The oil is reported to be antispasmodic in guinea pigs [1], and anti-diarrhoeal activity has been observed in mice and ascribed to the C9-aldehyde [6]. The hexane extract has been suggested to possess antagonistic activity on beta-adrenergic receptors and affect calcium metabolism in the rat [7].

SPECIFIC REFERENCES: 1. Killacky J *et al* (1976) *Planta Med.* 30:310. 2. Tomas-Barberan F *et al* (1987) *Phytochem.* 26:2281. 3. Skalta H *et al* (1988) *Planta Med.* 54:265. 4. Carnat A *et al* (1995) *Planta Med.* 61(5):490. 5. Carnat A *et al* (1999) *Fitoterapia* 70(1):44. 6. Salud-Peraz G *et al* (1997) *Phytother. Res.* 12(Suppl.)S:45. 7. Varga Solis R (2000) *Rev. Mex. Cien. Farm.* 31(3):23.

LETTUCE, WILD
LACTUCA VIROSA L.
Fam. Asteraceae

SYNONYMS: Lettuce Opium or Lactucarium is the name given to the dried latex. Garden (or Salad) Lettuce is *L. sativa* L., and Prickly Lettuce is *L. scariola* L.

HABITAT: Indigenous to central and southern Europe and northern Asia, cultivated elsewhere.

DESCRIPTION: Similar to garden lettuce, however the leaves are much narrower, with bristles on the undersurface of the midrib. The dried juice is less commonly used nowadays, it is dark reddish-brown externally and waxy internally. Taste: very bitter; odour: characteristic, heavy.

PART USED: Leaves, dried juice.

CONSTITUENTS: (i) Sesquiterpene lactones including lactucin, lactucopicrin, 8-desoxylactucin, jacquinelin, dihydrolactucin and lactuside A [1] (ii) Flavonoids; mainly based on quercetin [2] (iii) Coumarins; cichoriin and esculin [2] (iv) *N*-methyl-beta-phenethylamine [3] (disputed in [4]) (v) Hyoscyamine, a tropane alkaloid, (disputed in [4]). Very low amounts of morphine (i.e. nanogram concentrations) have been reported, although not confirmed, but are not thought to contribute to any pharmacological effect of wild lettuce [R7].

MEDICINAL USE: Mild sedative, hypnotic, analgesic, expectorant [R1]. Wild lettuce is used for bronchitis, irritable coughs and for insomnia and stress, especially in combination with other herbs such as Hops, Jamaica Dogwood and Valerian (q.v.). Therapeutically, a combination of constituents is thought to be the most effective [1]. Although widely used, there is little evidence for the efficacy of wild lettuce preparations, and the constituents are still disputed [4]. Sedative and analgesic effects have been confirmed in mice, measured using spontaneous locomotor activity, and the most active compounds found to be lactucin, its derivatives and lactuside A [R2,R7 and refs therein].

PREPARATIONS AND DOSE: Dried leaf, dose: 0.5–3 g or equivalent extract, three times daily.

SPECIFIC REFERENCES: 1. Gromek D *et al* (1992) *Phytother. Res.* 6(5):285. 2. Rees S *et al* (1984) *Bot. J. Linn.* Soc. 89:3313. 3. Marquardt P *et al* (1976) *Planta Med.* 30:68. 4. Huang Z *et al* (1982) *J. Pharm. Sci.* 71:270.

LIFE EVERLASTING
ANTENNARIA DIOICA (L.) GAERTN.
Fam. Asteraceae

SYNONYMS: Catsfoot, Cat's Ear, *Gnaphalium dioicum* L.

HABITAT: Northern Europe including Britain, Asia, North America.

DESCRIPTION: A low creeping perennial, with obovate leaves which are white and cottony on the undersurface. Flowers dioecious, in terminal clusters, rayless, pink or red, with red or white sepal-like bracts. Taste: astringent; odour: aromatic (stronger in the female flowers).

PART USED: Herb.

CONSTITUENTS: (i) Flavonoids including luteolin and its *O*-glycosides (ii) Volatile oil (iii) Triterpenes such as ursolic acid and sterols [R2,R4,1,2].

MEDICINAL USE: Astringent; used as a gargle or styptic as well as internally for diarrhoea [R1]. An extract has been shown to stimulate phagocytosis in mice inoculated with *Escherichia coli* [3].

SPECIFIC REFERENCES: 1. Didry N *et al* (1982) *Ann. Pharm. Fr.* 40:75. 2. Delaveau P *et al* (1980) *Planta Med.* 40:40. 3. Swiatek L *et al* (1982) *Planta Med.* 40:153.

LIFE ROOT
SENECIO AUREUS L.
Fam. Asteraceae

SYNONYMS: Squaw Weed, Golden Senecio.

HABITAT: Europe, including Britain, North America.

DESCRIPTION: Rhizome 2–5 cm long, with numerous roots; the root bark being hard and blackish surrounding a ring of whitish woody bundles and a large, dark, central pith. Root leaves up to 15 cm long, reniform; those on the stem shorter, incised and pinnatifid. Flower-heads few, in a loose corymb, up to about 2.5 cm broad, with yellow pistillate ray florets and hermaphrodite central tubular florets. Taste: bitter and astringent; odour: faint, slightly acrid.

PART USED: Rhizome, herb.

CONSTITUENTS: (i) Pyrrolizidine alkaloids; florosenine, otosenine, floridanine [1,2] (ii) Eremophilane sesquiterpenes, *trans*-9-oxofura-noeremophilane-8alpha-ethoxy-10alpha-*H*-eremophilane, cacalol and others [2].

MEDICINAL USE: Emmenagogue, diuretic, astringent, pectoral [R1]. Has been used as a uterine tonic and for amenorrhoea, and for menopausal symptoms. However, only samples with alkaloids absent should be taken internally.

SPECIFIC REFERENCES: 1. Roder E *et al* (1983) *Planta Med.* 49(1):57. 2. Resch J *et al* (1983) *Planta Med.* 47(4):252. 3. Zalkow L *et al* (1979) *J. Chem. Soc. Perkin Trans.* 1:1542.

LILY OF THE VALLEY
CONVALLARIA MAJALIS L.

Fam. Convallariaceae

SYNONYMS: May Lily, Muguet.

HABITAT: A common garden plant.

DESCRIPTION: Leaves broadly lanceolate, up to 15 cm long and about 5 cm wide, parallel-veined with entire margins. Flower stem carries 8–12 small, stalked, bell-shaped white flowers with six stamens. Rhizome cylindrical, slender, internodes about 5 cm apart bearing numerous slender rootlets, pale brown. Taste: sweet at first, then bitter; odour: pleasant.

PART USED: Leaves, whole plant.

CONSTITUENTS: (i) Cardiactive glycosides; the cardenolides convallatoxin, convalloside, convallatoxol, desglucocheirotoxin, lokunjoside, convallamaroside, glycosides of bipindogenin, sarmentologenin, sarmentosigenin A, rhodexin A, rhodexoside and others (ii) Flavonoid glycosides, in the leaves [R3;1,2].

MEDICINAL USE: Cardiac tonic [R1]. It has a similar action to digitalis (Foxglove, q.v.) but is less cumulative, and has been used to treat congestive heart failure. It is normally used as the isolated glycoside convallatoxin, either as a single extract or combined with other cardioactive drugs [3]. Lily of the Valley flowers are used in perfumery.

SPECIFIC REFERENCES: 1. Kopp B *et al* (1982) *Planta Med.* 45(4):195. 2. Saxena V *et al* (1992) *J. Nat. Prod.* 55(1):39. 3. Loew D (1997) *Z. Phytother.* 18:92.

LIME FLOWERS
TILIA PLATYPHYLLA SCOP.
T. CORDATA MILL, AND OTHERS
T. X EUROPEAEA L.
Fam. Tiliaceae

SYNONYMS: Lindenflowers, (*T. europaea* = *T. x vulgaris*).

HABITAT: Europe and North America.

DESCRIPTION: The flower-stalk bears about three to six yellowish-white, five-petalled flowers, on stalks half-joined to an oblong bract. The leaves are heart-shaped, greyish beneath and downy. The flowers are fragrant.

PART USED: Flowers, with or without the bract.

CONSTITUENTS: (i) Volatile oil, up to about 0.1%, containing farnesol, linalool, germacrene, geraniol, 1,8-cineole, 2-phenyl ethanol and others (ii) Flavonoids; hesperidin, quercetin, astralagin, tiliroside and others (iii) Mucilage (in the bract), consisting of polysaccharides based mainly on arabinose, galactose and rhamnose (iv) Phenolic acids such as chlorogenic and caffeic, tannins (v) Amino acids including GABA (gamma amino benzoic acid) [R2,R7;1,2,3,4].

MEDICINAL USE: Nervine, tonic, hypotensive, antispasmodic [R1]. They may be used for nervous disorders, catarrh, headaches including migraine, indigestion and other disorders, but the main use is for feverish colds, coughs and influenza. The polysaccharides are soothing and adhere to epithelial tissue [5]. The sedative usage is supported by evidence that components of the aqueous extract of the flowers bind to GABA receptors in rat brain, an effect not due entirely to the GABA content of the extract [4]. Sedative effects were confirmed using the elevated maze anxiety test in mice, although no anxiolytic effects were observed [6]. The extract is thought to act as an agonist of the peripheral benzodiazepine receptor and stimulated lymphocyte proliferation by this mechanism in a similar manner to a standard agonist [7]. Other activities described for Lime Flowers include inhibition of growth of fungi [8] and food-borne pathogens [9] and antispasmodic activity on isolated rat intestine [10].

PREPARATIONS AND DOSE: Dried flowers (with bract), dose: 2–4 g or equivalent extract, three times daily.

SPECIFIC REFERENCES: 1. Buchbauer G *et al* (1992) *Deutsche Apot. Ztg.* 132:748. 2. Kram G J *et al* (1985) *Pharmazie* 40(7):501. 3. Czygan F (1997) *Z. Phytotherapie* 18(4):242. 4. Cavadas C *et al* (1997) *Phytother. Res.* 11(1):17. 5. Schmidgall J *et al* (2000) *Planta Med.* 66(1):48. 6. Coleta M *et al* (2001) *Pharmacopsychiatry* 34(Suppl.1):S20. 7. Anesini C *et al* (1999) *Fitoterapia* 70(4):361. 8. Guerin J *et al* (1984) *Ann. Pharm. Franc.* 42(6):553. 9. Gonul E *et al* (1987) *Food Microbiol.* 4(1):97. 10. Lanza P *et al* (1986) *Fitoterapia* 57(3):185.

LIME FRUIT
CITRUS AURANTIFOLIA SWINGLE
Fam. Rutaceae

SYNONYMS: C. *medica* var *acida* Brandis, C. *acris* Mill., C. *limetta* Risso.

HABITAT: Indigenous to southern Asia and cultivated widely in the West Indies, Florida and Central America.

DESCRIPTION: Variable in appearance but usually resembling the lemon, except they are nearly globular, smaller and more greenish in colour.

PART USED: Fruit, juice.

CONSTITUENTS: (i) Volatile oil, consisting of about 75% limonene, with alpha-and beta-pinenes, sabinene, terpinolene, citral, alpha-terpineol, linalool, alpha-bergamotene, beta-bisabolene and others (ii) Coumarins; the major one being limettin, with bergamottin, bergapten (= 5-methoxypsoralen), dimethoxycoumarin, 8-geranoxy-psoralen, isoimperatorin, isopimpinellin and others (iii) Miscellaneous; flavonoids including hesperidin, vitamin C etc. [R2;1,2,3].

MEDICINAL USE: Anti-scorbutic, refrigerant [R1]. Limes are used more often for flavouring than medicinally. The juice is a traditional source of vitamin C and recent studies have shown that is also has immunomodulatory properties [4]. The coumarins such as bergapten are well-known for causing photosensitization, and allergies have been reported [5]. The extract of the rind is insecticidal to the mosquito, cockroach and housefly [6]. The expressed oil is used in perfumery.

SPECIFIC REFERENCES: 1. Slater C et al (1961) *J. Sci. Agric. Food* 12:732. 2. Tatum J *et al* (1977) *Phytochem.* 16:109. 3. Thompson H *et al* (1984) *J. Chromatog.* 314:323. 4. Gharagozloo M *et al* (2001) *J. Ethnopharmacol.* 77(1):85. 5. Rzeznik J (1997) *Novelles Dermatol.* 16(3):110. 6. Ezeonu F *et al* (2001) *Bioresource Tech.* 76(3):273.

LIPPIA
LIPPIA DULCIS TREV.
Fam. Verbenaceae

SYNONYMS: Yerba Dulce, Cimarron.

HABITAT: Mexico.

DESCRIPTION: Leaves, about 5 cm long, ovate, pointed, serrate above with prominent veins and glandular hairs. Taste and odour: aromatic, agreeable.

PART USED: Leaves.

CONSTITUENTS: (i) Volatile oil, containing camphor and 6-methyl-5-hepten-2-one (ii) Sesquiterpenes including hernandulcin, epihernandulcin, beta-hydroxyhernandulcin (iii) Acteoside (= verbascoside, a phenylpropanoid) is present in the flowers. Alkaloids and saponins have been shown to be absent [1,2].

MEDICINAL USE: Expectorant, demulcent [R1]. It is used mainly for respiratory ailments. Antibacterial effects against *Staphylococcus aureus*, *Streptococcus pneumoniae* and *S. pyogenes*, all of which are implicated in respiratory infections, have been observed [4]. The sesquiterpenes are very sweet in taste and the herb is used as a flavouring [2]. This and many other species of *Lippia* are also used as sedatives for the treatment of gastrointestinal complaints [5].

SPECIFIC REFERENCES: 1. Breitweiser K (1943) *Pharmazie Ind.* 10:76. 2. Kaneda N *et al* (1992) *J. Nat. Prod.* 55(8):1136. 3. Compadre C *et al* (1986) *J. Ethnopharmacol.* 15(1):89. 4. Caceres A *et al* (1991) *J. Ethnopharmacol.* 31(2):193. 5. Pascual M *et al* (2001) *J. Ethnopharmacol.* 76(3):201.

LIQUORICE
GLYCYRRHIZA GLABRA L.
Fam. Fabaceae

SYNONYMS: Licorice, Spanish or Italian liquorice is *G. glabra* var *typica* Reg. et Herd., Persian or Turkish Liquorice is *G. glabra* var *violacea* Boiss, Russian Liquorice is G. *glabra* var *glandulifera* Waldst. et Kit. Chinese or Manchurian Liquorice is from the closely related *G. uralensis* Fisch.

HABITAT: Native to the Mediterranean region and parts of Asia, cultivated worldwide.

DESCRIPTION: Liquorice root is well-known. The root and stolons vary in appearance depending on origin. They are usually found cut into lengths of up to 15–20 cm and of variable diameter, stolons normally being narrower than roots. The external surface when unpeeled is dark reddish-brown, longitudinally wrinkled with occasional root scars. Internally it is yellowish and fibrous, with a radiate structure; the stolons have a visible central pith. Liquorice is also found in commerce in the form of soft or hard extracts. Taste and odour: sweet, characteristic.

PART USED: Root, underground stem or stolon.

CONSTITUENTS: (i) Triterpenes of the oleanane type, mainly glycyrrhizin (= glycyrrhizic or glycyrrhizinic acid), and its aglycone glycyrrhetinic acid (= glycyrrhitic acid), liquiritic acid, glycyrrhetol, glabrolide, isoglabrolide, licoric acid, and phytosterols (ii) Flavonoids (isoflavonoids and chalcones); glabridin, liquiritigenin, liquiritin, rhamnoliquiritin, neoliquiritin, isoliquiritigenin, neoisoliquiritin, rhamnoisoliquiritin, licuraside, licochalcones A and B, echinatin, licoflavonol, licoisoflavones A and B, licoisoflavanone, formononetin, glabrol, glabrene, glabrone, glyzarin, kumatakenin, hispaglabridin A and B, shinpterocarpin, 1-methoxyphaseollin and maybe others (iii) Coumarins; liqcoumarin, umbelliferone, herniarin, glabrocoumarones A and B, glycyrin (iv) Polysaccharides, mainly glucans and galactans, e.g. glycyrrhizan GA, and glycoproteins (v) Volatile oil, containing fenchone, linalool, furfuryl alcohol, benzaldehyde and others (vi)

269

Miscellaneous; starch, sugars, amino acid etc. [R2,R7;1,2,3,4,5,6,7].

MEDICINAL USE: Demulcent, anti-inflammatory, expectorant, antitussive, spasmolytic [R1]. Other important uses are in the treatment of gastric and duodenal ulcers and for adrenocortical insufficiency. Liquorice has been used for thousands of years throughout the world for its medicinal properties, and recent pharmacological work has substantiated many of these, which will be summarized briefly. The major active ingredient is glycyrrhizin, which is responsible for the sweet taste. It is the main expectorant ingredient, and the 18-beta derivative of glycyrrhetinic acid has an antitussive activity comparable to that of codeine [8]. Both glycyrrhizin and glycyrrhetinic acid are anti-inflammatory and anti-allergic [8,9], helping to explain their efficacy in asthma. They have been shown to be hepatoprotective, mediating their activity through an antioxidative rather than a corticosteroid-like mechanism [9]. Liquorice has anti-ulcer activity and a derivative of glycyrrhetinic acid, carbenoxolone, is used clinically for ulcers, including aphthous (mouth) ulcers. Glycyrrhizin and glycyrrhetinic acid have mineralo-corticoid activity and this can limit their use in the long-term management of stomach ulcers. However, extracts of deglycyrrhizinized Liquorice have a similar protective effect against experimentally induced ulcers, and possess hepatoprotective effects in animals [10]. Glycyrrhizin has recently been found to have an anti-cariogenic activity by inhibiting bacterial growth and plaque formation; it has been suggested as a vehicle for topical oral medications [8]. It is also a thrombin inhibitor [11] and melanogenesis stimulator [12]. Liquorice has oestrogenic activity, ascribed to the isoflavonoids present. Liquiritigenin and isoliquiritigenin are monoamine oxidase inhibitors *in vitro* [13] and may therefore have anti-depressant activity, and glabridin and derivatives are antioxidants [14,15]. Glabridin is anti-fungal [16] Liquiritin also has significant anti-inflammatory activity in the rat paw oedema test. The polysaccharide fraction has anti-complement, immunostimulating, alkaline phosphatase inducing activity [7], and activates macrophages [17]. Adverse effects of liquorice are only seen after excessive consumption but can include hypertension and hypokalaemia [18] and slightly premature childbirth [19]. There is a vast amount of literature available on liquorice; for more detail, see reviews and references cited [R2,R5,R7,R8,R9,R13;8,9,10,11,12,13,14,15,16,17,18,19].

PREPARATIONS AND DOSE: Dried root, dose: 1–4 g, Liquorice Liquid Extract BP, dose: 2–5 ml.

SPECIFIC REFERENCES: 1. Saitoh T *et al* (1976) *Chem. Pharm. Bull.* 24:752, 991 and 1242. 2. Kinoshita T *et al* (1977) *Chem. Pharm. Bull.* 26:135 and 141. 3. Vaya J *et al* (1997) *Free Radical Biol. Med.* 23(2):302. 4. Kinoshita T *et al* (1997) *Nat. Prod. Lett.* 9(4):289. 5. Kinoshita T *et al* (1996) *Chem. Pharm. Bull.* 44(6):1218. 6. Kitagawa I *et al* (1994) *Chem. Pharm. Bull.* 42(5):1056. 7. Takada K *et al* (1992) *Chem. Pharm. Bull.* 40(9):2487. 8. Segal R *et al* (1985) *J. Pharm. Sci.* 74(1):79. 9. Kiso Y *et al* (1984) *Planta Med.* 50:298. 10. Al-Qarawi E *et al* (2001)

J. Herbs Spices Med. Plants 8(1):7–14. 11. Mauricio I *et al* (1997) *Biochem. Biophys. Res. Commun.* 235(1):259. 12. Jung G *et al* (2001) *Exp. Mol. Med.* 33(3):131. 13. Tanaka S *et al* (1987) *Planta Med.* 53(1):5. 14. Belinky P *et al* (1998) *Atherosclerosis* 137(1):49. 15. Haraguchi H *et al* (2000) *J. Pharm. Pharmacol.* 52(2):219. 16. Sato J *et al* (2001) *Biocontrol Sci.* 6(2):113. 17. Nose M *et al* (1998) *Biol. Pharm. Bull.* 21(10):1110. 18. Sigurjonsdottir H *et al* (2001) *J. Hum. Hypertens.* 15(8):549. 19. Strandberg T *et al* (2001) *J. Epidemiol.* 153(11):1085.

LIVERWORT, AMERICAN
HEPATICA NOBILIS GARS.
Fam. Ranunculaceae

SYNONYMS: Kidneywort, Liverleaf, *H. triloba* Chois, *Anemone hepatica* L. *H. nobilis* Mill.

HABITAT: North America, and cultivated as a garden plant elsewhere.

DESCRIPTION: Leaves long-stalked, leathery, smooth, dark green above, rounded with three broad, angular lobes. Taste: slightly astringent and bitter; odourless.

PART USED: Herb.

CONSTITUENTS: (i) Protoanemonin, in the fresh plant, which dimerizes on drying to produce anemonin (ii) Flavonoids including isoquercetrin, astragalin and quercimetrin (iii) Miscellaneous; anthocyanins, a saponin glycoside hepatrilobin [R2,R4,1].

MEDICINAL USE: Pectoral, astringent, tonic [R1]. Has been used in disorders of the liver and indigestion. Protoanemonin has antibiotic activity and causes irritation.

SPECIFIC REFERENCES: 1. Ruikgrok H (1963) *Planta Med.* 11:338.

LIVERWORT, ENGLISH
PELTIGERA CANINA (L.) WILL.
Fam. Peltigeraceae

SYNONYMS: Liverwort, Lichen Caninus.

HABITAT: Moist, shady places in Europe.

DESCRIPTION: Fronds foliaceous, coriaceous and lobed, attached to the ground, wall etc. directly.

PART USED: Plant.

CONSTITUENTS: Unknown; peltigeroside has been cited [R4]. The chlorine-containing metabolites nostoclide I and II have been isolated from a symbiotic cyanobacterium, *Nostoc* spp., found in the lichen [1]. The related species *P. aphthosa* contains the depsides methyl- and ethyl-orsellinate [2].

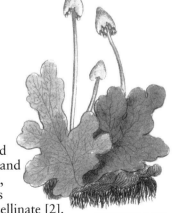

LIVERWORT

MEDICINAL USE: Mild purgative [R1]. Formerly used for liver complaints. *P. leucophlebia* shows potential cancer chemoprotective

271

activity and cytotoxicity in a number of *in vitro* assays [3].

SPECIFIC REFERENCES: 1. Yang X *et al* (1993) *Tet. Lett.* 34(5):761.
2. Ingolfsdottir K *et al* (1985) *Antimicrob. Agents Chemother.*
28(2):289. 3. Ingolfsdottir K *et al* (2000) *Pharm. Biol.* 38(4):313.

LOBELIA

LOBELIA INFLATA L.
Fan. Campanulaceae

SYNONYMS: Indian Tobacco, Pukeweed.

HABITAT: Eastern North America, cultivated elsewhere.

DESCRIPTION: Leaves pale green or yellowish, sessile, alternate, ovatelanceolate, 3–8 cm long, with a toothed margin and pubescent lamina. The fruit consists of an inflated, ovoid or flattened bilocular capsule containing numerous small, brown, reticulate seeds.
Taste: acrid; odour: faintly irritant.

PART USED: Herb, collected when the lower fruits are ripe.

CONSTITUENTS: (i) Piperidine alkaloids, mainly lobeline, with lobelanidine, lobelanine, and minor amounts of norlobelanine (= isolobelanine), lelobanidine, lobinine, isolobinine, lobinanidine and others (ii) Triterpenes including beta-amyrin palmitate (iii) Chelidonic acid [R2,R7;1,2,3].

MEDICINAL USE: Respiratory stimulant, expectorant, emetic, diaphoretic [R1]. Lobelia has been used for the treatment of asthma, bronchitis and as a tobacco deterrent; it is present in some anti-smoking mixtures. Lobeline has similar but less potent pharmacological properties to nicotine, which helps to alleviate the withdrawal symptoms associated with stopping smoking. Lobeline stimulates respiration in animals by stimulating the respiratory centre and at high doses stimulates the vomiting centre [R2,R7;4] and has recently been suggested as a treatment for psychostimulant abuse, because of its effects on the vesicular monoamine transporter (VMAT2) [5]. It has also been used as a poultice for treating boils and ulcers. Beta-amyrin palmitate isolated from Lobelia has been shown to have antidepressant effects in animals [3].

PREPARATIONS AND DOSE: Powdered leaf, dose: 200–600 mg daily, or equivalent extract, if prescribed by a herbalist. For general sales, 65 mg is the maximum, without a frequency restriction.

SPECIFIC REFERENCES: 1. Gross D (1971) *Forts. Chem. Org. Nat.* 29:1.
2. Schwarz H (1990) *Z. Phytother.* 11:159. 3. Subarnas A *et al* (1993)
J. Pharm. Pharmacol. 45(6):545. 4. Locock R (1992) *Can. Pharm. J.*
125(1):33. 5. Dwoskin L *et al* (2002) *Biochem. Pharmacol.* 63(2):89.

LOGWOOD
HAEMATOXYLON CAMPECHIANUM L.
Fam. Caesalpiniaceae

SYNONYMS: Peachwood.

HABITAT: Central America, naturalized in the West Indies.

DESCRIPTION: The wood is normally sold in chips for dyeing purposes; it has a dark, purplish-brown colour with a greenish iridescence which indicates it has been fermented. For medicinal use the unfermented chips are preferred; these have a bright reddish-brown tint.

PART USED: Wood.

CONSTITUENTS: (i) Isoflavones including haematoxylin and the related hematoxylol A and tetra-O-methyl hematoxylol B [1].

MEDICINAL USE: Astringent, anti-inflammatory [R1]. Formerly used for diarrhoea and haemorrhage. Haematoxylin is a red pigment used as a staining reagent; it has a sweet taste [1].

SPECIFIC REFERENCES: 1. Masuda H *et al* (1991) *Chem. Pharm. Bull.* 39(6):1382.

LOOSESTRIFE
LYSIMACHIA VULGARIS L.
Fam. Primulaceae

SYNONYMS: Yellow Loosestrife, Yellow Willowherb.

HABITAT: In wet places and by rivers in Britain and Europe.

DESCRIPTION: The herb reaches about 1 m, bearing short-stalked, oval to lanceolate leaves in whorls of two to four. The flowers are yellow, 1.5–2 cm in diameter, in axillary and terminal panicles. Taste: astringent, slightly acid; odourless.

PART USED: Herb.

CONSTITUENTS: (i) Saponosides A and B etc, based on primulagenin A and protoprimulagenin A (ii) Benzoquinones such as 2,5-dihydroxy-3-pentadecylbenzoquinone [1,2] (iii) Flavonoids based on kaempferol and quercetin, including rutin (iv) Phytosterols [R2].

MEDICINAL USE: Astringent, for nosebleeds, wounds and menorraghia; expectorant [R1]. Saponoside B exerts cytotoxicity, especially towards human melanoma cells and the benzoquinone pigment showed potent anti-fungal effects against *Candida albicans* [1,2].

SPECIFIC REFERENCES: 1. Janik I *et al* (1994) *Fitoterapia* 65(5):476. 2. Podolak I *et al* (1996) *Phytother. Res.* 12(Suppl.):S70.

LORENZO'S OIL
CONSTITUENTS: Glyceryl trierucate (a source of erucic acid, obtained from rapeseed or other oil) and glyceryl trioleate (a source of oleic acid) in the ratio 1 part to 4 parts respectively [R14;1,2,3,4].

273

MEDICINAL USE: Lorenzo's oil is used as a treatment for adrenoleu-codystrophy (ALD), an incurable, rare, genetic, X-linked metabolic disorder in which saturated very long chain fatty acids (VLCFA) accumulate and produce damage to the nervous system, adrenal cortex and testis [1]. The efficacy of the oil has been disputed, and it appears to show better effects in some forms of the disease or as a preventative treatment [2,3]. A recent study in Japanese patients with the disease, in which many of the early symptoms had already appeared, were promising and indicated that further trials should be instigated [5]. Thrombocytopenia and the production of giant platelets are common side effects [1] and lymphocytopenia has been reported [4].

SPECIFIC REFERENCES: 1. Konijnenberg A et al (1998) Platelets 9(1):41. 2. Girard S et al (2001) Ann. Med. Intern. 152(1):15. 3. Vargas C et al (2000) Genet. Mol. Biol. 23(4):697. 4. Barmaki P et al (2000) J. Inher. Metabol. Dis. 23(2):113. 5. Suzuki Y et al (2001) Brain Devel. 23(1):30.

LOVAGE
LEVISTICUM OFFICINALE KOCH
Fam. Apiaceae

SYNONYMS: *Ligusticum levisticum* L.

HABITAT: Native to the Mediterranean region, cultivated in Britain and North America.

DESCRIPTION: The plant is a large perennial herb. The leaves are divided into wedge-shaped segments, the stems hollow and the flowers yellow, borne on umbels. The fleshy rhizome has a greyish-brown external surface and bears numerous longitudinally furrowed rootlets. The root bark is thick, spongy and whitish, and the wood yellowish showing glistening oil glands in cross-section. Taste: sweet, then slightly bitter; odour: strongly aromatic, characteristic.

PART USED: Root and rhizome.

CONSTITUENTS: (i) Volatile oil, containing phthalides (about 70%), including E- and Z-butylidenephthalide, E- and Z-ligustilide, senkyunolide, isosenkyunolide, validene-4,5-dihydrophthalide, butylphthalide and others; and terpenes such as alpha- and beta-pinene, alpha- and beta-phellandrene, carvacrol (ii) Coumarins; bergapten, coumarin, psoralen, umbelliferone (iii) Miscellaneous; plant acids, beta-sitosterol, resins, gums etc. [R2;R19,1,2,3,4].

MEDICINAL USE: Sedative, carminative, spasmolytic, diaphoretic, expectorant, antimicrobial [R1]. Lovage is used for dyspepsia, colic, dysmenorrhoea and cystitis, and as a gargle or mouthwash for tonsillitis and aphthous ulcers. The phthalides have sedative and anticonvulsant activity in animals and Lovage extracts and oil are reportedly strongly diuretic in mice and rabbits [R2,R19;4]. Lovage is used as a flavouring in food products and alcoholic beverages.

PREPARATIONS AND DOSE: Dried root, dose: 0.5–2 g as an infusion or decoction in water or milk, or equivalent extract, three times daily.

SPECIFIC REFERENCES: 1. Gijbels M *et al* (1981) *Chromatographia* 14(8):451. 2. Gijbels M *et al* (1982) *Planta Med.* 44:207. 3. Cichy M *et al* (1994) *Leibigs Ann. Chem.* 2:397. 4. Vollmann C (1988) *Z. Phytother.* 9:128.

LUNGMOSS
LOBARIA PULMONARIA (L.) HOFFM.
Fam. Stictaceae

SYNONYMS: Oak Lungs, Lungwort, *Sticta pulmonaria* L.

HABITAT: Found on old trees and rocks throughout Europe.

DESCRIPTION: The lichen is flat, greyish or greenish-brown, leathery, forked, the lobes being about 1.5 cm broad at the widest part. The inner surface is reticulate with small depressions, which are evident on the upper surface as convexities. Taste: mucilaginous bitter, slightly acrid; odour: characteristic.

PART USED: Lichen.

CONSTITUENTS: (i) Lichen acids; stictinic, sticinic, norstictic, gyrophoric, thelophoric, constictic, connorstictic, cryptostictic and menegazziaic acids (ii) Fatty acids including palmitic, oleic and linoleic acids (iii) Mucilage (iii) Tannins (iv) Sterols; ergosterol, fucosterol etc. [1,2].

MEDICINAL USE: Astringent, demulcent, expectorant, mucolytic, orexigenic [R1]. It has been taken as an infusion for coughs, asthma and bronchitis.

PREPARATIONS AND DOSE: Dried lichen, dose: 1–2 g or equivalent extract, three times daily.

SPECIFIC REFERENCES: 1. Catalano S *et al* (1976) *Phytochem.* 15:22. 2. Zeybeck U *et al* (2000) *Sci. Pharm.* 68(3):317.

LUNGWORT
PULMONARIA OFFICINALIS L.
Fam. Boraginaceae

SYNONYMS: Lungwort Herb.

HABITAT: Shady places throughout Europe, cultivated in gardens.

DESCRIPTION: Leaves lanceolate, up to 60 cm long but usually much smaller, downy, spotted or blotched with white, abruptly narrowing at the base.

PART USED: Leaf.

CONSTITUENTS: (i) Allantoin (ii) Flavonoids; mainly glycosides of quercetin and kaempferol (iii) Mucilage, consisting of polysaccharides of galacturonic acid, arabinogalactans and rhamnogalactans (iv) Miscellaneous; vitamin C [1,2]. Pyrrolizidine alkaloids, which are common in other plants of the Boraginaceae, have been shown to be absent in one study, from all samples of *Pulmonaria officinalis* tested [3].

MEDICINAL USE: Emollient, expectorant, anti-haemorrhagic, astringent [R1]. It is used particularly for bronchitis, laryngitis and catarrh, but can also be used for diarrhoea and haemorrhoids and applied topically to aid wound healing.

PREPARATIONS AND DOSE: Dried leaf, dose: 2–4 g, or equivalent extract, three times daily.

SPECIFIC REFERENCES: 1. Brantner A *et al* (1995) *Planta Med.* 61(1):582. 2. Muller B *et al* (1990) *PZ Wissenschaft* 135(6):243. 3. Luthy J *et al* (1984) *Helv. Chim. Acta* 59:242.

MACE
MYRISTICA FRAGRANS HOUTT.
Fam. Myristicaceae

HABITAT: Native to the Molucca Islands, India and New Guinea, introduced into Sri Lanka and the West Indies.

DESCRIPTION: Mace is the arillus surrounding the nutmeg; it is a brittle, semi-translucent, net-like, bright reddish or orange-brown structure. When pressed with the nail it exudes oil. Taste and odour: aromatic, pungent, characteristic.

PART USED: Arillus (seed covering).

CONSTITUENTS: (i) Volatile oil, containing myristicin, elemene and safrole, together with monoterpene hydrocarbons such as camphene, alpha- and beta-pinene, sabinene, cymene, alpha-thujene and the monoterpene alcohols linalool, geraniol, borneol and others (ii) Resorcinols; malabaricone B and C (iii) Lignans such as dihydroguaretic acid (DHGA) [5]. This is similar in composition to that of Nutmeg (q.v.) but usually with higher concentrations of myristicin [1,2,3,4].

MEDICINAL USE: Stimulant, carminative [R1]. The lipophilic extract is anti-inflammatory, and myristicin is thought to be responsible [6]. The malabaricones are antimicrobial and anti-fungal [4]. Several studies have shown that extract of Mace increases glutathione S-transferase in the liver [7] and prevents DMBA-induced papillomagenesis in mouse skin [8]. Other chemopreventative effects of Mace include hepatic detoxification and antioxidant activity [9]. DHGA inhibits the formation of certain DNA adducts, which can indicate anti-cancer activity, and suppression of the growth of leukemia and lung cancer cell lines was seen [5]. High doses cause intoxication and hallucinations; see Nutmeg. Mace is used as a condiment and is reputed to be a constituent of a popular Cola (q.v.) drink [10].

SPECIFIC REFERENCES: 1. Sanford G *et al* (1971) *Pharm. Acta Helv.* 59(9–10):242. 2. Forrest T *et al* (1973) *Naturwissensch.* 60:257. 3. Baldry J *et al* (1976) *Int. Flav. Food. Add.* 7:28. 4. Orabi K *et al* (1991) *J. Nat. Prod.* 54(3):856. 5. Park S *et al* (1998) *Cancer Lett.* 127(1–2):23. 6. Ozaki Y *et al* (1989) *Jpn. J. Pharmacol.* 49(2):155. 7. Kumari M *et al* (1989) *Cancer Lett.* 46(2):87. 8. Jannu L *et al* (1991) *Cancer Lett.* 56(1):59. 9. Kumari M (1992) *Nutr. Res.* 12(3):385. 10. Randerath K et al (1993) *Biochem. Biophys. Res. Commun.* 192(1):61.

MADDER
RUBIA TINCTORUM L.
Fam. Rubiaceae

SYNONYMS: Dyer's Madder.

HABITAT: Native to southern Europe and parts of Asia, cultivated elsewhere.

DESCRIPTION: The root is normally found in commerce as short,

277

cylindrical pieces about 4 mm in diameter, with a thin, easily detached cork, leaving a red-brown, longitudinally furrowed inner bark. The transverse section shows a pinkish-red column marked with concentric striae. Taste: sweetish, then acrid; odour: slight.

PART USED: Root.

CONSTITUENTS: (i) Anthraquinone derivatives, at least 20 of which have been isolated, including ruberythric acid, and its primaveroside, alizarin, purpurin, mollugin, rubiadin and lucidin (ii) Asperuloside, an iridoid [1,2].

MEDICINAL USE: Formerly used for menstrual and urinary disorders, including kidney stones, and for liver diseases. Extracts are antimicrobial [3]. The rubiadins, especially lucidin, are now known to be genotoxic and mutagenic, and in many countries Madder has been removed from sale. Purpurin however is antimutagenic. [1,3,4,5,6].

SPECIFIC REFERENCES: 1. Kawasaki Y G et al (1992) Chem. Pharm. Bull. 40(6):1504. 2. Courchesne M et al (1993) J. Nat. Prod. 56:722. 3. Mehrabhian S et al (2000) Aerobiol. 16(3–4):455. 4. Westendorf J et al (1998) Carcinogenesis. 19(12):2161. 5. Marczylo T et al (2000) Mutagenesis 15(3):223. 6. Maree F et al (2001) Planta Med. 67(2):127.

MAGNOLIA
MAGNOLIA GLAUCA L.
Fam. Magnoliaceae

SYNONYMS: *M. virginiana* L. *M. acuminata*, *M. tripetata*.

HABITAT: North America, cultivated as a garden plant elsewhere.

DESCRIPTION: The inner bark occurs in long, fibrous strips, the outer surface rough, almost granular and pitted; the inner surface faintly striated. Fracture short with the inner part tough and fibrous.

PART USED: Bark.

CONSTITUENTS: Largely unknown, although (i) Lignans; magnolide has been reported (ii) Volatile oil [R2,R4]. *M. officinalis* contains (i) Lignans; magnolol, hinokiol and monoterpenyl magnolol and (ii) Sesquiterpenes such as eudesmol [1,2,3]. *M. grandiflora* also contains (i) Sesquiterpene lactones including costunolide and parthenolide [4,5].

MEDICINAL USE: Stimulant, tonic, aromatic, diaphoretic, and anti-inflammatory. This species is rarely employed, although *M. grandiflora* and *M. officinalis* are widely used in oriental medicine. Magnolol and hinokiol both inhibit Epstein-Barr virus early antigen activation (induced by phorbol ester) [1], and are antimicrobial [3]. Magnolol is known to reduce myocardial injury by inhibiting neutrophil activation in the rat [6] and experiments in cholesterol-fed rabbits indicates that it offers some protection against postangioplasty restenosis [7]. Costunolide has anti-inflammatory effects and inhibits NF-kappa B activation [4]. *M. officinalis* extracts potently inhibit growth of *Helicobacter pylori*, a causative organism for peptic ulcer [8]. For review of the genus, see [9].

SPECIFIC REFERENCES: 1. Konoshima T *et al* (1991) *J. Nat. Prod.* 54(3):816. 2. Kondo K *et al* (2000) *Natural Med.* 54(2):61. 3. Ho K *et al* (2001) *Phytother. Res.* 15(2):139. 4. Tae H *et al* (2001) *Planta Med.* 67(2):103. 5. Ganzera M *et al* (2001) *Chromatographia* 54(9–10):665. 6. Lee Y *et al* (2001) *Eur. J. Pharmacol.* 422(1–3):159. 7. Chen Y *et al* (2001) *Basic Res. Cardiol.* 96(4):353. 8. Bae E *et al* (1998) *Biol. Pharm. Bull.* 21(9):990. 9. Magnolia. Ed: Sarker R (2002) *Medicinal and Aromatic Plants* – Industrial Profiles. Taylor and Francis, London, UK.

MAIDENHAIR

ADIANTUM CAPILLUS-VENERIS L.
Fam. Polypodiaceae

SYNONYMS: Venus Hair, Rock Fern.

HABITAT: Southern Europe, occasionally found further north including Britain, and parts of North America and Canada.

DESCRIPTION: Fronds up to 30 cm long, two or three times pinnate, each leaflet or 'pinnule' up to about 1 cm, fan-shaped, with a toothed upper margin, narrowing at the base to a short petiolule. Veins prominent, converging at the base, and spore-cases (sori) visible at the edge of the undersurface. Stems shiny, dark brown. Taste: sweetish and astringent, odour: faint.

PART USED: Fern.

CONSTITUENTS: (i) Flavonoid glycosides; rutin, isoquercetin, astragalin, kaempferol 3,7-diglucoside and kaempferol 3-sulphate (ii) Triterpenoids including adiantone, and a number of hopane alcohols such as adian-5-en-3-ols and pterin-14-en-7-ol and others (iii) Hydroxycinnamic acid sulphate esters, four of which have been isolated [1,2].

PREPARATIONS AND DOSE: Dried herb, dose: 0.5–2 g or equivalent extract, three times daily.

MEDICINAL USE: Expectorant, antitussive, antipyretic, demulcent [R1]. Maidenhair is used as an ingredient of cough and bronchial medicines, and as a hair tonic. It may be used as an infusion. An extract of the plant has diuretic and hypoglycaemic activity in animals and is antimicrobial [3,4,5].

SPECIFIC REFERENCES: 1. Dewick P *et al* (1982) *Phytochem.* 20:2277. 2. Nakane T *et al* (1999) *Chem. Pharm. Bull.* 47(4):543. 3. Twaij H *et al* (1985) *Indian J. Pharmacol.* 17(1):73. 4. Jain S *et al* (1967) *Planta Med.* 4:439. 5. Neef H *et al* (1995) *Phytother. Res.* 9(1):45.

MALABAR NUT

ADHATODA VASICA NEES.
Fam. Acanthaceae

SYNONYMS: Arusa, Adulsa, *Justicia adhatoda* L.

HABITAT: India.

DESCRIPTION: Leaves up to 15 cm long, 4 cm broad, short-stalked, opposite, lanceolate, tapering to an acute apex with entire margins. *TASTE:* bitter, odour: tea-like.

PART USED: Leaves.

CONSTITUENTS: (i) Alkaloids; vasicine (= peganine) a quinazoline alkaloid, with vasicinone, 7-methoxyvasicinone, vasicinol, adhatodine, adhatonine, adhavasinone, anisotine, vasicoline, vasicol, 3-hydroxy-anisotine, desmethoxyaniflorine, vasicolinone and others (ii) Phytosterols and triterpenes; daucosterol alpha-amyrin, epitaraxerol (iii) Flavonoids; apigenin, astragalin, kaempferol, quercetin, vitexin, isovitexin, violanthin and others (iv) Essential oil; the flower volatile oil contains a ketone identified as 4-heptanone, with 3-methylheptanone and at least 36 other components (v) Fatty acids and hydrocarbons; decane, with 37-hydroxyhexatetracont-1-en-15-one and 29-methyltria-contan-1-ol, and linolenic, arachidonic, linoleic, palmitic and oleic acids [R16;1,2,3,4,5,6,7,8].

MEDICINAL USE: Expectorant, febrifuge, antispasmodic. In India the drug is highly esteemed in bronchitis, asthma and other pulmonary diseases. The activity is complex, for example vasicine is a bronchodilator both *in vitro* and *in vivo*, the activity being comparable to that of theophylline, but vasicinone is bronchodilatory *in vitro* but a bronchoconstrictor *in vivo*. However, the two alkaloids in combination had a more potent bronchodilatory activity than would be expected, and the combination of vasicinone with aminophylline also had an additive effect. *Adhatoda vasica* reduces ovalbumin and PAF-induced allergic reactions. The alkaloid fraction of the leaf is antibacterial, with a strong activity against *Pseudomonas aeruginosa, Streptococcus faecalis, Staphylococcus aureus, S. epidermidis,* and *E. coli.* Derivatives of vasicine such as bromhexine and ambroxol are used as mucolytics and have a growth inhibitory effect on *Mycobacterium tuberculosis.* Vasicine has a cholagogue action in dogs and is an abortifacient effect in guinea pigs (although not in rats) depending on the stage of pregnancy. Vasicine also has a uterotonic activity in humans, influenced by the degree of priming of the uterus by estrogens, and initiates rhythmic contractions of human myometrial strips from both non-pregnant and pregnant uteri, with an effect comparable to that of oxytocin. The alcoholic extract of the leaves also shows wound-healing activity. *Adhatoda vasica* leaves were found to control insect pests in oil seeds, both in laboratory and warehouse conditions. Due to the uterotonic effect the plant should not be used during pregnancy [R16;1,9,10,11,12].

SPECIFIC REFERENCES: 1. Claeson U *et al* (2000) *J. Ethnopharmacol.,* 72:1. 2. Thappa, R *et al* (1996) *Phytochemistry* 42(5):1485. 3. El-Megeed H *et al.* (1998) *Pharm. Pharmacol. Lett.* 8(4):167. 4. Jain M *et al* (1980) *Planta Med.* 46:250. 5. Dhar K *et al* (1981) *Phytochemistry* 20(2):319. 6. Bhartiya, H *et al* (1982) *Phytochemistry* 21(1):247. 7. El-Sawi S *et al* (1999) *Pharm. Pharmacol. Lett.* 9(2):52. 8. Singh R *et al* (1991) *Phytochem.* 30(11):3799. 9. Mullar A *et al* (1993)

Planta Med. 59(Suppl.):A586. 10. Brantner A *et al* (1998) *Pharm. Pharmacol. Lett.* 8(3):137. 11. Grange J *et al* (1996) *J. Ethnopharmacol.*, 1996, 50(1):49. 12. Gupta O. *et al* (1978) *Indian. J. Exp. Biol.* 16(10):1075.

MALE FERN

DRYOPTERIS FILIX-MAS (L.) SCHOTT.
D. ABBREVIATA (LAM & D.C.) NEWM.
D. BORREI NEWM. AND HYBRIDS AND VARIETIES
Fam. Polypodiaceae

SYNONYMS: Aspidium, *Aspidium filix-mas* Sw. American Aspidium or Marginal Fern is *D. marginalis* (L.) Gray.

HABITAT: Native to Europe and parts of Asia.

DESCRIPTION: The dried rootstock is reddish brown externally, about 4–6 cm in diameter and up to about 25 cm long, and consists of the rhizome with the bases of the fronds attached but trimmed of rootlets. The transverse section shows six to 10 vascular bundles in the rhizome and the frond bases, and should be greenish in colour. Taste: sweetish then astringent, bitter and nauseous; odour: slight but unpleasant.

PART USED: Rhizome.

CONSTITUENTS: (i) Phloroglucinol derivatives, the mixture is known as 'filicin' and is composed of aspidin, filicinic acid, filicylbutanone, aspidinol, albaspidin, flavaspidic acids, paraspidin, desaspidin and others (ii) Triterpenes such as 9(11)-fernene, 12-hopene and 11,13 (13)-hopadiene (iii) *n*-Alkanes, mainly C_{29} and C_{31} (iv) Volatile oil and resins. [1,2,3,4]. Other species like *D. fragrans* contain similar compounds, e.g. *D. fragrans* contains (i) Phloroglucinols including dryofragrin and aspidin PB and related compounds [5,6] (ii) Flavonoids based on kaempferol, such as sutchuenoside A and others [7]. *D. dickinsii* contains similar flavonoids [8]. *D. crassirhizoma* contains triterpenoids including trisnorhopane and fern-9,11-ene and others [9].

PREPARATIONS AND DOSE: Dried rhizome, 4–15g or equivalent extract, as a single dose.

MEDICINAL USE: Taenifuge, vermifuge [R1]. The main active constituents against intestinal worms are thought to be flavaspidic acid and desaspidin [1]. Male fern is often used in conjunction with a saline purgative to expel the parasites; however it should not be used with castor oil as this increases the absorption and toxicity. Symptoms of poisoning include nausea, vomiting, delirium, cardiac and respiratory failure. The phloroglucinols are fish poisons [5], and aspidinol, desaspidinol, aspidin, filixic acids and dryocrassin have anti-tumour promoting activity against Epstein-Barr induced activation induced by phorbol ester [10]. The kaempferol glycosides also inhibit the activities of HIV-1 reverse transcriptase [7].

SPECIFIC REFERENCES: 1. Calderwood J *et al* (1969) *J. Pharm. Pharmacol.* 21:55S. 2. Widen C *et al* (1971) *Helv. Chim. Acta*

281

54:2824. 3. Bottari F *et al* (1972) *Phytochem.* 11:2519. 4. Franchi G *et al* (1988) *Pharmacol. Res. Commun.* 20(Suppl.5):135. 5. Ito H *et al* (2000) *Chem. Pharm. Bull.* 48(8):1190. 6. Ito H *et al* (1997) *Chem. Pharm. Bull.* 45(10):1720. 7. Min S *et al* (2001) *Chem. Phar. Bull.* 49(5):546. 8. Fuchino H *et al* (1997) *Natural Med.* 51(6):537. 9. Shiojima K *et al* (1994) *Chem. Pharm. Bull.* 42(2):377. 10. Kapadia G *et al* (1996) *Cancer Lett.* 105(2):161.

MANACA

BRUNFELSIA HOPEANA (POHL) BENTH.
Fam. Solanaceae

SYNONYMS: Vegetable Mercury.

HABITAT: South America, the West Indies.

DESCRIPTION: The root has a papery, pale-brown epidermis, in transverse section showing several concentric rings of the xylem traversed by slender medullary rays. Taste: sweetish, odour: faintly aromatic.

PART USED: Root.

CONSTITUENTS: (i) Steroidal glycosides based on spirostanol and furastanol (ii) Coumarins such as scopoletin glucopyranoside and aesculetin (iii) Lignans including pinoresinol diglucoside and others [R4;1,2] (iv) Miscellaneous; an alkaloid manaceine and gelsemic acid [R4].

MEDICINAL USE: Alterative, diuretic, anti-rheumatic. Scopoletin isolated from *Brunfelsia hopeana* has an antispasmodic effect thought to be due to its ability to inhibit intracellular calcium mobilization [2].

SPECIFIC REFERENCES: 1. Ichiki H *et al* (1994) *Natural Med.* 48(4):314. 2. Oliviera E *et al* (2001) *Planta Med.* 67(7):605.

MANDRAKE, AMERICAN

PODOPHYLLUM PELTATUM L.
Fam. Berberidaceae

SYNONYMS: May Apple, Devil's Apple, Wild Lemon. Indian Podophyllum is *P. hexandrum* Royle (= *P. emodi* Wall.).

HABITAT: North America.

DESCRIPTION: The rhizome is a reddish-brown colour and occurs in pieces up to about 20 cm long and 0.5 cm in diameter. The outer surface can be smooth or wrinkled, depending on the time of collection. Nodes, visible as swellings with stem and leaf scars, occur at intervals of 3–5 cm. Fracture: starchy or horny, revealing a whitish interior; odour: unpleasant, acrid.

PART USED: Rhizome and the resin extracted from it.

CONSTITUENTS: (i) Lignans; the main one being podophyllotoxin, with the beta-D-glucoside, dehydropodophyllotoxin, 4-demethylpodophyllotoxin, and the beta-peltatins and their glucosides, picropodophyllin and its beta-D-glucoside and others (ii) Miscellaneous; flavonoids, mainly kaempferol and quercetin and their glucosides, resin, starch, gums etc. [1,2,3]. *P. hexandrum* contains similar lignans, with the exception of alpha-and beta-peltatins, which are reportedly absent; the concentration of podophyllotoxin and its dehydro and demethyl derivatives is very much higher [4].

MEDICINAL USE: Cathartic, purgative, anti-neoplastic, antiviral [R1]. The resin, known as podophyllin, is used as a topical application, as an ointment or frequently dispersed in alcohol or Compound Benzoin Tincture, for venereal warts, verrucae and similar conditions [5]. It is caustic and irritant and must be used with care. Internal administration is no longer advised, and even external application is not recommended during pregnancy, due to the cytotoxicity. Podophyllin and podophyllotoxin are embryocidal in animals and fatalities in humans have been recorded after ingestion. Derivatives of podophyllotoxin, for example etoposide and teniposide, are used clinically for the treatment of certain cancers [R14;6]. They also inhibit TNF (tumour necrosis factor) alpha m-RNA, and enhance IL-beta expression in lipopolysaccharide treated monocytes [7].

PREPARATIONS: Podophyllum Resin BP; Compound Podophyllum Paint BP.

SPECIFIC REFERENCES: 1. Dewick P *et al* (1982) *Phytochem.* 20:2277. 2. Graham N *et al* (1990) *Canadian Pharm. J.* 123(7):330. 3. Drew S *et al* (1987) *J. Pharm. Pharmacol.* 39:738. 4. Auterhoff H *et al* (1958) *Planta Med.* 6:240. 5. Livingstone C (1998) *Pharm. J.* 260(6990):556. 6. Dutcher J *et al* (2000) *J. Clin. Pharmacol.* 40(10):1079. 7. Pugh N *et al* (2001) *Immunopharmacol. Immunotoxicol.* 23(1):83.

MANGO

MANGIFERA INDICA L.
Fam. Anacardiaceae

HABITAT: Native to tropical Asia but cultivated widely for the fruit.

DESCRIPTION: A large evergreen tree, with linear or oblong leaves, a thick grey or brown bark which exfoliates in flakes, and the well-known fruit, which is a large drupe with yellow, juicy pulp and a single hard seed.

PART USED: Fruit, bark, leaves.

CONSTITUENTS: Bark: (i) Saponins and triterpenes, such as indicoside A and B, friedelin, mangsterol, manglupenone, manghopanol, mangoleanone, taraxerol and others (ii) Xanthones including mangiferin, 29-hydroxymangiferonic acid and mangostin. The leaf and flower contain (i) Essential oil composed of mono- and sesquiterpenes including humulene, elemene, ocimene, linalool, nerol and others (ii) Phenolic acids; several gallic acid derivatives have been isolated from the flower [R12,R16,1].

MEDICINAL USE: The fruit is a very popular food, and the juice and pulp used as a coolant and tonic. The bark and leaf extracts are

283

traditionally used to treat dysentery, asthma, constipation, worms, hypertension and various inflammatory disorders. Anti-inflammatory, antioxidant and cytotoxic effects have been shown for the bark [2,3,4]; as well as activity on alpha lipase [5]. The leaves are hypoglycaemic in animals [6]. Many of the effects are due to the presence of mangiferin, which is antiviral, hepatoprotective and activates peritoneal macrophages [R13,R16;7].

SPECIFIC REFERENCES: 1. Khan M *et al* (1993) *J. Nat. Prod.* 56(5):767. 2. Garrido G *et al* (2001) *Phytother. Res.* 15(1):18. 3. Martinez G *et al* (2000) *Phytother. Res.* 14(6):424. 4. Muanza D *et al* (1995) *Int. J. Pharmacog.* 33(2):98. 5. Prashanth D *et al* (2001) *Fitoterapia* 72(2):179. 6. Sharma S *et al* (1997) *Int. J. Pharmacog.* 35(2):130. 7. Guha S *et al* (1993) *Phytother. Res.*7:107.

MANNA
FRAXINUS ORNUS L.
Fam. Oleaceae

HABITAT: Southern Europe and parts of Asia.

DESCRIPTION: A saccharine exudate from the incised tree bark. Pale yellowish or whitish pieces, irregular on one side and smoother and curved on the other. Taste: sweet, honey-like; odour: slight.

PART USED: Exudation, bark.

CONSTITUENTS: The exudate (or 'manna') contains mainly mannitol, with oligosaccharides of mannitol, glucose and fructose. The bark contains: (i) Coumarins; esculin, esculetin, fraxin, fraxetin and others (ii) Secoiridoids including ligustrilide, isularoside, hydroxyornoside, oleuropein, framoside, and hydroxyframosides A and B (iii) Caffeic acid esters; calceolaroside B, verbascoside, isoacteoside, lugrandoside, and isolugrandoside (iv) Flavonoids based on quercetin [1,2,3].

MEDICINAL USE: Manna is a nutritive and mild laxative [R1]. The bark is used traditionally for wound-healing, and treatment of inflammation and dysentery. Antimicrobial effects have been demonstrated by extracts of the bark against a range of organisms [4], although antiviral effects tended to be weak [5]. Antioxidant activity was found, particularly in the coumarin fraction [6], and complement inhibition and other anti-inflammatory effects shown [7,8]. The wound-healing effects are supported by studies on skin regeneration, and protection against photodynamic damage has been shown, which was comparable to that of the sunscreen PABA (para-amino benzoic acid) [9]. Toxicological studies have shown the bark to be practically non-toxic: for further detail, see [1, and refs therein].

SPECIFIC REFERENCES: 1. Kostova I (2001) *Fitoterapia* 72:471. 2. Iossifova T *et al* (1997) *Biochem. Syst. Ecol.* 25:271. 2. Iossifova T *et al* (1998) *Phytochem.* 49:1329 and (1999) 50:297. 3. Kostova K *et al* (1992) *Planta Med.* 58:484. 4. Kostova I *et al* (1993) *J. Ethnopharmacol.* 39:205. 5. Galabov A *et al* (1996) *Z. Naturforsch.* 51C:558. 6. Marinova E *et al* (1994) *Food Chem.* 51:125. 7.

Ivanovska N *et al* (1996) *Phytother. Res.* 10:555. 8. Stefanova Z *et al* (1995) *J. Ethnopharmacol.* 46:101. 9. Lazarova G *et al* (1993) *Fitoterapia* 64:134.

MANUKA
LEPTOSPERMUM SCOPARIUM J R FORST ET G FORST.
Fam. Myrtaceae

SYNONYMS: New Zealand Tea Tree (not to be confused with Australian Tea Tree *Melaleuca alternifolia* q.v.).

HABITAT: New Zealand.

DESCRIPTION: An attractive, highly variable, evergreen shrub or small tree, which may range from a climber to a tree of 8 m in height. It produces prolific pink or whitish flowers in early summer.

PART USED: Oil distilled from the leaves and twigs.

CONSTITUENTS: Essential oil, the main components of which are (i) Beta-triketones including flavesone, leptospermone and isoleptospermone (ii) Mono- and sesquiterpenes including 1,8-cineole, terpinen-4-ol, alpha- and gamma-terpinene, *p*-cymene, alpha-pinene and others [1,2,3,4].

MEDICINAL USE: The tree is used traditionally by the Maori, for many different purposes. The timber, which is very hard and strong, is used for building; the leaves as an infusion for joint aches and pains; and the oil for sores, itching, lice and eczema. The oil is anti-fungal, antibacterial and antioxidant; it is now incorporated into creams, shampoos and mouthwashes. The antiseptic activity has been investigated in several studies [1,2,3,5] although variable since the composition depends on the source of the oil. Antispasmodic effects have been described on various types of isolated smooth muscle preparation [2,6]. For further detail, see [1,2 and refs therein].

SPECIFIC REFERENCES: 1. Porter N (2001) *HerbalGram* 53:26. 2. Lis-Balchin M *et al* (2000) *Phytother. Res.* 14(8):623. 3. Lis-Balchin M *et al* (1996) *Acta Hort.* 426:13. 4. Porter N *et al* (1998) *Phytochem.* 50:407. 5. Harkenthal M *et al* (1999) *Pharmazie* 54:460. 6. Lis-Balchin M *et al* (1998) *J. Pharm. Pharmacol.* 50:809.

MAPLE, RED
ACER RUBRUM L.
Fam. Sapindaceae

SYNONYMS: Swamp Maple.

HABITAT: America.

DESCRIPTION: Long, quilled pieces, externally blackish-brown, slightly polished, with numerous transverse lenticels and scattered, brownish, small warts. The inner bark very tough and fibrous, and pale reddish-brown or buff in colour. Taste: astringent and slightly bitter.

285

PART USED: Bark.

CONSTITUENTS: Unknown.

MEDICINAL USE: Formerly used by the American Indians as an application for sore eyes, because of its astringency. The leaves are toxic and have caused fatalities in horses due to hemolytic syndrome and hepatic degeneration [1,2].

SPECIFIC REFERENCES: 1. George L *et al* (1982) *Vet. Pathol.* 19(5):521. 2. Stair E *et al* (1993) *Vet. Hum. Toxicol.* 35(3):229.

MARIGOLD

CALENDULA OFFICINALIS L.
Fam. Asteraceae

SYNONYMS: Marybud, Calendula, Gold-bloom, *Caltha officinalis.*

HABITAT: A common garden plant.

DESCRIPTION: Flower-heads bright yellow or orange. Ligulate florets, usually detached from the ovary, are used; these are 15–25 mm long and about 3 mm broad, one to three toothed with four or five veins and an entire margin, with a short corolla tube containing the bifid stigma and style. Taste: saline, slightly bitter, odour: faint.

PART USED: Petals, flower-heads.

CONSTITUENTS: (i) Triterpenes; pentacyclic alcohols such as faradol, brein, arnidiol, erythrodiol, calenduladiol, heliantriols A1, B0, B1 and B2 etc., ursatriol, longispinogenine; the calendulosides A-D (in the root at least); calendasaponins A, B, C and D, alpha- and beta-amyrin, taraxasterol and lupeol (ii) Flavonoids; isorhamnetin glycosides including narcissin, and quercetin glycosides including rutin (iii) Sesquiterpene and ionone glycosides; officinosides A, B, C and D, loliolide, arvoside A (iv) Volatile oil containing menthone, isomenthone, caryophyllene, pedunculatine, alpha- and beta-ionone and others (v) Polysaccharides; PS-I, II and II based on a beta-D-galactan backbone with arabinose and rhamnose side chains (vi) Miscellaneous; chlorogenic acid and carotenoids [R7;1,2,3,4,5,6,7,8].

MEDICINAL USE: Anti-inflammatory, spasmolytic, anti-haemorrhagic, styptic, vulnerary, antiseptic [R1]. Internally it may be taken as an infusion for stomach disorders, gastric and duodenal ulcers and dysmenorrhoea; and externally as a lotion or ointment for cuts and bruises, nappy rash, sore nipples, burns, scalds etc. The anti-inflammatory effects are well-documented, both when taken internally and applied externally [9,10]. Many of the effects are due to the saponins, which are anti-inflammatory and anti-oedematous [11]; however the flavonoids are known to be lipoxygenase inhibitors [12], and the polysaccharides are immunomodulators [8] and are thought to be soothing to irritated mucosal membranes [13]. A methanolic extract is hypoglycaemic, gastroprotective and inhibits gastric emptying [4]. Cytotoxicity, uterotonic and other effects have been documented [R7], and genotoxicity in the *Aspergillus nidulans*, but not the Ames test, has been shown [14]. Extracts have anti-HIV activity *in vitro* [15]. Few clinical studies have been performed, although a recent open trial concluded that calendula extract was useful in treating burns and scalds [16]. The wound-healing properties are supported by evidence that Marigold extract induces vascularisation under experimental conditions [17].

PREPARATIONS AND DOSE: Dried florets, dose: 1–4g or equivalent extract, three times daily.

SPECIFIC REFERENCES: 1. Kaspryk Z et al (1973) *Phytochem.* 13:2299. 2. Wilkomirski B (1985) *Phytochem.* 24(12):3067. 3. Murukami T et al (2001) *Chem. Pharm. Bull.* 49(8):974. 4. Yoshikawa *et al* (2001) *Chem. Pharm. Bull.* 49(7):863. 5. Vidal-Olivier E *et al* (1989) *Planta Med.* 55:73. 6. Gracza L (1987) *Planta Med.* 53:227. 7. Willhun G *et al* (1987) *Planta Med.* 53:304. 8. Varljen J *et al* (1989) *Phytochem.* 28:2379. 9. Mascolo N *et al* (1987) *Phytother. Res.* 1(1):28. 10. Casely-Smith J *et al* (1983) *Lymphology* 16:150. 11. Zitterl-Eglseer K *et al* (1997) *J. Ethnopharmacol.* 57(2):139. 12. Bezakova L *et al* (1996) *Pharmazie* 51(2):126. 13. Schmidgall J *et al* (2000) *Planta Med.* 66:48. 14. Ramos A *et al* (1998) *J. Ethnopharmacol.* 61(1):49. 15. Kalvatchev Z *et al* (1997) *Biomed. Pharmacother.* 51(4):176. 16. Von Baranov A (1999) *Dtsch. Apott. Ztg.* 139:2135. 17. Patrick K *et al* (1996) *Phytomed.* 3:11.

MARIJUANA
CANNABIS SATIVA L.
Fam. Cannabinaceae

SYNONYMS: Cannabis, Marihuana, Indian Hemp, Hashish, Ganja, Bhang, Dagga, *C. indica* Lamk.

HABITAT: Indigenous to India and the Middle East, cultivated widely elsewhere, often illicitly. Varieties low in cannabinoids are being cultivated as a source of fibre.

DESCRIPTION: The flowering tops or 'herb' consists of the female flowers, seeds and upper leaves. The leaves are long-stalked, bearing usually five to seven lanceolate, pointed, sharply serrate leaflets. The seeds are globular, about 2 mm in diameter, often covered with the small leafy bracts; the whole head may be matted with resin. The resin itself, which may be separated from the rest, is found in greenish, yellowish or reddish-brown or black masses; it is usually hard and brittle. Taste and odour: aromatic and characteristic.

PART USED: Flowering tops, resin.

CONSTITUENTS: (i) Cannabinoids, about 70 of which have been isolated, the most important being delta$_9$-tetrahydrocannabinol (THC); with other isomers of TCH, cannabinol, cannabidiol, cannabigerol, cannabichromene, cannabipinol, cannabidivarin and others, and their corresponding carboxylic acids, such as THC-acid, which easily decarboxylate at high temperatures (e.g. when smoked). The

287

constituents vary widely depending on climate, cultivar, soil etc. (ii) Flavonoids; flavocannabiside, flavosativaside, glycosides of vitexin and isovitexin and others (iii) Essential oil, composed of olivetol, cannabene, myrcene (a sesquiterpene) (iv) Alkaloids; cannabisativine, muscarine and trigonelline (v) Miscellaneous; stilbene derivatives, e.g. 3,4'dihydroxy-bibenzyl and others [1,2,3,4,5,6,7,8]. For full review see [1,2].

MEDICINAL USE: Analgesic, anti-inflammatory, hypnotic, sedative, cataleptic, hallucinogenic. The herb and resin have been used for centuries both medicinally and recreationally, however the use is illegal in most countries except for certain medical and scientific purposes. The constituents of cannabis have been reinvestigated as therapeutic agents and pharmacological probes; they and their derivatives are being suggested for treating glaucoma, as anti-inflammatory and analgesic agents and a cannabinoid derivative is in clinical use as an anti-emetic in cancer chemotherapy. The medicinal uses have been well reviewed and the most important indications are for the pain, spasticity and tremor associated with multiple sclerosis, intractable pain and other neurological disorders such as Tourette's syndrome and epilepsy [3,4,9,10]. The anti-spastic, anti-tremor, cataleptic, hypotensive and analgesic effects have been confirmed in animals [3,4,5,6,8,11] and further work is continuing into their mode of action. The effects are not always predictable, and in some studies have not confirmed anti-spastic activity [12], although a study in a patient with pendular nystagmus correlated the relief of the spasms of eye muscles with increasing cannabinoid blood levels [13]. The effects of THC are due to the mimicking or potentiation of natural ligands known as endocannabinoids, the main ones are anandamide (arachidonyl ethanolamide) and its analogues, and a series of acyl glycerol derivatives. THC interacts with cannabinoid receptors in both the brain and periphery [3,8,11,14]. Other biochemical work has shown the basis for some of the analgesic effects to be an interaction with the enzymes involved in the inflammatory process, particularly cyclooxygenase, lipoxygenase and phospholipase A_2 [2,4,5,6]. Although THC is the major psychoactive agent it is less potent in other effects, such as anti-inflammatory activity, as for example cannabigerol and cannabidiol, or the non-cannabinoids olivetol and some of the flavonoids. Flavocannabiside and flavosativaside are lens aldose reductase inhibitors, which may augment the action of THC on lowering the intra-ocular pressure of the eye. It is increasingly apparent that synergistic interactions exist between the constituents of cannabis, for example an extract has a more potent effect on experimentally induced spasticity than a matched dose of THC alone [15]. Adverse effects include an increased risk of psychosis [16]. For further details of all aspects, see [2,3,9,12,17 and refs therein].

REGULATORY STATUS: CD. (Misuse of Drugs Act 1973). POM.

SPECIFIC REFERENCES: 1. Turner C et al (1980) *J. Nat. Prod.* 43:169. 2. McPartland J et al (2001) *J. Cannabis Ther.* 1(3–4):103. 3. Mechoulam R (1999) *Nat. Prod. Rep.* 16(2):131–143. 4. Formukong E *et al* (1989) *Phytother. Res.* (3–6):219. 5. Evans F (1991) *Planta Med.* 57 S60–67. 6. Evans F (1997) *Pharm. Sci.* 3:533. 7. Barrett M *et al* (1985) *Biochem. Pharmacol.* 34:2019. 8. Pertwee R (1997) *Pharm. Sci.* 3:539. 9. Williamson E *et al* (2000) *Drugs* 60(6):1303. 10. Mueller-Vahl K *et al* (2002) *Pharmacopsychiatry* 35(2):57. 11. Baker D *et al* (2000) *Nature* 404:84. 12. Killestein J *et al* (2002) *Neurology* 58(9):1404. 13. Schon *et al* (1999) *Neurology* 53:2209. 14. Consroe P *et al* (1998) *Neurobiol. Dis.* 5:534. 15. Williamson E (2001) *Phytomedicine* 8(5):401. 16. Van Os J *et al* (2002) *Am. J. Epidemiol.* 156(4):319. 17. Iversen L (2000) *The Science of Marijuana.* Oxford University Press, UK.

MARJORAM

ORIGANUM MAJORANA L.

Fam. Lamiaceae

SYNONYMS: Sweet Marjoram, *O. hortensis* Moensch. Wild Marjoram is Oregano (q.v.), *O. vulgare* L.

HABITAT: Native to the Mediterranean region, cultivated widely in gardens.

DESCRIPTION: The herb grows to about 25 cm high, branched above, with opposite, small, oval leaves up to about 1.5 cm long and 1 cm broad. The flowers are white or pink, small, almost hidden by green bracts, and arranged in small rounded spikes. Taste and odour: pleasant, characteristic.

PART USED: Herb.

CONSTITUENTS: (i) Volatile oil, composed of cis- and trans-sabinene hydrate, sabinene, linalool, carvacrol, 4-terpineol, alpha- and gamma-terpinene, estragole, eugenol, thymol, germacrene-D and others (ii) Flavonoids; luteolin-7-glucoside, diosmetin-7-glucoside and apigenin-7-glucoside (iii) Caffeic acid derivatives including rosmarinic acid (iv) Triterpenoids such as ursolic acid, oleanolic acid and phytosterols (v) Hydroquinones including methyl arbutin [1,2,3,4].

MEDICINAL USE: Stimulant, antispasmodic, emmenagogue, diaphoretic [R1]. Extracts have been shown to have antioxidant activity [5,6]; probably due to the flavonoids and rosmarinic acid. Marjoram is often used as a culinary flavouring. For a full review of the genus Origanum, see [7].

SPECIFIC REFERENCES: 1. Afshaypuor S *et al* (1997) *Planta Med.* 63:179. 2. Sarer E *et al* (1982) *Planta Med.* 46(4):236. 3. Vera R *et al* (1999) *Food Chem.* 66(2):143. 4. Lossner G (1968) *Planta Med.* 16:54. 5. Nakatani N *et al* (2000) *Biofactors* 13(1–4):141. 6. Woo J *et al* (2001) *Food Chem.* 75(4):439. 7. Oregano. Ed. Kintzios S (2002) *Medicinal and Aromatic Plants – Industrial Profiles.* Pub: Taylor and Francis, London, UK.

MARSHMALLOW
ALTHAEA OFFICINALIS L.
Fam. Malvaceae

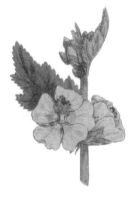

MARSHMALLOW

HABITAT: Europe including Britain, naturalized in the United States.

DESCRIPTION: A downy perennial reaching up to 2 m. Leaves broadly ovate or cordate, 10–20 cm long and about 10 cm wide, with 3–7 rounded lobes, palmate veins and a crenate margin. The flowers are pink, five-petalled, up to 3 cm in diameter. The root as it appears in commerce is dried, fibrous, cream-white when peeled, deeply furrowed longitudinally and with some root scars. Taste: sweet, mucilaginous, odour: slight.

PART USED: Leaves, root.

CONSTITUENTS: Root: (i) Mucilage, consisting of a number of polysaccharides composed of L-rhamnose, D-galactose, D-galacturonic acid and D-glucuronic acid; another is a highly branched L-arabifuranan etc., (ii) Flavonoids such as hypolaetin and isoscutellarin glycosides (iii) Coumarins such as scopoletin and *p*-coumaric acid (iv) Polyphenolic acids, including syringic, caffeic, salicyclic and vanillic acids. Leaf: (i) Mucilage; including a low molecular weight D-glucan (ii) Flavonoids such as kaempferol, quercetin and diosmetin glucosides (iii) Polyphenolics including chlorogenic and caffeic acids, also present in the flower [R2,R7;1,2,3,4,5,6,7,8,9].

MEDICINAL USE: Demulcent, emollient, expectorant [R1]. Both the leaves and root are used for coughs and bronchial complaints and for gastritis, enteritis, peptic ulcer and gastric inflammation in general, and for urinary inflammation and cystitis. They may be used externally as a soothing poultice and vulnerary, usually in the form of an ointment, for boils, ulcers and abscesses [10,11]. The mucilages have proven biological activity including the stimulation of phagocytosis *in vitro* [1] and hypoglycaemic activity in mice [2]. Antimicrobial and anti-inflammatory activities have also been documented [12,13]. Several of the polysaccharides isolated from the roots had antitussive activity [14]. Extracts of Marshmallow root are used to make confectionery.

PREPARATIONS AND DOSE: Dried leaf or root, dose: 2–5 g or equivalent extract, three times daily.

SPECIFIC REFERENCES: 1. Tomoda M *et al* (1980) *Chem. Pharm. Bull.* 28(3):824. 2. Tomoda M *et al* (1987) *Planta Med.* 53 (1):8. 3. Shimitzu N *et al* (1985) *Chem. Pharm. Bull.* 33:5539. 4. Gudej J *et al* (1991) *Planta Med.* 57(3):284. 5. Franz G *et al* (1987) *Planta Med.* 53:90. 6. Franz G *et al* (1989) *Planta Med.* 55:493. 7. Gudej J *et al* (1981) *Acta Pol. Pharm.* 38(3):385. 8. St. Nonov I *et al* (1992) *Fitoterapia* 63:474. 9. Didry N *et al* (1990) *Fitoterapia* 61(3):280. 10. Haln-Deinstrop E (1995) *Deutsche Apot. Ztg.* 135:1147. 11. Habrich C (1993) *Munch. Med. Woch.* 135(23):23. 12. Recio M *et al* (1989) *Phytother. Res.* 3:77. 13. Mascolo N *et al* (1987) *Phytother. Res.* 1(1):28. 14. Nosalova G *et al* (1992) *Pharmazie* 47(3):224.

MASTERWORT

PEUCEDANUM OSTRUTHIUM (L.) KOCH
Fam. Apiaceae

SYNONYMS: Imperatoria ostruthium L.

HABITAT: Parts of Europe but rare in Britain, Australia.

DESCRIPTION: Rhizome cylindrical, compressed, 5–10 cm long and 1–2 cm in diameter, with nodes at intervals of about 1.5 cm and a few scattered roots; some pieces terminating in slender, smooth, underground suckers. Taste and odour: aromatic, pungent.

PART USED: Rhizome.

CONSTITUENTS: (i) Volatile oil, containing about 95% terpenes, including alpha-pinene, *d*-phellandrene, *d*-limonene etc. (ii) Furocoumarins; peucedanin, oxypeucadanin, imperatorin, isoimperatorin and osthol (iii) Flavonoids, including hesperidin (iv) Miscellaneous; phthalides (unspecified) [1,2].

MEDICINAL USE: Stimulant, antispasmodic, carminative [R1]. Has been used for asthma, flatulence, dyspepsia and menstrual complaints. Extracts of the roots have been investigated for antiphlogistic and antipyretic activity and potent anti-inflammatory activity observed, which was attributable to the coumarin content [3]. Calcium antagonistic effects have also been seen using inhibition of contraction of aortic strips induced by potassium depolarisation [4]. Furocoumarins may cause photosensitization [2].

SPECIFIC REFERENCES: 1. Schimmer O *et al* (1980) *Planta Med.* 40(1):68. 2. Gijbels M *et al* (1985) *Fitoterapia* 61(1):17. 3. Hiermann A *et al* (1998) *Planta Med.* 64(5):400. 4. Rauwald H *et al* (1994) *Phytother. Res.* 8(3):135.

MASTIC

PISTACIA LENTISCUS L.
Fam. Anacardiaceae

HABITAT: Greece, Cyprus.

DESCRIPTION: The resin occurs in small, rounded or pear-shaped, transparent tears which, when masticated, form a dough-like mass. Taste and odour: cedar-like.

PART USED: Resin

CONSTITUENTS: (i) Volatile oil, about 2%, containing over 69 components. The major constituents are alpha-pinene, myrcene, caryophyllene and germacrene-D (ii) Resins; composed of polymers such as 1,4-poly-beta-myrcene, alpha- and beta-masticoresins and a polymeric proanthocyanidin [1,2].

MEDICINAL USE: Has been used in dentistry for filling teeth. The essential oil has antimicrobial effects against several bacteria and fungi [1,4,5]. The resin (mastic) has preventative effects against gastric and duodenal ulcer [6] and is also hypotensive [7]. This effect has been

291

shown to be due to the polymeric proanthocyanidin [8].

SPECIFIC REFERENCES: 1. Magiatis P (1999) *Planta Med.* 65(8):749. 2. Van den Berg K *et al* (1998) *Tet. Lett.* 39(17):2645. 3. Sanz M *et al* (1992) *Pharmazie* 47(6):466. 4. Bonsignore L *et al* (1998) *Fitoterapia* 69(6):537. 5. Iauk L *et al* (1996) *J. Chemother.* 8(3):207. 6. Al-Said M *et al* (1986) *J. Ethnopharmacol.* 15(3):271. 7. Villar A *et al* (1987) *Int. J. Crude Drug Res.* 25(1):1. 8. Sanz M *et al* (1993) *Pharmazie* 48 (2):152.

MATE
ILEX PARAGUARIENSIS ST. HIL.
Fam. Aquifoliaceae

SYNONYMS: Paraguay Tea, Yerba Mate, Jesuit's Brazil Tea.

HABITAT: South America, especially Brazil and Argentina.

DESCRIPTION: The leaves appear in commerce either broken or as coarse powder. They are ovate, up to 15 cm long, with a crenate or serrate margin and a leathery texture. Taste: astringent, bitter; odour: characteristic, aromatic.

PART USED: Leaves.

CONSTITUENTS: (i) Xanthine derivatives; mainly caffeine and theobromine (theophylline is present in minor amounts) (ii) Triterpenoid saponins; matesaponins (MSP)-1,2,3 and 4, based on ursolic acid, and nudicaucin C and guaiacin B based on oleanolic acid, and ilexoside A and B derivatives (iii) Polyphenolics, tannins and caffeic acid derivatives; chlorogenic, and dicaffeoylquinic acids, (iv) Flavonoids: quercetin, rutin and kaempferol (v) Miscellaneous; volatile oil, vanillin, menisdaurin, a nitrile glucoside, and vitamin C [1,2,3,4,5,6].

MEDICINAL USE: Stimulant, diuretic, mild analgesic [R1]. Used for mild depression and rheumatic pains in combination with other remedies, and gastrointestinal disorders. Mate is used to make the most popular tea-like beverage in South America. The stimulant effects are due mainly to the caffeine and theobromine content. Mate has antioxidant effects, mainly due to the caffeic acid derivatives [7,8] and also increases bile flow [9]. Although generally non-toxic, mutagenic and clastogenic effects have been observed for the extract [10] and it is thought that a high consumption of Mate may potentiate carcinogenesis in the human oropharynx and oesophagus, which is a public health problem in Uruguay [11].

PREPARATIONS AND DOSE: Dried leaf, dose: 2–4 g or equivalent extract, three times daily.

SPECIFIC REFERENCES: 1. Filip R *et al* (2001) *Fitoterapia* 72:774. 2. Gosmann G *et al* (1995) *J. Nat. Prod.* 58(3):438. 3. Martinet A *et al* (2001) *Phytochem. Anal.* 12(1):48. 4. Ohem N *et al* (1988) *Planta Med.* 54:576. 5. Willems M (1989) *Planta Med.* 55:114. 6. Hikada K *et al* (1987) *Chem. Pharm. Bull.* 35:524. 7. Filip R *et al* (2000) *Nutr. Res.* 20(10):1437. 8. Gugliucci A (1996) *Biochem. Biophys. Res.*

Comm. 224(2):338. 9. Gorzalczany S *et al* (2001) *J. Ethnopharmacol.* 75(2–3):291. 10. Fonseca C *et al* (2000) *J. Environ. Pathol. Toxicol. Oncol.* 19(4):333. 11. Vassallo A *et al* (1985) *J. Natl. Cancer Inst.* 75:1005.

MATICO
PIPER ELONGATUM VAHL.

Fam. Piperaceae

SYNONYMS: Matica, *Piper angustifolia* Ruiz and Pavon. *Artanthe elongata* Miq.

HABITAT: South America.

DESCRIPTION: Leaves usually occur broken in commerce, recognizable by the reticulate surface, convexly on the upper surface due to deeply sunk veins, which are prominent on the lower surface. The undersurface is also hairy. Taste and odour: aromatic, tea-like.

PART USED: Leaves.

CONSTITUENTS: (i) Essential oil containing camphor, borneol, azulene, dill apiol, asarone (ii) Tannins, resins etc. [R2,R4].

MEDICINAL USE: Astringent, stimulant, diuretic, styptic [R1]. Used for leucorrhoea, haemorrhage and piles, and to stimulate the libido.

MAYWEED
ANTHEMIS COTULA L.

Fam. Asteraceae

SYNONYMS: Stinking Mayweed, Dog Chamomile, *Maruta cotula* D.C., *M. foetida* Cass.

HABITAT: Europe, including Britain.

DESCRIPTION: The herb resembles Chamomile in appearance, but the flowers have no membranous scales at the base and the outer florets have no styles. Taste and odour: unpleasant, acrid.

PART USED: Herb.

CONSTITUENTS: (i) Sesquiterpene lactones; anthecotulide and several of its dehydro and dihydro derivatives (ii) Flavonoids [1,2].

MEDICINAL USE: Antispasmodic, emmenagogue, emetic. Has been used for amenorrhoea and sick headaches. Anthecotulide is a potent allergen, and this species, when misidentified as Chamomile, has been responsible for causing allergies in humans. The flavonoid extract exhibits antimicrobial activity [2].

SPECIFIC REFERENCES: 1. Baruah R *et al* (1985) *Planta Med.* 51(6):531. 2. Quarenghi M *et al* (2000) *Fitoterapia* 71(6):710.

MEADOW LILY
LILIUM CANDIDUM L.
Fam. Liliaceae

SYNONYMS: White Lily, Madonna Lily.

HABITAT: Native to southern Europe, cultivated in gardens in Britain and North America.

DESCRIPTION: The bulb consists of free, fleshy scales, lanceolate and curved, about 3 cm long and 1 cm broad in the centre. Taste: mucilaginous, bitter and unpleasant.

PART USED: Bulb.

CONSTITUENTS: (i) Steroidal saponins based on diosgenin (ii) Flavonoids, including kaempferol glycosides (iii) Pyroline derivatives: jatropham and its glucoside (iv) Miscellaneous; carboxylic acids, beta-sitosterol, methyl palmitate etc. [1,2,3].

MEDICINAL USE: Demulcent, astringent [R1]. Has been used internally for female complaints and dropsy, and externally as a poultice for ulcers, inflammation etc. The extract is anti-fungal and shows inhibitory activity towards tumour promotion and carcinogenesis [3].

SPECIFIC REFERENCES: 1. Haladova M *et al* (1999) *Pharmazie* 54(2):159. 2. Eisenreichova E *et al* (2000) *Pharmazie* 55(7):549. 3. Vachalkova A *et al* (2000) *Neoplasma* 47(5):313.

MEADOWSWEET
FILIPENDULA ULMARIA (L.) MAXIM
Fam. Rosaceae

SYNONYMS: Queen-of-the-Meadow, Bridewort, *Spiraea ulmaria* L.

HABITAT: A common wild plant throughout Europe, parts of Asia and cultivated in North America.

DESCRIPTION: Leaves long-stalked, pinnate, with 2–5 pairs of toothed leaflets more than 2 cm long, and small leaflets in between. Stipules green above, downy beneath. Flowers in dense clusters, creamy, with 5–6 petals, 25 mm across. Taste: astringent and slightly aromatic.

PART USED: Herb.

CONSTITUENTS: (i) Volatile oil; containing salicylaldehyde (up to 75%), ethylsalicylate, methylsalicylate, methoxybenzaldehyde and others (ii) Phenolic glycosides; spiraein, monotropin, gaultherin (iii) Flavonoids; spiraeoside, rutin, hyperoside, avicularin (iv) Tannins, mainly hydrolysable tannides (v) Miscellaneous; phenylcarboxylic acids, traces of coumarin, ascorbic acid [R2,R7;1,2,3,4].

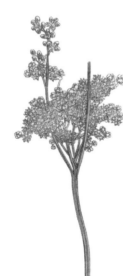

MEADOWSWEET

MEDICINAL USE: Stomachic, antacid, astringent, anti-rheumatic [R1]. Decoctions of Meadowsweet have anti-ulcer effects against a variety of experimental ulcerogenic procedures, including aspirin and ethanol (but not histamine) induced ulceration, in rats [4], despite the content of salicylates. Extracts also have other properties including lowering of motor activity, increasing the tonus of isolated guinea pig and rabbit intestine and uterus [1]. The tannins are bactericidal *in vitro* against a number of bacteria [5,6,7] and also inhibit the enzyme elastase [6]. Anti-inflammatory activity can be ascribed partly to the salicylate content, and a complement inhibiting substance has been described, which was not identified but was shown not to be one of the known constituents [8]. Extracts also have immunomodulating [9] and anticoagulant activity [10].

PREPARATIONS AND DOSE: Dried herb, dose: 4–6 g, or equivalent extract, three times daily.

SPECIFIC REFERENCES: 1. Lindemann A *et al* (1982) *Lebens. Wiss. Technol.* 15(5):286. 2. Scheer T *et al* (1987) *Planta Med.* 53:573. 3. Valle M *et al* (1988) *Planta Med.* 54:181. 4. Barnaulov O *et al* (1977) *Rastit. Resur.* 13:661. 5. Csedo K *et al* (1993) *Planta Med.* 59(Suppl.)A675. 6. Lamaison J *et al* (1990) *Ann. Pharm. Francais.* 46(6):335. 7. Rauha J *et al* (2000) *Int. J. Food. Microbiol.* 56(1):3. 8. Halkes S *et al* (1997) *Pharm. Pharmacol. Lett.* 7(2–3):79. 9. Kudryashov B *et al* (1990) *Farm. Toksicol* 53(4):39. 10. Halkes S *et al* (1997) *Phytother. Res.* 11(7):518.

MELILOT

MELILOTUS OFFICINALIS (L.) PALLAS.
Fam. Fabaceae

SYNONYMS: Ribbed Melilot, King's Clover, Yellow Sweet Clover, *M. arzensis* Willd.

HABITAT: Grows on bare and waste ground throughout Europe.

DESCRIPTION: An erect biennial reaching up to about 1 m. Leaves pinnately trifoliate, the upper ones being longer and narrowed at both ends. The yellow flowers are in axillary racemes, typically papilionaceous with the keel shorter than the wings, 5–6 cm long. The pod is 3–5 mm long, ribbed and hairless. Odour: like new-mown hay, due to the coumarin content.

PART USED: Herb.

CONSTITUENTS: (i) Coumarin derivatives; the glycoside melilotoside, which hydrolyses on drying to produce free coumarin, dihydro-coumarin, melilotin, melilotic acid, melilotol, and the hydroxy-coumarins scopoletin, umbelliferone and others. Dicoumarol (= melitoxin) is produced when Melilot has spoiled and fermentation has taken place (ii) Flavonoids; robinin, quercetin, clovine (iii) Phenolic acids and glycosides, including melilotosides (iv) Triterpene saponins such as the melilotus saponins, azuki saponins, soya sapogenols, astragaloside VIII and wisteriasaponin D [R2,R17;1,2,3,4,5,6].

MEDICINAL USE: Aromatic, carminative, spasmolytic [R1]. The herb is used particularly for oedematous and inflammatory conditions such as

295

burn injuries and lymphoedema, post-operative oedema and to improve venous return. Clinical studies have shown benefit in many of these conditions, including in post-mastectomy lymphoedema and rosacea [7,8,9; for full detail see R17 and refs therein]. The flower and leaf extracts have shown analgesic activity, prolongation in pentobarbital induced hypnosis time and smooth muscle relaxant activity in mice; they are also hypotensive and vasodilatory in rabbits. Melilot extract containing 0.25% coumarin gave positive results in several models of acute inflammation [10]. Dicoumarol is a potent anticoagulant and should be present only at very low levels. In general however, Melilot herb does not act as an anticoagulant and is considered safe [R17].

SPECIFIC REFERENCES: 1. Hammouda F et al (1983) Fitoterapia 54:249. 2. Bos R et al (1995) Planta Med. 61(S):68. 3. Dombrowicz E et al (1991) Pharmazie 46(2):156. 4. Khodakov G et al (1996) Adv. Exp. Med. Biol. 405:211. 5. Udayama M et al (1998) Chem. Pharm. Bull. 46(3):526. 6. Hirakawa T et al (2000) Chem. Pharm. Bull. 48(2):286. 7. Muraca M et al (1999) Gazz. Med. Ital. 158(4):133. 8. Aloisi D et al (1999) Minerva Cardioangiol. 47(11):496. 9. Iruassich S et al (1999) Ann. Ital. Dermatol. Clin. Sper. 53(1):28. 10. Plesca-Manea L et al (2003) Phytother. Res. (in press).

MESCAL BUTTONS
LOPHOPHORA WILLIAMSII (LEMAIRE) COULT.
Fam. Cactaceae

SYNONYMS: Peyote, Peyotl, Pellote, Anhalonium.

HABITAT: Mexico, parts of the southern North America.

DESCRIPTION: The dried cactus is cut into slices about 2–5 cm in diameter and 0.5–1 cm thick, hence the name mescal 'buttons'. Fracture: short and horny, pale brown; taste: gritty, mucilaginous, pungent and bitter.

PART USED: Cactus stem.

CONSTITUENTS: Alkaloids, the main one being mescaline; with N-acetyl mescaline, N-methyl mescaline, anhalamine, anhalidine, lophophorine and many others. See [1,2,3 and refs therein].

MEDICINAL USE: Hallucinogen, emetic. This is the Sacred Mushroom of the Aztecs. It is of medicinal value but is used illicitly as a narcotic and hallucinogen. See [2,3] for full review.

REGULATORY STATUS: CD. (Misuse of Drugs Act 1973).

SPECIFIC REFERENCES: 1. Willaman J (1970) Lloydia 33(3A):1. 2. Anderson E (1996) Peyote, the Divine Cactus. Univ. Arizona Press, Tucson, USA. 3. Richardson P (1988) Encyclopedia of Psychoactive Drugs: Flowering Plants – Magic in Bloom. Burke Publishing Co. London, UK.

MEZEREON

DAPHNE MEZEREUM L.
D. GNIDIUM L.
Fam. Thymeliaceae

SYNONYMS: Spurge Olive, Spurge Laurel. Other species have also been used medicinally.

HABITAT: Native to Europe, cultivated elsewhere as an ornamental.

DESCRIPTION: The root is brownish, very tough, with the outer bark peeling off easily to leave the fibrous inner bark. Taste: acrid and caustic; odour: unpleasant when fresh.

PART USED: Root, root bark, bark.

CONSTITUENTS: (i) Diterpene ortho esters; daphnetoxin, mezerein and related compounds (ii) Coumarins including daphnetin, daphnoretin, daphnin, triumbellin and umbelliferone [R2;1,2]. *D. gnidium* contains (i) Diterpene esters including mezerein and daphnetoxin (ii) Coumarins including daphnetin, daphnin (iii) Flavonoids; luteolin, orientin, isoprientin, genkwanin and others [3,4].

MEDICINAL USE: The orthoesters are highly inflammatory and co-carcinogenic, and mezerein has anti-leukaemic activity [1,2]; they are currently of great scientific interest but cannot be recommended for medicinal use. Mezereon was formerly taken as a stimulant, alterative and anti-rheumatic. Mezerein activates protein kinase C but daphnetoxin does not [3]. The coumarin and flavonoid extract from *D. gnidium* is antibacterial but not anti-fungal [4], although anti-mycobacterial effects have been reported [5]. *D. gnidium* is less irritant to the skin than *D. mezereum* but the coumarins are still phototoxic [6], and the presence of any diterpene esters means that it should not be applied to the skin or taken internally in any event.

SPECIFIC REFERENCES: 1. Evans F *et al* (1983) *Prog. Chem. Org. Nat. Prod.* 44:1. 2. Kreher B *et al* (1990) *Planta Med.* 56(6):572. 3. Saraiva L *et al* (2001) *Planta Med.* 67(9):787. 4. Cottiglia F *et al* (2001) *Phytomed.* 8(4):302. 5. Iauk L *et al* (1996) *Phytother. Res.* 10(S):S166. 6. Rapisarda A *et al* (1998) *Phytother. Res.* 12(1):49.

MILK THISTLE

SILYBUM MARIANUM (L.) GAERTN.

Fam. Asteraceae

SYNONYMS: Marian Thistle, Mediterranean Milk Thistle, *Carduus marianus.*

HABITAT: Throughout Europe, rare in Britain.

DESCRIPTION: Leaves spiny, dark green with a crenate margin and conspicuous white veins. Flower-heads rayless, purple, solitary with sepal-like bracts ending in sharp yellow spines. Taste and odour: slight.

PART USED: Seeds, aerial parts.

CONSTITUENTS: (i) Flavolignans; the mixture of these is known as silymarin and is composed mainly of silybin (= silibinin), with isosilybin, dihydrosilybin, silydianin, silychristin, and in some varieties at least, silandrin, silymonin, silyhermin and neosilyhermin (ii) Flavonoids based on apigenin, kaempferol, and luteolin (iii) Triterpenes; beta-sitosterol etc [R17;1,2,3,4 and references therein].

MEDICINAL USE: Hepatoprotective. Milk Thistle was formerly used in the UK for nursing mothers, as a bitter tonic, demulcent, as an antidepressant, for liver complaints, and for the same purposes as Holy Thistle (q.v.). In Germany and other parts of Europe it was used extensively for liver diseases and jaundice and this is the most important use today. Silymarin has been shown conclusively to exert an anti-hepatotoxic effect in animals against a variety of toxins, particularly those of the death cap mushroom *Amanita phalloides.* This fungus contains some of the most potent liver toxins known, the amatoxins and the phallotoxins, both of which cause haemorrhagic necrosis of the liver. Pre-treatment of animals with silymarin and silybin can give 100% protection against this type of poisoning, and when silybin was given by intravenous injection to human patients up to 48 hours after ingestion of the death cap it was found to be highly effective in preventing fatalities. Silymarin has been used successfully to treat patients with chronic hepatitis and cirrhosis; it is active against hepatitis B virus, is hypolipidaemic and lowers fat deposits in the liver in animals. It also has anti-inflammatory effects via inhibition of lipoxygenase. Antioxidant effects have been described and these are thought to contribute to a beneficial effect in experimental cholestasis and doxorubicin-induced cardiotoxicity in rats [5,6,7]. There is a vast amount of information on Milk Thistle: see [R17,1,2,4,8 and refs therein].

PREPARATIONS AND DOSE: Silymarin, dose: 420 mg daily.

SPECIFIC REFERENCES: 1. Wellington K *et al* (2001) *BioDrugs* 15(7):466. 2. Morazzoni P *et al* (1995) *Fitoterapia* 66(1):3. 3. Ahmed A *et al* (1989) *Phytochem.* 28:1751. 4. Saller R *et al* (2001) *Drugs* 61(14):2035. 5. Kosina P *et al* (2002) *Phytother. Res.* 16:S33. 6. Psotova J *et al* (2002) *Phytother. Res.* 16:S63. 7. Hagymasi K *et al* (2002) *Phytother. Res.* 16:S78. 8. Boerth J *et al* (2002) *J. Herbal Pharmacother.* 2(2):11.

MISTLETOE
VISCUM ALBUM L.
Fam. Loranthaceae

HABITAT: A parasite growing on deciduous trees, particularly fruit trees and poplars, throughout Europe.

DESCRIPTION: Woody, regularly branched, with elliptical, yellowish-green, leathery leaves in pairs; monoecious, inconspicuous four-petalled flowers, followed by sticky, white, globular berries in winter.

PART USED: Young leafy twigs.

Constituents: (i) Glycoproteins; the mistletoe lectins and viscumin (ii) Polypeptides; known as the viscotoxins (iii) Flavonoids; usually quercetin-derived and dependent on the host tree to some extent (iv) Polyphenolic acid derivatives; caffeic, *p*-coumaric, ferulic, gentisic and other acids (v) Polysaccharides, especially in the berries (vi) Triterpenes; betulinic acid, lupeol, oleanolic and ursolic acids and others (vii) Lignans; syringin, syringaresinol, eleutheroside E and others (viii) Alkaloids, in some (for example Korean) varieties [R7;1,2].

Medicinal Use: Hypotensive, cardiac tonic, immunostimulant, anti-neoplastic, sedative, antispasmodic [R1]. Mistletoe was formerly used for high blood pressure and tachycardia, and as a nervine; however the anti-cancer effects are now the most important. The cardiotonic activity is thought to be due to the lignans, which show significant cAMPphosphodiesterase inhibitory activity. The polysaccharides stimulate the immune response in mice and a commercial preparation of Mistletoe increased antibody production in rats stimulated with antigen after irradiation. The viscotoxins bind to DNA and viscumin inhibits protein synthesis. Several other mechanisms of action have been documented; for example mistletoe lectin-1 (ML-1) increases tumour necrosis factor alpha release [3] and viscotoxin-free extracts stimulate human granulocyte activity [4]. The anti-neoplastic activity of Mistletoe is well-documented, and many clinical trials have been carried out (for example for bladder, head and neck, and other cancers). The trials are of variable quality and the results are not always conclusive; but in general Mistletoe appears to be a useful adjunct to cancer chemotherapy. Recently mistletoe extract has shown promise in treating hepatitis C; however the number of patients was rather low (five) [5]. See [R7;6,7,8,9,10,11 and refs therein]. The genus has recently been comprehensively reviewed [12].

Specific References: 1. Fukunaga T *et al* (1987) *Chem. Pharm. Bull.* 35:3292. 2. Franz H *et al* (1981) *Biochem. J.* 195:481. 3. Boneberg E *et al* (2001) *J. Pharmacol. Exp. Ther.* 298(3):996. 4. (Kleijnen J *et al* (1994) *Phytomed.* 1:255. 5. Tusenius K *et al* (2001) *Comp. Ther. Med.* 9:12. 6. Stein G *et al* (1999) *Anticancer Res.* 19(4B):2925 and (5B):3907. 7. Grossarth-Maticek R *et al* (2001) *Alt. Ther. Health Med.* 7:57. 8. Ernst E (2000) *Fortschr. Med.*142(45):52. 9. Consensus Group. Iscador prescribing guidance 2001. *Weleda, Ltd, Ilkeston, UK.* 10. Steuer-Vogt M *et al* (2001) *Eur. J. Cancer* 37(1):23. 11. Stein G (2001) *Deutsch. Med. Wochensr.* 1126(28-29):833. 12. Mistletoe. Ed. Bussing A (2000) *Medicinal and Aromatic Plants – Industrial Profiles.* Pub: Taylor and Francis, London, UK.

MONSONIA

Monsonia ovata Cav.
Fam. Geraniaceae

Habitat: South Africa.

Description: Leaves opposite, very small, stalked, ovate, serrate, with filiform stipules. Flowers white, axillary, geranium-like, either solitary or occasionally in pairs on one peduncle. Stems branched, with slender spreading hairs, up to 30 cm long. Taste: astringent, slightly aromatic.

PART USED: Whole plant.

CONSTITUENTS: Undetermined.

MEDICINAL USE: Astringent; formerly used for acute and chronic diarrhoea and ulcerated lower bowel [R1].

MOTHERWORT
LEONURUS CARDIACA L.
AND OTHER SPECIES OF *LEONURUS*
Fam. Lamiaceae

SYNONYMS: Lion's Tail.

HABITAT: Grows in waste places throughout Europe and central Asia.

DESCRIPTION: Leaves stalked, palmately 5–7 lobed, serrate, downy on the undersurface with prominent, reticulate veins. Stems unbranched, quadrangular. Flowers downy, pinkish-purple or white, the lower lip spotted purple, about 12 mm long, in axillary whorls. Taste: very bitter; odour: slight.

PART USED: Herb.

CONSTITUENTS: (i) Iridoids; leonuride, ajugol, ajugoside, galiridoside and others (ii) Diterpenes of the labdane type, such as leocardin, which is a mixture of two epimers (iii) Flavonoids; rutin, quinqueloside, genkwanin, quercetin, quercitrin, isoquercitrin, hyperoside, and apigenin and kaempferol glucosides (iv) Alkaloids; stachydrine, betonicine, leonurine, leonurinine and others (v) Phenolics such as caffeic acid 4-rutinoside, tannins, plant acids etc. [R2,R7;1,2,3].

MEDICINAL USE: Cardiac tonic, sedative, nervine, antispasmodic, emmenagogue [R1]. Studies in China have shown that extracts have anti-platelet aggregation actions and decrease the levels of blood lipids [4,5]; they also have an inhibitory effect on pulsating myocardial cells *in vitro* [6]. Leonurine causes a vaso-relaxation independent of endothelium [7]. A preparation containing Motherwort together with other sedative herbs was investigated: studies on the individual components indicated that the *Leonurus* extract reduced hexobarbital sleeping time and increased exploratory behaviour in mice, which was the opposite of the effect produced by the mixture [8]. No further clinical data appears to be available.

PREPARATIONS AND DOSE: Dried herb, dose: 2–4 g, or equivalent extract, three times daily.

SPECIFIC REFERENCES: 1. Malakov P *et al* (1985) *Phytochem.* 24(10):2341. 2. Kartnig T *et al* (1985) *J. Nat. Prod.* 48(3):494. 3. Knoss W *et al* (1998) *Planta Med.* 64(4):357. 4. Chang C *et al* (1986) *Chung Hoi I Tsa Chih* 6(1):39. 5. Peng Y (1983) *Bull. Chin. Mat. Med.* 8:41. 6. Xanxing X (1983) *J. Trad. Chin. Med.* 3:185.

7. Chen C *et al* (2001) *Life Sci.* 168(8):953. 8. Weischer M *et al* (1994) *Z. Phytother.* 15(5):257.

MOUNTAIN ASH
SORBUS AUCUPARIA L.
Fam. Rosaceae

SYNONYMS: Rowan Tree, Witchen, *Pyrus aucuparia* (L.) Gaertn.

HABITAT: Europe, western Siberia, temperate Asia and northern North America.

DESCRIPTION: A well-known tree. The fruit is scarlet, globular, 6–9 mm in diameter, with calyx teeth at the apex. The bark is greyish, smooth, with a soft, spongy outer layer and a short, granular fracture.

PART USED: Berries, bark.

CONSTITUENTS: (i) Cyanogenetic glycosides, in the seeds and fruit pulp, including amygdalin and prunasin (ii) Parasorbic acid, an alpha, beta- unsaturated lactone, and its glycosides; mainly in the fresh plant [R2;1,2].

MEDICINAL USE: Astringent, antimicrobial [R1]. It has been used for infections of the urinary tract, menstrual disorders and rheumatism, although little clinical or pharmacological work is available. The ripe berries have been used as a gargle in sore throats and tonsillitis, and a decoction of the bark for diarrhoea.

SPECIFIC REFERENCES: 1. Fikenscher L *et al* (1981) *Planta Med.* 41:313. 2. Sticher O *et al* (1980) *Planta Med.* 39:269.

MOUNTAIN FLAX
LINUM CATHARTICUM L.
Fam. Linaceae

SYNONYMS: Purging Flax.

HABITAT: A wild European plant growing in meadows.

DESCRIPTION: Leaves opposite, small, the lower ones obovate, the upper lanceolate, with entire margins. Flowers small, white, with five pointed petals, serrate sepals, arranged in a loose panicle. Taste: bitter and acrid; odourless.

PART USED: Herb.

CONSTITUENTS: (i) Volatile oil, about 0.15% (ii) Lignans and tannins are thought to be present [R2].

MEDICINAL USE: Laxative, diuretic, anti-rheumatic [R1].

MOUNTAIN LAUREL
KALMIA LATIFOLIA L.
Fam. Ericaceae

SYNONYMS: Sheep Laurel, Lambkill, Spoonwood.

301

HABITAT: North America.

DESCRIPTION: An evergreen shrub. Leaves broadly lanceolate, leathery, about 6 cm long and 3 cm broad, with narrowly reflexed margins and a prominent midrib. Taste: astringent and slightly bitter; odour: slight.

PART USED: Leaves.

CONSTITUENTS: (i) Diterpenes; andromedan derivatives including andromedatoxin, asebotoxin, rhodotoxin, lyonol A, kalmiatoxins I-VI, and grayanoids such as the grayanotoxins I, II, III and XVIII (ii) Acylphloroglucinols such as phloretin and acetophenone derivatives (iii) Flavonoids; asebotin and hyperoside [R2;1,2,3].

MEDICINAL USE: Cardiac sedative, astringent [R1]. Has been used for febrile conditions, inflammation, diarrhoea and haemorrhage. Large doses are toxic. The grayanotoxins are cytotoxic [1] and act as insect anti-feedants [2]. Extracts are antimicrobial against *Candida albicans, Trichophyton rubrum* and *Streptococcus mutans* [4].

SPECIFIC REFERENCES: 1. Mancini S *et al* (1979) *J. Nat. Prod.* 42(5):483. 2. El-Naggar S *et al* (1980) *J. Nat. Prod.* 43(5):617 and (6):739. 3. Wolters B (1997) *Deutsch.* Apot. Ztg. 137:2253. 4. Heisey R *et al* (1992) *Lett. Appl. Microbiol.* 14(4):136.

MOUSE EAR
PILOSELLA OFFICINARUM L.
Fam. Asteraceae

SYNONYMS: Mouse Ear Hawkweed, *Hieraceum pilosella* L.

HABITAT: A common plant growing in sandy soil in Europe, North America and temperate Asia.

DESCRIPTION: A small creeping plant giving off leafy runners. The leaves are lanceolate, about 3 cm long, greyish above with scattered slender hairs and whitish underneath due to the dense covering of branched hairs. Flowers solitary, pale yellow, composite, about 2–3 cm diameter, outer florets often reddish underneath. Taste: bitter; odour: faint.

PART USED: Herb.

CONSTITUENTS: (i) Umbelliferone, a coumarin (ii) Flavonoids including luteolin and its glycosides (iii) Caffeic and chlorogenic acids [R2].

MEDICINAL USE: Expectorant, diuretic, spasmolytic, sialogogue, vulnerary [R1]. It is used mainly for whooping cough, bronchitis and asthma as an infusion, and for wounds as a compress. An extract shows weak anti-fungal activity [1] and has diuretic and anti-inflammatory effects in animals [2,3].

PREPARATIONS AND DOSE: Dried herb, dose: 2–4 g or equivalent extract, three times daily.

SPECIFIC REFERENCES: 1. Guerin J *et al* (1985) *Ann. Pharm. Francais.* 43(1):77. 2. Bolle P *et al* (1993) *Pharm. Res.* 27(Suppl.1):29. 3. Beaux D *et al* (1999) *Phytother. Res.* 13(3):222.

MUGWORT
ARTEMISIA VULGARIS L.

Fam. Asteraceae

SYNONYMS: Felon Herb.

HABITAT: Grows in waste places throughout Europe.

DESCRIPTION: A downy perennial reaching about 1.5 m in height. Leaves pinnatisect, with five to seven lobes, deeply incised, serrate, dark green and almost hairless on the upper surface and silvery and downy underneath. Flowers yellowish or purplish brown, rayless, in branched spikes. Taste: bitter; odour: aromatic.

PART USED: Herb.

CONSTITUENTS: (i) Volatile oil, containing linalool, 1,8-cineole, alpha- and beta-thujone, borneol, cineole, alpha- and beta-pinene, nerol, neryl acetate, linalyl acetate, myrcene, vulgarole, cadinol, cadinenol, muurolol, spathulenol and others (ii) Sesquiterpene lactones; vulgarin, yomogin, pilostachyn and others (iii) Flavonoids; quercetin-3-glucoside, quercetin-3-rhamnoglucoside and 5,3' dihydroxy-3,7,4'-trimethoxyflavone (iv) Coumarin derivatives; umbelliferone, esculetin, 7,8-methylendioxy-9-methoxycoumarin (v) Caffeic acid derivatives including dicaffeoylquinic acids (vi) Triterpenes such as 3-beta-hydroxurs-12-en-27,28-dionic acid, beta-amyrin, beta-sitosterol etc. [R2;1,2,3,4].

MUGWORT

MEDICINAL USE: Emmenagogue, diaphoretic, choleretic, anthelmintic, diuretic, stomachic, orexigenic [R1]. Mugwort is taken as an infusion for amenorrhoea, anorexia and dyspepsia, and less often for threadworm or roundworm infestation. Used in Chinese medicine for nausea and vomiting. The oil is antimicrobial [8], but irritates the skin. Anti-inflammatory effects have been observed, and a reduction in tissue injury brought about by ischaemia and reperfusion, and it also exerts antihypertensive activity [7]. Mugwort should not be taken during pregnancy.

PREPARATIONS AND DOSE: Dried herb, dose: 0.5–2 g or equivalent extract, three times daily.

SPECIFIC REFERENCES: 1. Marco J et al (1993) *Phytochem.* 32:460 and (1991)30:2403. 2. Micaelis K et al (1982) *Z. Naturforsch.* 37:152. 3. Wallnofer B et al (1989) *Phytochem.* 28:2687. 4. Murrar R et al (1986) *J. Nat. Prod.* 49(3):550. 5. Carnat A et al (1985) *Ann. Pharm. Francais.* 43(4):397. 6. Carnat A et al (2000) *Fitoterapia* 71(5):587. 7. Tigno X et al (2000) *Clin. Hemorheol. Microcirc.* 23(204):159 and 167. 8. Kaul V et al (1976) *Indian J. Pharm.* 38:21.

MUIRA-PUAMA
PTYCHOPETALUM OLACOIDES BENTH.

Fam. Olacaceae

SYNONYMS: Liriosma ovata Miers.

HABITAT: Brazil.

303

DESCRIPTION: The root in commerce usually occurs as hard, tough fibrous, light brown, woody splinters, 5–8 cm long and about 0.5 cm across, without any root bark. Taste: slightly astringent; odourless.

PART USED: Root.

CONSTITUENTS: (i) Triterpenes; esters of behenic and lignoceric acids, lupeol and other phytosterols (ii) Volatile oil, containing alpha- and beta-pinene, alpha-copaene, camphor, camphene, elixene, alpha-humulene, beta-caryophyllene, caryophyllene oxide, limonene and others (iii) Miscellaneous; flavonoids, alkaloids and saponins (unspecified)[R2;1,2,3].

MEDICINAL USE: Aphrodisiac, astringent [R1]. Used for treating male impotence and as a general tonic for fatigue. The plant extract has been shown to possess both motor depressant and stimulant properties, depending on the test model used, and an alpha-adrenergic receptor agonist effect was inferred [4]. This is not consistent with aphrodisiac activity, although vasodilation of erectile tissues has been suggested as a possible mechanism for this effect [5]. Muira puama potentiates yohimbine-induced lethality, reverses reserpine-induced ptosis and prevents apomorphine-induced stereotypy in mice [6]. A study recently showed an apparent increase in female libido, produced by a mixture of Muira Puama and Ginkgo (q.v.). It also has an anxiogenic effect in animals consistent with stimulant activity [7].

PREPARATIONS AND DOSE: Dried root, dose: 0.5–2g or equivalent extract, three times daily.

SPECIFIC REFERENCES: 1. Auterhoff H *et al* (1968) *Arch. Pharm.* 301:481 and (1971) 304:223. 2. Uber Bucek E *et al* (1987) *Planta Med.* 53(2):231 3. Ito Y *et al* (1995) *Natural Med.* 49(4):486. 4. Paiva L et al (1998) *Phytother. Res.* 12:294. 5. Antunes E *et al* (2001) *Phytother. Res.*15(5):416. 6. Siquiera I *et al* (1998) *Pharm. Biol.* 36:327. 7. Da Silva A *et al* (2002) *Phytother. Res.* 16(3):223.

MULBERRY
MORUS NIGRA L.
M. ALBA L.
Fam. Moraceae

SYNONYMS: Black or Purple Mulberry (= *M. nigra*), White Mulberry, (= *M. alba*).

HABITAT: Both are cultivated worldwide in temperate regions.

DESCRIPTION: The fruit of the black mulberry resembles that of the blackberry, except that the remains of the calyx can be seen on each fleshy lobe of the fruit. Taste and odour: pleasant, characteristic.

PART USED: Fruit, leaves, root bark.

CONSTITUENTS: *M. nigra* fruit: Invert sugar, pectin, fruit acids, vitamin C. No information on other parts of this species. *M. alba* leaves: (i) Flavonoids; rutin, moracetin, skimmin, roseoside II, astragalin and

others (ii) Anthocyanins; cyanidin and delphinidin glucosides (iii) Phytosterols; beta-sitosterol, beta-amyrin (iv) Coumarins including umbelliferone, bergapten, artocarpin and scopoletin [1,2,3,4,5,6].
Roots: (i) Stilbene glucosides including oxyresveratrol glucoside, the sangennons, kuwanons, mulberrosides and mulberrofurans [7,8] (ii) Nitrogen-containing sugars such as calystegins A3, B1, B2 and C1, which are tropane-based [8] (iii) Polysaccharides containing rhamnose, arabinose, xylose, mannose, galactose and glucose [9].

MEDICINAL USE: The fruits are a popular nutrient, refrigerant, and mild laxative. The leaves are diuretic, hypotensive and expectorant [R1]. Extracts of *M. alba* are hypoglycaemic, slightly antispasmodic and hypotensive in rats [7,11], and both *M. alba* and *M. nigra* leaf extracts reduce blood sugar levels in experimentally diabetic (but not normoglycaemic) mice [12]. A small clinical trial of 24 patients with type 2 diabetes showed that Indian Mulberry (*M. indica* L.) reduced fasting blood sugar, as well as serum cholesterol and triglyceride levels [13]. Externally applied extracts appeared to shorten the telogen phase of hair growth in rabbits, and clinical studies suggested a potential use in male pattern baldness [14]. Inhibition of various types of enzyme activities has been reported; for example the mulberrosides and sangennons inhibit platelet cyclooxygenase and lipoxygenase [7] and the nitrogen-containing sugars are glucosidase inhibitors [9]. The flavonoids induce differentiation of human promyelocytic leukemia cell lines *in vitro* [4] and are free-radical scavengers, also inhibiting low density lipoprotein oxidation [5]. The polysaccharides are immunomodulators [10]. Mulberry leaf extracts are essentially non-toxic in animals [15].

BIBLICAL REFERENCES: 2 Samuel 5: 230-24; 1 Chronicles 14:14–15; Luke 17: 6.

SPECIFIC REFERENCES: 1. Nomura T *et al* (1983) *Planta Med.* 47:151. 2. Kimura Y *et al* (1986) *J. Nat. Prod.* 94(4):639. 3. El-Khrisy E *et al* (1992) *Fitoterapia* 63(1):92. 4. Sun S-Y *et al* (2000) *Biol. Pharm. Bull.* 23(4):451. 5. Doi K *et al* (2001) *Chem. Pharm. Bull.* 49(2):151. 6. Onogi A *et al* (1994) *Jpn. J. Pharmacog.* 74(4):423. 7. Qiu F *et al* (1996) *Planta Med.* 62(6):559. 8. Shin N-H *et al* (1998) *Biochem. Biophys. Res. Commun.* 243(3):801. 9. Asano N *et al* (1994) *Carbohydr. Res.* 259(2):243. 10. Shuxiu W *et al* (1995) *Phytother. Res.* 9(6):448. 11. Lemus I *et al* (1999) *Phytother. Res.* 13(2):91. 12. Hosseinzadeh H *et al* (1999) *Pharm. Pharmacol. Lett.* 9(2):63. 13. Andallu B *et al* (2001) *Clin. Chim. Acta* 314(1–2):47. 14. Kuwana R *et al* (1996) *Nishinihon J. Dermatol.* 58(4):619. 15. Mitsuya M *et al* (2001) *Pharmacometrics* 61(1):169.

MULLEIN
VERBASCUM THAPSUS L.
V. THAPSIFORME SCHRAD.
V. PHLOMOIDES L.
Fam. Scrophulariaceae

SYNONYMS: Aaron's Rod. Great Mullein is *V. thapsus*; Orange Mullein is *V. phlomoides. V. densiflorum Bertol.* = *V. thapsiforme* Schrad.

HABITAT: V. thapsus is native to Britain, the other species to Europe, North America and temperate Asia.

DESCRIPTION: V. thapsus: a stout perennial, covered with thick, woolly down, usually unbranched. Leaves broadly lanceolate, crenate, with a decurrent base, stems winged. Flowers yellow, almost flat, 15–30 mm in diameter. Taste: mucilaginous and slightly bitter; odour: faint.

PART USED: Herb, flowers.

CONSTITUENTS: V. thapsus: (i) Iridoids including ajugol, and catalpol glycosides (ii) Flavonoids such as verbascoside, hesperidin, (iii) Saponins, volatile oil, tannins, Mucilage [R4,1]. *V. thapsiforme:* (i) Iridoids; harpagoside, verbenalin, aucubin, catalpol, isocatalpol, methylcatalpol and their glycosides (ii) Saponins called mullein-saponins I-V, which are saikosaponins based on saikogenin, together with verbascosaponins, songarosaponins and many others (iii) Flavonoids; rutin, hesperidin and others [2,3,4,5].

MEDICINAL USE: Expectorant, demulcent, diuretic, emollient, vulnerary [R1]. Mullein is used particularly for bronchitis and catarrh and externally for inflammation and to aid wound-healing. Gerard has an interesting recipe: "the yellow flowers being steeped in oil and set in warm dung until they be washed into the oil and consumed away, to be a remedy for piles". It is also used in a more conventional formulation for influenza, and recently it was shown that an extract was effective against the herpes simplex and influenza viruses, especially in conjunction with the antiviral agent amantadine [6,7]. Inhibition of protein biosynthesis was also shown by the aqueous extract and saponin fractions, both of which had a similar effect in isolated rat liver ribosomes [8].

PREPARATIONS AND DOSE: Dried herb, dose: 4–8 g or equivalent extract, three times daily.

SPECIFIC REFERENCES: 1. Washarina T *et al* (1991) *Chem. Pharm. Bull.* 39(12):3261. 2. Gryzbek J *et al* (1996) *Z. Phytother.* 17(6):389. 3. Swiatek L *et al* (1982) *Planta Med.* 45(3):12P. 4. Siefert K *et al* (1985) *Planta Med.* 5. Miyase T *et al* (1997) *Chem. Pharm. Bull.* 45(12):2029. 6. Zgorniak-Nowosielska I *et al* (1991) *Arch. Immunol. Exp. Ther.* 39:103. 7. Serkedjieva J (2000) *Phytother. Res.* 14(7):571. 8. Paszkiewicz-Gadek A *et al* (1990) *Phytother. Res.* 4(5):177.

MUSTARD

BLACK MUSTARD

WHITE MUSTARD

BRASSICA NIGRA (L.) KOCH.
B. JUNCEA (L.) CZERN ET COSS.
SINAPIS ALBA L.
Fam. Brassicaceae

SYNONYMS: Black Mustard; Brown Mustard (= Indian Mustard,
S. juncea); White Mustard: *B. alba* L., *B. hirta* Moench.

HABITAT: *B. nigra* and *S. alba* are cultivated in Europe and North
America, *B. juncea* in India.

DESCRIPTION: The seeds are globular, 1–2 mm in diameter, with white
mustard seeds being slightly larger at up to 2.5 mm diameter. Taste
and odour: when ground, strong, pungent, characteristic.

PART USED: Seed, leaf for production of oil.

CONSTITUENTS: (i) Glucosinolates; black mustard contains sinigrin,
which on hydrolysis by the enzyme myrosin produces allyisothio-
cyanate, and white mustard sinalbin, which produces *p*-hydroxybenzyl
isothiocyanate (ii) Miscellaneous; sinapine, sinapic acid, fixed oil,
protein, mucilage etc. [R2,R19]. *B. juncea* has been re-investigated
more recently and the oil shown to contain (i) Sulphur-containing
compounds such as allyl isothiocyanate, 2-phenyl ethyl isothiocyanate,
5-methyl isothiazole, benzene acetaldehyde and benzene propane
nitrile, beta ionone and others (ii) Phytoalexins such as brassilexin,
a new sulphur-containing phytoalexin (iii) Flavonoids based on
isorhamnetin [1,2,3].

MEDICINAL USE: The oil has been used as a rubefacient, counter-
irritant, stimulant, diuretic and emetic [R1]. It is usually used
medicinally as an external application for rheumatic pains and
bronchitis, but must be used with caution. The seed oil of *B. juncea*
is antimicrobial [4]. Black mustard powder given to rats inhibited
mutagenicity induced by benzo[a]pyrene [5]. All types of mustard
are used as condiments and flavourings.

BIBLICAL REFERENCES: Matthew 13:31 and 17:20; Mark 4:31;
Luke 13:19 and 17: 6.

SPECIFIC REFERENCES: 1. Shin S-W *et al* (2001) *Korean J. Pharmacog.*
32(2):140. 2. Devys M *et al* (1988) *Tet. Lett.* 29(49):6447. 3. Choi J
et al (2000) *Nat. Prod. Sci.* 6(4):199. 4. Rajendra Prasad Y *et al* (1993)
Fitoterapia 64(4):373. 5. Polasa K *et al* (1994) *Food Chem. Toxicol.*
32(8):777.

MYROBALAN
TERMINALIA CHEBULA RETZ.

Fam. Combretaceae

SYNONYMS: Black Chebulic, Inknut.

HABITAT: India and other parts of Asia.

DESCRIPTION: A large deciduous tree with glabrous, ovate or elliptic leaves up to 20 cm long. The flowers are white or yellow, in terminal spikes, with an unpleasant odour. The fruits are ovoid, pendulous drupes, up to 5 cm long, yellow or orange brown in colour when ripe.

PART USED: Fruit, leaves, stem.

CONSTITUENTS: (i) Triterpene glycosides; chebulosides I and II, arjunin, arjunglycoside and others (ii) Tannins and polyphenols; chebulinic acid, chebulin, punicalagin, punicalin, hydroxymicromeric acid, terflavins A, B, C and D, ellagic and gallic acids [R16;1,2,3,4].

MEDICINAL USE: Astringent, laxative, cardiotonic, anti-asthmatic, febrifuge and carminative. Myrobalan is highly regarded in Ayurvedic medicine and is used to strengthen the brain and enrich the blood [R16]. Some of these uses have been substantiated; for example an extract of the fruit rind increased the contractile force of the frog heart [5] and the water-soluble fraction inhibited anaphylaxis and reduced blood histamine levels [6]. An aqueous extract of the fruit has antimutagenic and anti-tumour activity [7,3]. The extract is also antiviral [8], and antioxidant effects have been observed [9]. Gallic acid and its methyl ester inhibited cytotoxicity against cultured human tumour cell lines [3], and exerted strong antibacterial activity against MRSA (methicillin-resistant *Staphylococcus aureus*) and other organisms. The extract is generally considered to be non-toxic [R16].

PREPARATIONS AND DOSE: Powdered herb or leaf: dose: 1–6 g, or equivalent extract.

SPECIFIC REFERENCES: 1. Singh C et al (1990) *Phytochem.* 29(7):2438. 2. Kundu A et al (1993) *Phytochem.* 32(4):999. 3. Lee S et al (1995) *Arch. Pharm. Res.* 18(2):118. 4. Sato Y et al (1997) *Biol. Pharm. Bull.* 20(4):401. 5. Reddy V et al (1990) *Fitoterapia* 61(6):517. 6. Shin T et al (2001) *J. Ethnopharmacol.* 4(2):133. 7. Grover I et al (1992) *Indian J. Exp. Biol.* 30(4):399. 8. Kurokawa M et al (1995) *Chem. Pharm. Bull.* 43(4):641. 9. Fu N et al (1992) *Chin. Trad. Herbal Drugs* 23(1):26.

MYROBALAN, BELERIC
TERMINALIA BELERICA (GAERTN) ROXB.

Fam. Combretaceae

SYNONYMS: Belleric Myrobalan.

HABITAT: Common throughout Asia.

DESCRIPTION: A large deciduous tree with a characteristic blue-grey, cracked bark. The leaves are broadly elliptical up to 25 cm long and directed towards the apex of the branches. The flowers are pale greenish yellow, in axillary spikes, with an unpleasant odour. The fruits are globular, hairy and grey, up to 2 cm in diameter.

PART USED: Fruit.

CONSTITUENTS: (i) Triterpenes; belleric acid and the saponins bellericoside and bellericanin, with beta sitosterol and others (ii) Tannins and polyphenols; phyllemblin, ethyl gallate, and chebulagic, ellagic and gallic acids [R16;1,2].

MEDICINAL USE: Tonic, liver protective, antiviral, astringent and anti-diarrhoeal. Beleric Myrobalan is used in Ayurvedic medicine to strengthen the immune system, especially as part of a formulation known as 'Triphala', which contains other species of *Terminalia*. Hepatoprotective and hypolipidemic activity has been demonstrated [3,4,5] and partly ascribed to the gallic acid content [6]. Several clinical studies have been carried out in India, mainly on the preparation Triphala, with encouraging results against obesity, ulcers, hypergly-caemia and inflammatory disorders see [R16 and refs therein].

PREPARATIONS AND DOSE: Powdered dried fruit, dose: 1–3 g or equivalent extract.

SPECIFIC REFERENCES: 1. Nandy A *et al* (1989) *Phytochem.* 28(10):2769. 2. Ali M *et al* (1991) *Indian J. Nat. Prod.* 7(1):16. 3. Anand K *et al* (1994) *Phytother. Res.* 8(5):287. 4. Shaila H *et al* (1998) *Int. J. Cardiol.* 67(2):119. 5. Anand K *et al* (1997) *Pharmacol. Res.* 36(4):315. 6. Ahmad I *et al* (1998) *J. Ethnopharmacol.* 62(2):183.

MYRRH

COMMIPHORA MOLMOL ENGL.
C. ABYSSINICA (BERG.) ENGL.
AND POSSIBLY OTHER *COMMIPHORA* SPP.

Fam. Burseraceae

SYNONYMS: *Balsamodendron myrrha* Nees. *Commiphora myrrha* Holm.

HABITAT: Northeast Africa and Arabia.

DESCRIPTION: The oleo-gum resin exudes from fissures or incisions in the bark and is collected as irregular masses or tears, varying in colour from yellowish to reddish brown, often with white patches. The surface may be oily or covered with fine dust. Taste: bitter and acrid; odour: aromatic.

PART USED: Oleo-gum Resin.

CONSTITUENTS: (i) Volatile oil, containing heerabolene, elemol, eugenol, cuminaldehyde, numerous furanosesquiterpenes including furanodiene, furaneudesma-1,3-diene, furanodienone, curzerene, curzerenone, lindestrene, 2-methoxy furanodiene and other derivatives (ii) Resins including alpha-, beta- and gamma-commiphoric acids, commiphorinic acid, heeraboresene, alpha- and beta-heerabomyrrhols

309

and commiferin (iii) Gums, composed of arabinose, galactose, xylose and 4-O-methylglucuronic acid (iv) Sterols etc. [R2,R7;1,2,3,4].

MEDICINAL USE: Stimulant, expectorant, antiseptic, anti-inflammatory, antispasmodic, carminative [R1]. Myrrh is used internally for stomach complaints, tonsillitis, pharyngitis and gingivitis, and externally for ulcers, boils and wounds. It is analgesic, anti-inflammatory [5], antithrombotic [6], anti-ulcerogenic [7] and has an anti-carcinogenic effect on solid tumours in mice [8]. Furaneudesma-1,3-diene interacts with opioid receptors and shows structural similarities with morphiceptin and other opioid agonists [3]. A product containing myrrh has been shown to be effective against fascioliasis in human patients and schistosomiasis in mice [9,10]. Few signs of toxicity or adverse events were noted [9]. The extract is reportedly antimicrobial *in vitro* [R19]. Myrrh is reasonably safe, although very large doses produced disturbances in haematological parameters and other signs of toxicity, and even lethality, in the rat [11].

PREPARATIONS AND DOSE: Tincture of Myrrh BPC 1973, dose: 1–2.5 ml three times daily, or by topical application.

BIBLICAL REFERENCES: Exodus 30:23; Esther 2:12; Psalm 45:8; Proverbs 7:17; Song 1:13, 3: 6, 4:6 and 14; 5:1 and 13; Matthew 2:11; John 19:39.

SPECIFIC REFERENCES: 1. Zhu N *et al* (2001) *J. Nat. Prod.* 64(11):1460. 2. Brieskorn C *et al* (1982) *Planta Med.* 44(2):87. 3. Dolara P *et al* (1996) *Phytother. Res.* 10(Suppl.1):S81. 4. Ubillas R *et al* (1999) *Planta Med.* 65(8):778. 5. Tariq M *et al* (1986) *Agents Actions* 17(3–4)381. 6. Olajide O (1999) *Phytother. Res.* 13(3):231. 7. Al-Harbi M *et al* (1997) *J. Ethnopharmacol.* 55(2):141. 8. Al-Harbi M *et al* (1994) *Chemother.* 40(5):337. 9. Massoud A *et al* (2001) *Am. J. Trop. Med. Hyg.* 65(2):96. 10. Badria F *et al* (2001) *Pharm. Biol.* 39(2):127. 11. Omer S *et al* (1999) *Vet. Hum. Toxicol.* 4 1(4):193.

MYRTLE

MYRTUS COMMUNIS L.

Fam. Myrtaceae

HABITAT: Indigenous to southern Europe, cultivated elsewhere.

DESCRIPTION: An evergreen shrub with ovate, smooth, glossy leaves.

PART USED: Leaves, fruit.

CONSTITUENTS: (i) Volatile oil, containing alpha-pinene, cineole, myrtenol, nerol, geraniol, geranyl actetate, limonene, linalool and dipentene (ii) Acylphloroglucinol derivatives; myrtocommulon A and B (iii) Tannins, epigallocatechin, epicatechin gallate and other derivatives (iv) Flavonoids such as myricetin (about 90%) with kaempferol and quercetin glycosides [R2;1,2,3].

MEDICINAL USE: Antiseptic, anti-parasitic. Used for urinary infections as a substitute for Buchu (q.v.). Leaf extracts show antimicrobial activity *in vitro* [4], insecticidal activity against lice [5], molluscicidal

[6] and other anti-parasitic effects [7]. An ointment containing Myrtle extracts has been used to treat herpes simplex infection with some success [8].

BIBLICAL REFERENCES: Nehemiah 8:15; Isaiah 41:9 and 55:13; Zechariah 1:8 and 11.

SPECIFIC REFERENCES: 1. Joseph M *et al* (1987) *Pharmazie* 42(2):142. 2. Martin T *et al* (1999) *Pharm. Biol.* 37(1):28. 3. Romani A *et al* (1999) *Chromatographia* 49(1–2):17. 4. Mansouri S (1999) *Pharm.Biol.* 37(5):357. 5. Gauthier R *et al* (1989) *Plantes Med. Phytother.* 23(2):95. 6. Deruaz D *et al* (1993) *Phytother. Res.* 7(6):428. 7. Martin T *et al* (1997) *Fitoterapia* 68(3):276. 8. Zolfaghari M *et al* (1997) *Iranian J. Med. Sci.* 22(3–4):134.

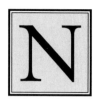

NEEM

AZADIRACHTA INDICA A JUSS.
Fam. Meliaceae

SYNONYMS: Nim, Margosa, Indian Lilac.

HABITAT: Indigenous to India and Southeast Asia, naturalized in West Africa, cultivated widely.

DESCRIPTION: A large deciduous tree. The bark is greyish-brown, externally fissured, with a buff inner surface and fibrous fracture. Taste: bitter; odourless.

PART USED: Bark, leaves, seeds.

CONSTITUENTS: (i) Limonoids; azadirachtin and various hydro-, hydroxy- and methoxy- derivatives, nimbanal, nimbolides A and B, margocin, margocinin, margocilin and many others (ii) Triterpenes including nimbin, nimbidin, nimbinin, nimbolone, nimbionone, gedunin, margosinone and others (iii) Fixed oil, in the seeds, containing many of the above (iv) Polysaccharides, in the bark and fruit pulp [R13,R16;1,2,3,4,5,6 and refs therein].

MEDICINAL USE: Anti-inflammatory, antipyretic, antimalarial, insecticide, anthelmintic [R1]. The seed oil and leaf extract are used in the treatment of skin diseases and as a hair dressing, but Neem is a very important medicinal plant in Asia and is used for a wide variety of ailments [R13,R16]. An extract of the leaves and bark has been found to have significant anti-inflammatory and antipyretic activity, coupled with low toxicity, in animals [7]; both the nimbidin derivatives and the polysaccharides may contribute to this activity [6,8]. Antifungal, antibacterial and antiviral properties have been documented [R16;9]. Neem is also used to treat malaria; nimbolide, nimbinin and gedunin derivatives are antimalarial *in vitro* and in mice, against *Plasmodium berghei* [4,10]. Anti-ulcer, contraceptive, radioprotective, hepatoprotective, CNS depressant, hypotensive, hypoglycaemic and anxiolytic effects and many other activities have been reported [11,12]. The limonoids are insect anti-feedants and have been used as repellents and to treat parasitic infections such as lice, as well as to preserve stored crops from insect damage. Neem appears to be relatively safe; however there are unsubstantiated reports of renal toxicity in human patients who have treated themselves for malaria with this plant. For further information see [R13,R12;13 and refs therein].

SPECIFIC REFERENCES: 1. Majumdar P *et al* (1987) *Phytochem.* 26(11):3021. 2. Ara I *et al* (1990) *Phytochem.* 29(3):911. 3. Ara I *et al* (1989) *J. Nat. Prod.* 51(6):1054. 4. Khalid S *et al* (1989) *J. Nat. Prod.* 52(5):922. 5. Kurokawa Y *et al* (1990) *Shoyakugaku Zasshi* 44(1):29. 6. Fujiwara T *et al* (1984) *Chem. Pharm. Bull.* 32:1385. 7. Okpanyi S *et al* (1981) *Planta Med.* 41:34. 8. Pillai N *et al* (1981) *Planta Med.* 43:59. 9. Sairam M *et al* (2000) *J. Ethnopharmacol.* 71(3):377. 10. MacKinnon S *et al* (1997) *J. Nat. Prod.* 60(4):336. 11. Garg S *et al* (1998) *J. Ethnopharmacol.* 60(3):235. 12. Kumar A *et al* (2002) *Phytother. Res.* 16(1):74. 13. Neem. Ed. Puri H (1999) *Medicinal and Aromatic Plants – Industrial Profiles.* Pub: Taylor and Francis, London, UK.

NETTLE
URTICA DIOICA L.

Fam. Urticaceae

SYNONYMS: Stinging Nettle.

HABITAT: Nettles grow in waste places everywhere.

Description: Stems quadrangular, with opposite, cordate or lanceolate leaves, serrated at the margin and bearing stinging cells. Flowers green with yellow stamens, male and female on separate plants.

'Tender-handed, grasp the nettle

And it stings you for your pains

Grasp it like a man of mettle

And it soft as silk remains'

PART USED: Root, herb.

CONSTITUENTS: Root: (i) Lignans, including pinoresinol, secoisolariciresinol, dehydrodiconiferyl alcohol, neo-olivil, and others [1,2,3] (ii) Lectins, the mixture known as UDA (Urtica Dioica Agglutinin) which is composed of at least 6 isolectins [4] (iii) Triterpenes; oleanolic and ursolic acid derivatives [5]. Leaf: (i) Flavonoids, mainly isorhamnetin, kaempferol and quercetin glycosides (ii) Glycoprotein (iii) Miscellaneous; indoles such as histamine and serotonin, betaine, acetylcholine, vitamin C and other vitamins, ionyl glucoside, caffeic acid derivatives, chlorophyll in high yields, protein and dietary fibre [R7;3,6,7].

MEDICINAL USE: Nettle root extracts are being used increasingly for mild, benign prostate hyperplasia (BPH), and associated difficulties in micturition. Nettles also have a long history of use as an anti-allergenic and anti-inflammatory, in rheumatic disorders and skin eruptions, and are reputed to be diuretic, astringent, tonic, and anti-haemorrhagic [R1]. Many of these uses are now being substantiated [6]. The effects on the prostate have been investigated in a number of ways, for example using experimental BPH in mice [8], by measuring sex hormone-binding globulin (SHBG) to human prostate membranes [9,2], and by inhibition of proliferation of human prostatic epithelial and stromal cells [10]. In all cases, activity was found, and in addition several compounds from the roots are known to be aromatase inhibitors [5]. The anti-inflammatory use can also be supported by a post-marketing surveillance study, which showed efficacy in rheumatism with few (if any) adverse events [11]. Leaf extracts inhibit the pro-inflammatory transcription factor NF-kappaB [12], partially inhibit cyclooxygenase and lipoxygenase, and inhibit tumour necrosis factor and interleukin 1-beta secretion stimulated by lipopolysaccharide [13]. A trial of nettle sting (rather than an extract) for osteoarthritic pain at the base of the thumb or finger also produced alleviation of some of the pain [14]. Diuretic activity has been confirmed in the rat [15] and immunomodulation also described [16]; and recently anti-fungal activity shown *in vitro* [17]. Nettles are consumed as food, and used as a source of chlorophyll. For more details, see [R2,R17;3,6 and refs therein].

313

PREPARATIONS AND DOSE: Dried herb, dose: 2–4 g, or equivalent extract, three times daily.

BIBLICAL REFERENCES: Job 30:7; Proverbs 24:31; Isaiah 34:13; Hosea 9:6; Zephaniah 2: 9.

SPECIFIC REFERENCES: 1. Chaurasia N *et al* (1986) *Deutsch. Apot. Ztg.* 126:1559. 2. Schottner M *et al* (1997) *Planta Med.* 63(6):529. 3. Bombardelli E *et al* (1997) *Fitoterapia* 68(5):387. 4. Damme E *et al* (1988) *Plant Physiol.* 86:598. 5. Gansser D *et al* (1995) *Planta Med.* 61(2):138. 6. Koch E (2001) *Planta Med.* 67(7):489. 7. Neugerbauer W *et al* (1995) *Nat. Prod. Lett.* 6(3):177. 8. Lichius J *et al* (1997) *Planta Med.* 63(4):307. 9. Hryb D *et al* (1995) *Planta Med.* 61(1):31. 10. Konrad L *et al* (2000) *Planta Med.* 66(1):44. 11. Chubrasik S *et al* (1999) *Pain Clinic* 11(3):179. 12. Riehemann K *et al* (1999) *FEBS Lett.* 442(1):89. 13. Obertreis B *et al* (1996) *Arzneim. Forsch.* 46(1):52 and 46(4):389. 14. Randall C *et al* (2000) *J. Royal Soc. Med.* 93(6):305. 15. Tahri A *et al* (2000) *J. Ethnopharmacol.* 73(1–2):95. 16. Basaran A *et al* (1997) *Phytother. Res.* 11(8):609. 17. Yongabi K *et al* (2000) *J. Phytomed. Therap.* 5(1):39.

NIGHT-BLOOMING CEREUS
SELENICEREUS GRANDIFLORUS BRITT. ET ROSE
Fam. Cactaceae

SYNONYMS: Sweet-scented Cactus, *Cereus grandiflorus* Mill., *Cactus grandiflorus.*

HABITAT: West Indies.

DESCRIPTION: The stems and flowers are often preserved in spirit. Stems fleshy, five to seven angled, about 1–2 cm in diameter. The flowers are large, 10–13 cm in diameter, with oblong-lanceolate white petals and linear, orange, hairy calyx segments; numerous stamens and a many-rayed stigma.

PART USED: Fresh or preserved plant.

CONSTITUENTS: (i) Alkaloids and amines, including hordenine (formerly called cactine), tyramine, and others as yet unidentified (ii) Flavonoids, including rutin, hyperoside, and others based on isorhamnetin [1,2,3].

MEDICINAL USE: Cardiac stimulant, diuretic, tonic [R1]. Used for palpitations and angina. Hordenine (cactine) and tyramine have a mild positive inotropic activity on the heart and the herb is often used in conjunction with Hawthorn and Valerian (q.v.) [4]. There is little data available on toxicity: the juice of the plant is irritant to the nasal mucosa and the herb causes diarrhoea in large doses [R2].

SPECIFIC REFERENCES: 1. Brown S *et al* (1968) *Phytochem.* 7:2031. 2.Wagner H *et al* (1982) *Planta Med.* 44:36. 3. Petershofer-Halmeyer H *et al* (1982) *Sci. Pharm.* 50:29. 4. Busanny-Caspari E *et al* (1986) *Therapiewoche* 36(23):2545.

NUTMEG

MYRISTICA FRAGRANS HOUTT.

Fam. Myristicaceae

SYNONYMS: Myristica fragrans L.

HABITAT: Native to the Indonesia, Molucca Islands and New Guinea, introduced into Sri Lanka and the West Indies.

DESCRIPTION: The seed is ovoid, about 3 cm long and 2 cm broad, with a pale brown surface reticulately patterned with grooves, lines and specks. The internal structure is variegated brown and white, due to the in-folding of the darker perisperm into the endosperm. Odour: aromatic, characteristic; taste: bitter, aromatic.

PART USED: Seed.

CONSTITUENTS: (i) Volatile oil, about 10% but variable, containing camphene, eugenol and pinene as the major constituents, with cymene, alpha-thujene, gamma-terpinene, linalool, terpineol, myristicin, safrole, elemicin, copaene, isoeugenol, methyleugenol and others (ii) Lignans and neolignans, such as myrisfragransin, fragnasols A, B, C etc.; licarin-B (iii) Diarylpropanoids and diterpenes such as dihy-droisoeugenol and sclareol (iv) Fixed oil containing myristic, palmitic and other acids, and protein [R2,R19;1,2,3,4,5,6].

MEDICINAL USE: Carminative, spasmolytic, anti-emetic, orexigenic, topical anti-inflammatory [R1]. Nutmeg is used medicinally for nausea and vomiting, flatulence, indigestion and diarrhoea. Extracts of Nutmeg decrease kidney prostaglandin levels in rats, inhibit contractions of rat stomach strips produced by prostaglandin E2 and decrease levels of prostaglandin-like material produced by isolated human colon [7]. They also inhibit platelet aggregation; this activity was found to be due to eugenol and isoeugenol [2] and is a result of inhibition of prostaglandin synthesis [8]. Extracts of Nutmeg are anti-inflammatory in rodents [9], probably by a similar mechanism, and exert hypolipidemic properties [10]. The neolignans are anti-fungal [4]. Nutmeg extracts have anti-diarrhoeal activity, shown by inhibition of secretion induced by *E. coli* enterotoxins in isolated ileal loop preparations [11] and have been used in the treatment of Crohn's disease [12]. Large doses of Nutmeg oil decreases fertility in rats and some constituents are carcinogenic [13] and mutagenic [14]. Large doses cause intoxication, hypnosis and tachycardia; these actions are thought to be due to myristicin, which is thought to be metabolised to a hallucinogenic amphetamine-like moiety; however in normal doses Nutmeg is considered safe [15]. Nutmeg is a popular culinary spice. See also Mace.

PREPARATIONS AND DOSE: Dried seed, dose: 0.3–1 g.

SPECIFIC REFERENCES: 1. Gottleib O (1979) *J. Ethnopharmacol.*1:309. 2. Rasheed A *et al* (1984) *Planta Med.* 50(2):222. 3. Sarath-Kumara S *et al* (1985) *J. Sci. Food Agric.* 36(2):93. 4. Miyazawa M *et al* (1996) *Nat. Prod. Lett.* 8(1):25. 5. Bae-Kim Y *et al* (1991) *Arch. Pharm. Res.* 14(1):1. 6. Juhasz L *et al* (2000) *J. Nat. Prod.* 63(6):866. 7. Bennett A *et al* (1971) *New Eng. J. Med.* 290:110. 8. Bennett A *et al* (1988) *Phytother. Res.* 2(3):124. 9. Oljide O *et al* (1999) *Phytother. Res.* 13(4):344. 10. Ram A *et al* (1996) *J. Ethnopharmacol.* 55(1):49. 11. Gupta S *et al* (1992) *Int. J. Pharmacog.* 30(3):179. 12. Shafkan I *et al* (1977) *New Eng. J. Med.* 296:694. 13. Miller E *et al* (1983) *Cancer Res.* 43:1124. 14. Mahmoud I *et al* (1992) *Int. J. Pharmacog.* 30(2):81. 15. Hallstrom H *et al* (1997) *Nat. Toxins* 5(5):186.

NUX VOMICA

STRYCHNOS NUX VOMICA L.
Fam. Loganiaceae

SYNONYMS: Poison Nut.

HABITAT: India to northern Australia.

DESCRIPTION: The seeds are disc-shaped, up to about 2 cm in diameter and about 0.5 cm thick, usually flattened, often with a keeled margin, greyish-green with a satiny sheen due to the closely appressed hairs. On the convex side the raphe is visible as a line going from the central hilum to the micropyle. Fracture: extremely hard and horny, showing the white cotyledons, straight radicle and small embryo. Taste: very bitter; odourless.

PART USED: Seeds.

CONSTITUENTS: (i) Indole alkaloids, the main one being strychnine, accounting for approximately 50% of the alkaloids, with strychnine n-oxide, brucine and its n-oxide, alpha- and beta-colubrine, condylo-carpine, diaboline, geissoschizine, icajine, isostrychnine, normacusine, novacine, pseudobrucine, pseudo-alpha-colubrine, pseudo-beta-colubrine, pseudostrychnine, strychnocrysine, strychnopentamine, isostrychnopentamine, vomicine and others [1,2,3,4,5] (ii) Iridoids; mainly loganin [6] (iii) Miscellaneous; chlorogenic acid, fixed oil [R2,R3].

MEDICINAL USE: Stimulant, bitter, tonic [R1]. The action is mainly due to strychnine, which is a potent CNS stimulant. Nux Vomica has been used as a tonic and analeptic but this cannot really be justified; its therapeutic properties are limited and recorded fatalities from deliberate or accidental ingestion are numerous. Poisoning causes muscle stiffness and spasm, resulting in the fixed grinning expression known as 'risus sardonicus', due to clamping of the jaw; contraction of the abdominal muscles and the diaphragm arrests respiration and death may easily result [R14]. The alkaloids are anti-malarial, with activity against *Plasmodium falciparum* [5]. The root bark is anti-diarrhoeal in mice [7] and loganin has hepatoprotective properties [6].

SPECIFIC REFERENCES: 1. Bissett N *et al* (1976) *J. Nat. Prod.* 39:263. 2. Baser K *et al* (1982) *Phytochem.* 21:1423. 3. Cai B-C *et al* (1990) *Chem. Pharm. Bull.* 38:1295. 4. Biala R *et al* (1998) *J. Nat. Prod.* 61(1):138. 5. Frederich M *et al* (1999) *Antimicrob. Agents Chemother.* 43(9):2328. 6. Visen P *et al* (1998) *Phytother. Res.* 12(6):405. 7. Shoba F *et al* (2001) *J. Ethnopharmacol.* 76(1):73.

OAK

QUERCUS ROBUR L.
Q. PETRAEA (MATT.) LEIB. AND OTHER SPECIES OF
QUERCUS.

Fam. Fagaceae

SYNONYMS: Tanner's Bark.

HABITAT: Throughout Europe, planted elsewhere.

DESCRIPTION: The bark has a greyish external surface with occasional brown lenticels, a reddish brown inner surface with longitudinal striations. Fracture fibrous, showing projecting medullary rays. Taste: astringent; odour: slightly aromatic.

PART USED: Bark.

CONSTITUENTS: Tannins 15–20%, consisting of (i) Ellagitannins including castalagin, peducnulagin, vesvalagin, acutissimins A and B, eugenigrandin, guajavacin B, stenophyllanin C (ii) Catechins; monomeric and dimeric catechins; catechin tannins and oligo-proanthocyanidins (iii) Gallotannins and gallic acid [R2,R8,R9;1,2,3,4].

MEDICINAL USE: Astringent, haemostatic, antiviral, antiseptic [R1]. It has been used as a decoction in small doses for diarrhoea, and as an enema for haemorrhoids and gargle for throat problems. Externally it may be used in compresses or added to baths for skin diseases such as eczema [4]. It should not be applied to large areas of broken skin or taken internally in large doses.

BIBLICAL REFERENCES: Genesis 35:4, 8; Joshua 24:26; Judges 6:11, 19; 2 Samuel 18:9–14; Kings 13:14; 1 Chronicles 10:12; Isaiah 1:29–30, 2:13, 6:13, 44:14; Ezekiel 6:13, 27:6; Hosea 4:13; Amos 2:9; Zechariah 11:2.

SPECIFIC REFERENCES: 1. Konig M *et al* (1994) *J. Nat. Prod.* 57:1411. 2. Pallenbach E *et al* (1993) *Planta Med.* 59:264. 3. Scalbert A *et al* (1988) *Phytochem.* 27:3483. 4. Willuhn G (1992) *Deutsche Apoth. Ztg.* 132:1873.

OATS

AVENA SATIVA L.

Fam. Graminae

SYNONYMS: Groats.

HABITAT: Widely distributed as a cereal crop.

DESCRIPTION: The seeds with the husks removed are found crushed, as a coarse powder of flakes, creamy white and buff coloured with a mealy taste.

PART USED: Seeds.

CONSTITUENTS: (i) Proteins, prolamines known as avenin, avenalin and gliadin (ii) Starch and soluble polysaccharides; mainly beta-glucans

317

and arabinogalactans (iii) Saponin glycosides, including avenacosides A and B, and soyasaponin I (iv) Phytosterols; cholesterol, beta-sitosterol, delta-5-avenasterol (v) Flavonoids such as the tricin glycosides, and vitexin, isovitexin and others, in the leaves (vi) Amines; gramine in grain; avenic acids in the leaves (vii) Fatty oil, composed of avenoleic, oleic, ricinoleic and linoleic acids (viii) Miscellaneous; vitamin E, vitamin B etc. [R2;1,2,3,4].

MEDICINAL USE: Anti-depressant, thymoleptic, cardiac tonic [R1]. Used for debility, menopausal symptoms and depression. Ingestion of oats lowers cholesterol levels: the effect is attributed to the saponins and polysaccharides [R2,1,4,5]. The sedative effect has not been proven, and reports that extracts of oats counteract dependence on cigarettes and morphine have been disputed [6,7]. Oats are externally emollient and a colloidal fraction is used in bath preparations for eczema or dry skin.

SPECIFIC REFERENCES: 1. Onning G *et al* (1996) *Adv. Exp. Med. Biol.* 405:365. 2. Hamberg M (1997) *Adv. Exp. Med. Biol.* 433:69. 3. Hamber M *et al* (1998) *Lipids* 33(4):355. 4. Willuhn G (1992) *Deutsch. Apot. Ztg.* 132:1873. 5. Davy B *et al* (2002) *J. Am. Clin. Nutr.* 76(2):351. 6. Griffiths E *et al* (1992) *J. Clin. Pharmacol.* 33(2):244P. 7. Connor J *et al* (1975) *J. Pharm. Pharmacol.* 27:92.

OLIVE
OLEA EUROPEA L.
Fam. Oleaceae

HABITAT: Native to the Mediterranean region.

DESCRIPTION: An evergreen shrub, from the fruit of which is expressed the oil. Virgin, or cold expressed oil, has a greenish tinge and is used as a food, refined oil is yellowish. Both have a characteristic odour.

PART USED: Oil, leaves.

CONSTITUENTS: Oil; Glycerides of oleic acid, about 70–80%, with smaller amounts of linoleic, palmitic and stearic acid glycerides. Leaf: (i) Iridoids; the most important being oleuropein, with oleuroside, ligustroside and oleoside dimethyl ether (ii) Triterpenes; oleanolic and maslin acids (iii) Chalcones such as olivin and its glycosides (iv) Flavonoids; mainly apigenin and luteolin glycosides [R2;1,2,3].

MEDICINAL USE: The oil is nutritive, emollient, and a mild aperient [R1]. Apart from the widespread food use, olive oil may be used externally as an emollient in liniments and embrocations, as an enema in chronic constipation, to soften ear wax and for numerous other purposes. The unsaturated fatty acids are anti-inflammatory and lower blood cholesterol levels, and have been shown to reduce the incidence of colonic carcinogenesis in rats [4]. Recently a high intake of olive oil (54g/day) was associate with a reduced risk of myocardial infarction [5]. The leaves have a hypoglycaemic, hypotensive and vasodilatory action in rats and have anti-arrhythmic effect both *in vitro* and *in vivo*

[6,7,8,9,10]. These effects are attributed to oleuropein, which has calcium antagonistic activity [11] and also enhances nitric oxide production by mouse macrophages [12]. A leaf extract has been shown to stimulate the thyroid, in a mechanism unrelated to the pituitary gland [13].

PREPARATIONS: Olive Oil BP.

BIBLICAL REFERENCES: Genesis 8:11; Exodus 27: 20 and 30: 24; Leviticus 24:2; Kings 18: 32; Job 15: 33, Psalm 52:8 and 128: 3; Micah 6:15 and others.

SPECIFIC REFERENCES: 1. Bianchi G *et al* (1994) *Phytochem.* 35:1335. 2. Kuwajima H *et al* (1988) *Phytochem.* 27:1757. 3. Bianco A *et al* (1992) *J. Nat. Prod.* 55:760. 4. Bartoli R *et al* (2000) *Gut* 46:191. 5. Fernandez-Jarne E *et al* (2002) *Int. J. Epidemiol.* 31(2):474. 6. Lassere B *et al* (1983) *Naturwissensch.* 70:95. 7. Duarte J *et al* (1993) *Planta Med.* 59:318 365. 8. Zarzuelo A *et al* (1991) *Planta Med.* 57:417. 9. Occhiuto F *et al* (1990) *Phytother. Res.* 4:140. 10. Gonzalez M *et al* (1992) *Planta Med.* 58:513. 11. Rauwald H *et al* (1994) *Phytother.* Res. 8(3):135. 12. Visioli F *et al* (1998) *Life Sci.* 62:541. 13. Al-Qarawi A *et al* (2002) *Phytother. Res.* 16(3):286.

OLIVER BARK

CINNAMOMUM OLIVERI BAILL.

Fam. Lauraceae

SYNONYMS: Australian Cinnamon, Black Sassafras.

HABITAT: New South Wales and Queensland, Australia.

DESCRIPTION: The bark occurs in flat strips, with a coarsely granular, brown outer surface with white cork patches. Odour: reminiscent of sassafras and cinnamon.

PART USED: Bark.

CONSTITUENTS: Volatile oil, containing mainly methyleugenol, with safrole, camphor and alpha-pinene [R4].

MEDICINAL USE: Stimulant [R1]. As safrole is carcinogenic, it would be better avoided.

ONION

ALLIUM CEPA L.

Fam. Alliaceae

HABITAT: Widely cultivated throughout the world.

DESCRIPTION: Such a common vegetable hardly requires description.

PART USED: Bulb.

CONSTITUENTS: (i) Essential oil, composed of volatile, sulphur containing, compounds such as allylpropyldisulphide, dimethylsulphide, methylpropyldisulphide, thiopropanal-S-oxide; (ii) Non-volatile sulphur compounds such as allicin, alliin, methylalliin, cycloalliin, trans-S-(1-propenyl) cysteine sulphoxide, S-methylcysteine and its

319

sulphoxide and many others (iii) Triterpenes including alliospirosides A, B, C and D; cepasides, oleanolic acid, campesterol, and others (iv) Flavonoids; kaempferol, quercetin, isorhamnetin, cyanidin and paeonidin glycosides (v) Miscellaneous; phenolic acids, fixed oil, sugars, vitamins etc. [R13;1,2,3,4,5,6]. Onion has been widely investigated. For a more comprehensive account see [R13;6 and refs therein].

MEDICINAL USE: Expectorant, diuretic, carminative, antispasmodic [R1]. Like Garlic (q.v.) onion is the subject of intensive research. Extracts of onion are hypoglycaemic in humans when taken orally; this is attributable to the allylpropyldisulphide, S-methylcysteine sulphoxide, allicin and probably others [7]. Onion extracts have been shown to have anti-asthmatic effects, acting at least in part by antagonizing platelet-activating factor [8] and alliin and allicin have an inhibitory effect on platelet aggregation [9], possibly by the same mechanism as well as by inhibiting thromboxane production [10]. Anti-hypertensive and anti-hyperlipidemic effects have been documented [11]. Onions have well-known antibiotic and anti-fungal activity, and anti-inflammatory, anti-oxidant, anti-mutagenic, chemopreventant and many other effects have been reported. For a recent, very comprehensive review, which includes clinical data on onion and other species of *Allium,* see [6].

BIBLICAL REFERENCES: Numbers 11:5.

SPECIFIC REFERENCES: 1. Bayer T *et al* (1989) *Phytochem.* 28(9):2373. 2. Kravets S *et al* (1988) *Chem. Nat. Comp.* 23(6):700. 3. Urushibara S *et al* (1992) *Tetrahedron* 33(9):1213. 4. Tokitomo Y *et al* (1992) *Biosci. Biotech. Biochem.* 56(11):1865. 5. Thomas D *et al* (1994) *J. Agric. Food Chem.* 42(8):1632. 6. Griffiths G *et al* (2002) *Phyther. Res.* 16(7):603. 7. Kumari K *et al* (1995) *Planta Med.* 61(1):72. 8. Dorsch W *et al* (1984) *Eur. J. Pharmacol.* 107(1):17. 9. Liakopoulou-Kyriakides M *et al* (1985) *Phytochem.* 24:600 and 1593. 10. Srivastava K (1989) *Prostagland. Leukotr. Ess. Fatty Acids* 35(3):183. 11. Kiviranta J *et al* (1989) *Phytother. Res.* 3(4):132.

ORANGE

BITTER ORANGE

SWEET ORANGE

CITRUS AURANTIUM VAR *AMARA* L.

C. AURANTIUM VAR *SINENSIS* L.

Fam. Rutaceae

SYNONYMS: Bitter Orange: Seville Orange; Sweet Orange: *C. sinensis* (L.) Osbeck, *C. dulcis* Pers.

HABITAT: Cultivated worldwide in warm temperate countries.

DESCRIPTION: The orange is too well known to require description.

PART USED: Peel, oil, juice, fruit.

CONSTITUENTS: (i) Volatile oil, both types of fairly similar composition, containing about 90% limonene with aldehydes such as octanal and decanal. Sweet orange oil generally contains more aldehydes (ii) Flavonoids; hesperidin (major), neohesperidin, naringin, tangeretin, nobiletin and others (iii) Coumarins; umbelliferone, 6,7-dimethoxycoumarin and bergapten (iv) Miscellaneous; triterpenes such as limonin, vitamin C (in the juice), carotenoids, pectin etc. [R19;1,2,3,4].

MEDICINAL USE: Carminative, aromatic, stomachic [R1]. The flavonoids are anti-inflammatory, antibacterial and anti-fungal. An extract of the rind is often referred to as 'citrus bioflavonoids', and many of the observed pharmacological effects of orange peel are due to the hesperidin content. These include reducing vascular permeability in chronic venous insufficiency, calcium channel blocking activity, hypotensive and anti-hypercholesterolemic effects, as well as anti-inflammatory analgesic, antimicrobial and many other properties. Orange peel and oils are used widely as flavouring in foods, drinks and medicine, and the juice is a well-known source of vitamin C. For a comprehensive review of the chemistry and pharmacology of hesperidin, see [1, and refs therein].

SPECIFIC REFERENCES: 1. Garg A et al (2001) Phytother. Res. 15(8):655. 2. Lund E et al (1977) J. Food Sci. 42:385. 3. Natarajan S et al (1976) Econ. Bot. 30:38. 4. Tatum J et al (1977) Phytochem. 16:1091.

OREGANO
ORIGANUM VULGARE L.
Fam. Lamiaceae

SYNONYMS: Wild Marjoram. Sweet Marjoram (q.v.), is O. majorana L.

HABITAT: Common throughout the Mediterranean region, North Africa, and other parts of Europe and temperate Asia; cultivated widely in gardens.

DESCRIPTION: A perennial woody herb reaching up to about 90 cm high, branched above, with opposite, small, oval leaves up to about 1.5 cm long and 1 cm broad. The flowers are white or purplish-pink, small, tubular, with a darker purple calyx, and arranged in cyme-like panicles. Taste and odour: aromatic, characteristic.

PART USED: Herb.

CONSTITUENTS: (i) Volatile oil, with a widely varying composition, usually containing carvacrol as the major constituent, with thymol, germacrene-D, caryophyllene, linalool, myrcene, borneol, terpinen-4-ol, alpha-pinene and gamma-terpinene (ii) Monoterpene glycosides based on thymoquinone, thymol, benzyl alcohol and carvacrol, usually with glucose and galactose (iii) Flavonoids, including naringin, with diosmetin, luteolin and apigenin glycosides (iv) Caffeic and rosmarinic acids (v) Tocopherols (= vitamin E) [1,2,3,4,5,6].

321

MEDICINAL USE: Used particularly for coughs, bronchitis and other respiratory tract conditions, and also for dyspepsia, rheumatism and menstrual and urinary tract disorders [R1]. Extracts have antioxidant activity [5]; probably due to a combination of the tocopherols, flavonoids and rosmarinic acid. Oregano is more frequently used as a culinary flavouring rather than a medicine.

SPECIFIC REFERENCES: 1. Hristova R *et al* (1999) *Acta Pharm.* 49(4):299. 2. Mastelic J *et al* (2000) *Flav. Frag. J.* 15(3):190. 3. Kulevanova S *et al* (2001) *J. Liq. Chrom. Rel. Tech.* 24(4):589. 4. Zgorka G *et al* (1997) *Pharm. Pharmacol. Lett.* 7(4):187. 5. Lagouri V *et al* (1996) *Int. J. Food Sci. Nutr.* 47(6):493. 6. Oregano. Ed. Kintzios S (2002) *Medicinal and Aromatic Plants – Industrial Profiles.* Pub: Taylor and Francis, London, UK.

OREGON GRAPE
MAHONIA AQUIFOLIUM (PURSH.) NUTT.
Fam. Berberidaceae

SYNONYMS: Mountain Grape, Holly-leaved Berberis, *Mahonia aquifolia* Nutt. *Berberis aquifolium* Pursh., *Odostemon aquifolium* Pursh.

HABITAT: North America, widely cultivated as an ornamental elsewhere.

DESCRIPTION: The plant grows to about 2 m in height, producing bright green, spiny, leathery leaves and small yellow flowers. The root is about 1–4 cm in diameter, with a thin, yellowish or brownish-grey bark, longitudinally wrinkled, greenish-yellow internally; and a hard, yellowish wood with numerous medullary rays. Taste: bitter; odourless.

PART USED: Root, rhizome, stem bark.

CONSTITUENTS: Alkaloids: (i) Benzylisoquinolines; berberine, oxyberberine, jatrorrhizine, columbamine (ii) Bisbenzylisoquinolines; berbamine, oxyacanthine, armoline, baluchistine, obamegine, aquifoline (iii) Aporphines; isocorydine, magnoflorine, corytuberine and isothebaine [1,2,3,4] (iv) Polysaccharides, in the stem bark [5].

MEDICINAL USE: Alterative, tonic, cholagogue, anti-diarrhoeal [R1]. Mountain Grape is used particularly for gastritis and skin diseases such as psoriasis and eczema. Anti-proliferative effects on keratinocytes have been reported for the extract; this activity together with anti-lipoxygenase and antioxidant effects [6] contribute to the anti-psoriatic activity, which has been confirmed clinically [7,8,9]. Generally, the alkaloids are responsible for these effects: for example berberine, oxyacanthine and berbamine are antioxidants [2]; corytuberine, columbamine, oxyberberine and especially berbamine and oxyacan-thine are lipoxygenase inhibitors [3,4]; and oxyacanthine and berbamine are very potent keratinocyte proliferation inhibitors [5]. Anti-inflammatory effects are supported by the anti-complement activity of the bisbenzylisoquinolines. The extract inhibits interleukin-8 production, although the polysaccharide fraction induced production of IL-8 in human monocyte THP-1 cells [5]. Other pharmacological effects described for the plant include relaxation of the rat aorta by isothebaine and isocorydine, by a mechanism involving calcium channel antagonism and possibly alpha-adrenergic receptor blocking [11]. The extract is also anti-fungal against a number of fungal species [12] and antibacterial in vitro against bacterial species isolated from patients with acne [13].

SPECIFIC REFERENCES: 1. Willaman J et al (1970) Lloydia 33:1. 2. Muller K et al (1994) Planta Med. 60(5):421. 3. Misik V et al (1995) Planta Med. 61(4):372. 4. Bezakova L et al (1996) Pharmazie 51(10):758. 5. Kostalova D et al (2001) Fitoterapia 72(7):802. 6. Muller K et al (1995) Planta Med. 61(1):74. 7. Gieler U et al (1995) J. Dermatol. Treatment 6(1):31. 8. Augustin M et al (1996) Z. Phytother. 17(1):44. 9. Augustin M et al (1999) Forsch. Komplement. 6(Suppl.2):19. 10. Kostalova D et al (2001) Cesk. Farm. 50(6):286. 11. Sotnikova R et al (1997) Meth. Find. Exp. Clin. Pharmacol. 19(9):589. 12. McCutcheon A et al (1994) J. Ethnopharmacol. 44(3):157. 13. Slobodnikova L et al (2000) Cesk. Dermatol. 75(3):99.

ORRIS

IRIS FLORENTINA L.
I. GERMANICA L.
I. PALLIDA LAM.
AND OTHER SPP
Fam. Iridaceae

SYNONYMS: Florentine Orris, Orris Root.

HABITAT: Cultivated Italy and Morocco and grown in many countries, including Britain, as ornamentals.

DESCRIPTION: The rhizome may be peeled or unpeeled. The better quality rhizome is peeled, creamy-white, irregular in shape, often flattened or constricted in places and bearing small marks where the rootlets have been removed. Fracture: very hard; odour: characteristic, like violets.

PART USED: Rhizome.

CONSTITUENTS: (i) Essential oil, about 0.1–2%, known as 'orris butter', consisting of about 85% myristic acid, with irone, ionone, methyl myristate (ii) Isoflavones; irilone (in *I. germanica* and *I. florentina*, irilone-4'-glucoside, irisolone-4'-bioside, irigenin, iristectogenin-B, irisflorentin, irifloside and iridin (in *I. florentina*) (iii) Triterpenes; the iridals, (e.g. alpha-irigermanal), iristectorone K, beta-sitosterol, alpha- and beta-amyrin [R2;1,2,3,4,5].

MEDICINAL USE: Demulcent, aromatic, expectorant, anti-diarrhoeal [R1]. It has been taken for coughs and diarrhoea as an infusion. Spasmolytic and anti-ulcer properties have been described [R2]. Iris species are known to have piscicidal, cytotoxic, insecticidal and other effects; many of which are attributable to the isoflavones [1]. Orris is used in dental preparations, in cachous and in

323

perfumery, due to the pleasant odour of violets of the essential oil.

SPECIFIC REFERENCES: 1. Miyake Y *et al* (1997) *Can. J. Chem.* 75:734. 2. El-Moghazy A *et al* (1980) *Fitoterapia* 5:237. 3. Morita N *et al* (1973) *Chem. Pharm. Bull.* 21:600. 4. Tsukida K *et al* (1973) *Phytochem.* 12:2318. 5. Orhan I *et al* (2002) *Fitoterapia* 73(4):316.

OSIER, RED, AMERICAN
CORNUS SERICEA L.
Fam. Cornaceae

SYNONYMS: Rose Willow, Red Willow, Silky Cornel.

HABITAT: North America.

DESCRIPTION: Bark in thin, irregular pieces or short quills, purplish externally, somewhat warty; inner surface brown and finely striated. Fracture: short; taste: astringent and bitter; odour: slight.

PART USED: Bark, root-bark.

CONSTITUENTS: No information available.

MEDICINAL USE: Astringent, bitter, tonic [R1]. Has been used for diarrhoea, dyspepsia and vomiting.

OX-EYE DAISY
LEUCANTHEMUM VULGARE LAM.
Fam. Asteraceae

SYNONYMS: Moon Daisy, Marguerite, Dog Daisy, *Chrysanthemum leucanthemum* L.

HABITAT: Europe, including Britain, and parts of Asia and Russia.

DESCRIPTION: The leaf stem is angular, up to about 60 cm, bearing dark green, serrate, spatulate leaves. The white, yellow-centred solitary flowers are 25–50 mm in diameter, with an involucre of green bracts with membranous black edges. Taste: bitter; odour: reminiscent of Valerian.

PART USED: Herb.

CONSTITUENTS: (i) Flavonoids including niviaside and apigenin-7-O-glucuronide (ii) Polyynes including trideca-3,5,7,9,11-pentayn-1-ole and its acetate (iii) Cyclitols [R2].

MEDICINAL USE: Antispasmodic, diuretic, tonic [R1]. It has been used as an infusion in a similar way to Chamomile (q.v.), and externally in the form of a compress for wounds and swellings. It is emetic in large doses and the polyynes are strongly sensitizing [R2;1].

SPECIFIC REFERENCES: 1. Zeller W *et al* (1985) *Arch. Dermatol.* 277(1):28.

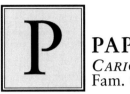

P PAPAYA
CARICA PAPAYA L.
Fam. Caricaceae

SYNONYMS: Pawpaw, Papaw.

HABITAT: Cultivated in most tropical countries.

DESCRIPTION: The fruit is the size of a small melon, and when ripe is a greenish-yellow or orange colour. The flesh is a yellow sweet pulp with numerous black seeds.

PART USED: Leaf, seeds, fruit pulp, latex.

CONSTITUENTS: (i) Proteolytic enzymes; the mixture from the latex is known as 'papain' and consists of papain, chymopapain, caricain, chitinase, papaya peptidases A and B, and others; the fruit also contains beta-galactidases I, II and III and many others (ii) Alkaloid; carpaine, pseudocarpine and carpanine are found in the seeds and leaf, and traces in the fruit (iii) Monoterpenes; linalool, linalool oxide and alpha-terpineol in the fruit (iv) Glucosinolates; benzyl isothiocyanate is present in the seeds (v) Carotenoids; mainly beta-carotene, violaxan-thin, kryptoxanthin and zeaxanthin, in the fruit (vi) Flavonoids, mainly myricetin, quercetin, kaempferol and apigenin glycosides (vii) Miscellaneous; vitamins and minerals [R12,R16;1,2,3,4,5].

MEDICINAL USE: The ripe fruit is an important part of the diet in many tropical countries. The unripe fruit and other parts of the plant are used as a digestive, anthelmintic, diuretic and abortifacient [R1]. The enzymes from the latex hydrolyse polypeptides, amides and esters, particularly when used in an alkaline environment, and are used to aid digestion. The extract inhibits experimental ulcer formation in rats [6]. The dried latex has been used to induce abortion, sometimes applied to the neck of the womb for this purpose, and it has been shown to be uterotonic in rats [7]. Other anti-fertility effects have been supported by several animal studies. The latex extract interrupts the oestrus cycle in females, and reduces spermatogenesis, and the seeds have similar anti-fertility properties [R13,R16;7,8,9,10 and refs therein]. Anthelmintic activity has also been described in a number of studies using mice and pigs [11], the activity being due almost entirely to the benzyl isothiocyanate content [5,12]. Other antimicrobial effects such as antibacterial, anti-amoebic and anti-fungal properties have also been found [13,14]. The roots and leaves are used as a diuretic, and diuretic activity has been demonstrated in rats for root extracts [15], as well as antihypertensive activity by the fruit juice [16]. Papaya enzymes have also found other uses: for their action on scar tissue and to aid wound-healing, for example in chronic ulcers where de-sloughing is required [17], and in the treatment of burns in children [18]. Inhalation of the enzyme powder has caused allergies but otherwise it is usually non-toxic when taken orally; however care should be taken with high doses [R14]. Papain is used to tenderize meat and for other dubious purposes in the 'fast food' industry.

SPECIFIC REFERENCES: 1. Azarkan M *et al* (1997) *Phytochem.*

46(8):1319. 2. Oberg K *et al* (1998) *Eur. J. Biochem.* 258(1):214. 3. Keil U *et al* (1989) *Phytochem.* 28(9):2281. 4. Khuzhaev V *et al* (2001) *Chem. Nat. Compounds* 36(4):418. 5. Kermanshai R *et al* (2001) *Phytochem.* 57(3):427. 6. Chen F *et al* (1981) *Am. J. Chin. Med.* 9(3):205. 7. Cherian T (2000) *J. Ethnopharmacol.* 70(3):205. 8. Pathak N *et al* (2000) *Phytomed.* 7(4):325. 9. Lohiya N *et al* (1994) *Planta Med.* 60(5):400. 10. Udoh P *et al* (1999) *Phytother. Res.* 13(3):226. 11. Satrija F *et al* (1995) *J. Ethnopharmacol.* 48(3):161. 12. Kumar D *et al* (1991) *Fitoterapia* 62(5):403. 13. Tona L *et al* (1998) *J. Ethnopharmacol.* 61(1):57. 14. Emeruwa A *et al* (1982) *J. Nat. Prod.* 45(2):123. 15. Sripanidkulchai B *et al* (2001) *J. Ethnopharmacol.* 75(2–3):185. 16. Eno A *et al* (2000) *Phytother. Res.* 15(4):235. 17. Hewitt H *et al* (2000) *West Indian Med. J.* 49(1):32. 18. Starley I *et al* (1999) *Burns* 25(7):636.

PAREIRA
CHONDRODENDRON TOMENTOSUM RUIZ ET PAV.
AND OTHER SPECIES
Fam. Menispermaceae

SYNONYM: Pareira Brava

HABITAT: South America.

DESCRIPTION: The root is about 2–5 cm in diameter, tortuous, black, longitudinally furrowed with transverse ridges and some constrictions. Internally it is greyish-brown, and the transverse section shows three or four concentric rings, traversed by wide medullary rays. The stem pieces are similar but the external surface is greyish and marked with numerous round, warty lenticels. Taste: bitter then slightly sweet; odourless.

PART USED: Root, stem.

CONSTITUENTS: Alkaloids, *d*-tubocurarine, *l*-curarine, *l*-beebirine, chondrocurine and others [1,2].

MEDICINAL USE: Formerly used as a tonic, diuretic and aperient [R1]. Pareira is mainly used as a source of tubocurarine, a potent neuromuscular blocker, used to paralyse muscles during surgical operations. Tubocurarine has been used as a template for the development of many new muscle relaxant drugs such as atracurium [R3]. Species of *Chondrodendron*, often combined with *Strychnos* spp. (q.v.) were used to prepare 'curare', the famous South American arrow poisons. Tubocurarine is ineffective (i.e. non-toxic) when administered orally. For review, see [R3;1,2 and refs therein].

SPECIFIC REFERENCES: 1. Bisset N (1992) *J. Ethnopharmacol.* 36(1):1. 2. Benakis A *et al* (1999) *Epith. Klin. Farmakol. Farmakokinetikes* 17(3):177.

PARSLEY
PETROSELINUM CRISPUM (MILL) NYMAN.
Fam. Apiaceae

SYNONYMS: P. sativum Hoffm., *Carum petroselinum* Benth. and Hook., *Apium petroselinum* L.

HABITAT: Native to the eastern Mediterranean, cultivated worldwide.

DESCRIPTION: Parsley is a well-known plant, easily distinguished by its dissected leaves and distinctive taste. The root is yellowish white, up to 10 cm long and 2 cm wide, usually found chopped in commerce, longitudinally wrinkled with occasional root scars. Taste and odour: characteristic, aromatic.

PART USED: Root, seeds, leaves.

CONSTITUENTS: (i) Volatile oil, containing apiole, myristicin, beta-phellandrene, *p*-mentha-1,3,8-triene, 4-isopropenyl-1-methylbenzene, 2-(*p*-toluyl)propan-2-ol, limonene, eugenol, alpha-thujene, alpha- and beta-pinene, camphene, alpha-terpinene, osthole, carotol, pyrazines, hex-3-enal and others (ii) Coumarins; oxypeucedanin, bergapten, xanthotoxin, isopimpinellin, psoralen, 8- and 5-methoxy-psoralen, imperatorin and isoimperatorin (iii) Flavonoids; apiin, 6"-acetylapiin, luteolin, apigenin-7-glucoside, luteolin-7-glucoside and others (iv) Phthalides; Z-ligustilide, cnidilide, neocnidilide and senkyunolide (v) Miscellaneous; petroside, a monoterpene glucoside, polyacetylenes, proteins, fats, vitamins etc. [R7;1,2,3,4,5].

MEDICINAL USE: Diuretic, spasmolytic, carminative, aperient, antiseptic, expectorant, antirheumatic, sedative [R1]. The flavonoids, particularly apigenin, have been shown to be anti-inflammatory, to inhibit histamine release and to act as free-radical scavengers [6]. Parsley extract has been shown to lower blood pressure in animals [7] and has calcium antagonistic activity [8]. It has a uterotonic effect in animals [R7;7] and the flavonoids apiin and apigenin are phytoestrogens [4]. In some countries Parsley is used to treat diabetes, and hypoglycemic properties have in fact been shown in rats [9,10]. Antioxidant activity in rat brain homogenates has been reported for the extract [11] and in human subjects, as measured by activity of superoxide dismutase and other enzyme markers [12]. Apiin and apigenin are also antimutagenic [13]. The coumarins are weakly antimicrobial [14] and the phthalides are sedative in mice [15]. The leaves are used as a common culinary herb.

PREPARATIONS AND DOSE: Dried root, dose: 2–4 g or equivalent extract, three times daily.

SPECIFIC REFERENCES: 1. Masanetz C *et al* (1998) *Flav. Frag. J.* 13(2):115. 2. Gijbels M *et al* (1985) *Fitoterapia* 56(1):17. 3. Chaudhary S A *et al* (1986) *Planta Med.* 52(6):1986. 4. Yoshikawa M *et al* (2000) *Chem. Pharm. Bull.* 48(7):1039. 5. Warncke D (1994) *Z. Phytother.* 15(1):50. 6. Middleton E *et al* (1984) *Biochem. Pharmacol.* 33:3333. 7. Opdyke D (1975) *Food Cosm. Toxicol.* 13(Suppl.):897.

8. Neuhaus-Carlisle K *et al* (1993) *Planta Med.* 59(Suppl.7):A582.
9. Tunah T *et al* (1999) *Phytother. Res.* 13(2):138. 10. Yarat A *et al*
(2001) *Pharm. Biol.* 39(3):230. 11. Fejes S *et al* (2000) *Phytother. Res.*
14(5):362. 12. Nielsen S *et al* (1999) *Br. J. Nutr.* 81(6):447. 13. Milic
B *et al* (1998) *Phytother. Res.* 12(Suppl.1):S3. 14. Ojala T *et al* (2000)
J. Ethnopharmacol. 73(1–2):299. 15. Bjeldanes L *et al* (1977) *J. Org.
Chem.* 42:2333.

PARSLEY PIERT

APHANES ARVENSIS L.

Fam. Rosaceae

SYNONYMS: *Alchemilla arvensis* Scop.

HABITAT: Native to Europe.

DESCRIPTION: A more or less prostrate, hairy annual, with three-
lobed, fan-shaped, serrate leaves and small, insignificant green
flowers with no petals, found in axillary clusters, surrounded by
toothed, leaf-like stipules. Taste: astringent; odourless.

PART USED: Herb.

CONSTITUENTS: Largely unknown. Tannins are reported to be
present [R7].

MEDICINAL USE: Diuretic, demulcent [R1]. Used particularly for
kidney and bladder complaints, often taken as an infusion.

PREPARATIONS AND DOSE: Dried herb, dose: 2–4 g or equivalent
extract, three times daily.

PASSION FLOWER

PASSIFLORA INCARNATA L.
Fam. Passifloraceae

SYNONYMS: Maypop.

HABITAT: Native to North America, cultivated elsewhere.

DESCRIPTION: The plant is a climber, reaching up to about 9 m in
length, bearing ovate or cordate leaves, palmately three-lobed, coiled
tendrils and white, cross-shaped flowers.

PART USED: Leaves, whole plant.

CONSTITUENTS: (i) Alkaloids; harman, harmine, harmaline, harmol
and harmalol are present in low amounts, but the presence of the
latter four has been disputed. Beta-carboline alkaloids: 1,2,3,4-
tetrahydrocarboline and its methyl derivative (ii) Flavonoids;
apigenin and various glycosides, chrysin, schaftoside, isoschaftoside,
homoorientin, isovitexin, kaempferol, luteolin, orientin, quercetin,
rutin, saponaretin, saponarin and vitexin (iii) Miscellaneous; an 8-
pyrone derivative, sterols, sugars, gums etc. [1,2,3,4,5]. *P. edulis*
contains similar types of compounds [6] and cycloartane triterpenoids
such as the cyclopassifloic acids and cyclopassiflosides [7] but has not

been well-characterized. It is more usually used as the source of edible passion fruit.

MEDICINAL USE: Sedative, hypnotic, antispasmodic, hypotensive, anodyne [R1]. Recent studies have begun to confirm these effects. Passiflora extracts have CNS-depressant activities and are hypotensive; they are used for their sedative and soothing properties, to lower blood pressure, prevent tachycardia and for insomnia. Anxiolytic activity has been reported in mice, using the elevated plus maze test [5,6,8]. Sedative effects are also well-documented [9,10] and attributed at least in part to the flavonoid, particularly chrysin, content [5,9]. Although extracts of *P. edulis* were found to be devoid of anxiolytic effects in one study [6], other reports were positive in the same model [11,12]. Anti-inflammatory activity of the extract has been shown in rats [13] and apigenin is known for its antispasmodic and anti-inflammatory activity [14]. Recent research has demonstrated other pharmacological actions in animals, which may lead to new indications; for example aphrodisiac, antitussive and anti-asthmatic activities [15,16]. Clinical studies of passiflora are sparse, but those that are available seem to show positive results. In a double-blind randomized trial using 36 patients with generalized anxiety, the extract was as effective as oxazepam but with a lower incidence of impairment of job performance. As a result of another study in 65 opiate addicts, it has been advocated as an adjunctive therapy with clonidine for opiate with-drawal symptoms [17]. Generally Passiflora is well-tolerated with few side effects; however isolated reactions involving nausea and tachycardia in one case, and vasculitis in another, have been reported [18,19]. Experiments in animals suggest that Passiflora has synergistic effects with other herbs such as Kava (q.v.) [20].

PREPARATIONS AND DOSE: Dried herb, dose: 0.25–1 g or equivalent extract, three times daily.

SPECIFIC REFERENCES: 1. Meier B (1995) *Z. Phytother.* 16(20):115. 2. Rehwald A *et al* (1995) *Phytochem. Anal.* 6:96. 3. Chimichi S *et al* (1998) *Nat. Prod. Lett.* 11(3):225. 4. Tsuchiya H *et al* (1999) *Chem. Pharm. Bull.* 47(3):440. 5. Zanoli P *et al* (2000) *Fitoterapia* 71:S117. 6. Dhawan K *et al* (2001) *Fitoterapia* 72:698 and 921. 7. Yoshikawa K *et al* (2000) *J. Nat. Prod.* 63(10):1377. 8. Dhawan K *et al* (2001) *J. Ethnopharmacol.* 78(2–3):165. 9. Speroni E *et al* (1996) *Phytother. Res.* 10(Suppl.1):S92. 10. Soulimani R *et al* (1997) *J. Ethnopharmacol.* 57(1):11. 11. Maluf E *et al* (1991) *Phytother. Res.* 5(6):262. 12. Petry R *et al* (2001) *Phytother. Res.* 15(2):162. 13. Borrelli F *et al* (1996) *Phytother. Res.* 10(Suppl.1):S104. 14. Middleton E *et al* (1984) *Biochem. Pharmacol.* 33:3333. 15. Dhawan K *et al* (2003) *Phytother. Res.* (in press). 16. Dhawan K *et al* (2002) *Fitoterapia* 73(5):397. 17. Akhondzadeh S *et al* (2001) *J. Clin. Pharm. Ther.* 26(5):363 and 369. 18. Fisher A *et al* (2000) *J. Toxicol. Clin. Toxicol.* 38(1):63. 19. Smith G *et al* (1993) *Br. J. Rheumatol.* 32(1):87. 20. Capasso A *et al* (1995) *Acta Pharm.* 21(2):12.

PATCHOULI

POGOSTEMON CABLIN (BLANCO) BENTH.
Fam. Lamiaceae

SYNONYMS: Patchouly, *P. patchouli* Pell., *P. heyneanus* Benth.

HABITAT: Tropical Asia.

DESCRIPTION: A perennial herb with ovate leaves, which give a strong, characteristic odour when rubbed.

PART USED: Leaves.

CONSTITUENTS: (i) Volatile oil, containing sesquiterpenes, mainly patchouli alcohol, with pogostol, norpatchulenol, beta-patchoulene, alpha-guaiene and others (ii) Flavones including pachypodol, ternatin, licochalcin A, ombuin, 4,5,-dihydroxy-3,3,6,7,8-pentamethoxyflavone and 5,7-dihydroxy-3,4,-dimethoxyflavanone [1,2,3].

MEDICINAL USE: Rarely used in medicine, although an extract has calcium antagonist activity [4]. The flavones are anti-aggregatory against rabbit platelets *in vitro*, [3], and have cell differentiation and cytotoxic properties in promyelocytic leukaema HL-60 cells. The oil is widely used in perfumery.

SPECIFIC REFERENCES: 1. Akhila A *et al* (1984) *Fitoterapia* 55(6):363. 2. Park E *et al* (1998) *Planta Med.* 64(5):464. 3.Tasi W-J *et al* (1995) *Chin. Pharm. J.* 47(5):431. 4. Ichikawa K *et al* (1989) *Chem. Pharm. Bull.* 37(2):345.

PAWPAW, AMERICAN

ASIMINA TRILOBA (L.) DUR.
Fam. Annonaceae

SYNONYMS: Custard Apple.

HABITAT: North America.

DESCRIPTION: Seeds flat, brown, slightly polished with darker brown lines on the surface, oblong-oval, with a greyish hilum at one end. Taste and odour: resinous.

PART USED: Seeds.

CONSTITUENTS: (i) Acetogenins including annonacin, asimin, asiminacin, asiminecin, asimicin, asimilobin, asimicinone, bullatacin, bullatacinone, bullatetrocin, trilobacin, trilobin, murisolin A, murisolinone, asitrocin, asitrocinones, gigantitrocins and asitrilobins, and various hydroxy derivatives (ii) Lignans such as syringaresinol (iii) Fatty acids; cis-delta-9- and cis-delta-11 hexadecanoates and octadecanoates and others [1,2,3,4,5,6,7,8,9,10,11].

MEDICINAL USE: The fruit is edible. The acetogenins are lethal to brine shrimp (the method of screening used to isolate them), and are cytotoxic in a number of human tumour cell lines [1,2,3,4,5,6,7,8, 9,10]. They also display insecticidal and other pesticidal activities [12]. Asimicin is weakly irritant and skin sensitizing [12].

SPECIFIC REFERENCES: 1. Zhao G *et al* (1992) *J. Nat. Prod.* 55(3):347. 2. Zhao G *et al* (1994) *J. Med. Chem.* 37(13):1971. 3. Zhao G *et al* (1995) *Tetrahedron* 51(26):7149. 4. Woo M *et al* (1995) *Bioorg. Med. Chem.* 5(11):1135. 5. Woo M *et al* (1995) *J. Nat. Prod.* 58(10):1533. 6. Zhao G *et al* (1996) *Nat. Toxins* 4(3):128. 7. He K *et al* (1996) *J. Nat. Prod.* 59(11):1029. 8. He K *et al* (1997) *Bioorg. Med. Chem.* 5(3):510. 9. Woo M *et al* (2000) *Bioorg. Med. Chem.* 8(1):285. 10. Kim E-J *et al* (2000) *J. Nat. Prod.* 63(11):1503. 11. Wood R *et al* (1999) *Lipids* 34(10):1099. 12. Avalos J *et al* (1993) *Contact Derm.* 29(1):33.

PEACH

PRUNUS PERSICA STOKES
Fam. Rosaceae

SYNONYMS: *Persica vulgaris* Nutt., *Amygdalus persica* L.

HABITAT: Cultivated in many parts of the world.

DESCRIPTION: The peach tree and its fruit are well known.

PART USED: Leaves, oil expressed from the seeds. Peaches are normally grown for the fruit.

CONSTITUENTS: Leaves: (i) Cyanogenetic glycosides based on mandelic acid (ii) Flavonoids based on quercetin (iii) Triterpenes; sitogluside, beta-sitosterol and ursolic acid [1]. Fruit: Polyphenols such as caffeic and chlorogenic acids [2]. Oil: mainly glycerides of oleic acid, with some palmitic and stearic acid glycerides, some benzaldehyde and cyanhydrin. [R4].

MEDICINAL USE: Sedative, diuretic, expectorant [R1]. The leaves have been used to treat constipation; and a crude extract has been shown to contain spasmogens as well as spasmolytic compounds, when applied to isolated guinea pig ileum. The spasmogenic effect was found to be cholinergic, and more potent than the spasmolytic effect, which was calcium antagonistic in nature [3]. An extract of the flowers protected against UV-induced DNA damage in skin fibroblast cells [4]. The oil may be used as an emollient and in toilet preparations. The fruit is a prized item of diet.

SPECIFIC REFERENCES: 1. Chandra S *et al* (1990) *Fitoterapia* 61(4):379. 2. Carbonaro G *et al* (2001) *Food Chem.* 72(4):419. 3. Gilani A *et al* (2000) *J. Ethnopharmacol.* 73(1–2):87. 4. Heo M *et al* (2001) *Mutat. Res. Gen. Toxicol.* 496(1–2):47.

PELLITORY

ANACYCLUS PYRETHRUM (L.) LINK.
Fam. Asteraceae

SYNONYMS: *Anthemis pyrethrum* L. *Matricaria pyrethrum* Baill.

HABITAT: Spain and other Mediterranean countries.

DESCRIPTION: The root occurs in dark brown, cylindrical pieces, longitudinally furrowed, often with a tuft of soft, woolly hairs at the crown. Taste: acrid, pungent, causing a flow of saliva; odour: characteristic.

PART USED: Root.

CONSTITUENTS: (i) Essential oil, containing eugenol (ii) Alkamides such as isobutylamide [1,2].

MEDICINAL USE: Rubifacient, counter-irritant, used externally for toothache. A trial in 200 dental patients showed efficacy of the root extract compared with xylocaine [3] and anti-inflammatory activity has also been found in various animal experimental models [4]. Many of the actions are probably due to the eugenol present, which is antimutagenic [1] and anti-inflammatory (see also Cloves). The alkamides are also anti-inflammatory, and inhibit cyclo-oxygenase and lipoxygenase *in vitro* [2].

SPECIFIC REFERENCES: 1. Sukumaran K *et al* (1995) *Mutat. Res. Gen. Toxicol.* 343(1):25. 2. Muller-Jakic B *et al* (1994) *Planta Med.* 60(1):37. 3. Patel V *et al* (1992) *Phytother. Res.* 6(3):158. 4. Rimbaud V *et al* (1996) *Phytother. Res.* 10(5):421.

PELLITORY-OF-THE-WALL

PARIETARIA OFFICINALIS L.
AND OTHER SPP.
Fam. Urticaceae

SYNONYMS: *P. diffusa* Mert. et Koch.

HABITAT: Native to Europe.

DESCRIPTION: A perennial herb with slender, lanceolate-ovate leaves and brittle, reddish, ridged stalks. The flowers are unisexual, green with yellow stamens; the female flowers are terminal and the male flowers in axillary clusters. Taste: and odour: slight.

PART USED: Herb.

CONSTITUENTS: (i) Flavonoids; 3-glucosides and 3-rhamnosides of quercetin, kaempferol and isorhamnetin; 3-sophorosides of quercetin and kaempferol and 3-neohesperidosides of kaempferol and isorhamnetin (ii) Phenolic acids including chlorogenic, isoferulic, gallic, and *p*-coumaric acids [1,2].

MEDICINAL USE: Diuretic, demulcent. It has been used to treat cystitis, pyelitis and dysuria as well as kidney stones [R1]. Little pharmacological or other information is available.

PREPARATIONS AND DOSE: Dried herb, dose: 1–5 g or equivalent extract, three times daily.

SPECIFIC REFERENCES: 1. Ollivier B *et al* (1985) *J. Pharm. Belg.* 40(3):173. 2. Budzianowski J *et al* (1985) *J. Nat. Prod.* 48(2):336.

PENNYROYAL
MENTHA PULEGIUM L.
Fam. Lamiaceae

SYNONYMS: European Pennyroyal. *Mentha pulegioides* Sieber, *Pulegium erectum* Mill., *P. vulgare* Mill. American Pennyroyal is *Hedeoma pulegioides* (L.) Pers.

HABITAT: A common wild or garden plant.

DESCRIPTION: A prostrate, or sometimes erect perennial, with ovate leaves up to about 2–3 cm long and only slightly serrate; lilac flowers in axillary clusters with a hairy, ribbed calyx tube. Taste and odour: mint-like but characteristic.

PART USED: Herb.

CONSTITUENTS: (i) Volatile oil, consisting mainly of pulegone, with isopulegone, menthol, isomenthol, isomenthone, piperitone, neomenthol, menthyl acetate, alpha- and beta-pinene, camphene, beta-phellandrene, *p*-cymene, 2-octanol, limonene (ii) Polyphenolic acids and flavonoids such as hesperidin and diosmin [R2,R7;1,2,3]. American Pennyroyal contains similar constituents.

MEDICINAL USE: Carminative, diaphoretic, stimulant, emmenagogue [R1]. The oil has been principally used for delayed menstruation; however in effective doses it is abortifacient and toxic. In small doses and as an infusion, the herb is used for colds, colic and dyspepsia. Pulegone is antibacterial against *Staphylococcus aureus*, *Escherichia coli* and *Listeria* and *Salmonella* species, and fungi such as *Candida albicans* and other pathogens [4]. Topically it may be used for skin eruptions, itching and gout. The oil is irritant, hepatotoxic and nephrotoxic and must not be used during pregnancy. It is also an insect repellant [R7;5].

PENNYROYAL

PREPARATIONS AND DOSE: Dried herb, dose: 1–4 g or equivalent extract, three times daily.

SPECIFIC REFERENCES: 1. Montes M *et al* (1986) *Ann. Pharm. Francaises.* 44(2):135. 2. Reis-Vasco E *et al* (1999) *Flav. Frag. J.* 14(3):156. 3. Hurrell R *et al* (1999) *Br. J. Nutr.* 81(4):289. 4. Flamini G *et al* (1999) *Phytother. Res.* 13(4):349. 5. Briggs C (1989) *Can. Pharm. J.* 122(7):369.

PEONY
PAEONIA OFFICINALIS L.
P. LACTIFLORA PALLAS
P. SUFFRUCTICOSA ANDREWS.
Fam. Ranunculaceae

SYNONYMS: Common Peony. *P. albiflora* Pallas(= *P. lactiflora*). Moutan (= *P. suffructicosa*). The botanical name of this plant is in some doubt. Several species are used in Oriental medicine.

HABITAT: A common garden plant.

DESCRIPTION: The root is spindle-shaped, furrowed, and pinkish-grey or whitish externally when scraped. Taste: sweet then bitter; odourless.

PART USED: Root.

CONSTITUENTS: Little or no information is available for *P. officinalis.*
P. lactiflora: (i) Monoterpenoid glycosides; paeoniflorin, albiflorin, paeonol, oxypaeoniflorin, benzoylpaeoniflorin, benzoylalbiflorin, palbinone, paenonilactones and beta-pinene vicianoside (ii) Benzoic acid (iii) Polysaccharides; peonans SA, SB and PA composed mainly of hexa-uronic acid residues (iv) Acetophenones; 2,5-dihydroxy-4-methoxyacetophenone and 2,5-dihydroxy-4-methylacetophenone (v) Penta-, hexa- and octa-galloyl glucose [1,2,3,4,5,6,7,8,9].
P. suffructicosa: (i) Monoterpene glucosides including paeoniflorin, galloyl paeoniflorin, paeonolide, apiopaeonoside, galloyl oxypaeoniflorin, suffructicosides A, B, C, D and E, paeonisuffrone, paeonisuffral, mudanpiosides A, G, H and I, mudanoside B (ii) Stilbene derivatives; resveratrol, and trimers of resveratrol called suffructicosols A, B and C (iii) Triterpenes; betulinic and oleanolic acids, betasitosterol etc. (iv) Caffeic and benzoic acids (v) Pentagalloylglucose [10,11,12,13, 14,15,16,17].

MEDICINAL USE: Antispasmodic, tonic [R1]. Little information for *P. officinalis;* however *P. lactiflora* and *P. suffructicosa* are widely used to improve blood flow and as an ingredient of many traditional Oriental formulae. Few clinical results are available but there is a large amount of data on the pharmacological effects of the extract and their constituents. Effects on the cardiovascular system include an endothelium-dependant vasodilator effect in isolated rat aorta, and an increase in superoxide dismutase activity in rats administered a high fat diet, for extracts of *P. lactiflora* [8,18]. The acetophenones and paeonol are anti-platelet aggregatory [7]. Paeoniflorin is vasodilatory but reverses guanethidine-induced hypotension in rats [19], has a smooth muscle relaxant activity and is anti-hyperglycaemic in rats [2]. Peoniflorin also attenuates age-related learning deficiency in rats [20]. The peonans are immunostimulatory in the reticulo-endothelial system and have anti-complement activity [5,6] and palbinone inhibits human monocyte interleukin 1-beta [9]. Both *P. lactiflora* and *P. suffructicosa* inhibit oxidative DNA damage induced by phenylhydroquinone [15]. The suffructicosides are antioxidative with potent free-radical scavenging effects [10,13]. The constituent pentagalloyl glucose is antiviral *in vitro* against *Herpes simplex* and HIV-transcriptase [21] and also inhibits the growth of human hepatocellular carcinoma SK-HEP-1 cells [12]. Extracts of Peony have an immunomodulatory effect on experimentally induced adjuvant arthritis in rats [22] and an open trial of the total glucosides of Peony showed similar results and improved clinical symptoms in 29 rheumatoid arthritis patients [23]. Anticonvulsant activity has also been attributed to the glucosides [24] and the extract shown to protect against neurone damage, using an experimental model of epilepsy [25].

SPECIFIC REFERENCES: 1. Kadota S *et al* (1993) *Chem. Pharm. Bull.* 41(3):487. 2. Hsu F *et al* (1997) *Planta Med.* 63(4):323. 3. Chuang W-C *et al* (1996) *Planta Med.* 62(4):347. 4. Huiying L *et al* (1984) *Planta Med.* 50(6):501. 5. Tomoda M *et al* (1993) *Biol. Pharm. Bull.* 16(12):1207. 6. Tomoda M *et al* (1994) *Biol. Pharm. Bull.* 17(9):1161. 7. Lin H-C *et al* (1999) *Planta Med.* 65(7):595. 8. Goto H *et al* (1996) *Planta Med.* 62(5):436. 9. Kadota S *et al* (1995) *Phytother. Res.* 9(5):379. 10. Yoshikawa M *et al* (1992) *Chem. Pharm. Bull.* 40(8):2248. 11. Lin H-C *et al* (1999) *J. Nat. Prod.* 61(3):343. 12. Oh G-S *et al* (2001) *Cancer Lett.* 174(1):17. 13. Matsuda H *et al* (2001) *Chem. Pharm. Bull.* 49(1):69. 14. Yoshikawa M *et al* (2000) *Chem. Pharm. Bull.* 48(9):1327. 15. Okubo T *et al* (2000) *Biol. Pharm. Bull.* 23(2):199. 16. Ding H-Y *et al* (1999) *Chem. Pharm. Bull.* 47(5):652. 17. Sarker S *et al* (1999) *Tetrahedron* 55(2):513. 18. Goto H *et al* (1999) *Phytotherapy Res.* 13(6):526. 19. Cheng J-T *et al* (1999) *Clin. Exp. Pharmacol. Physiol.* 26(10):815. 20. Ohta H *et al* (1994) *Pharmacol. Biochem. Behav.* 49(1):213. 21. Xu H-X *et al* (1996) *Phytother. Res.* 10(3):207. 22. Ge Z-D *et al* (1995) *Chinese Pharmacol. Bull.* 11(4):303. 23. Wang Z-J *et al* (1994) *Chinese Pharmacol. Bull.* 10(2):117. 24. Zhang Y *et al* (1994) *Chinese Pharmacol. Bull.* 10(5):372. 25. Tsuda T *et al* (1997) *Exp. Neurol.* 146(2):518.

PEPPER
PIPER NIGRUM L.
Fam. Piperaceae

SYNONYMS: Black Pepper, White Pepper.

HABITAT: Cultivated widely in the tropics, especially in India, Indonesia and South America.

DESCRIPTION: Black pepper consists of the unripe fruit, which is globular, about 3–6 mm in diameter, with a wrinkled, reticulated dark brown or greyish-black surface. White pepper is prepared from riper fruit with the outer pericarp removed; it has therefore a slightly smaller diameter and the vascular bundles are visible as longitudinal lines on the yellowish-white surface. Taste and odour: pungent, characteristic; white pepper is more pungent than black but less aromatic.

PART USED: Fruit.

CONSTITUENTS: (i) Volatile oil, about 2–4% in Black Pepper but very little in white pepper, containing sabinene as the major component, with beta-bisabolene, camphene, guaiacol, beta-caryophyllene, alpha-cubebene, beta-farnesene, hydrocarveol, limonene, myrcene, myristicin, alpha- and beta-pinene, safrole, alpha- and beta-selinene, alpha-thujene, piperonal, and others (ii) Alkaloids and amides in both types, the major pungent principle being piperine, with piperanine, piperylin, piperettine, piperolein A and B, cumaperine, sarmentine, piperidine and others (iii) Miscellaneous; fixed oil, vitamins and amino acids etc. [R16;1,2,3,4].

MEDICINAL USE: Carminative, stimulant. Pepper has been used for indigestion and flatulence [R1]. It is used throughout the world as a condiment. The oil is antimicrobial [1,2] and extracts have antibacterial effects against *Staphylococcus aureus, S. faecalis, Escherichia coli* and other pathogens [R16;5]. Pepper also has antioxidant activity [6]. Extracts stimulate secretion of gastric acid in animals via a cholinergic mechanism and increase absorption from the intestine [R16;7]. Extracts of Black Pepper and piperine increase proliferation of melanocytes *in vitro* and are inhibited by protein kinase-C inhibitors [8]. Piperine is a hepatic enzyme inducer, indicating a possible detoxifying effect on dietary carcinogens [9], and protects the liver against damage by carbon tetrachloride and other toxins [10]. A protective effect against induction of experimental colon cancer has also been noted [11]. Other effects demonstrated for piperine include anticonvulsant and anti-inflammatory properties [R16;12]. Black Pepper is an ingredient of the preparation 'Trikatu' which is an important part of many Ayurvedic formulations; it has synergistic effects with other drugs and may enhance their absorption [13]. For a recent comprehensive review of Black Pepper, see [14].

PREPARATIONS AND DOSE: Dried fruits, dose: 300–600 mg; oleoresin, dose: 15–20 mg.

SPECIFIC REFERENCES: 1. Dorman H *et al* (2000) *J. Appl. Microbiol.* 88(2):308. 2. Jain S *et al* (1971) *Planta Med.* 20:118. 3. Jain S *et al* (1972) *Planta Med.* 22:136. 4. Sengupta S *et al* (1987) *Fitoterapia* 58(3):147. 5. Nakatarni N *et al* (1986) *Environ. Health Persp.* 67:135. 6. Annis S *et al* (2000) *J. Agric. Food Chem.* 48(10):5072. 7. Johri R *et al* (1992) *Biochem. Pharmacol.* 43(7):1401. 8. Lin Z *et al* (1999) *Planta Med.* 65(7):600. 9. Singh A *et al* (1993) *Cancer Lett.* 72(1–2):5. 10. Koul I *et al* (1993) *Planta Med.* 59(5):413. 11 Nalini N *et al* (1998) *J. Ethnopharmacol.* 62(1):15. 12. D'Hooge R *et al* (1996) *Arzneim. Forsch.* 46(6):557. 13. Williamson E (2001) *Phytomed.* 8(6):1. 14. Black Pepper. Ed. Ravindran P (2000) *Medicinal and Aromatic Plants – Industrial Profiles.* Taylor and Francis, London, UK.

PEPPER, LONG
PIPER LONGUM L.
Fam. Piperaceae

HABITAT: Native to South Asia, and cultivated widely, especially in India.

DESCRIPTION: Long Pepper is a slender, perennial climber, with the inflorescence consisting of a cylindrical spike which bears the unripe fruits, which are small globular berries, black or greenish surface, embedded in the fleshy spike. Taste and odour: pungent, characteristic, aromatic.

PART USED: Fruit, root.

CONSTITUENTS: (i) Volatile oil containing beta-bisabolene, beta-caryophyllene and pentadecane as the major constituents, together with dihydrocarveol, alpha-thujene, piperonal, terpinolene, zingiberene and others (ii) Alkaloids and amides, the most abundant being piperine, with methylpiperine, tetrahydropiperine, piperlongumine, piperettine, pipernonaline, asarinine, pelleterine, longamide, piperidine and others and their derivatives (iii) Lignans; sesamin, pulviotol, fargesin, and others (iv) Fixed oil composed of esters of tridecanoic, octadecenoic and eicosapentaenoic acids (v) Miscellaneous vitamins and amino acids etc. [R16;1,2,3,4,5,6,7].

MEDICINAL USE: Carminative, stimulant, laxative, anti-asthmatic. Long Pepper is used for similar purposes to Pepper (q.v.) and is widely used to flavour food. The oil is antimicrobial, and piperine and piperlongumine have antibacterial effects against *Staphylococcus aureus* and *Bacillus subtilis* [R16;8]. Amoebicidal activity has also been reported *in vitro* and *in vivo* [9]. Long Pepper, and isolated piperine, protect the liver against damage by carbon tetrachloride and other toxins [10]. Other effects described for Long Pepper include anti-inflammatory properties and decrease in serum cholesterol levels in rats fed a high fat diet [R16]. Long Pepper is also an ingredient of 'Trikatu', used in Ayurvedic medicine. Piperine is a hepatic enzyme inducer, indicating a possible detoxifying effect on dietary carcinogens, and a bioavailability enhancer; see Pepper [R16;6, and refs therein].

PREPARATIONS AND DOSE: Dried fruits or root, dose: 500 mg–1 g.

SPECIFIC REFERENCES: 1. Parmar V *et al* (1998) *Phytochem.* 49(4):1069. 2. Shankaracharya N *et al* (1997) *J. Food Sci. Technol.* 34(1):73. 3. Lee S *et al* (2001) *Crop Protection* 20(6):523. 4. Das B *et al* (1996) *Planta Med.* 62(6):582. 5. Koul I *et al* (1988) *Phytochem.* 27(11):3523. 6. Sengupta S *et al* (1987) *Fitoterapia* 58(3):147. 7. Shoji N *et al* (1986) *J. Pharm. Sci.* 75(12):1188. 8. Reddy P *et al* (2001) *Pharm. Biol.* 39(3):236. 9. Ghosal S *et al* (1996) *J. Ethnopharmacol.* 50(3):167. 10. Koul I *et al* (1993) *Planta Med.* 59(5):413.

PEPPERMINT

MENTHA X *PIPERITA* L.
(A HYBRID BETWEEN *M. SPICATA L.* AND *M. VIRIDIS*)
Fam. Lamiaceae

SYNONYMS: Black Mint: *M. piperita* var *vulgaris* Sole; White Mint: *M. piperita* var *officinalis* Sole.

HABITAT: Cultivated widely, particularly in Europe and America.

DESCRIPTION: Stems quadrangular, those of black mint are purplish. Leaves up to 9 cm long, 3 cm broad, petiolate, with a serrated margin. Those of the Black Mint are tinged with purple. The flowers are small, lilac or reddish-purple, in tight whorls at the base of the leaves. Taste and odour: very characteristic.

PART USED: Herb, distilled oil.

CONSTITUENTS: (i) Essential oil, containing menthol, menthone

337

and menthyl acetate as the major components, with isomenthone, menthofuran, isomenthol, neomenthol, piperitone, alpha- and beta-pinene, limonene, cineole, pulegone, viridiflorol, ledol and others (ii) Flavonoids; rutin, menthoside, luteolin and eryodictiol rutinosides, and others (iii) Phenolic acids and lactones; rosmarinic acid, dimethylheptanolides and others (iv) Miscellaneous: azulenes, choline, carotenes etc. [R9,R17;1,2,3,4 and refs therein].

MEDICINAL USE: Spasmolytic, carminative, antiemetic, diaphoretic, antiseptic [R1]. The herb is used in herbal teas and Peppermint oil is used in many indigestion and colic mixtures. It is an ingredient of some cough and cold remedies, and the herb extract inhibits histamine release in experimental allergic rhinitis in rats [5]. Menthol is used in similar preparations, for both oral ingestion and inhalation. Menthol and Peppermint oil can be applied externally to treat headache, with some success [6]. The spasmolytic and carminative effects have been shown experimentally *in vivo* and *in vitro* and shown to be post-synaptic and probably mediated via a rise in c-AMP levels [7], thus confirming what has been common knowledge for centuries. Several clinical studies support the efficacy of Peppermint oil in irritable bowel syndrome, although a meta-analysis of these concludes that it is not proven, since many trial designs were of poor quality [8]. The extracted oil is considered safe, as long as the constituent pulegone (which is present in higher concentrations in very young plants) is not above 1% [9]. Peppermint is a popular flavouring for confectionery, ice cream, sauces and liqueurs, as well as for cosmetics, dentifrices, mouthwashes and medicines.

PREPARATIONS AND DOSE: Powdered Herb, dose: 2–4 g; Peppermint Oil BP, dose: 0.05–2 ml; Concentrated Peppermint Water BPC 1973, dose: 0.25–1 ml.

SPECIFIC REFERENCES: 1. Taddei I *et al* (1988) *Fitoterapia* 59(6):463. 2. Duband F *et al* (1992) *Ann. Pharm. Francaises* 50(3):146. 3. Naf R *et al* (1998) *Flav. Frag. J.* 13(3):203. 4. Kazura L *et al* (1996) *Acta Pharm.* 46(4):315. 5. Inoue T *et al* (2001) *Biol. Pharm. Bull.* 24(1):92. 6. Gobel H *et al* (1995) *Phytomedicine* 2:93. 7. Lis-Balchin M *et al* (1999) *Med. Sci. Res.* 27(5):307. 8. Pittler M *et al* (1998) *Am. J. Gastroenterol.* 93(7):1131. 9. Anderson F (2001) *Int. J. Toxicol.* 20(Suppl.3):61.

PERILLA

PERILLA FRUTESCENS (L.) BRITT AND VARIETIES.
Fam. Lamiaceae

SYNONYMS: Wild Coleus, Beefsteak Plant, Purple Mint, Chinese Basil. *P. ocimoides*, L., *P. crispa* Thunb.

HABITAT: Indigenous to mountainous Asia, widely grown in China, Korea, Japan and India.

DESCRIPTION: A short-day annual plant resembling basil or coleus, reaching up to 1.5 m in height. The stems are branching, purplish to brown in colour, quadrangular in cross-section. The leaves are oval with an acute apex and dentate margin, up to about 12 cm. The inflorescence is a terminal raceme, the flower purple or white. Taste: characteristically pungent and aromatic.

PART USED: Herb.

CONSTITUENTS: (i) Volatile oil, containing perillaldehyde, perilla ketone, perillene, shisool, limonene, p-menthadiene, p-menthadienal, limonene, naginataketone, escholtziaketone, elemicin, myristicin, dillapiole, rosefuran, eugenol and others (ii) Triterpenes and sterols, including beta-sitosterol, stigmasterol, and ursolic, oleanolic and tormentic acids (iii) Phenolic acids; rosmarinic, cinnamic and caffeic acids and their esters (iv) Monoterpene glycosides such as the perillosides and jasmonoid glucosides, based on perillic acid, and various volatile oil components (v) Cyanogenetic glycosides including prunasin and sambunigrin (vi) Flavonoids; apigenin, luteolin and others [1 and refs therein].

MEDICINAL USE: Antidote and anti-allergic, particularly for shellfish poisoning. It is also anti-inflammatory and antipyretic, and used for coughs, colds and other chest complaints, as well as nausea and vomiting and to improve the blood circulation. It may be applied externally in the form of a cream or lotion to treat dermatitis and eczema. Perilla is very important in Chinese, Japanese and Korean medicine and is part of many traditional formulae, as well as being an important flavouring for food. Many of the uses have been substantiated, for example the anti-allergic and anti-inflammatory activities have been demonstrated in mice, and clinically in several small open studies. All aspects of perilla are well-reviewed in [1]. More recently perilla extracts have been shown to induce nitric oxide production in murine cultured vascular smooth muscle cells, which supports the ancient use as a tonic for the blood and circulation [2].

SPECIFIC REFERENCES: 1. Perilla. Eds: Yu H-C *et al* (1997) *Medicinal and Aromatic Plants – Industrial Profiles.* Taylor and Francis, London, UK. 2. Makano T *et al* (2002) *Phytother. Res.* 16(Suppl.1):S19.

PERIWINKLE

VINCA MAJOR (L.) PICH.

Fam. Apocynaceae

SYNONYMS: Greater Periwinkle, *V. pubescens* Urv.

HABITAT: Indigenous to southern Europe, grown widely elsewhere as an ornamental.

DESCRIPTION: A semi-procumbent shrub with stems up to about 1 m; leaves dark green, broadly lanceolate, up to about 8 cm long and 5 cm broad, with entire margins. Flowers blue, solitary, with five joined petals, up to 5 cm in diameter. Taste: slightly bitter and acrid; odourless.

PART USED: Herb.

CONSTITUENTS: Indole alkaloids; majdine, isomajdine, majoridine, akuammine, akuammicine, carpanaubine, ervine, reserpinine, serpentine, sarpagine, tetrahydroalstonine, vincamajine, vincamajoreine, 10-hydroxy-cathofoline and others [1,2]. The cytotoxic dimeric alkaloids present in the Rosy (Madagascar) Periwinkle (q.v.), which are used to treat certain types of cancer, have not been found in *V. major*. For more information on reserpine-type indole alkaloids, see Rauwolfia.

MEDICINAL USE: Astringent, anti-haemorrhagic. It is used particularly to treat menorrhagia and leucorrhoea, and for nose bleeds, mouth ulcers and sore throats.

SPECIFIC REFERENCES: 1. Balsevich J *et al* (1992) *Planta Med.* 44(2):91. 2. Kaul J *et al* (1966) *Lloydia* 29:25.

PERIWINKLE, ROSY
CATHARANTHUS ROSEUS (L.) G DON.
Fam. Apocynaceae

SYNONYMS: Madagascar Periwinkle, *Vinca rosea* L.

HABITAT: Thought to originate in the West Indies or Madagascar, but now a pan-tropical naturalized and cultivated plant.

DESCRIPTION: An erect, bushy perennial reaching 75 cm, with stems containing milky latex; leaves ovate or broadly lanceolate, with a rounded apex and entire margins. Flowers white or pink, with a yellow or crimson 'eye', solitary, with a tubular calyx flaring into five petals, up to 5 cm in diameter. Taste: bitter; odourless.

PART USED: Herb.

CONSTITUENTS: (i) Dimeric indole alkaloids: about 20 have been isolated, including vincristine (leurocristine), vinblastine (vincaleuroblastine), vingramine and methylvingramine (ii) Monomeric indole alkaloids including ajmaline, akuammine, akuammicine, reserpine, serpentine, alstonine, vincamine, vincaline, yohimbine, and others [R3,R12;1,2,3] (iii) Cyclitols such as bornesitol [4] (iv) Volatile oil containing alkanes, phenylpropanoids, ketones etc. [5]. For further details, see [R12 and refs therein].

MEDICINAL USE: The bisindole alkaloids, particularly vicristine and vinblastine, are used to treat certain types of cancer, particularly leukemias and lymphomas. The herb is used mainly as a source of these, rather than as a herbal medicine and investigations are ongoing into their production by cell and tissue cultures of the plant. The alkaloids are also used to make semi-synthetic derivatives such as vindesine and vinorelbine [R14]. The traditional use of herb is as an anti-diabetic and anti-fertility agent; the hypoglycaemic effects have been confirmed in animals [6] and other actions such as hypolipidemic properties demonstrated [7], although it cannot be recommended for this use.

SPECIFIC REFERENCES: 1. Czygan F-C (1995) *Z. Phytother.* 16(3):178. 2. Jossang A *et al* (1998) *J. Org. Chem.* 44(2):91. 3. Kaul J *et al* (1966) *Lloydia* 29:25. 4. Nishibe S *et al* (2001) *Natural Med.* 55(5):268. 5. Brun

G *et al* (2001) *Flav. Frag. J.* 16(2):116. 6. Singh S *et al* (2001) *J. Ethnopharmacol.* 76(3):269. 7. Mukherjee B *et al* (1995) *Fitoterapia* 66(6):483.

PERSIAN LILAC

MELIA AZEDARACH L.
Fam. Meliaceae.

SYNONYMS: Persian Lilac, Bead or China Tree.

HABITAT: Many parts of Asia, the Middle East; cultivated as an ornamental.

PART USED: Root bark.

CONSTITUENTS: Root bark: (i) Limonoids and protolimonoids, melianon, melianol, melianodiol and meliantol; the meliatoxins and trichilins and their dehydro and acetyl derivatives; meliacins such as gedunin, nimbolins A and B, melianins A and B, and their decomposition products fraxinellose and azedainic acid; meliacarpins and meliocarpinins (ii) Triterpenoids and steroids, including 24-methylene-cycloartanone, cycloeucalenone, cycloeucanol and others (iii) Miscellaneous substances including vanillic acid and aldehyde, and an alkaloid paraisine (ocaziridine) [1,2,3,4,5,6,7]. Leaf: a glycopeptide, meliacine, has been isolated [8].

MEDICINAL USE: Anthelmintic, anti-parasitic, cytotoxic. It is used for much the same purposes as Neem (q.v.). Many of the limonoids are cytotoxic to various cancer cell lines *in vitro* [1,2,3,4]. Meliacine, a glycopeptide, is active against replication of the foot and mouth disease virus (FMDV) *in vitro* [8], and inhibits interferon production in mouse fibroblast cultures, also *in vitro* [7]. The leaf extract possesses activity against pseudorabies virus in cultured Vero cells [9]. Intensive research is still being directed at the pharmacology of this plant.

SPECIFIC REFERENCES: 1. Takeya K *et al* (1996) *Bioorg. Chem.* 4(8):1355. 2. Takeya K *et al* (1996) *Phytochem.* 42(3):709. 3. Fukuyama Y *et al* (2000) *Chem. Pharm. Bull.* 48(2):301. 4. Itokawa H *et al* (1995) *Chem. Pharm. Bull.* 43(7):1171. 5. Ekong D *et al* (1971) *Chem. Commun.* 1177 and (1967):808. 6. Lavie D *et al* (1969) *Tet. Lett.* 3525. 7. Kraus W *et al* (1981) *Chemische Berichte* 114:267. 8 Andrei G *et al* (1990) *J. Interferon Res.* 10(5):469. 9. Wachsman M *et al* (1998) *Arch. Virol.* 143(3):581.

PERUVIAN BALSAM

MYROXYLON BALSAMUM VAR *PEREIRAE* (ROYLE) HARMS.
Fam. Fabaceae

SYNONYMS: Balsam of Peru, *M. peruiferum.*

HABITAT: Central America.

DESCRIPTION: The balsam is a dark brown to black, oily fluid, which exudes from the tree after the bark has been beaten and scorched. It is soaked up with rags and boiled with water to separate the balsam, which sinks to the bottom. Taste: acrid and bitter; odour: sweet, balsamic, vanilla-like.

PART USED: Balsam.

CONSTITUENTS: (i) Essential oil, about 50–65%, comprised mainly of benzyl benzoate, benzyl cinnamate (= cinnamein), cinnamyl cinnamate (= styracin), free benzoic and cinnamic acids, vanillin, farnesol, styrene, nerolidol and coumarin (ii) Resins, about 25–30%, consisting of peruresinotannol combined with cinnamic and benzoic acids (iii) Isoflavones including cabreuvin [R2,R3,1,2].

MEDICINAL USE: Stimulant, expectorant, antiseptic[R1]. It is used to treat catarrh and diarrhoea and externally for wounds, ulcers, pruritis, nappy rash, eczema and ringworm. The isoflavone cabreuvin is active against *Helicobacter pylori*, a causative organism of gastrointestinal ulcers. It is an ingredient of cough syrups, some soaps and cosmetics and used as a perfume fixative. Peruvian balsam is known to cause allergies in sensitive individuals [3].

SPECIFIC REFERENCES: 1. Wolf J et al (1996) *Pharm. Ztg.* 141(41):56. 2. Ohsaki A et al (1999) *Bioorg. Med. Chem. Lett.* 9(8):1109. 3. Worhl S et al (2001) *Br. J. Dermatol.* 145(2):268.

PHYSIC NUT

JATROPHA CURCAS MIERS.
Fam. Euphorbiaceae

SYNONYMS: Purging nut, vomiting nut. *J. gossypifolia* L. is a separate species, but often included as 'Physic Nut' or 'Bellyache Bush' and used in the same manner.

HABITAT: A pan-tropical weed, originating in America, found mainly on waste ground.

DESCRIPTION: An erect shrub reaching up to 5 m in height, with orbicular three- or five-lobed leaves, green or purplish. The 'nuts' are fleshy, up to 4 cm in diameter, becoming dry, with two or three loculi-containing black seeds. The whole plant contains a viscous, milky latex, and the seeds contain an irritant fixed oil.

PART USED: Capsules, leaves, latex.

CONSTITUENTS: (i) Diterpenes, including phorbol and 12-phorbol esters, particularly in the seed oil; curculathyrones A and B and others (ii) Triterpenes such as oleanolic acid, taraxasterol, friedelin, beta-sitosterol (iii) Miscellaneous; a series of jatropholones and curcusones, flavonoids, proteins and fatty acids [R12 and refs therein; 1,2].

MEDICINAL USE: The leaf is used to treat diarrhoea, and to increase milk flow after childbirth. Anti-fungal, antibacterial, anthelminthic and other activities have been described; however the latex and seed oil are too toxic to recommend the plant for medicinal use, mainly because of the phorbol derivatives. The seed oil is purgative, caustic and abortifacient [R12 and refs therein].

SPECIFIC REFERENCES: 1. Adolf W *et al* (1982) *Phytochem.* 23(1):129. 2. Kafagy S *et al* (1977) *Planta Med.* 31:273.

PICHI

FABIANA IMBRICATA RUIZ ET PAV.
Fam. Solanaceae

HABITAT: South America.

DESCRIPTION: Stem irregularly branched, the twigs covered with closely overlapping heath-like leaves, which are fleshy, obtuse, and keeled with a prominent midrib beneath. Flowers, if present, white, tubular, constricted at the throat. Taste: bitter; odour: faint, agreeable.

PART USED: Leaves, twigs.

CONSTITUENTS: (i) Sesquiterpenes, of the amorphane and cadinane type, such as fabianane, 3,11-cadinadiene, 4-amophen-11-ol, fabiaimbricatan-15-oic acid and others (ii) Coumarins; mainly scopoletin, beta-methylesculetin and their glycosides (iii) Triterpenes such as oleanolic acid (iv) Miscellaneous flavonoids (rutin), *p*-hydroxyacetophenone [1,2,3,4,5,6].

MEDICINAL USE: Diuretic, tonic, hepatic, stimulant [R1]. It has been used for dyspepsia and jaundice, and for kidney complaints. The extract, and several constituents (including oleanolic acid and fabiaimbricatan-15-oic acid) have insect antifeedant activity [2]. The related *F. patagonia* is diuretic in rats [7].

SPECIFIC REFERENCES: 1. Schmeda-Hirschmann G *et al* (1994) *Phytochem.* 36:1439. 2. Schmeda-Hirschmann G *et al* (1995) *Phytother. Res.* 9(3):219. 3. Brown G (1994) *J. Nat. Prod.* 57(2):328. 4. Brown G (1994) *Planta Med.* 60(5):495. 5. Ngo K-S *et al* (1999) *Tetrahedron* 55(52):15099 and 15109. 6. Razmillic I *et al* (1994) *Planta Med.* 60(2):140. 7. Alvarez M *et al* (2002) *Phytother. Res.* 16:71.

PILEWORT

RANUNCULUS FICARIA L.
Fam. Ranunculaceae

SYNONYMS: Lesser Celandine, *Ficaria ranunculoides* Moench.

HABITAT: Common in Europe, including Britain, and western Asia.

DESCRIPTION: Leaves mostly radical, the petioles up to about 15 cm long, the lamina up to 4 cm long and 5 cm broad, ovate, cordate or reniform. The flowers are solitary, on long peduncles, bright yellow with three sepals and 8–12 lanceolate petals each with a nectary at the base. Roots fleshy, oblong or club-shaped, up to about 3 cm long. Taste: slightly bitter; odour: faint.

PART USED: Herb.

CONSTITUENTS: (i) Saponins based on hederagenin and oleanolic acid, the most abundant being hederagenin glucoside, and others with rhamnose, arabinose and glucose as the sugar moieties

343

(ii) Protoanemonin and anemonin (iii) Tannins [R7;1,2,3,4].

MEDICINAL USE: Anti-haemorrhoidal, astringent [R1]. As the name denotes, it is used chiefly for piles, taken internally and also applied externally in the form of an ointment or suppository. The saponins have a local anti-haemorrhoidal effect [3] which is increased by the astringency of the tannins. The saponins are also fungicidal [4]. Protoanemonin has antibiotic activity; however it easily dimerizes to anemonin which is inactive.

PREPARATIONS AND DOSE: Dried herb, dose: 2–5 g or equivalent extract, three times daily.

SPECIFIC REFERENCES: 1. Texier O *et al* (1984) *Phytochem.* 23:2903. 2. Pourrat H *et al* (1979) *Ann. Pharm. Francaises* 237:441. 3. Pourrat H *et al* (1982) *Ann. Pharm. Francaises* 40:373. 4. Bonora A *et al* (1987) *Phytochem.* 26:2277.

PIMPERNEL, SCARLET
ANAGALLIS ARVENSIS L.
Fam. Primulaceae

SYNONYMS: Poor Man's Weatherglass.

HABITAT: Europe including Britain, parts of Asia and Russia.

DESCRIPTION: A prostrate annual; leaves opposite, about 1–2 cm long and 1 cm broad, ovate, sessile, with black dots on the undersurface. Flowers small, scarlet, star-like, finely toothed at the tip with hairs along the margins. The flowers open in sunshine and close when humid, hence the synonym. Taste: mucilaginous, acrid; odourless.

PART USED: Herb.

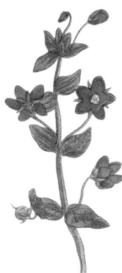

PIMPERNEL

CONSTITUENTS: (i) Saponins: anagallisins A,B,C,D and E, based on anagalligenin (a derivative of oleanolic acid); anagallosaponins I-V, anagallosides and their desgluco derivatives; and other glycosides of protoprimulagenin A (ii) Cucurbitacins B, D, E, I, L and R, and the related arvenins I, II, III and IV [R2;1,2,3,4,5].

MEDICINAL USE: Diuretic, diaphoretic, expectorant. The saponins are antiviral *in vitro*, [1,6,7], and *in vivo* against experimental herpes simplex in rabbits [7] and molluscicidal [5]. The cucurbitacins are cytotoxic (see Bryony, White). This herb is poisonous [8] and cannot be recommended. For a review of the pharmacology of the cucurbitacins, see [9 and refs therein].

SPECIFIC REFERENCES: 1. Amoros M *et al* (1977) *Phytochem.* 16:787. 2. Yamada Y *et al* (1978) *Phytochem.* 17:1798. 3. Shashi B *et al* (1991) *Tetrahedron* 47(28):5212. 4. Shoji N *et al* (1994) *Chem. Pharm. Bull.* 42(9):1750. 5. Abdel-Gawad M *et al* (2000) *Jpn. J. Infect Dis.* 53(1):17. 6. Amoros M *et al* (1987) *Antiviral Res.* 8(1):13. 7. Amoros M *et al* (1988) *Planta Med.* 54(2):128. 8. Rivero R *et al* (2001) *Vet. Hum. Toxicol.* 43(1):27. 9. Miro M (1995) *Phytother. Res.* 9(3):159.

PINE OILS

PUMILIO PINE

SCOTCH PINE

PINUS SPP.
P. MUGO L., AND VARIETIES
P. SYLVESTRIS L.
Fam. Pinaceae

SYNONYMS: Swiss Mountain Pine, Dwarf Pine (*P. mugo*).

HABITAT: P. mugo is native to central and southern Europe,
P. sylvestris to Europe and Asia, and cultivated in North America.

PART USED: Oil distilled from the needles.

CONSTITUENTS: P. mugo: alpha- and beta-pinene, d-limonene,
anethole, dipentene, camphene, myrcene, borneol, bornyl acetate,
hexanal, cuminaldehyde, cadinene, terpineol, and others [1,2,3,4].
P. sylvestris: Volatile oil composed of alpha-pinene (the major
constituent), with beta-pinene, d-limonene, alpha- and gamma-
terpinene, beta-ocimene, myrcene, camphene, sabinene, terpinolene,
bornyl acetate, borneol, cineole, caryophyllene, chamazulene,
3-beta-oxytrans-biformene and its acetate, and others [5,6].

MEDICINAL USE: Antiseptic, decongestant, expectorant [R1]. The
pine oils are commonly used in cough and cold remedies, particularly
inhalations, and in rubefacients for use in muscle stiffness and
rheumatism. They are also used as flavour and fragrance ingredients
in toiletries, detergents and disinfectants. Extracts of *P. sylvestris*
inhibit prostaglandin synthesis [5] and are antimicrobial [7] and
cytotoxic to human lymphocytes in vitro [8].

SPECIFIC REFERENCES: 1. Ikeda M *et al* (1962) *J. Food Sci.* 27:455.
2. Kartnig T *et al* (1996) *Sci. Pharm.* 64(3–4):487. 3. Kartnig T *et al*
(1997) *Sci. Pharm.* 65(4):289. 4. Reichling J *et al* (1998) *Deutsche
Apot. Ztg.* 138(38):47. 5. Wagner H *et al* (1986) *Planta Med.*
52(3):1844. 6. Roschin V *et al* (1985) *Khim. Prir. Soedin* 1:122. 7.
Rauha J-P *et al* (2000) *Int. J. Food Microbiol.* 56(1):3. 8. Lazuka J
et al (2001) *Food Chem. Toxicol.* 39(5):485.

PINE, WHITE

PINUS STROBUS L.
Fam. Pinaceae

SYNONYMS: Eastern White Pine, Deal Pine.

HABITAT: Native to North America, found widely in the northern
hemisphere.

DESCRIPTION: The inner bark occurs in pieces about 2–3 mm thick,
bright buff coloured on the inner surface, smooth and finely striated;

on the outer surface there are numerous scattered, small oil glands. Fracture: tough, shortly fibrous. Taste: mucilaginous, astringent; odour: slight.

PART USED: Inner bark.

CONSTITUENTS: (i) Coniferin, coniferyl alcohol (ii) Diterpenes; strobol, strobal, abienol (iii) Triterpenes, e.g. 3-beta-methoxyserrat-14-en-21-one (iv) Essential oil, mucilage [1].

MEDICINAL USE: Expectorant, demulcent, diuretic [R1]. Mainly used in the form of a syrup, for coughs and colds.

SPECIFIC REFERENCES: 1. Zinkel D et al (1972) Phytochem. 11:425 and 3387.

PINK ROOT
SPIGELIA MARILANDICA L.
Fam. Loganiaceae

SYNONYMS: Indian Pinkroot, Wormgrass, Maryland Pink.

HABITAT: North America.

DESCRIPTION: It is a perennial herb growing to about 45 cm, bearing bright red flowers.

PART USED: Herb, rhizome.

CONSTITUENTS: (i) Spigeleine, an alkaloid (ii) Essential oil (iii) Tannin [R4]. S. anthelmia L. contains similar alkaloids, including spiganthine [1,2].

MEDICINAL USE: Vermifuge, taken as an infusion morning and evening with a purgative such as Senna (q.v.). S. anthelmia contains cardiotonic principles, particularly spiganthine [2,3].

SPECIFIC REFERENCES: 1. Achenbach H et al (1995) J. Nat. Prod. 58(7):1092. 2. Wagner H et al (1993) Int. J. Pharmacog. 31(1):7. 3. Wagner H et al (1986) Planta Med. 52(3):378.

PINUS BARK
TSUGA CANADENSIS CARR.
Fam. Pinaceae

SYNONYMS: Hemlock Spruce, Hemlock bark, Pinus canadensis L., Abies canadensis Michx.

HABITAT: North America.

DESCRIPTION: The bark occurs in pieces of very variable size and up to 2 cm thick. Outer surface of older pieces with rhizome, deeply fissured; younger bark with exfoliating cork, reddish coloured. Inner surface light yellowish-brown, longitudinally striated. Fracture: short, fibrous; taste: astringent; odour: reminiscent of turpentine.

PART USED: Bark.

CONSTITUENTS: (i) Essential oil, containing apinene, bornyl acetate, cadinene (ii) Stilbene derivatives; picea tannols (iii) Tannins, 10–14% [R2,R4].

MEDICINAL USE: Astringent, tonic, diuretic, diaphoretic, antiseptic. Used for diarrhoea, cystitis, colitis, leucorrhoea; and for gingivitis and laryngitis as a gargle or mouthwash. The oil is considered to be non-toxic and it is recommended that it should be used fresh [R18]. Although called Hemlock Bark, it should not be confused with the highly toxic plant Hemlock, *Conium maculatum* (q.v.).

PREPARATIONS AND DOSE: Dried bark, dose: 1–2 g or equivalent extract, three times daily.

PIPSISSEWA
CHIMAPHILA UMBELLATA NUTT.
Fam. Pyrolaceae

SYNONYMS: Prince's Pine, Ground Holly, Umbellate Wintergreen.

HABITAT: Parts of Europe (not including Britain) and northern North America.

DESCRIPTION: A short perennial. Leaves leathery, oblanceolate, about 3 cm long and 1 cm across, with a serrate margin and rounded apex.

PART USED: Leaves.

CONSTITUENTS: (i) Quinones; including the hydroquinones arbutin and isohomoarbutin, and the naphthaquinones renifolin and chimaphilin (ii) Flavonoids; hyperoside, avicularin, kaempferol etc. (iii) Triterpenes; ursolic acid, taraxasterol, beta-sitosterol etc. (iv) Miscellaneous; methyl salicylate, epicatechin gallate, tannins etc [R19;1,2,3].

MEDICINAL USE: Astringent, alterative, tonic [R1]. Used for kidney disorders in a similar manner to Uva-Ursi (q.v.), which also contains hydroquinones. These are responsible for the urinary antiseptic properties. It is also used for rheumatism, and extracts have been reported to have hypoglycaemic activity in animals [2]. Chimaphilin can cause dermatitis in sensitive individuals [3].

SPECIFIC REFERENCES: 1. Walewska E *et al* (1969) *Pharmazie* 24:423. 2. Bolkart K *et al* (1968) *Naturwissensch.* 55:445. 3. Hausen B *et al* (1988) *Contact Derm.* 19(3):180.

PITCHER PLANT
SARRACENIA PURPUREA L.
S. FLAVA L.
Fam. Sarraceniaceae

HABITAT: North America.

DESCRIPTION: A carnivorous plant with 'pitchers' reaching 5–20 cm or more long, formed from the leaf-stalks and stipules, the latter forming a sharp wing on the inner side, the leaf blade forming a rounded, heart-shaped hood. Taste: bitter and astringent; odourless.

PART USED: Root, leaves.

CONSTITUENTS: Not well investigated. Reported to contain glycosides named as sarracenin and sarracenic acid, of unknown structure [R4]. *S. flava* L contains alkaloids: coniine and gamma-coniceine, mainly in the liquid in the pitcher [1].

MEDICINAL USE: Stomachic, diuretic, laxative [R1], usually as an infusion. At one time this plant had a great (but obviously undeserved) reputation as a prophylactic against smallpox.

SPECIFIC REFERENCES: 1. Foder G *et al* (1985) *The Alkaloids Vol 3,* Ed. Pelletier, S. Pub: John Wiley, UK.

PLANTAIN
PLANTAGO MAJOR L.
Fam. Plantaginaceae

SYNONYMS: Greater Plantain.

HABITAT: A common weed in Britain and many other parts of the world.

DESCRIPTION: Leaves strongly veined, in a basal rosette, broadly oval, with a blunt apex, abruptly narrowing at the base into a long petiole. Flowers tiny, yellowish-green with purple then yellowish anthers, in a long, dense, spike. Taste: astringent; odourless.

PART USED: Leaves, seeds.

CONSTITUENTS: (i) Iridoids; aucubin, 3,4-dihydroaucubin, 6'-*O*-beta-glucosylaucubin, catalpol, melittin and geniposide (ii) Flavonoids; apigenin and its 7-glucoside, luteolin, scutellarin, baicalein, nepetin, hispidulin and plantagoside (iii) Triterpenes based on oleanolic and ursolic acids, (iv) Polysaccharides composed mainly of arabinose, galactose and xylose (v) Plant acids such as chlorogenic, neochlorogenic, fumaric, hydroxycinnamic and benzoic acids and their esters (vi) Fatty acids; eicosapentaenoic, pentadecanoic, docosahexaenoic, oleic and other acids [1,2,3,4,5,6,7,8].

MEDICINAL USE: Anti-inflammatory, analgesic, diuretic, anti-haemor-rhagic [R1]. Many of these uses are supported by recent pharmacological tests. The leaves have been used for wound-healing and other skin conditions, as well as for infections, bleeding and circulatory problems. Extracts have been shown to have anti-inflammatory and analgesic effects, as well as immunomodulating, antioxidant [2,9], and hypogly-caemic activity [10]. The polysaccharides activate complement [5,7] and ursolic acid, together with some of the fatty acids, is a selective cyclooxygenase (COX-2) inhibitor [3]. The leaf extract enhances immune properties in a number of test systems [11]. Aucubin is a mild aperient; it also stimulates the secretion of uric acid by the kidneys [12]. Apigenin is an anti-inflammatory agent [13] and baicalein is anti-inflammatory and anti-allergic (see Scullcap). Both of these, and the other flavonoid constituents, inhibit HIV-transcriptase activity [14]. Plantain is also used widely in Chinese medicine to treat urinary diseases, tuberculous ulcers, bacillary dysentery, hepatitis and other conditions.

PREPARATIONS AND DOSE: Dried leaf, dose: 2–4 g or equivalent extract, three times daily.

SPECIFIC REFERENCES: 1. Ringbom T *et al* (2001) *J. Nat. Prod.* 64:745. 2. Samuelssen A (2000) *J. Ethnopharmacol.* 71:1. 3. Ringbom T *et al* (1998) *J. Nat. Prod.* 61:1212. 4. Murai M *et al* (1996) *Natural Med.* 50(4):306. 5. Samuelssen A (1995) *Phytother. Res.* 9(3):211. 6. Samuelssen A (1999) *Carbohyd. Res.* 315(3–4):312. 7. Michaelson T *et al* (2000) *Scand. J. Immunol.* 52(5):483. 8. Hetland G *et al* (2000) *Scand. J. Immunol.* 52(4):348. 9. Nunez Guillen M *et al* (1997) *Int. J. Pharmacog.* 35(2):99. 10. Rodriguez J *et al* (1994) *Phytother. Res.* 8(6):372. 11. Gomez-Flores R *et al* (2000) *Phytother. Res.* 14(8):617. 12. Inoue H *et al* (1974) *Planta Med.* 25:285. 13. Middleton E *et al* (1984) *Biochem. Pharmacol.* 33:3333. 14. Nishibe S *et al* (1997) *Natural Med.* 51(6):547.

PLEURISY ROOT

ASLEPIAS TUBEROSA L.
Fam. Asclepiadaceae

SYNONYMS: Butterfly Weed.

HABITAT: North America.

DESCRIPTION: The rootstock is slightly annulate, with a knotty crown. Roots longitudinally wrinkled, greyish-brown externally, whitish internally, composed of concentric cylinders of tissue which can easily be separated. Fracture: uneven, tough, short, starch; taste: nutty, bitter; odour: faint.

PART USED: Root.

CONSTITUENTS: (i) Cardenolides; e.g. asclepiadin. Related species such as *A. curassavica*, *A. subulata* and *A glaucescens* are better investigated and were found contain similar cardiac glycosides including asclepin, afroside, uscharin, calotropin, calactin, syrioside, frugoside, glucofrugoside and their aglycones (ii) Flavonoids; rutin, kaempferol, quercetin and isorhamnetin (iii) Triterpenes; friedelin, alpha- and beta-amyrin, viburnitol, and lupeol (iv) Miscellaneous; essential oil etc. [R2,R7;1,2,3,4].

MEDICINAL USE: Expectorant, tonic, diaphoretic, antispasmodic [R1]. It is also reputed to be mildly aperient and carminative. The main use is in the treatment of pleurisy, as the name implies, to relieve the pain and ease breathing. It has also been used for uterine disorders, and abortifacient and oestrogenic activity has been demonstrated in rats [5,6]. The cardenolides have positive inotropic and cardiotonic effects [7] and have been suggested as possible anti-cancer agents [8]. Little further information is available and because of the potential toxicity should be used with caution [R7].

SPECIFIC REFERENCES: 1. Pagani F (1975) *Boll. Chim. Farm.* 114(8):450. 2. Abe F *et al* (2000) *Chem. Pharm. Bull.* 48(7):1017. 3. Jolad S *et al* (1986) *Phytochem.* 25:2581. 4. Seiber J *et al* (1982)

Phytochem. 21:2343. 5. Conway G *et al* (1979) *J. Ethnopharmacol.* 1:241. 6. Costello C *et al* (1950) *J. Am. Pharm. Ass. Sci. Ed.* 39:233. 7. Patnaik G *et al* (1978) *Arzneimittelforsch.* 28:1095 and 1368. 8. Koike K *et al* (1980) *Chem. Pharm. Bull.* 28:401.

POISON OAK
POISON IVY

TOXICODENDRON DIVERSILOBIUM (L.) KUNTZ
T. RADICANS (L.) KUNTZ AND OTHER SPECIES
Fam. Anacardiaceae

SYNONYMS: Poison Ivy: *Rhus toxicodendron* L., T. (Michx) Greene, *T. pubescens* Mill.

HABITAT: North America.

DESCRIPTION: Leaves trifoliate, about 10 cm long with a downy undersurface. Taste: acrid and astringent; odourless.

PART USED: Leaves.

CONSTITUENTS: (i) Urushiols, a series of alkyl catechols of varying chain length and double bond position. (ii) Pentadecylcatechols, and heptadecylcatechols, a series. Poison Ivy contains mainly pentadecylcatechols with some heptadecylcatechols, and poison oak *vice versa* [R2;1,2,3,4].

MEDICINAL USE: The only medicinal use is as a homoeopathic remedy. *Toxicodendron* species are contact allergens, causing sensitization on initial exposure, and dermatitis of varying severity on subsequent exposure. It is possible to build up some sort of immune tolerance using usual techniques in highly sensitive individuals. The extract has both genotoxic and anti-genotoxic effects *in vitro*, depending on the dilution [6]. Cross reactivity exists between species of *Toxicodendron,* but not necessarily with *Philodendron* species, which also contain alkyl resorcinols [7].

SPECIFIC REFERENCES: 1. Millet S *et al* (1976) *Phytochem.*15:553. 2. Gross M *et al* (1984) *Phytochem.* 24:2263. 3. Lepoittevin J-P *et al* (1986) *J. Med. Chem.* 29(2):287. 4. Baer H (1975) In: 'Toxic Plants', Ed. A Kinghorn; pub: Columbia Press, US. 5. El Sohly M *et al* (1982) *J. Nat. Prod.* 45(5):532. 6. Wenqing L. *et al* (2000) *Biol. Med.* 29(6):300. 7. Knight T *et al* (1996) *Am. J. Contact Dermatitis* 7(3):138.

POKEWEED

PHYTOLACCA AMERICANA L.
Fam. Phytolaccaeae

SYNONYMS: Pokeroot, P. *decandra* L.

HABITAT: North America.

DESCRIPTION: The root is usually sold in transverse slices or split lengthways. The outer surface is yellowish- to brownish-grey, wrinkled longtidinally and marked with transverse bars of cork. The inner surface is whitish or buff, very hard, and shows characteristic concentric rings of vascular tissue separated by parenchyma. The berries are subglobular, purplish black, fleshy, about 8 mm in diameter and composed of 10 carpels, each containing one lens-shaped seed. The powder is strongly sternutatory; taste: slight.

PART USED: Root, berries.

CONSTITUENTS: (i) Triterpenoid saponins; the phytolaccosides A-I etc., based on the aglycones phytolaccagenin and phytolaccic acid, and cerebrosides based on phytosphingosine ceramides (ii) Lectins; the mixture known as pokeweed mitogen, consisting of a series of glycoproteins (iii) Proteins such as phytolacain R, and peptides such as PAFP-s (iv) Alkaloids of the betalain type, such as phytolaccine, betaine, isobetanine, betanidine and isobetanidine (v) Lignans including isoamericanin A (vi) Polyphenols and flavonoids based on kaempferol and quercetin (vii) Gamma-amino butyric acid and histamine [R7;1,2,3,4,5,6,7,8,9].

MEDICINAL USE: Anti-rheumatic, anti-inflammatory, alterative, emetic, cathartic [R1]. The phytolaccosides are potent anti-inflammatory agents in the rat paw oedema test [10], and a saponin extract has a comparable anti-dexudative and anti-granulomatous activity to that of hydrocortisone in mice. It had no effect on the adrenal gland but high doses caused thymolysis. Phytolaccosides B and E inhibited exudate formation after sponge pellet and carrageenan-induced oedema in rats [R7]; the cerebrosides are inhibitors of cyclooxygenase-2 (COX-2) enzyme, and isoamericanin A has been shown to induce prostacyclin formation [9], all of which support the anti-inflammatory usage. The proteins are antiviral; they inhibit the replication of the influenza and HSV-1 viruses and poliovirus, and the peptide PAFP-s has anti-fungal activity [3]. The lectins are agglutinating, and Pokeweed mitogen (PWM) is used as a tool in biochemical research. Pokeweed has caused toxic (particularly gastrointestinal) symptoms and heart block, when accidentally eaten by mistake for parsnip or horseradish, or as a freshly made herbal tea [11]. No toxic effects have been observed from other types of products, possibly because the proteins and lectins are denatured during processing. The related species *P. dodecandra* (endod) is used as a molluscicide [12]. For further information on both species, see [R2 and R7, and refs therein].

PREPARATIONS AND DOSE: Dried root, dose: 0.06–0.3 g or equivalent extract, three times daily.

SPECIFIC REFERENCES: 1. Takahasha H *et al* (2001) *Chem. Pharm. Bull.* 49(2):246. 2. Sam S *et al* (2001) *Chem. Pharm. Bull.* 49(3):321. 3. Shao F *et al* (1999) *Biochim. Biophys. Acta Protein Structure Mol. Enzymol.* 1430(2):262. 4. Uchikoba T *et al* (2000) *Biochim. Biophys. Acta. Gen. Subj.* 1523(2–3):254. 5. Yonezawa H *et al* (1999) *J. Biochem.* 126(1):26. 6. Bylka W *et al* (2001) *Acta Pol. Pharm.* 58(1):69. 7. Kang S *et al* (1987) *Planta Med.* 53:338. 8. Kang S *et al* (1980) *J. Nat. Prod.* 43:510. 9. Hasegawa T *et al* (1987) *Chem. Lett.*

2:329. 10. Woo W *et al* (1978) *Planta Med.* 34:87. 11. Hamilton R *et al* (1995) *Vet. Hum. Toxicol.* 37(1):66. 12. Parkhurst R *et al* (1989) *Biochim. Biophys. Res. Comm.* 158:436.

POLYPODY ROOT
POLYPODIUM VULGARE L.
Fam. Polypodiaceae

HABITAT: Grows on old walls and trunks of trees throughout Europe.

DESCRIPTION: The rhizome is slender, about 3 mm in diameter, striated longitudinally, knotty, with cup-shaped leaf base scars on the upper side at intervals of about 1 cm and rootlet scars on the undersurface. Transverse section horny, greenish-brown, with an irregular circle of vascular bundles near the circumference. Taste: very sweet, faintly acrid; odourless.

PART USED: Rhizome.

CONSTITUENTS: (i) Saponin glycosides, based on polypodosapogenin, including osladin and polypodoside A (ii) Ecdysteroids; polypodins A and B, inokosterone, pterosterone and abutasterone (iii) Phloroglucin derivatives [1,2,3]. Other species such as *Polypodium decumanum* (Calaguala) contain similar compounds, as well as flavonoids and coumarins including rutin and melilotoside, and the anthocyanin selligueain [4].

MEDICINAL USE: Expectorant, pectoral, alterative [R1]. It has been used in coughs and chest disorders, as a tonic in dyspepsia and loss of appetite, and in skin diseases such as psoriasis. The sweet taste is due to osladin [2]. It occasionally produces a rash after ingestion; the reason for this is unknown and it appears to be harmless. Calaguala is also used for psoriasis and has been shown to have immunosuppressive effects [5] and inhibit elastase release form neutrophils [4]. Selligueain inhibits elastase activity [4], and is anti-inflammatory and analgesic *in vitro* [6].

SPECIFIC REFERENCES: 1. Coll J *et al* (1994) *Tetrahedron* 50(24):7247. 2. Yamada H *et al* (1995) *J. Org. Chem.* 60(2):386. 3. Camps F *et al* (1990) *J. Chromatog.* 514(2):199. 4. Vasange M *et al* (1997) *Planta Med.* 63(6):511. 5. Tuominen M *et al* (1991) *Phytother. Res.* 5(5):234. 6. Subarnas A *et al* (2000) *Phytomedicine* 7(5):401.

POMEGRANATE
PUNICA GRANATUM L.
Fam. Punicaeae

HABITAT: Indigenous to North-western India and the Middle East, cultivated in the Mediterranean region and elsewhere.

DESCRIPTION: The tree is very beautiful with scarlet flowers; it is said to have flourished in the Garden of Eden, and the fruit is well-known. The rind of the fruit occurs in concave fragments, brownish-red externally and yellowish internally with depressions left by the seeds. The bark, mainly stem bark, occurs in flat or quilled pieces, externally yellowish-grey, furrowed, occasionally with patches of lichen; internally finely striated. Taste: astringent; odourless.

PART USED: Bark, rind of fruit.

CONSTITUENTS: (i) Piperidine alkaloids: pelletierine, isopelletierine, methylisopelletierine, pseudopelletierine and norpseudopelletierine, sedridine, hygrine and norhygrine (ii) Ellagitannins; punicacorteins A-D, punicalin, punicalagin, punigluconin, tellamagrandin, granatin, corilagin, casuanin and casuarinin (iii) Flavonoids based on quercitrin (iv) Anthocyanins; pelagonidin glucoside (v) Triglycerides, including di-O-punicyl-O-octadecatrienylglycerol [R16;1,2,3,4,5,6].

MEDICINAL USE: Taenifuge, astringent [R1]. This is a very old remedy, being mentioned in the papyrus Ebers (Egypt, ca. 1550 BC). It is taken by decoction, followed by a purgative. The alkaloids are anthelmintic; pelletierine in particular causes the tapeworm to relax its grip on the wall of the intestine so it can be expelled by a cathartic [7]. If systemic absorption of pelletierine occurs it may give rise to toxic symptoms such as muscle cramps and dizziness. The ellagitannins are responsible for the astringency and are known to inhibit carbonic anhydrase [4]. Extracts of the fruit rind are antimicrobial, including against *Salmonella typhi* [8,9,10], and anti-fungal [11]. They inhibit diarrhoea in animals [12,13] and show anti-implantational effects in rats [14]. The aqueous extract inhibited gastric mucosal damage induced by ethanol, attributed to the tannin content [15], and reduced blood glucose levels in experimentally diabetic rats [16,17]. Recently, alpha-amylase inhibition [18], hepatoprotective [19] and immunomodulatory activity have been identified in extracts of the fruit rind [20]. The fruit juice appears to confer cardiovascular health benefits, possibly due to anti-oxidant activity [21].

PREPARATIONS AND DOSE: Dried bark or root powder, dose: 1.5–3 g; fruit powder: 4–8 g.

BIBLICAL REFERENCES: Exodus 39:24–24; Numbers 13:23 and 20:5; Deuteronomy 8:8; 1 Samuel 14:2; Song of Solomon 4:3 & 13, 6:7 & 11, 7:12, 8:2 and others.

SPECIFIC REFERENCES: 1. Tanaka T *et al* (1986) *Chem. Pharm. Bull.* 34(2):656. 2. Neuhofer H *et al* (1993) *Pharmazie* 48(5):389. 3. Tanaka T *et al* (1992) *Chem. Pharm. Bull.* 40(11):2975. 4. Satomi H *et al* (1993) *Biol. Pharm. Bull.* 16(8):787. 5. Chauhan D *et al* (2001) *Pharm. Biol.* 39(2):155. 6. Yusuph M *et al* (1997) *Phytochem.* 44(7):1391. 7. Hukkeri V *et al* (1993) *Fitoterapia* 64(1):69. 8. Prashanth D *et al* (2001) *Fitoterapia* 72(2):171. 9. Perez C *et al* (1994) *J. Ethnopharmacol.* 44(1):41. 10. Navarro V *et al* (1996) *J. Ethnopharmacol.* 53(3):143. 11. Dutta B *et al* (2000) *Biomedicine* 20(3):187. 12. Pillai N (1992) *Int. J. Pharmacog.* 30(3):201. 13. Das A *et al* (1999) *J. Ethnopharmacol.* 68(1–3):205. 14. Prakash A *et al* (1985) *Acta Eur. Fert.* 16(6):441. 15. Gharzouli K *et al* (1999)

Phytother. Res. 13(1):42 . 16. Jafri M *et al* (2000) *J. Ethnopharmacol.* 70(3):309. 17. Das A *et al* (2001) *Phytother. Res.* 15(7):628. 18. Prashanth D *et al* (2001) *Fitoterapia* 72(2):179. 19. Asockson C *et al* (2001) *Indian Drugs* 38(4):183. 20. Gracious R *et al* (2001) *J. Ethnopharmacol.* 78(1):85. 21. Aviram M *et al* (2000) *Am. J. Clin. Nutr.* 71:1062.

POPLAR

POPULUS ALBA L.
P. TREMULOIDES MICHX.
P. NIGRA L. AND OTHER SPP.
Fam. Salicaceae

SYNONYMS: White Poplar (= *P. alba*), Quaking Aspen, American Aspen (= *P. tremuloides*), Black Poplar (= *P. nigra*).

HABITAT: P. alba and *P. nigra* are European species, *P. tremuloides* is North American.

DESCRIPTION: The bark occurs as curved or flattened pieces or may be shredded. The outer layer is usually removed, leaving a dull brown surface. The inner surface is smooth and varies in colour from nearly white to brown. Taste: bitter; odourless.

PART USED: Bark.

CONSTITUENTS: (i) Phenolic glycosides; salicin, populin (salicin 6-benzoate), salicortin, tremulacin, tremuloidin, cinnamrutinosides A and B (ii) Lignans including (+)-isolariciresinol mono-beta-D-glucopyranoside (iii) Flavonoids based on quercetin, including rutin [R2,R7;1,2,3,4].

MEDICINAL USE: Anti-inflammatory, anodyne, astringent, diuretic, stimulant [R1]. The salicyl glycosides are anti-inflammatory (see Willow) and the flavonoids are thought to contribute to the activity of the extract [4]. Poplar is an ingredient of a preparation also containing *Solidago virgaurea* and *Fraxinus excelsior* (Golden Rod and Ash, q.v.) for inflammatory disorders, which has been shown to have clinical efficacy [5]. This product is also analgesic, antipyretic and antioxidant [6]. Poplar has also been used traditionally to treat urinary complaints, such as cystitis, stomach, and liver disorders, and debility and anorexia.

BIBLICAL REFERENCES: Genesis 30: 37; Hosea 4:13.

SPECIFIC REFERENCES: 1. Jossang A *et al* (1994) *Phytochem.* 35:547. 2. Picard S *et al* (1994) *J. Nat. Prod.* 57:808. 3. Thieme H *et al* (1969) *Pharmazie* 24:567. 4. Albrecht M *et al* (1990) *Planta Med.* Proc. Biol. Chem. Active Nat. Subs, Bonn, July 17–22, P32. 5. Klein-Galczinsky C (1999) *Wien. Med. Wochenschr.* 149(8–10):248. 6. Schempp H *et al* (2000) *Arzneim. Forsch.* 50(4):362.

POPPY
PAPAVER SOMNIFERUM L.
Fam. Papaveraceae

SYNONYMS: Opium Poppy.

HABITAT: Native to Asia, cultivated widely elsewhere for food and medicinal purposes and as a garden ornamental.

DESCRIPTION: The flowers vary in colour from white to reddish-purple, but are usually pale lilac with a purple base spot. The capsules are subspherical, depressed at the top with the radiating stigma in the centre, below which are the valves through which the seeds are dispersed. There is a swollen ring just above where the capsule joins the stem. The seeds are small, greyish, reniform and attached to the internal projections or placentae.

PART USED: Capsule, latex exuded from the unripe capsule (Opium), seeds.

CONSTITUENTS: (i) Alkaloids; the major one is morphine, with codeine and thebaine and lesser amounts of very many others including narceine, narcotine, papaverine, salutaridine, oripavine and sanguinarine (ii) Meconic acid [R3,R14;1,2]. The seeds contain a fixed oil [3].

MEDICINAL USE: Narcotic, analgesic, antispasmodic, anti-diarrhoeal, antitussive, diaphoretic [R1]. The total alkaloidal extract is known as papaveretum and is used routinely for preoperative analgesia and relaxation, now with the narcotine removed due to its genotoxicity. Morphine is a very potent analgesic; however, due to its potential for inducing dependence is used only for severe pain in the short term, or for terminal illness. Semi-synthetic derivatives are often used in its place and many, such as oxycodone, have been developed from the morphinane nucleus. Papaverine and oripavine are spasmolytic [4] and have been used in cough mixtures for this purpose. Opium is the starting material for the production of heroin. For further details see [R3;1,2 and refs therein]. Poppy seeds are used in the food industry to produce oil and to flavour bread. They contain the same alkaloids but in much smaller amounts [5]. The seed oil has chemopreventive properties as measured by an increase in glutathione-S-transferase activity [3]. For a recent review, see [6].

PREPARATIONS: Papaveretum BPC, Opium Tincture BP 2002 and others, see [R3,R14].

REGULATORY STATUS: Depending on strength, P, POM, or CD (Misuse of Drugs Act 1973).

SPECIFIC REFERENCES: 1. Calixto J *et al* (2000) *Phytother. Res.* 14(6):401. 2. Calixto J *et al* (2001) *Emerging Drugs* 6(2):261. 3. Aruna K *et al* (1996) *Phytother. Res.* 10(7):577. 4. Gomez-Serranillos P *et al* (1996) *Phytother. Res.* 10(Suppl.1):S116. 5. Paul B S *et al* (1996) *Planta Med.* 62(6):544. 6. Poppy. Ed: Bernath J (1999) *Medicinal and Aromatic Plants – Industrial Profiles.* Taylor and Francis, London, UK.

POPPY, RED

PAPAVER RHOEAS L.
Fam. Papaveraceae

SYNONYMS: Corn Poppy.

HABITAT: Common throughout Europe and Britain, especially in fields and disturbed ground.

DESCRIPTION: Flowers solitary, with four, silky, bright red petals often with a dark centre. The stamens are numerous with blue-black anthers, and the stigma is radiate. The two sepals, which fall off soon after opening, and the stalk are covered with bristly hairs.

PART USED: Flowers.

CONSTITUENTS: (i) Alkaloids, the papaverrubines, rhoeadine, isorhoeadine, stylopine, protopine and many others, variable in composition due to the existence of chemical races (ii) Meconic acid (iii) Mecocyanin, a red anthocyanin pigment (iv) Mucilage, tannin [R3;1,2,3].

MEDICINAL USE: Anodyne, expectorant [R1]. It was formerly used as an infusion or in the form of a syrup. For a recent review of the genus, see [4].

SPECIFIC REFERENCES: 1. El-Masry S J *et al* (1981) *Planta Med.* 41:61. 2. Williamson E *et al* (1978) *Phytochem.* 17:2087. 3. Willaman J *et al* (1970) *Lloydia* 33(3A):1 4. Poppy. Ed. Bernath J (1999) *Medicinal and Aromatic Plants – Industrial Profiles.* Taylor and Francis, London, UK.

PRICKLY ASH, NORTHERN

ZANTHOXYLUM AMERICANUM MILL
Fam. Rutaceae

SYNONYMS: Toothache Tree, Yellow Wood.

HABITAT: Canada and North America.

DESCRIPTION: Northern prickly ash bark occurs in curved or quilled fragments, about 1 mm thick, externally brownish-grey, faintly furrowed with whitish patches and flattened spines about 5 mm long. Taste: bitter and pungent, causing salivation.

PART USED: Bark, berries.

CONSTITUENTS: (i) Isoquinoline alkaloids; alpha-fagarine (= allocryptopine) and beta-fagarine (= skimmianine), magnoflorine, laurifoline, nitidine, chelerythrine, tambetarine and candicine (ii) Coumarins, including xanthyletin, xanthoxyletin, xanthotoxin, alloxanthyletin, isoorientin, cnidilin, dipetalin, psoralen and imperatorin (iii) Lignans; sesamin and asarinin (iv) Resin, tannin, volatile oil [R7;1,2,3,4]. The related West African species, *Z. zanthoxyloides* (Lam.) Watson contains alkaloids including pellitorine [5], piperonyl-4-acrylic isobutyl amide [6] and zanthoxylol [7].

MEDICINAL USE: Anti-rheumatic, analgesic, diaphoretic, carminative, antipyretic, anti-diarrhoeal [R1]. It is used both internally and externally to treat rheumatism and toothache, for fevers and as a tonic, and for circulatory insufficiency. Chelerythrine is antimicrobial. The coumarins are cytotoxic *in vitro* to human leukaemia cells and are lethal to brine shrimp [4,3]. *Z. zanthoxyloides* has been used for similar purposes, and as a chewing stick for cleaning the teeth. It has anti-sticking activity ascribed to the zanthoxylol [7]. Piperonyl-4-acrylic isobutyl amide is anti-inflammatory [6].

PREPARATIONS AND DOSE: Dried bark, dose: 1–3 g or equivalent extract, three times daily.

SPECIFIC REFERENCES: 1. Fish F *et al* (1975) *Lloydia* 38:268. 2. Fish F *et al* (1973) *J. Pharm. Pharmacol.* 25S:115. 3. Saqib Q *et al* (1990) *Phytother. Res.* 4(6):216. 4. Ju Y *et al* (2001) *Phytother. Res.* 15(5):441. 5. Adesina S (1986) *J. Nat. Prod.* 49(4):715. 6. Oriowo M (1982) *Planta Med.* 44(1):54. 7. Elujoba A *et al* (1985) *J. Pharm. Biomed. Anal.* 3(5):447.

PRICKLY ASH, SOUTHERN
ZANTHOXYLUM CLAVA-HERCULIS L.
Fam. Rutaceae

HABITAT: Southern parts of North America.

DESCRIPTION: Similar to Northern Prickly Ash (q.v.), but the bark is about 2 mm thick, with conical, corky spines up to 2 cm long. Fracture: short, green in the outer and yellow in the inner part; taste: bitter and pungent, causing salivation.

PART USED: Bark, berries.

CONSTITUENTS: (i) Alkaloids; magnoflorine, laurifoline, nitidine, chelerythrine, tambetarine, N-acetylannonaine and candicine (ii) Amides, including cinnamamide, herculin and neoherculin (iii) Lignans including asarinin and sesamin (iv) Miscellaneous; coumarins, tannin, etc. [1,2,3,4,5].

MEDICINAL USE: Similar to Northern Prickly Ash (q.v.), i.e. as an antirheumatic, analgesic, diaphoretic, carminative, antipyretic and anti-diarrhoeal [R1]. It is used as a fish poison, the activity attributed at least in part to the N-acetylannonaine content [3]. The alkaloids have various actions including hypotensive properties for nitidine [5], anti-inflammatory effects for chelerythrine [R7] and the extract has neuromuscular blocking activity [6].

PREPARATIONS AND DOSE: Dried bark, dose: 1–3 g or equivalent extract, three times daily.

SPECIFIC REFERENCES: 1. Fish F *et al* (1975) *Lloydia* 38:268. 2. Fish F *et al* (1973) *J. Pharm. Pharmacol.* 25S:115. 3. Rao K *et al* (1986) *J. Nat. Prod.* 49(2):340. 4. Krane B *et al* (1984) *J. Nat. Prod.* 47:1. 5. Addae-Mensah I *et al* (1986) *Planta Med.* 52(Suppl.1):58. 6. Bowen J *et al* (1981) *Fed. Proc.* 40:696.

PRIMROSE
PRIMULA VULGARIS HUDS.
Fam. Primulaceae

HABITAT: A well-known wild flower growing in woods and grassy banks in Britain and parts of Europe, Asia and North Africa.

DESCRIPTION: The leaves are up to about 12 cm long and 3 cm broad, oblanceolate, with a rounded apex and tapering to a decurrent base. The margin is irregular and the lamina shows a characteristic, reticulate venation, depressed above and prominent and hairy beneath. Rootstock knotty, with successive leaf-base scars and cylindrical, branched, rootlets. Taste: insipid; odourless.

PART USED: Root, herb.

CONSTITUENTS: (i) Saponins, including primulaveroside (ii) Phenolic glycosides (iii) Flavonoids [1].

MEDICINAL USE: Anti-inflammatory, antispasmodic, vermifuge, emetic, vulnerary [R1]. Seldom used today but formerly used for rheumatism, gout, insomnia, and as a poultice to heal wounds.
For information on primula saponins, see Cowslip.

SPECIFIC REFERENCES: 1. Thieme H *et al* (1971) *Pharmazie* 7:434.

PRUNE
PRUNUS DOMESTICA L.
Fam. Rosaceae

SYNONYMS: Plum Tree.

HABITAT: Widely cultivated.

DESCRIPTION: The prune, or dried plum, is too well-known to require description.

PART USED: Fruit.

CONSTITUENTS: Pulp: Anthocyanins, sugars, malic acid. Kernel: fixed oil, about 45%, amygdalin and benzoic acid [R3;1].

MEDICINAL USE: Laxative, refrigerant, nutritive [R1]. Prunes are either eaten as a food or added to other preparations for their laxative effect.

SPECIFIC REFERENCES: 1. Wesche-Ebeling P *et al* (1996) *Food Chem.* 57(3):399.

PSYLLIUM
PLANTAGO PSYLLIUM L.
P. INDICA L.
Fam. Plantaginaceae

SYNONYMS: P. psyllium: Flea Seeds, Dark Psyllium, Spanish or French Psyllium, Brown Psyllium. *P. indica:* Black Psyllium, *P. arenaria* Waldst et Kit. The seeds of *P. major* (see Plantain) have been used as a substitute, and *P. asiatica* L. is used in the Far East.

HABITAT: Native to the Mediterranean region, cultivated widely throughout the world. *P. indica* is native to Asia but cultivated in Europe and Egypt.

DESCRIPTION: P. psyllium seeds are deep brown and glossy, *P. indica* seeds are blackish-brown and slightly smaller.

PART USED: Seeds. The whole plant, as well as the seeds, of *P. asiatica* is used in Oriental medicine.

CONSTITUENTS: Similar to Ispaghula, q.v. (i) Mucilage, consisting of a mixture of polysaccharides composed of mainly of D-xylose units, with smaller amounts of L-arabinose (ii) Phenyl-ethanoids including acteoside and forsythoside (iii) Monoterpene alkaloids (+)-boschni-akine and its acid derivative (= indicaine and plantagonine) (iv) Triterpenes such as stigmasterol, beta-sitosterol, campesterol (v) Fixed oil rich in polyunsaturated fatty acids etc. The herb contains the iridoid plantarenaloside. *P. asiatica* contains 3'4 dihydroaucubin and other iridoids [R3;1,2,3].

MEDICINAL USE: Bulk laxative [R1]. The seeds swell when moistened into a gelatinous mass, but to a lesser extent than Ispaghula [R3]. Psyllium is a source of soluble dietary fibre, with beneficial effects on serum glucose and cholesterol levels. *P. psyllium*, at a dose level of 5 g three times daily, was shown to be hypoglycaemic in 125 patients with type II (non-insulin dependent) diabetes mellitus (NIDDM) [4], and also lowered the glycaemic index of bread in a study of 12 patients with NIDDM [5]. An intake of 8 g per day of psyllium seed reduced serum cholesterol levels in a randomized controlled crossover study of 68 adults with hyperlipidaemia [6].

PREPARATIONS AND DOSE: Seeds, dose: 6–12 g daily.

SPECIFIC REFERENCES: 1. Oshio H *et al* (1982) *Planta Med.* 44:204. 2. Tomoda M *et al* (1987) *Planta Med.* 53(1):8. 3. Nishibe S *et al* (2001) *Natural Med.* 55(5):258. 4. Rodriguez-Moran M *et al* (1998) *J. Diabetes Comp.* 12(5):273. 5. Frati Munari A *et al* (1998) *Arch. Med. Res.* 29(2):137. 6. Jenkins D *et al* (2002) *J. Am. Clin. Nutr.* 75(5):834.

PUFFBALL

LYCOPERDON PERLATUM PERS
L. PYRIFORME SCHAEEF EX PERS AND OTHER SPP.
CALVATIA LILACINA (BERK) HENN AND OTHER SPP.
Fam. Lycoperdaceae

HABITAT: Europe mainly.

DESCRIPTION: The fungus forms a globose or depressed ball, varying in size from 10 cm to 30 cm in diameter, sometimes furrowed at the base. Whitish when young, with a white internal mass containing yellow spores, darkening with age and when ripe, discharging brownish or blackish spores by rupturing the skin.

PART USED: Fungus.

CONSTITUENTS: Not well-investigated. *L. perlatum* contains lycoperdic acid [1]. *L. bovista* L. contains a glycoside lycoperdin, xanthine derivatives and amino acids [R4]. *L. pyriforme* contains azo- and azoxyformamides [2]. *C. lilacina* contains *p*-carboxyphenyl-azoxycyanide [3].

MEDICINAL USE: Haemostatic [R1]. *L. perlatum* contains anti-fungal substances active against *Candida albicans, C. tropicalis* and other pathogens [4].

SPECIFIC REFERENCES: 1. Yoshifuji S *et al* (1995) *Chem. Pharm. Bull.* 43(10):1617. 2. Kopke B *et al* (1999) *Nat. Prod. Lett.* 13(1):41. 3. Gasco A *et al* (1974) *Tet. Lett.* 38:3431. 4. Pujol V *et al* (1990) *Ann. Pharm. Francaises* 48(1):17.

PULSATILLA
ANEMONE PULSATILLA L. AND OTHER SPP.
Fam. Ranunculaceae

SYNONYMS: Pasque Flower, Wind Flower, Meadow Anemone, *Pulsatilla vulgaris* Mill.

HABITAT: Europe and parts of Russia.

DESCRIPTION: Leaves feathery, hairy, stalked, up to about 15 cm long, 8 cm broad, bipinnate, the leaflets opposite, each segment trifid, narrow, with acute points. Leaf-stalks cylindrical, channelled on the upper surface, purplish at the base. Flowers large, solitary, purple, with numerous stamens with bright yellow anthers. Sepals are hairy, purplish. Taste: when fresh, acrid and burning; odourless.

PART USED: Herb.

CONSTITUENTS: (i) Lactones; protoanemonin, which dimerizes on drying to anemonin, ranunculin (ii) Triterpenoids, the pulsatilla saponins based on hederagenin (iii) Miscellaneous; anemone camphor, tannins, volatile oil [R2;1,2].

MEDICINAL USE: Nervine, antispasmodic, alterative. Used for nervous exhaustion and amenorrhoea in women, as a sedative and for catarrh [R1]. Protoanemonin is antibacterial and irritant; however it is not found in dried plant material so the irritancy does not constitute a practical problem [1,3]. Many of the pulsatilla saponins are anti-fungal [3].

PREPARATIONS AND DOSE: Dried plant, dose: 0.12–0.3 g or equivalent extract. Should not be used fresh.

SPECIFIC REFERENCES: 1. Pourrat A *et al* (1980) *J. Pharm. Belg.* 35(4):277. 2. Evans F *et al* (1980) *Planta Med.* 38:289. 3. Ekabo O *et al* (1996) *J. Nat. Prod.* 59(4):431.

PUMPKIN
CUCURBITA MAXIMA DUCHESNE.
C. PEPO L. AND OTHER SPP.
Fam. Cucurbitaceae

SYNONYMS: Squash, Gourd.

HABITAT: Cultivated widely throughout the world.

DESCRIPTION: The seeds are broadly ovate, about 2 cm long, whitish, with a shallow groove, and flat ridge round the margin. The hilum is near the pointed end. Taste: nutty; odourless.

PART USED: Seeds.

CONSTITUENTS: (i) Fixed oil, the main component of which is linoleic acid, with oleic, palmitic and to a lesser extent stearic acids (ii) Sterols and triterpenes, including cholestanol and lathostanol derivatives, spirostanol, alpha- and beta-amyrin; also present in the flowers (iii) Cucurbitacins, to a variable extent depending on variety etc. (iv) Proteins and peptides [R8;1,2,3,4,5,6]. The herb contains flavonols including astragalin, quercetin, rutin and nicoflorin [7].

MEDICINAL USE: Taenicide, diuretic, demulcent, anti-fertility agent. It has been taken for tapeworm with a saline purgative. The seeds are now widely used clinically, primarily to treat enlargement of the prostate gland, often in combination with Pygeum Bark, Saw Palmetto and Nettle (q.v.) [R8;4,8]. Extracts of the seed appear to reduce sperm motility in rats [9] and have spasmolytic activity [10]. Spinasterol is anti-genotoxic in an *in vivo* micronucleus test [3]. The proteins present include a trypsin inhibitor and a ribosome-inactivating protein [5,6] The cucurbitacins are known to be toxic (see Bryony) but are normally present in negligible amounts and a total extract of the seed showed no toxic effects when given over several weeks to rats and swine [11]. Extracts of other parts, such as the fruit, leaves and flowers, were antimicrobial against *Bacillis subtilis* and general sedative effects [12]. Pumpkins and other variety of squash are popular and important vegetables. For further information see [R8;4 and refs therein].

SPECIFIC REFERENCES: 1. Schabort J (1978) *Phytochem.* 17:1062. 2. Cattel L *et al* (1979) *Planta Med.* 37(3):264. 3. Villasenor I *et al* (1996) *Mut. Res.* 360(2):89. 4. Bombardelli E *et al* (1997) *Fitoterapia* 68(4):291. 5. Yoshinari S *et al* (1996) *Eur. J. Biochem.* 242(3):585. 6. Mutambe F *et al* (1991) *J. Pharm. Pharmacol.* 43(Suppl.1):P62. 7. Krauze-Baranowska M *et al* (1996) *Acta Pol. Pharm.* 53(1):53. 8. Odenthal K (1996) *Phytother. Res.* 10(Suppl.1):S141. 9. Tupala E *et al* (1998) *Pharm. Pharmacol. Lett.* 8(4):178. 10. Hill R *et al* (1990) *J. Pharm. Pharmacol.* 42(Suppl.1):P179. 11. De Quieroz-Neta A *et al* (1994) *J. Ethnopharmacol.* 43(1):45. 12. Villasenor I *et al* (1995) *Phytother. Res.* 9(5):376.

PYCNOGENOL
PINUS PINASTER AITON.

Fam. Pinaceae

SYNONYMS: French Maritime Pine, *P. maritimus* Lam.

HABITAT: Indigenous to south-western France, Spain, southern Italy and Portugal, on forested sand dunes.

DESCRIPTION: A typical pine, reaching 40 metres in height.

PART USED: Bark extract.

CONSTITUENTS: Pycnogenol is a standardized water extract containing (i) Monomeric polyphenols such as catechin, epicatechin and taxifoliin (ii) Simple and condensed flavonoids including procyanidins and proanthocyanidins [1,2,3,4]. The bark also contains resin, which is a source of Turpentine and Colophony (q.v.).

MEDICINAL USE: Antioxidant. Pycnogenol is used particularly for chronic venous insufficiency (CVI), and neurodegenerative diseases of ageing. The antioxidant properties have been demonstrated in a number of *in vitro* and *in vivo* systems [1,2,3,4]. Studies have also shown that it has vaso-active properties, including inhibition of platelet aggregation induced by cigarette smoke [5], a relaxant effect upon blood vessels [6] and a reduction in capillary fragility, perivascular inflammation and oedema [2]. The mechanism of action appears to involve nitric oxide [4] as well as free-radical-scavenging ability [3]. Several clinical trials have demonstrated an improvement in pain and leg 'heaviness' and oedema, and an improvement in blood flow in patients with CVI when compared with placebo [7,8,9]. It is also useful in the treatment of vascular retinopathies such as those associated with diabetes [10] and the results of recent pilot trials suggest a role in managing the inflammation associated with systemic lupus erythematosus (SLE) [11] as well as chloasma (melasma) [12]. The extract possesses anti-inflammatory effects when used both topically and orally [13] and inhibits inflammatory transcription factors such as NFkappa-B *in vitro* [1]. Further investigations are currently underway to assess the effect of Pycnogenol in protecting against Alzheimer's and other dementias. It has been already shown to protect vascular endothelial cells against beta amyloid-induced injury [14] and glutamate-induced cytotoxicity [15]. Oral administration was found to reduce serum cholesterol levels in some patients taking the preparation for other purposes [9].

SPECIFIC REFERENCES: 1. Packer L *et al* (1999) *Free Rad. Biol. Med.* 27(5/6):704. 2. Gulati O (1999) *Eur. Bull. Drug. Res.* 7:8. 3. Virgili F *et al* (1998) *Free Rad. Biol. Med.* 24(7/8):1120. 4. Virgili F *et al* (1998) *FEBS Lett.* 431(3):315. 5. Putter M *et al* (1999) *Thromb. Res.* 95(4):155. 6. Fitzpatrick D *et al* (1998) *J. Cardiovasc. Pharmacol.* 32(4):509. 7. Archangeli P (2000) *Fitoterapia* 71:236. 8. Petrassi C *et al* (2000) *Phytomed.* 7(5):383. 9. Koch R (2002) *Phytother. Res.* 16(1):S1. 10. Spadea L *et al* (2001) *Phytother. Res.* 15(3):219. 11. Stefanescu M *et al* (2001) *Phytother. Res.* 15(8):698. 12. Ni Z *et al*

(2002) *Phytother. Res.* 16(6):567. 13. Blazso G *et al* (1997) *Pharmazie* 52:380. 14. Liu F *et al* (2000) *Biol. Pharm. Bull.* 23(6):735. 15. Kobyashi M *et al* (2000) *Free Rad. Res.* 32(2):115.

PYGEUM BARK
PRUNUS AFRICANA (HOOK F.) KALKM.
Fam. Rosaceae

SYNONYMS: African Prune, *Pygeum africanum* Gaert.

HABITAT: Central and southern Africa.

DESCRIPTION: A tropical evergreen tree.

PART USED: Bark.

CONSTITUENTS: (i) Sterols and pentacyclic triterpenes, including abietic, oleanolic, ursolic and crataegolic acids (ii) Ferulic acid esters [R8;1,2,3].

MEDICINAL USE: Traditionally used for micturition problems and now for benign prostatic hyperplasia (BPH) and prostatitis [R8,R11;1,3,4]. Clinical studies have shown the extract to be effective: in a trial of more than 100 patients over two months, significant improvements in urinary parameters were observed [5]. A preparation also containing Nettle (q.v.) showed synergistic activity in the inhibition of aromatase and 5-alpha reductase *in vitro*, both of which are implicated in the development of BHP [6]. Pygeum extract also antagonized testosterone in the prostate and seminal vesicles of the rat [3] and inhibited leukotriene synthesis, indicating a role in preventing inflammatory cells from infiltrating the prostate [7]. Acute and chronic toxicity and mutagenicity tests have shown no adverse effects, and the extract appears to be well-tolerated in men when administered over long periods [8]. For further details see [R8;R11;1,8,9 and refs therein].

SPECIFIC REFERENCES: 1. Bombardelli E *et al* (1997) *Fitoterapia* 68(3):205. 2. Ganzera M *et al* (1999) *J. Med. Food* 2(1):21. 3. Cristoni A *et al* (2000) *Fitoterapia* 71:S21. 4. Odenthal K (1996) *Phytother. Res.* 10(Suppl.1):S141. 5. Barlet A *et al* (1990) *Wien Klin. Wochenschr.* 102:667. 6. Hartmann R *et al* (1996) *Phytomedicine* 3(2):121. 7. Paubert-Braquet M *et al* (1994) *J. Lipid Mediators Cell Signal.* 9:285. 8. Pepping J (2001) *Am. J. Health-Syst. Pharm.* 58(11):120. 9. Wilt T *et al* (2002) *Cochrane Database Syst. Rev.* (1):CD001044.

PYRETHRUM
CHRYSANTHEMUM CINERARIAEFOLIUM (TREV) VIS.
C. COCCINEUM WILLD.
C. MARSHALLII ASCHERS.
Fam. Asteraceae

SYNONYMS: Insect Flowers, Dalmation Insect Flowers, *Pyrethrum cinerariifolium* Trev. *Tanacetum cinerariifolium* (Trev.) Sch. Bip. *C. coccineum* and *C. marshallii* are known as Persian and Causasian Insect Flowers, respectively.

HABITAT: Indigenous to the Balkans but widely cultivated elsewhere.

Description: The unopened flower-heads are preferred; they are about 7 cm in diameter, with two or three rows of lanceolate greenish-yellow, hairy bracts. The receptacle is nearly flat, without paleae; the ligulate florets are creamy-white and the tubular florets yellow. Taste: slightly acrid; odourless.

PART USED: Flowers.

CONSTITUENTS: (i) Pyrethrins; esters of chrysanthemic and pyrethric acids, known as pyrethrins I and II, cinerins I and II, jasmolins I and II etc. (ii) Sesquiterpene lactones (iii) Pyrethrol, a triterpenoid [R3;1,2,3,4].

MEDICINAL USE: Insecticide [R1]. The natural pyrethrins are used to treat lice and scabies infestations, and have been used to develop semi-synthetic derivatives such as permethrin, phenothrin, tetramethrin, cypermethrin and decamethrin, which can be more potent and offer more chemical stability. Pyrethrin I is the most potent of the naturally occurring compounds, although all have a knock-down effect on the insect. All have been shown to have clinical efficacy [1,3], although the semi-synthetic compounds are more likely to lead to resistance arising because of the longer persistence. Pyrethrum is relatively harmless to humans and animals, and may be used as a spray, lotion or powder, or for fumigation.

SPECIFIC REFERENCES: 1. Haustein U-F *et al* (1991) *Hautzart* 42(1):9. 2. Kasaj D F *et al* (1999) *Chromatographia* 50(9–10):607. 3. Dewick P (2002) In: *Medicinal Natural Products* 2nd ed. Pub Wiley, UK:188. 4. Verma K *et al* (1984) *J. Commun. Dis.* 16(2):144.

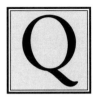

QUASSIA
PICRASMA EXCELSA (SW.) PLANCH
QUASSIA AMARA L.
Fam. Simaroubaceae

SYNONYMS: Bitter Wood. Jamaica Quassia, *Picraenia excelsa* Lindl.,
(= *P. excelsa*); Surinam Quassia (= *Q. amara*). Japanese Quassia is
Picrasma ailanthoides Planch., (= *P. quassinoides* Bennett).

HABITAT: P. excelsa is native to the West Indies, *Q. amara* to South
America and *P. ailanthoides* to the Far East.

DESCRIPTION: Quassia occurs in commerce as logs, chips or shredded.
The wood is whitish, becoming yellow on exposure to the air. Cork
may be present, with blackish or greyish markings due to fungus,
in inferior samples. Taste: intensely bitter; odourless.

PART USED: Wood.

CONSTITUENTS: (i) Quassinoids; quassin, isoquassin (= picrasmin),
neoquassin, 18-hydroxyquassin, paraine and nigakilactone A in
P. excelsa; and quassin, quassinol, neoquassin, quassialactol, quassimarin
and similikalactone in *Q. amara. P. ailanthoides* contains nigakilactones
A–N and nigakihemiacetals A–F [1,2,3,4,5,6] (ii) Alkaloids; beta-
carbolines, in *P. excelsa* and *Q. amara;* including canthin-6-one,
2-methoxycanthin-6-one, 5-methoxycanthin-6-one, 4-methoxy-5-
hydroxycanthin-6-one and N-methyl-1-*vinyl*-beta-carboline [7,8,9].
P. ailanthoides contains a series of picrasidine alkaloids [10].

MEDICINAL USE: Tonic, bitter, insecticide, anthelmintic, febrifuge, antimalarial [R1]. Quassia has been used clinically as a fresh infusion to treat
head lice [11]. The quassinoids are responsible for the bitterness and most
of the pharmacological activity; many of them are amoebicidal *in vitro*
and *in vivo* [6,12,13]. The alkaloids do not appear to contribute to the
anti-malarial activity [14]. Anti-fertility effects have been reported for the
crude methanol extract, which inhibited both basal and LH (luteinizing
hormone)-stimulated steroidogenesis in rat Leydig cells *in vitro* [15]. It
also caused a reduction in the weight of testis, epididymis and seminal
vesicles, and a decrease in serum levels of testosterone and LH [16].
Quassimarin has been reported to have anti-leukaemic properties [2].
Quassia extracts have been used to expel threadworms, administered as
an enema. Some of the quassinoids are anti-tuberculous *in vitro* [17] and
the nagakilactones have anti-ulcer activity in rats [18]. Quassia has long
been used as a bitter flavouring in alcoholic and soft drinks.

PREPARATIONS AND DOSE: Powdered wood, dose: 0.3–0.6 g

SPECIFIC REFERENCES: 1. Wagner H *et al* (1980) *Planta Med.* 38:204.
2. Kupchan S *et al* (1976) *J. Org. Chem.* 41:3481. 3. Murae T *et al*
(1973) *Tetrahedron* 29:1515. 4. Murae T *et al* (1975) *Chem. Pharm.
Bull.* 23(9):2191. 5. Dou J *et al* (1996) *Int. J. Chromatog.* 34(5):349. 6.
Polonsky J (1973) *Fortschr. Chem. Org. Nat.* 30:101. 7. Wagner H *et al*
(1979) *Planta Med.* 36:113. 8. Barbetti P *et al* (1987) *Planta Med.*
53(3):289 and (1990)56(2):216. 9. Njar V *et al* (1993) *Planta Med.*

59(3):259. 10. Li H-Y *et al* (1993) *Chem. Pharm. Bull.* 41(10):1807. 11. Jensen O *et al* (1978) *Acta Dermatol. Venereol.* 58:557. 12. Harris A *et al* (1982) *J. Pharm. Pharmacol.* 34(Supple.1)P43. 13. Ajaiyeoba E *et al* (1999) *J. Ethnopharmacol.* 67(3):321. 14. Bray D *et al* (1987) *Phytother. Res.* 1(1):22. 15. Njar *et al* (1995) *Planta Med.* 61(2):180. 16. Raji Y *et al* (1997) *Life Sci.* 61(11):1067. 17. Rahman S *et al* (1997) *Chem. Pharm. Bull.* 45(9):1527. 18. Niiho Y *et al* (1994) *Natural Med.* 48(2):116.

QUEBRACHO

ASPIDOSPERMA QUEBRACHO-BLANCO SCHLECHT.
AND OTHER SPECIES
Fam. Apocynaceae

SYNONYMS: White Quebracho. Red Quebracho is *Schinopsis quebracho-colorado* (Schlecht) Barkl. et T Meyer.

HABITAT: Argentina.

DESCRIPTION: The bark occurs in curved or flat pieces up to about 2.5 cm thick, greyish and deeply fissured externally. The inner surface is yellowish-brown, often with a reddish tint, and striated. The transverse fracture shows a coarsely granular outer layer and a fibrous or splintery, darker inner layer. Taste: bitter; odourless.

PART USED: Bark.

CONSTITUENTS: (i) Indole alkaloids; aspidospermine, aspidospermatine, akuammicine, yohimbine (= quebrachine), eburnaminine, quebrachamine, pyrifolidine and others [1,2,3]. Cell cultures have also yielded aspidochibine and 3-oxo-14,15-dehydrorhazinilam [4] (ii) Cyclitols such as quebrachitol [5] (iii) Tannins, including tannic acid [6,7,8].

MEDICINAL USE: Anti-asthmatic, tonic, febrifuge [R1]. The alkaloids are alpha adrenergic receptor blockers, and have hypotensive (but arterial hypertensive), spasmolytic and diuretic effects, with respiratory stimulant and peripheral vasoconstricting actions. Yohimbine has been used to treat erectile dysfunction in men and an extract of Quebracho improved this, and also libido, in a small study in males [9]. For actions of yohimbine, see Yohimbe. The tannin extract has been used as a drench to treat parasitic infections in sheep, with some success [7], although dietary administration was less effective and may lead to toxicity [8]. Large doses have toxic effects, including nausea and vomiting. The tannins have astringent and antimicrobial activity [4].

REGULATORY STATUS: POM.

SPECIFIC REFERENCES: 1. Lyon R *et al* (1973) *J. Pharm. Sci.* 62:218. 2. Deutsch H *et al* (1994) *J. Pharm. Biomed. Anal.* 12(10):1283. 3. Wolf J (1996) *Pharm. Ztg.* 141(35):34. 4. Aimi N *et al* (1991) *Tet. Lett.* 32(37):4949. 5. Nishibe S *et al* (2001) *Natural Med.* 55(5):268. 6. Makkar H *et al* (1995) *Br. J. Nutr.* 73(6):897. 7. Athanasiadou S *et al* (2001) *Br. J. Nutr.* 86(6):697. 8. Athanasiadou S *et al* (2001) *Vet. Parasitol.* 99(3):205. 9. Sperling H *et al* (1999) *Urologie – Ausgabe A* 38(1):56.

QUEEN'S DELIGHT

STILLINGIA SYLVATICA L.
Fam. Euphorbiaceae

SYNONYMS: Queen's Root, Yaw Root.

HABITAT: North America.

DESCRIPTION: The root usually occurs in tapering, tough, fibrous pieces. It is greyish-brown externally with a pinkish-white wood, showing numerous small resin glands. Taste: bitter and acrid; odour: characteristic and unpleasant.

PART USED: Root.

CONSTITUENTS: (i) Diterpene esters of the daphnane and tigliane type, including prostatin and gnidilatin (ii) Fixed oil, composed mainly of gamma-tocotrienol [1,2].

MEDICINAL USE: Alterative, laxative, tonic, diuretic [R1]. It is generally given as a tonic and 'blood purifier' in combination with other remedies. The diterpene esters are irritant [1], however they are unstable and unlikely to be present in most extracts and preparations. The extract is sometimes used homoeopathically and is not thought to pose any risk [3]

SPECIFIC REFERENCES: 1. Adolph A *et al* (1980) *Tet. Lett.* 21:2887. 2. Aitzetmuller K *et al* (1992) *J. Chromatog.* 603(1–2):165. 3. Zahn P *et al* (1993) *Planta Med.* 59(7S.):A683.

QUINCE

CYDONIA OBLONGATA MILL.
Fam. Rosaceae

HABITAT: Native to the Middle East but cultivated elsewhere for its fruit.

DESCRIPTION: The seeds are usually clumped in a double row by the dried mucilage contained in the testa. In appearance and size they resemble apple pips but have been pressed into a more angular shape.

PART USED: Seeds, fruit.

CONSTITUENTS: Seeds: (i) Mucilage and pectin about 20% (ii) Amygdalin, about 0.4% (iii) Fixed oil, containing mainly oleic, capric, linoleic, and palmitic acids [R4;1,2]. Fruit: (i) Volatile flavour components such as the marmelo oxides and lactones, and quince oxepine [3,4] (ii) Sesterterpene esters based on vulgarosides [5].

MEDICINAL USE: Demulcent. The seeds have been used in diarrhoea and in the form of a lotion to soothe the eyes. The mucilage extracted from them has been shown to accelerate wound healing in experimental injuries in the rabbit [6]. The fruit is used to make jam.

SPECIFIC REFERENCES: 1. Karawya M *et al* (1980) *Planta Med.* 40(Suppl.1):68. 2. Turkoz S *et al* (1998) *Acta Pharm. Turc.* 40(1):39. 3. Winterhalter P *et al* (1991) *Tet. Lett.* 32(30):3669. 4. Naf R *et al* (1991) *Tet. Lett.* 32(35):4487. 5. De Tommasi N *et al* (1996) *J. Nat. Prod.* 59(3):267. 6. Hemmati A *et al* (2000) *J. Herbs Spices and Med. Plants* 7(4):41.

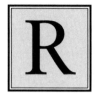

RAGWORT
SENECIO JACOBAEA L.
Fam. Asteraceae

SYNONYMS: Common Ragwort, Tansy Ragwort.

HABITAT: Grows as a common weed in many parts of the world.

DESCRIPTION: A medium or tall perennial, usually hairless. Leaves alternate, pinnately lobed, with the end lobe small and blunt, the segments deeply and irregularly toothed. Flowers rayed, 15–25 mm in diameter, daisy-like bright golden yellow, in dense, flat-topped clusters.

PART USED: Herb.

CONSTITUENTS: (i) Volatile oil, containing germacrene D and 1-undecene as the major components, with 1-nonene, myrcene, *trans*-ocimene and beta-caryophyllene [1] (ii) Pyrrolizidine alkaloids; seneciphylline, senecionine, jacoline, jaconine, jacobine, jacozine and others [2,3].

MEDICINAL USE: Formerly used as a diaphoretic, in coughs and colds and for rheumatism and gout [R1]. These alkaloids are hepatotoxic and also deplete vitamin A levels in animals [3]. Ragwort should not be taken internally or applied to broken skin. It has occasionally been used externally as an ointment or lotion for rheumatic pains, myalgia and other similar conditions.

SPECIFIC REFERENCES: 1. Matsuda H *et al* (1986) *Chem. Pharm. Bull.* 34(3):1153. 2. Segall H *et al* (1979) *Toxicol. Lett.* 4:193. 3. Moghaddam M *et al* (1989) *Toxicol. Lett.* 45(2–3):149.

RASPBERRY
RUBUS IDAEUS L.
Fam. Rosaceae

HABITAT: Cultivated in most temperate countries.

DESCRIPTION: Leaves stalked, pinnate with 3–5 leaflets, up to 12 cm in length, the terminal leaflet being longer than the others. Leaflets ovate, acuminate, rounded at the base, with an irregularly dentate, mucronate, toothed margin, green on the upper surface, white and densely tomentose on the lower. Taste: astringent; odourless. The fruits are well-known.

PART USED: Leaves. The fruit is very widely consumed as a dessert.

CONSTITUENTS: The leaves have not been well investigated, but contain: (i) Polypeptides (unspecified) (ii) Flavonoids, mainly glycosides of kaempferol and quercetin, including rutin (iii) Tannins [1,2,3]. The fruit contains: (i) Anthocyanins based on cyanidin [4] (ii) Monoterpene glycosides such as linalool arabinoglucoside [5]. The seed oil is composed of (i) Polyunsaturated neutral lipids and fatty acids (ii) Phospholipids (iii) Tocopherols, (up to a vitamin E equivalent of 97 mg/100 g) [6].

MEDICINAL USE: Raspberry leaf tea has been used for centuries to facilitate childbirth, and it is usually recommended that it be drunk freely before and during confinement for maximum benefit [R1]. A retrospective observational study on 108 mothers in Australia indicated that a shortening of labour and reduction in medical intervention occurred, with no untoward effects apart from a single case of diarrhoea and anecdotal reports of strong Braxton Hicks contractions [7]. However, a larger, randomized placebo-controlled trial of 192 women by the same authors did not confirm such benefits, although no adverse effects for either mother or baby were noted [8]. Uterine relaxant effects have been demonstrated in animals on several occasions [1,2,9], but despite attempts to fractionate the extract [8] no further identification of the active principle(s) has been made. The extract appears to affect only the pregnant uterus from both rats and humans, with no activity on the non-pregnant uterus [10]. Smooth muscle relaxant effects have also been documented for the extract using guinea pig ileum *in vitro* [11]. The leaf extract has been used as an astringent for diarrhoea and sore throat and is antimicrobial [12], and the cyanidin glycosides from the fruit are cyclo-oxygenase inhibitors and antioxidants [5].

PREPARATIONS AND DOSE: Dried leaf, dose: 4–8 g, three times daily as an infusion.

SPECIFIC REFERENCES: 1. Henning W (1981) *Leibens. Unters. Forsch.* 173:180. 2. Beckett A *et al* (1954) *J. Pharm. Pharmacol.* 6:785. 3. Czygan F-C (1995) *Z. Phytother.* 16(6):366. 4. Pabst A *et al* (1991) *Tet. Lett.* 32(37):4885. 5. Seeram N *et al* (2001) *Phytomedicine* 8(5):362. 6. Oomah B *et al* (2000) *Food Chem.* 69(2):187. 7. Parsons M *et al* (1999) *Austral. Coll. Midwives Inc. J.* 9:20. 8. Simpson M *et al* (2001) *J. Midwifery Womens Health* 46(2):51. 9. Patel A *et al* (1995) *J. Pharm. Pharmacol.* 47:1129. 10. Bamford D *et al* (1970) *Br. J. Pharmacol.* 40(1):161P. 11. Rojas-Vera J *et al* (2002) *Phytother. Res.* 16(7):665. 12. Rauha J-P *et al* (2000) *Int. J. Food Microbiol.* 56(1):3.

RAUWOLFIA

RAUWOLFIA SERPENTINA (L.) KURTZ.
R. VOMITORIA AFZ. AND OTHER SPECIES.
Fam. Apocynaceae

SYNONYMS: Snakeroot, Indian Snakeroot. *R. vomitoria* is African Rauwolfia.

HABITAT: R. serpentina is indigenous to India; *R. vomitoria* to Africa.

DESCRIPTION: R. serpentina root occurs in commerce as cylindrical or tapering, tortuous pieces, about 2 cm in diameter, with few branches or rootlets. The outer surface is yellowish-brown and wrinkled. *R. vomitoria* root is larger, with a greyish-brown exterior. Taste: very bitter; odourless.

PART USED: Root.

CONSTITUENTS: (i) Indole alkaloids, the most important being reserpine, with rescinnamine, reserpinine, ajmaline (rauwolfine),

369

isoajmaline (isorauwolfine), ajmalinine, ajmalicine, rauwolfinine, sarpagine, serpentine, reserpiline, serpentinine, and many others; in *R. vomitoria*, similar compounds occur as well as yohimbine, reserpoxidine, *epi*-rescinnamine and seredine [R3,R14 and refs therein;1,2].

MEDICINAL USE: Used since time immemorial in India to treat insomnia and various forms of mental illness. A small study in India of a preparation containing Rauwolfia (with other herbs) has suggested potential for treating insomnia [3]. Many of the effects are due to the presence of reserpine, which has antihypertensive and antipsychotic effects. It depletes noradrenaline stores in peripheral sympathetic nerve terminals and reduces catecholamines and serotonin in the brain, and for this reason it can cause severe depression. It is very potent and causes toxicity in overdose. There are reports that the incidence of breast cancer is higher in women taking reserpine, but these are controversial [4,5]. The use of Rauwolfia in schizophrenia has been superceded by more modern antispychotic agents; and reserpine is now used more often as a biochemical tool in scientific research because of its properties of depleting neurotransmitters. It is also an efflux inhibitor, and reduces multi-drug resistance in bacteria. Ajmaline is an anti-arrhythmic drug used clinically in Japan [R3].

REGULATORY STATUS: POM.

SPECIFIC REFERENCES: 1. Court W *et al* (1982) *Planta Med.* 45:105 and (1983)48:228. 2. Lovati M *et al* (1996) *Fitoterapia* 67(5):422. 3. Rani P *et al* (1998) *Phytomedicine* 5(4):253. 4. Labarthe D *et al* (1980) *JAMA* 243:2304. 5. Friedman G (1983) *J. Chronic Dis.* 36:367.

RED CLOVER
TRIFOLIUM PRATENSE L.
Fam. Fabaceae

HABITAT: Widely distributed throughout Europe including Britain, naturalized in North America and many other parts of the world.

DESCRIPTION: The flower-heads are globular or egg-shaped, sometimes paired, usually unstalked, reddish-purple, about 2–3 cm long and 2 cm broad, composed of numerous individual, typically papilionaceous keeled flowers. Leaflets trefoil, often with a whitish crescent; stipules triangular.

PART USED: Flower-heads.

CONSTITUENTS: (i) Isoflavones; afrormosin, biochanin A, daidzein, formononetin, genistein, pratensein calyconin, pseudobaptigenin, orobol, irilone, and trifoside and their glycoside conjugates (ii) Other flavonoids, including pectolinarin and trifoliin (= isoquercitrin) (iii) Coumarins; coumestrol, medicagol and coumarin (iv) Volatile oil, containing furfural (v) Miscellaneous; Clovamides, L-dopa-caffeic acid conjugates, minerals, vitamins and phytoalexins etc. [R7;1,2,3].

MEDICINAL USE: Alterative, antispasmodic, expectorant, sedative, dermatological agent [R1]. It is traditionally used mainly as a tonic and for skin complaints such as psoriasis and eczema, and as an expectorant in coughs and bronchial conditions. More recently red clover has been used as a source of isoflavones, as a form of hormone replacement therapy. These are oestrogenic in animals [4], but the clinical use for menopausal women has not yet been well supported by clinical studies [5,6] apart from a beneficial effect on hot flushes [7]. An extract was found to reduce pain in a small, randomized, placebo controlled trial of women with cyclical mastalgia [8] and research continues. Biochanin A was shown to inhibit metabolic activation of the carcinogen, benzo(a)pyrene, in a mammalian cell culture, which suggests chemopreventive properties [3,9]. Red Clover extracts also inhibit cytochrome P450 3A4 *in vitro* [10].

PREPARATIONS AND DOSE: Dried flowers, dose: 4 g or equivalent extract, three times daily.

REGULATORY STATUS: GSL.

SPECIFIC REFERENCES: 1. Dewick P (1977) *Phytochem.* 16:93. 2. Klejdus B *et al* (2001) *Anal. Chim. Acta* 450(1–2):81. 3. Chae Y-H *et al* (1991) *Cancer Lett.* 60(1):15. 4. Burdette J *et al* (2002) *J. Nutr.* 132(1):27. 5. Fugh-Berman A *et al* (2001) *Menopause* 8(5):333. 6. Hale G *et al* (2001) *Menopause* 8(5):338. 7. Van der Weijer P *et al* (2001) *N. Am. Menopause Soc.* 12th Ann. Meeting Oct 4–6 New Orleans P077. 8. Ingram D *et al* (2001) *Breast* 10:1054. 9. Cassady J *et al* (1988) *Cancer Res.* 48(22):6257. 10. Budzinski J *et al* (2000) *Phytomed.* 7(4):273.

RED ROOT
CEANOTHUS AMERICANUS L.
Fam. Rhamnaceae

SYNONYMS: Jersey Tea Root.

HABITAT: North America.

DESCRIPTION: Root tough, woody, dark brown, striated or finely wrinkled longitudinally. Bark thin, brittle, deep brown; wood, reddish, with obscure concentric rings. Taste: astringent; odourless.

PART USED: Root.

CONSTITUENTS: Little information available (i) Flavonoids based on quercetin and kaempferol [1]. The related species *C. integerrimus* and *C. sanguineus* contain cyclopeptide alkaloids including ceanothin B, discarine, frangufoline, and myrianthine [2].

MEDICINAL USE: Astringent, expectorant, antispasmodic [R1]. *C. integerrimus* has been shown to have antiviral and anti-tumour activities *in vitro* [3].

SPECIFIC REFERENCES: 1. Pinchon-Prum N *et al* (1985) *Ann. Pharm. Francaises* 43(1):27. 2. Lagarias J *et al* (1979) *J. Nat. Prod.* 42:220 and 663. 3. Nakanishi T *et al* (1993) *Jpn. J. Pharmacog.* 7:295.

REHMANNIA

REHMANNIA GLUTINOSA (GAERTN.) LIBOSCH.
Fam. Scrophulariaceae

SYNONYMS: Chinese Foxglove, Di Huang (Chinese), Shojio (Japanese).

HABITAT: China, Japan and other parts of Southeast Asia.

DESCRIPTION: A perennial herb reaching about 40 cm, with light reddish-purple tubular flowers. The root is orange, thick and tuberous, with a sweetish taste. In Chinese medicine it is used fresh, dried and cured.

PART USED: Root.

CONSTITUENTS: (i) Iridoid glycosides including the rehmanniosides A-D, jioglutosides and rehmaglutins A-D, aucubin, ajugol and catalpol (ii) Phenethyl alcohol glycosides called jionosides A,B etc.; acetoside, isoacetoside, purpureaside C, cistanoside A and F and others [R17;1,2]

MEDICINAL USE: Antipyretic, anti-inflammatory, anti-haemorrhagic, restorative to the adrenal glands. The uncured root is used traditionally in China for skin rashes, diabetes and bleeding, the cured root for disorders of menstruation and anaemia. Rehmannia is also used to support normal adrenal function during corticosteroid therapy and (unlike liquorice for example) it is not hypertensive. Administration to rabbits raised serum corticosteroid levels, which had been depressed after treatment with dexamethasone [3], and abolished immunosup-pressive effects induced by both dexamethasone and cyclophos-phamide, in mice. The jionosides demonstrated aldose reductase activity [4]. Other tests in which Rehmannia showed beneficial properties include experimental arthritis in rats, protective effects on various organs during chemotherapy of tumour-bearing mice [R17;5] and an increase in nitrogen excretion in rats with renal failure [6]. See [R17].

SPECIFIC REFERENCES: 1. Tang W *et al* (1992) *In: Chinese Drugs of Plant Origin.* Pub Springer-Verlag, Berlin. 2. Sasaki H *et al* (1989) *Planta Med.* 55:458. 3. Cha L *et al* (1988) *Chin. J. Integr. Trad. West. Med.* 8(2):95. 4. Nishimura H *et al* (1990) *Planta Med.* 56:684. 5. Kubo M *et al* (1994) *Biol. Pharm. Bull.* 17(9):1282. 6. Yokozawa T *et al* (1995) *Phytother. Res.* 9(1):1.

REISHI MUSHROOM

GANODERMA LUCIDUM (CURTIS FR.) P KARST.
G. JAPONICUM (FR. LLOYD) AND OTHER SPECIES
Fam. Polyporaceae

SYNONYMS: Ling Zhi, Chi Zhi (Chinese), Mannentake (Japanese).
G. japonicum = *G. chinensis* Zhao, Xu et Zhang.

HABITAT: China, Japan and North America, growing on tree stumps, mainly of conifers. It is now cultivated for commerce.

DESCRIPTION: Reishi takes several widely varying forms, including a more rare, branched or 'antler' type, in addition to the usual mushroom shape. The colour varies from red to black, through yellow, orange and brown. Generally, the red and antlered varieties are more highly prized. The cap is circular, semi-circular, kidney or fan-shaped, leathery with either a smooth or rippled upper surface. The undersurface shows the spore tubes.

PART USED: Mature fruiting body of the fungus.

CONSTITUENTS: (i) Triterpenes, mainly lanostane type, such as the ganoderic acids A-Z, with ganoderals A and B, ganoderiols A and B, epoxyganoderiols A-C, ganolucidic acids A-E, lucidones A-C, lucidenic acids A-M and others, over (ii) Polysaccharides, mainly glucans and arabino-oxyglucans (iii) Peptidoglycans known as ganoderans A-C [1,2,3,4].

MEDICINAL USE: Classically used as an adaptogen and general tonic, to prolong life, prevent ageing and generally improve well-being and mental faculties, Reishi is one of the most thoroughly researched of all Chinese medicines. It was immortalized in Chinese and Japanese paintings and statues and was used by Taoist monks. It is now widely used in cancer patients as an adjunct to chemotherapy and radiation treatment, to support immune resistance, and as a sedative, liver protectant and cholesterol-lowering agent. The active principles are considered to be the triterpenes and polysaccharides. Antihypertensive effects have been observed, due to inhibition of angiotensin converting enzyme inhibition [4], and cholesterol-lowering effects were noted in animals [5]. The most important application is still as an immune-system enhancer, and various animal and clinical studies support such a use; many of these are in literature not easily available but are well-reviewed in [1]. The antioxidant, hepatoprotective and radioprotective effects are supported by clinical and other studies [6,7] and are well-reviewed in [1].

PREPARATIONS AND DOSE: Dried powder, dose: 6–12 g or equivalent extract daily.

SPECIFIC REFERENCES: 1. Reishi Mushroom. *American Herbal Pharmacopoeia and Therapeutic Compendium* 2000. Ed. Upton R. Pub: AHP, Santa Cruz, US. 2. Nishitoba T *et al* (1985) *Agric. Biol. Chem.* 49(6):1793, (5):1547, (12):3637; (1986) 50(3):809, (1988) 52(1):211, 52(2):367. 3. Sato H *et al* (1997) *Agric. Biol. Chem.* 50(11):2887. 4. Morigiwa A *et al* (1986) *Chem. Pharm. Bull.* 34(7):3025. 5. Shiao M *et al* (1994) *J. Am. Chem. Soc.* 547:432. 6. Chen W *et al* (1995) *Phytother. Res.* 9(7):533. 7. Lee J-M *et al* (2001) *Phytother. Res.* 15(3):245.

REST HARROW

ONONIS SPINOSA L.
Fam. Fabaceae

SYNONYMS: Cammock, Spiny Rest Harrow.

HABITAT: Common on arable and wasteland throughout Europe and Russia.

DESCRIPTION: A woody perennial, with roundish leaves, oval or trefoil spines, flowers in leafy spikes, pink, papilionaceous, with the wings equalling the keel. The root is more or less flattened, twisted and branched, deeply wrinkled and brown in colour. Taste: sweet and mucilaginous at first, then rather bitter; odour: resembling that of liquorice.

PART USED: Root, aerial parts.

CONSTITUENTS: (i) Volatile oil, containing *trans*-anethole as the major component, with menthone, isomenthone, camphor, linalool, menthol, estragole, borneol, carvone and *cis*-anethole (ii) Phenolics; trifolirfizin and other pterocarpans, tannins etc. (iii) Lectins and phytohaemaglutinins (iv) Triterpenes; alpha-onocerin, beta-sitosterol etc. In the aerial parts: Flavonoids, isoflavones and pterocarpans; rutin, hyperoside, cosmosiin, myricetrin, and apigenin, vitexin, luteolin, kaempferol, quercetin, faceidin, penduletin, formononetin, tectorigenin, and biochanin A glycosides [1,2,3,4].

MEDICINAL USE: Diuretic, anti-lithic, anti-inflammatory, expectorant [R1]. Rest Harrow is used mainly for its effects on the urinary system, as an infusion. Recent studies in animals have supported these uses to some extent [5].

SPECIFIC REFERENCES: 1. Hilp K *et al* (1975) *Arch. Pharm.* 308:429. 2. Koster J *et al* (1983) *Planta Med.* 48:131. 3. Kartnig T *et al* (1985) *Helv. Chim. Acta* 60(9–10):253. 4. Kirmizigul S *et al* (1997) *J. Nat. Prod.* 60(4):378. 5. Bolle P *et al* (1993) *Pharmacol. Res.* 27 (Suppl.1):27.

RHATANY

KRAMERIA TRIANDRA RUIZ ET PAVON
Fam. Krameriaceae

SYNONYMS: Peruvian Rhatany. Para Rhatany is *K. argentea* Mart.

HABITAT: Peru, Bolivia.

DESCRIPTION: Root woody, cylindrical, deep reddish-brown and rough externally, with a coarsely fibrous bark and hard, tough, woody centre. Taste: very astringent; odourless.

PART USED: Root.

CONSTITUENTS: (i) Tannins, exclusively condensed tannins composed of procyanidins and propelargonidins (ii) Lignans, neolignans and norlignans, including kramentosan, conocarpan and decurrenal (iii) Benzofurans such as ratanhiaphenols I and II (iv) Phlobaphene; a pigment known as krameria red [R3;1,2,3,4].

MEDICINAL USE: Astringent. Rhatany is used as an anti-diarrhoeal, styptic, anti-haemorrhagic and vulnerary. It may be used as an infusion or decoction internally for diarrhoea or haemorrhage, including menorrhagia, as an ointment or suppository for haemorrhoids, topically for chilblains and wounds, as a lozenge, gargle or mouthwash for gingivitis and pharyngitis. The astringency is due to those polyphenols (tannins) with a degree of polymerization of more than five units [1]. The extract is antiviral against *Herpes simplex* type I [5] and antibacterial against *Yersinia enterocolitica, Staphylococcus aureus,* and others [6].

PREPARATIONS AND DOSE: Dried root, dose: 0.5–2 g or equivalent extract, three times daily.

SPECIFIC REFERENCES: 1. Scholz R *et al* (1986) *Planta Med.* 52(6):58P. 2. Williams V *et al* (1983) *Phytochem.* 22:569. 3. De Bellis O *et al* (1994) *Fitoterapia* 65(6):503. 4. Silva S *et al* (2001) *Nat. Prod. Lett.* 15(5):323. 5. Lohezic F *et al* (1999) *Pharm. Pharmacol. Res. Comm.* 5(3):249. 6. Djipa C *et al* (2000) *J. Ethnopharmacol.* 71(1–2):307.

RHUBARB
CHINESE RHUBARB
INDIAN RHUBARB
JAPANESE RHUBARB
ENGLISH RHUBARB

RHEUM OFFICINALE BAILL.
R. PALMATUM L. AND OTHER VARIETIES AND HYBRIDS.
R. EMODI WALL.
R. PALMATUM (= R. COREANUM)
R. RHAPONTICUM WILLD.
Fam. Polygonaceae

SYNONYMS: Chinese Rhubarb; Dahuang; Indian Rhubarb; Himalayan Rhubarb; English Rhubarb; Rhapontic Rhubarb; Garden Rhubarb.

HABITAT: Most Rhubarb is cultivated, the origin being shown by the name.

DESCRIPTION: Chinese Rhubarb comes in different grades and sizes; the older rhizome is larger and occurs in peeled flats or rounds, often with circular holes made for hanging by a string during the drying process. The cut surface has a bright yellow, marbled or reticulate appearance due to the reddish-brown medullary rays; when freshly cut it is pinkish. Poorer quality grades are paler and less carefully peeled. English Rhubarb, not normally found in commerce, is unpeeled, in smaller pieces and has red veins. Taste: bitter; odour: aromatic and characteristic.

PART USED: Rhizome. The young leaf stalks of English rhubarb are used for food.

CONSTITUENTS: (i) Anthraquinone derivatives; Chinese Rhubarb contains chrysophanic acid (= chrysophanol), emodin (= rheum emodin), aloe-emodin, rhein and physcion, with their O-glycosides (mainly monoglucosides) such as glucorhein, chrysophanein, glucoemodin; lesser amounts of the sennosides A-E, reidin C, rheinosides a, b, c and d, and others [1,2,3,4]. Both Indian and Japanese Rhubarbs contain similar anthraquinones, but English Rhubarb contains only chrysophanic acid and some of its glycosides [1] (ii) Tannins and procyanidins; in Chinese Rhubarb, d-catechin and epicatechin gallate, with various cinnamoyl and coumaroyl galloyl glucosides and fructoses [5] (iii) Stilbene derivatives; in English Rhubarb: rhaponticin (= rhapontin), and in *R. undulatum* L. and others, rhaponticin and its gallates, and rhapontigenin, piceatannol and resveratrol [6].

MEDICINAL USE: Astringent, aperient, tonic, stomachic [R1]. In large doses Rhubarb is a laxative. English Rhubarb is similar but milder in action. It has been shown to have both astringent and cathartic properties [7]; the tannins are astringent and the anthraquinones are laxative (see also Senna). Emodin and aloe-emodin are cytotoxic to some cultured tumour cell lines, to a greater extent than to normal cells, and constituents such as resveratrol are known to be chemoprotectants [8]. Emodin is also a selective inhibitor of casein kinase II [9] and a potent antioxidant [10]. Several of the constituents, in all categories, are anti-inflammatory and inhibit 5-lipoxygenase [11], and the stilbenes are also known to inhibit NFkappaB activation, which helps to explain the anti-inflammatory activity [12]. They are anti-allergic, particularly rapontigenin and piceatannol [13]. In Chinese medicine Rhubarb is very highly regarded; it is used for jaundice, abdominal pains, indigestion, amenorrhoea, kidney disease, scalds and burns. It was shown to have some protective effects on the progression of experimental chronic renal failure in rats [14] and the tannins, especially epicatechin gallate, reduced blood levels of urea nitrogen in rats with adenine-induced renal failure [15]. The galloyl esters interfere with the biosynthesis of cholesterol [5]. Very few clinical trial results are available for Rhubarb; however, haemostatic effects were shown in a double blind, randomized trial of 175 patients with bleeding peptic ulcer [16], and beneficial effects in severe acute pancreatitis (including a reduction in multiple organ failure) have been described [17].

PREPARATIONS AND DOSE: Dried root and rhizome, dose: 0.2–1 g or equivalent extract, three times daily.

SPECIFIC REFERENCES: 1. Zwaving J et al (1972) *Planta Med.* 21:254. 2. Oshio H et al (1974) *Chem. Pharm. Bull.* 22:823. 3. Kashiwada Y et al (1984) *Chem. Pharm. Bull.* 32(9):3461. 4. Yamagishi T et al (1987) *Chem. Pharm. Bull.* 35(8):3132. 5. Abe I et al (2000) *Planta Med.* 66(8):753. 6. Matsuda H et al (2001) *Bioorg. Chem. Lett.* 9(1):41. 7. Fairbairn J et al (1976) *Pharmacol.* 14(Suppl.1):48. 8. Shi Y-Q et al (2001) *Anticancer Res.* 21(4A):2847. 9. Yim H et al (1999) *Planta Med.* 65(1):9. 10. Yuan Z et al (1997) *Pharm. Pharmcol. Lett.* 7(1):9. 11. Miyamoto H et al (2001) *Natural Med.* 55(4):159. 12. Kageura T et al (2001) *Bioorg. Chem. Lett.* 9(7):1887. 13. Matsuda H et al (2001) *Biol. Pharm. Bull.* 24(3):264. 14. Zhang G et al (1996) *Nephrol. Dialysis Trans.* 11(1):186. 15. Yokozawa T et al (1991) *Nephron* 58(2):155. 16. Peigen X et al (1988) *Phytotherapy Res.* 2(2):55. 17. Yan M et al (2001) *Chin. J. Gastroenterol.* 6(2):94.

RICE
ORYZA SATIVA L.
Fam. Gramineae

HABITAT: Widely cultivated in wet, tropical areas.

DESCRIPTION: The grains hardly require description.

PART USED: Seeds; oil.

CONSTITUENTS: The fixed oil, expressed from the bran contains (i) Fatty acids; mainly unsaturated: oleic, linoleic and alpha-linolenic acids, with some saturated (palmitic and stearic) acids (ii) Sterols and triterpenes including beta-sitosterol, campesterol, stigmasterol, squalene and gamma-oryzanol (a mixture of ferulic acid esters of triterpene alcohols) (iii) Tocotrienols and alpha-tocopherol [1, and refs therein]. The seed also contains starch.

MEDICINAL USE: Nutritive, demulcent [R1]. Boiled Rice is easily digested in gastric upsets and rice-water, similar to barley water, can be made. It is included in several oral rehydration products for treating diarrhoea. Rice bran oil has numerous beneficial effects on health, the most important probably being the lowering of blood cholesterol levels and anti-atherosclerotic effects. These are due mainly to the gamma-oryzanol and phytosterol fraction and have been confirmed in several clinical studies, and mechanisms of action have been postulated. There do not appear to be any toxicity issues. The chemistry, pharmacology and clinical uses of rice bran oil have been well reviewed recently [1]. Fermented rice bran is now being suggested as a nutritional supplement, as it contains many essential amino acids, and has recently been shown to have an anti-stress and anti-fatigue effect in rodents [2].

SPECIFIC REFERENCES: 1. Cicero A *et al* (2001) *Phytother. Res.* 15(4):277. 2. Kim K *et al* (2002) *Phytother. Res.* 16(7):700.

RINGWORM BUSH
CASSIA ALATA L.
Fam. Caesalpiniaceae

HABITAT: Native to tropical America, widely naturalized and cultivated in moist tropical areas.

SYNONYMS: Ringworm Shrub, Kinkeliba, Candelabra Bush, Candle Tree.

DESCRIPTION: A small tree or large shrub, reaching up to 3 m, with compound pinnate leaves up to 40 cm long. The flowers are attractive, golden yellow, terminal racemes, up to 30 cm long, developing into long, dark brown, winged pods containing up to 50 quadrangular seeds.

PART USED: Leaves.

CONSTITUENTS: (i) Anthraquinone glycosides, mainly aloe-emodin, chrysarobin, chrysophanol and rhein (ii) Triterpenes including daucosterol, beta-sitosterol (iii) Flavonoids; kaempferol, lutein and their glycosides [R12,1,2,3].

377

MEDICINAL USE: Traditionally used to treat skin diseases such as ringworm, it is anti-fungal, antibacterial [1], analgesic and anti-inflammatory [2]. It is also taken internally for stomach complaints, and the anthraquinones are laxative (see Senna, Rhubarb). Several clinical studies have supported the traditional use for ringworm, other fungal infections and ezcema [3,4].

SPECIFIC REFERENCES: 1. Ogunti E *et al* (1991) *Fitoterapia* 62(2):537. 2. Palanichamy S *et al* (1990) *Fitoterapia* 61(1):442. 3. Palanichamy S *et al* (1990) *J. Ethnopharmacol.* 29(1):73 and 29(3):337. 4. Damodaran S *et al* (1994) *J. Ethnopharmacol.* 42(1):19.

ROSE
ROSA GALLICA L.
R. DAMASCENA MILL. AND OTHER SPP.
Fam. Rosaceae

HABITAT: Cultivated throughout the world.

DESCRIPTION: A common, thorny, garden shrub needing no description.

PART USED: Flowers.

CONSTITUENTS: Volatile oil, containing beta-phenethyl alcohol, geraniol, nerol, citronellol, geranic acid, eugenol, myrcene and many other constituents [R3,R19;1].

MEDICINAL USE: Rarely used medicinally, but the oil is an important ingredient of many cosmetics and perfumes, and used as a flavouring agent. It is generally non-sensitising and non-irritant. The fruits of the Dog Rose (q.v.) are used as an astringent and source of vitamin C [R1,R18].

PREPARATIONS: Concentrated Rose Water BPC 1949, Rose Oil BPC 1949.

ROSEMARY
ROSMARINUS OFFICINALIS L.
Fam. Lamiaceae

HABITAT: Native to the Mediterranean region, cultivated widely elsewhere.

DESCRIPTION: Stem woody, quadrangular, branched; bearing linear leaves about 1.5–3.5 cm long, green above and whitish beneath, with strongly revolute margins. Flowers if present, bluish-lilac, two-lipped, with two stamens only. Taste and odour: aromatic, characteristic.

PART USED: Herb.

CONSTITUENTS: (i) Volatile oil, composed of borneol, camphene, camphor, cineole, limonene, linalool, isobornyl acetate, 3-octanone, terpineol, verbenol and others (ii) Flavonoids; apigenin, diosmetin, diosmin, genkwanin, 6-methoxygenkwanin, hispidulin, sinensetin, luteolin and derivatives (iii) Rosmarinic acid, caffeic, chlorogenic neochlorogenic and labiatic acids (iv) Diterpenes such as picrosalvin

(= carnosol), carnosolic acids and rosmariquinone (v) Triterpenes such as ursolic and oleanolic acids and their derivatives [R7;1,2,3,4].

MEDICINAL USE: Anti-inflammatory, tonic, astringent, diaphoretic, stomachic, nervine, anodyne, antiseptic [R1]. The anti-inflammatory properties of Rosemary extracts may be due to the rosmarinic acid, ursolic acid and apigenin, all of which have this effect [5]; rosmarinic acid has also been suggested as a possible potential treatment for septic shock, since it suppresses the endotoxin-induced activation of complement, the formation of prostacyclin, thrombocytopaenia and the concomitant release of thromboxane A2 [6]. Diosmin is also reported to be more effective in decreasing capillary fragility than rutin (see Rue). Antimicrobial activity is well known for Rosemary oil [2] and Rosemary extracts acid are antiviral, at least partly due to the rosmarinic and carnosolic acids content [4]. These compounds are also inhibitors of skin tumourigenesis [7], and Rosemary extract also inhibits DMBA-induced mammary tumourigenesis [8] and benzo(a)pyrene-induced genotoxicity in human bronchial cells [9]. The essential oil has spasmolytic and anticonvulsant effects on smooth muscle and cardiac muscle, due in part to anticholinesterase activity [10]. This also gives a mechanism by which the traditional use of Rosemary as 'the herb of remembrance' may help to improve the memory, and a possible use as an adjunctive treatment in dementia [11]. Other properties described include anti-hepatotoxic and cholagogic activity [12,13], and antioxidant effects [14]. Rosemary extracts are hyperglycaemic in animals and inhibit the release of insulin [15]. Rosemary has long been a popular ingredient of hair preparations, shampoos and tonics. It is a well-known culinary herb.

PREPARATIONS AND DOSE: Dried herb, dose: 2–4 g or equivalent extract, three times daily; Rosemary oil BPC 1973 and BP 2002.

SPECIFIC REFERENCES: 1. Panizzi L *et al* (1993) *J. Ethnopharmacol.* 39:167. 2. Collin M *et al* (1987) *Food Microbiol.* 4:311. 3. Litvinenko V *et al* (1970) *Planta Med.* 18:243. 4. Paris A *et al* (1993) *J. Nat. Prod.* 56:1426. 5. Parnham M (1985) *Drugs Future* 10:756. 6. Rampart M *et al* (1986) *Biochem. Pharmacol.* 35:1397. 7. Huang M-T *et al* (1994) *Cancer Res.* 54:701. 8. Singletary K (1991) *FASEB J.* 5:5A927. 9. Offord E *et al* (1995) *Carcinogenesis* 16(9):2057. 10. Hof S *et al* (1989) *Planta Med.* 55:106. 11. Howes M-J *et al* (1999) *J. Pharm. Pharmacol.* 51:S238. 12. Joyeux M *et al* (1995) *Phytother. Res.* 9:228. 13. Hoefler C *et al* (1987) *J. Ethnopharmacol.* 19:133. 14. Haraguchi H *et al* (1995) *Planta Med.* 61:333. 15. Al-Hader A *et al* (1994) *J. Ethnopharmacol.* 43:217.

ROSINWEED

SILPHIUM LACINIATUM L.
Fam. Asteraceae

SYNONYMS: Compass Weed.

HABITAT: Northern Europe.

DESCRIPTION: Fragments of leaves stiff, papery, brittle, hairless, with a faintly reticulate surface. Root up to about 5 cm long, 2–3 cm in diameter, laterally branched at the base, dark greyish-brown, striated longitudinally; the transverse section showing concentric lines and a radiate structure, variegated dark grey and white with a small central pith. Taste: bitter then acrid; odourless.

PART USED: Herb, root.

CONSTITUENTS: Inulin, in the root; terpenes, resin acids [R4]. Little information is available.

MEDICINAL USE: Formerly used as an antispasmodic, diuretic, expectorant, emetic [R1].

RUE
RUTA GRAVEOLENS L.
Fam. Rutaceae

SYNONYMS: Garden Rue, Herb of Grace, Herbygrass.

HABITAT: Native to southern Europe, cultivated in Britain and elsewhere as an ornamental.

DESCRIPTION: Leaves blue green, alternate, bipinnate, with oblanceolate segments, wedge-shaped below, with numerous translucent, small, punctate oil glands. Flowers yellow with five concave petals incurved at the tip, stem cylindrical, smooth and branched. Taste: pungent; odour: strong and characteristic.

PART USED: Herb.

CONSTITUENTS: (i) Volatile oil, containing 2-undecanone, 2-heptanol, 2-nonanol, 2-nonanone, limonene, pinene, anisic acid, phenol, guaiacol, linalyl acetate, menthol and others (ii) Rutin and other flavonoids such as quercetin (iii) Coumarins; bergapten, daphnoretin, isoimperatorin, naphthoherniarin, psoralen, pangelin, rutamarin, rutarin, rutaciltin, scopoletin, gravelliferone, and umbelliferone (iv) Alkaloids; arborine, arborineine, gamma-fagarine, graveoline, graveolinine, kokusaginine, rutacridine, skimmianine, 1-hydroxy-3-methoxy-N-methylacridone (v) Lignans, in the root; savinin and helioxanthin [1,2,3,4,5,6].

MEDICINAL USE: Stimulant, antispasmodic, emmenagogue [R1]. Rue is usually used as a uterine stimulant; it should only be taken in small doses and not by pregnant women. The volatile oil is reportedly anthelmintic. The furocoumarins can cause phototoxicity; this property is utilized in the treatment of psoriasis by psoralen derivatives. Rutin has been extensively investigated for its ability to reduce capillary fragility and is often taken as a food supplement. Its other properties include anti-oedema effects and it may be partly responsible for the anti-inflammatory effect of the herb observed in a number of animal tests [7,8]. The extract has antimicrobial activity [9] and calcium antagonistic activity when measured against potassium depolarization-induced contraction of guinea pig aortic strips [10].

It has also been shown to inhibit tumour formation on mouse skin induced by benzo(a)pyrene [11] and increase survival times of rats fed a thrombogenic diet [12].

PREPARATIONS AND DOSE: Dried herb, dose: 0.5–1 g or equivalent extract, three times daily.

BIBLICAL REFERENCES: Luke 11:42.

SPECIFIC REFERENCES: 1. Novak I *et al* (1967) *Planta Med.* 15:132.
2. Rosza Z *et al* (1980) *Planta Med.* 39:218 . 3. Schimmer O (1991)
Z. Phytother. 12:151. 4. Reisch J *et al.* (1967) *Pharmazie* 22:220
and (1975)25:435. 5. Varga E *et al* (1976) *Fitoterapia* 47:107.
6. Becela-Deller C (1995) *Z. Phytother.* 16:275. 7. Mascolo N
et al (1987) *Phytother. Res.* 1(1):28. 8. Atta A *et al* 91998)
J. Ethnopharmacol. 60(2):117. 9. Ojala T *et al* (2000)
J. Ethnopharmacol. 73(1–2):299. 10. Rauwald H *et al* (1994)
Phytother. Res. 8(3):135. 11. Van Duren B *et al* (1971) *J. Natl.
Cancer Inst.* 46:1039. 12. Robbins R (1967) *J. Atheroscler. Res.* 7:3.

RUPTUREWORT

HERNIARIA GLABRA L.
H. HIRSUTE L.
Fam. Caryophyllaceae

SYNONYMS: Smooth Rupturewort, Herniary.

HABITAT: Grows throughout Europe but is rare in Britain.

DESCRIPTION: A prostrate, bright green, more or less hairless plant.
Flowers green, sessile, in clusters at the base of the small, oval,
opposite leaves. Taste: insipid; odourless.

PART USED: Herb.

CONSTITUENTS: (i) Coumarins; herniarin, scopoletin, umbelliferone
(ii) Flavonoids; isorhamnetin, hyperoside and various quercetin
glycosides (iii) Phenolic acids; salicylic, ferulic, vanillic, p-coumaric,
caffeic and protocatechiuc (iv) Triterpene saponins, herniaria saponins
I-VII, based on medicagenic, 16-hydroxymedicagenic, and gypsogenic
acids [R2;1,2,3].

MEDICINAL USE: Astringent, diuretic, mild spasmolytic [R1]. Used
principally for bladder complaints in the form of an infusion, and,
as the name suggests, for ruptures. Gerard writes: "it is singular good
for Ruptures and that very many that have been bursten were restored
to health by the use of this herbe also the powder thereof taken with
wine... wasteth away the stone in the kidney and expelleth them".
Despite this, little pharmacological work has been described for this herb.

SPECIFIC REFERENCES: 1. Franck H *et al* (1975) *Deutsch Apot. Ztg.*
115:1206. 2. Freiler M *et al* (1996) *Planta Med.* 61:S66. 3. Krolikoswka
M *et al* (1979) *Acta Pol. Pharm.* 36:469.

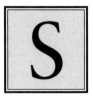

SABADILLA
SCHOENOCAULON OFFICINALE A. GRAY
Fam. Liliaceae

SYNONYMS: Cevadilla.

HABITAT: Mexico and parts of South America.

DESCRIPTION: The seeds are linear, about 6 mm long, pointed, brownish-black, shiny and wrinkled.

PART USED: Seeds.

CONSTITUENTS: (i) Alkaloids, of the ceveratrum type, including veracevine, sabadilline, sabadine, cevine, cevadine, cevagenine, germidine and neogermidine. The mixture is known as 'veratrine' [R14;1,2] (ii) Fixed oil, containing tiglic and angelic acids and their esters [R4].

MEDICINAL USE: Insecticide [R1]. The seeds have been used in the form of an ointment for topical use as parasiticide for lice and fleas, but the alkaloids are too toxic to recommend for this use (see Hellebore, American), as they may be absorbed through the skin. Veratrine resembles Aconite (q.v.) in action; it is an irritant and acts as a direct stimulant on peripheral nerve endings and muscle tissue. Ingestion causes an intense burning sensation, violent vomiting, purging, and muscle weakness or even death [R14].

REGULATORY STATUS: POM.

SPECIFIC REFERENCES: 1. Kupchan S *et al* (1961) *Lloydia* 24(1):17. 2. Ujvary I *et al* (1997) *Phytochem.* 44(7):1257.

SAFFLOWER
CARTHAMUS TINCTORIUS L.
Fam. Asteraceae

SYNONYMS: False Saffron, Dyer's Saffron, Honghua (Chinese).

HABITAT: Indigenous to parts of Asia, cultivated elsewhere.

DESCRIPTION: The florets are usually separated from the flowerheads, either loose or compressed into circular masses. The florets are cylindrical, slender, orange, about 1 cm long, with five teeth. Taste: slightly bitter; odour: faint.

PART USED: Flowers, seed oil

CONSTITUENTS: Flowers: (i) Carthamone, 'Safflower Yellow', a benzoquinone pigment (ii) Dihydroflavones and chalcones; carthamin, neocarthamin and tinctormine (ii) Lignans; tetracheloside, matairesinoside and 2-hydroxyarctiin (iii) Triterpene alcohols (iv) A polysaccharide composed of xylose, fructose, galactose, glucose, arabinose, rhamnose and uronic acid residues (v) Cartorimine, a cycloheptanone oxide. Seed: Serotonin derivatives including N-(p-coumaroyl)serotonin. Seed oil: Polyunsaturated fatty acids; mainly linoleic acid (ca. 74%) with lesser amounts of oleic acid and traces of alpha-linolenic acid [1,2,3,4,5,6,7,8,9,10].

MEDICINAL USE: Laxative, diuretic [R1]. Safflowers were formerly used as an infusion for children's complaints such as measles, fevers and eruptive skin conditions. The polysaccharide induces antibody formation in mice following peritoneal injection; these antibodies cross react with antisera specific for *Streptococcus pneumoniae* type III and type VIII [4]. Safflower is used widely in Chinese medicine for injuries, contusions and strains and for amenorrhoea, and has been shown to have anti-inflammatory activity [5,7]. Extracts have also been tested on blood coagulation, where a prolongation of clotting time was observed and platelet aggregation inhibited. Other properties included an increase in the tolerance of mice to hypoxia and a stimulant effect on the uterus, particularly the pregnant uterus, in animals [11]. Clinically Safflower is used in China to treat coronary disease, thrombotic disorders and menstrual disturbances, and alcoholic extracts are applied topically to ulcers and wounds [R20]. Carthamone is immunosuppressive, and lowers blood pressure in spontaneously hypertensive rats [12]. Extracts of the flowers are anti-mycotic [13] Tinctormine is a calcium antagonist [3] and the serotonin derivatives are antioxidants [7,8]. For effects of the lignans, see Burdock. The oil is used in cooking.

SPECIFIC REFERENCES: 1. Rao C (Ed.) *In: The Chemistry of Lignans* (1978) Pub: Andhra University Press, Andhra Pradesh, India. 2. Amling R (1991) *Z. Phytother.* 12:9. 3. Zhang H *et al* (1997) *Chem. Pharm. Bull.* 45:3355. 4. Caldes G *et al* (1981) *J. Gen. Appl. Microbiol.* 27:157. 5. Akihisa T *et al* (1996) *Phytochem.* 12:1255. 6. Boik J In: *Natural Compounds in Cancer Therapy* (2001) Oregon Medical Press USA, p. 216. 7. Zhang H *et al* (1997) *Chem. Pharm. Bull.* 45:1910. 8. Takii T *et al* (1999) *J. Biochem.* 125(5):910. 9. Xu S (1986) *Chung Yao Tung Pao* 11(2):42. 10. Yin H *et al* (2000) *J. Nat. Prod.* 63(8):1164. 11. Shi M *et al* (1995) *Chung Kuo Chung Yao Tsa Chi* 20:173. 12. Liu Z *et al* (1992) *Yao Hsueh Hsueh Pao* 12:537. 13. Blaszczyk T *et al* (2000) *Phytother. Res.* 14(3):210.

SAFFRON

CROCUS SATIVUS L.
Fam. Iridaceae

SYNONYMS: Hay Saffron.

HABITAT: Native to the Mediterranean region, cultivated in Spain, France, Italy and the Middle East.

DESCRIPTION: Saffron consists of the three filiform, deep orange-red stigmas attached to the upper part of the style. These give the appearance of a loose mass of threads, about 2.5 cm long. Each stigma is tubular, slit at the end and toothed at the apex. Taste: characteristic and bitter; odour: aromatic, characteristic.

PART USED: Flower pistils gathered in the autumn.

CONSTITUENTS: (i) Volatile oil, containing 2-butenoic acid lactone, cineole, isophorone, oxysafranal, safranal, 3,5,5-trimethyl-4-hydroxy-1-cyclohexanone-2-ene and others (ii) Crocins; which are carotenoid

383

glycosides including picrocrocin, which decomposes to safranal, crocins 1,2,3 and 4 which are glucose and gentiobiose esters of crocetin (= alpha-crocin) and methylcrocetin (= beta-crocetin) and other related compounds (iii) Vitamins B1 and B2 (iv) Fixed oil [R2,R5;1,2,3,4].

MEDICINAL USE: Formerly used as a carminative, diaphoretic and emmenagogue [R1]. In Chinese medicine it is used for depression, shock and menstrual difficulties. It is used mainly as a colouring and flavouring for food. The spicy, warm odour is due to the safranal, and the bright yellow colour imparted to food is due to the crocin [R19;4]. Safranal, crocin and picrocrocin inhibit tumour cell growth *in vitro* [5] and in mice [6], and a role for chemoprevention by Saffron has been proposed [7,8,9]. Crocin and crocetin also inhibit skin tumour promotion in mice induced by the phorbol ester TPA and Epstein-Barr virus activation [10], and antimicrobial activity against *Staphylococcus epidermidis* and *Micrococcus luteus* has been described [11]. More recently Saffron has been shown to improve ethanol-induced impairment of learning behaviour in experimental mice, an effect attributed to the crocin content [12], and it is being further investigated as a possible treatment for neurodegenerative disorders. For further detail and reviews, see [1,4 and refs therein].

BIBLICAL REFERENCES: Song of Solomon 4:14.

SPECIFIC REFERENCES: 1. Abe K *et al* (2000) *Phytother. Res.* 14(3):149. 2. Dhingra V *et al* (1975) *Indian J. Chem.*13:339. 3. Morimoto S *et al* (1994) *Planta Med.* 60:438. 4. Saffron. Negbi M (Ed.) (1999) *Medicinal and Aromatic Plants – Industrial Profiles.* Pub: Taylor and Francis, London, UK. 5. Escribano J *et al* (1997) *Cancer Lett.* 100:23. 6. Salomi M *et al* (1991) *Nutr. Cancer* 16:67. 7. Nair S *et al* (1991) *Cancer Lett.* 57:109. 8. Nair S *et al* (1995) *Cancer Biother.* 5:257. 9. Nair S *et al* (1991) *J. Ethnopharmacol.* 16:75. 10. Konoshima T *et al* (1998) *Phytother. Res.* 12(6):400. 10. Kamalinejad M *et al* (1999) *J. Pharm. Pharmacol.* 51S:240. 11. Sugiura M *et al* (1995) *Phytother. Res.* 9(1):100.

SAGE

SALVIA OFFICINALIS L.
Fam. Lamiaceae

SYNONYMS: Garden Sage, Red Sage. Spanish Sage is *S. officinalis* subspp. *lavandulifolia* (Vahl) Gams, and Greek Sage is *S. triloba* L. fil.

HABITAT: Native to the Mediterranean region, cultivated worldwide.

DESCRIPTION: Leaves stalked, 3–5 cm long and 1–2.5 cm broad, oblong lanceolate and rounded at the base and at the apex, crenulate at the margin. The venation is finely but distinctly reticulated, depressed on the upper surface, prominent on the lower. Taste: pungent; odour: strong, aromatic.

PART USED: Leaves.

CONSTITUENTS: (i) Volatile oil, containing alpha- and beta-thujone as the major components, usually about 50%, with cineole, borneol, camphor, 2-methyl-3-methylene-5-heptene and others. Spanish sage does not contain thujone, and Greek sage contains only small amounts. (ii) Diterpene bitters; picrosalvin (= carnosol), carnosolic acid, abietane derivatives called royleanones, such as horminone, and others (iii) Flavonoids; salvigenin, genkwanin, 6-methoxygenkwanin, hispidulin, luteolin and derivatives (iv) Phenolic acids; salvianolic, rosmarinic, caffeic, labiatic etc. (v) Salviatannin, a condensed catechin [R3,R7;1,2,3,4,5,6,7].

MEDICINAL USE: Aromatic, astringent, antiseptic, spasmolytic, reputed memory enhancer [R1]. It may be used as an infusion to reduce perspiration, and also as a gargle or mouthwash for pharyngitis, tonsillitis, sore gums, mouth ulcers and other similar disorders. Rosmarinic acid and other components are anti-inflammatory (see Rosemary). Sage extracts and oil have been reported to be antimicrobial [7] and antispas- modic in animals [8]. The flavonoids and phenolic acid derivatives are antioxidants, which inhibit lipid peroxidation [9] and scavenge free radicals [3,4,5,6,10]. A product containing Sage and Alfalfa (q.v.) has shown promise in alleviating some menopausal symptoms in women [11]. Carnosol and carnosolic acid inhibit the binding affinity of [35S]TBPS (a ligand of the GABA/benzodiazepine receptor complex) in rat brain membrane tissue [12], although the clinical significance of this is not yet apparent. Sage oil, and monoterpenes isolated from it, have anticholinesterase activity *in vitro* and *in vivo*, [9], which may help to explain the reputed memory-enhancing effects. See [13] for full review. Sage is a popular culinary herb.

PREPARATIONS AND DOSE: Dried herb, dose: 1–4 g or equivalent extract, three times daily.

SPECIFIC REFERENCES: 1. Brieskorn C et al (1971) *Deutsch Apot. Ztg.* 111:141. 2. Murko D et al (1978) *Planta Med.* 25:295. 3. Lu Y et al (2001) *Food Chem.* 75(2):197. 4. Lu Y et al (2001) *Tetrahedron* 42(6):8223. 5. Ho C-T et al (2000) *Biofactors* 13(1–4):161. 6. Wang M et al (1999) *J. Nat. Prod.* 62(3):454. 7. Recio M et al (1989) *Phytother. Res.* 43:77. 8. Taddei I et al (1988) *Fitoterapia* 59:463. 9. Zupko I et al (2001) *Planta Med.* 67(4):366. 10. Perry N et al (2001) *J. Pharm. Pharmacol.* 53(10):1347. 11. De Leo V et al (1998) *Minerva Ginecol.* 50(5):207. 12. Rutherford D et al (1992) *Neurosci. Lett.* 135(2):224. 13. Sage. Ed. Kintzios S (2000) *Medicinal and Aromatic Plants – Industrial Profiles.* Pub: Taylor and Francis, London, UK.

SAGO
METROXYLON RUMPHII MART.
Fam. Palmae

SYNONYMS: Pearl Sago.

HABITAT: Cultivated in the tropics.

DESCRIPTION: The starch grains are shortly cylindrical, with one flat end and the opposite end rounded.

PART USED: Prepared pith-starch.

MEDICINAL USE: Demulcent, nutritive [R1]. Used as an easily digested food for convalescents.

SALEP
ORCHIS SPP.
Fam. Orchidaceae

HABITAT: Central and southern Europe.

DESCRIPTION: Salep is the dried tuberous root of many species of *Orchis*, imported from Europe. Tubers whitish or pale brownish-yellow, about 23 cm long and 8–15 mm in diameter, oblong-oval or elliptical, sometimes compressed, with a stern scar at one end and tapering at the other.

PART USED: Root.

CONSTITUENTS: Mucilage, consisting of salep mannans, about 50%, starch etc. [R2].

MEDICINAL USE: Demulcent, nutritive [R1]. Has been used similarly to Arrowroot (q.v.).

SAMPHIRE
CRITHMUM MARITIMUM L.
Fam. Apiaceae

SYNONYMS: Sea Fennel.

HABITAT: Grows on rocks on the coast of East Anglia and other parts of Britain.

DESCRIPTION: A succulent plant, reaching about 25 cm, with glaucous, alternate leaves.

PART USED: Herb.

CONSTITUENTS: (i) Polyacetylenes including falcarinol and falcarindiol (ii) Volatile oil containing O-geranylvanillin, dillapiole, sabinene, limonene, beta-phellandrene,thymol methyl ether and gamma-terpinene (iii) Vitamin C: ascorbic acid, dehydroascorbic acid [1,2,3].

MEDICINAL USE: Anti-obesity agent, diuretic [R1]. The polyacetylenes and O-geranylvanillin are cytotoxic *in vitro* against brine shrimp [1] and the essential oil is insecticidal [3], antioxidant and antimicrobial [4]. Samphire was formerly used as a protection against scurvy because of the ascorbic acid content, and is an item of food, often pickled.

SPECIFIC REFERENCES: 1. Cunsolo F *et al* (1993) *J. Nat. Prod.* 56(9):1598. 2. Francke W (1982) *Econ. Bot.* 36(2):163. 3. Tsoukatou M *et al* (2001) *Z. Naturforsch.* C 56(3–4):211. 4. Ruberto G *et al* (2000) *Planta Med.* 66(8):687.

SANDALWOOD
SANTALUM ALBUM L.
Fam. Santalaceae

SYNONYMS: Santalwood, East Indian Sandalwood. Australian Sandalwood is *Eucarya spicata*; West Indian Sandalwood is *Amyris balsamifera.*

HABITAT: Native to, and cultivated in, tropical Asia.

DESCRIPTION: The wood is sold for medicinal purposes as fine raspings, yellowish in colour, and with a characteristic fragrant odour.

PART USED: Heartwood and the oil distilled from it.

CONSTITUENTS: Volatile oil, containing at least 90% of the sesquiterpene alcohols alpha- and beta-santalol; with the sesquiterpene hydrocarbons alpha- and beta-santalene, alpha- and beta-curcumene; santene, borneol, etc. [1,2,3].

MEDICINAL USE: Rarely used medicinally. The oil is reportedly diuretic and antiseptic [R1] and used to treat urinary disorders, and has antioxidant activity [4]. It is a common ingredient of perfumes and cosmetics and the wood much prized for carving aromatic ornaments.

SPECIFIC REFERENCES: 1. Adams D *et al* (1975) *Phytochem.* 14:1459. 2. Patnikar S *et al* (1975) *Tet. Lett.* 15:1293. 3. Demole D *et al* (1976) *Helv. Chim. Acta* 59:737. 4. Scartezzini P *et al* (2000) *J. Ethnopharmacol.* 71(1–2):23.

SANDERSWOOD, RED
PTEROCARPUS SANTALUS L.
Fam. Caesalpiniaceae

SYNONYMS: Red Sandalwood, Rubywood.

HABITAT: Southern India and the Philippines.

DESCRIPTION: Usually met with in commerce as shavings or raspings, with a deep purplish red tint. Taste and odour: very slight.

PART USED: Wood.

CONSTITUENTS: (i) Isoflavones known as pterocarpans; pterocarpin; isopterocarpin, homopterocarpin, and santal, and also liquiritigenin and isoliquiritigenin and others (ii) Terpenoids such as pterocarpol, cedrol (= cedar camphor) and eudesmol (iii) Pterostilbene (iv) Lignans; savinin and calocedrin (v) Benzxanthrenone pigments; santalins A and B, which are red, and C and Y, which are yellow [R2;1,2,3,4,5,6].

MEDICINAL USE: Little used medicinally here but in India it is occasionally used for diabetes [R1]; the anti-diabetic constituent is pterostilbene [1,7], which also has insecticidal activity [1]. The lignans are anti-inflammatory and inhibit TNF-alpha production in lipopolysaccharide-stimulated cells and T-cell proliferation elicited by concanavalin-A, but are not generally cytotoxic [6]. It is sometimes used as a colouring agent.

SPECIFIC REFERENCES: 1. Seshadri T (1972) *Phytochem.* 11:881. 2. Singh S *et al* (1992) *Fitoterapia* 63:555. 3. Singh S *et al* (1993) *Fitoterapia* 64:84. 4. Krishnaveni K *et al* (2000) *Phytochem.* 53(5):605. 5. Krishnaveni K *et al* (2000) *Chem. Pharm. Bull.* 48(9):1373. 6. Cho J *et al* (2001) *Biol. Pharm. Bull.* 24(2):167. 7. Kameswara R *et al* (2001) *J. Ethnopharmacol.* 74(1):69.

SANICLE

SANICULA EUROPEA L.

Fam. Apiaceae

HABITAT: Grows in shady places throughout Europe, including Britain.

DESCRIPTION: Leaves long-stalked, green above and paler below, rounded in outline, 5–8 cm in diameter, deeply divided into five irregularly trifid and serrate lobes which are broadly wedge-shaped below. Flowers white, small, in simple umbels. Taste: bitter, then acrid; odourless.

PART USED: Herb.

CONSTITUENTS: (i) Saponins, including the saniculosides and acylsaniculosides (e.g. saniculoside-N and R-1) based on the saniculogenins; barrigenol, and barringtogenol (ii) Chlorogenic and rosmarinic acids (iii) Flavonoids such as rutin and isoquercetin (iv) Miscellaneous; allantoin, traces of essential oil, vitamin C [R2,R4;1,2,3].

MEDICINAL USE: Astringent, alterative, vulnerary [R1]. It has been taken as an infusion and applied topically. Extracts are antiviral against the human parainfluenza virus type 2 [4].

SPECIFIC REFERENCES: 1. Engel S *et al* (1972) *Dermat. Mschr.* 158:22. 2. Arda N *et al* (1997) *J. Nat. Prod.* 60(11):1170. 3. Schopke T *et al* (1998) *Planta Med.* 64(1):83. 4. Karagoz A *et al* (1999) *Phytother. Res.* 13(5):436.

SARSAPARILLA

SMILAX ARISTOLOCHIAEFOLIA MILL

S. REGELII KILLIP ET MORTON

S. SIEBOLDII MIQ.

S. GLABRA ROXB.

S. FEBRIFUGA KUNTH

Fam. Smilacaceae

SYNONYMS: *S. aristolochiaefolia:* American, Mexican, Vera Cruz or Grey Sarsaparilla, *S. medica* Schlecht; *S. regelii:* Jamaican, Honduras or Brown Sarsaparilla; *S. febrifuga:* Ecuadorian or Guayaquil Sarsaparilla. Indian Sarsaparilla is *Hemidesmus indicus* Brown (Aristolochiaceae).

HABITAT: The origins are not always easy to determine but some indication is apparent from the names. The plants are climbing vines native to tropical America and the West Indies.

DESCRIPTION: The roots are narrow, very long, cylindrical, up to about 6 mm in diameter and usually found in commerce folded and bound into bundles. Pieces of rhizome, if present, are much thicker and are cut. The external surface varies from greyish- to yellowish- or reddish-brown; ridges, furrows and scars may or may not be present. The transverse section also shows highly variable features. Taste: sweetish and acrid; odourless.

PART USED: Roots, rhizome.

CONSTITUENTS: (i) Saponins, based on the aglycones sarsapogenin and smilagenin; the major one being parillin (= sarsaponin), with smilasaponin (= smilacin) and sarsaparilloside [R2,R7;1,2]. *S. sieboldii* contains smilaxin A, B and C, and sieboldins A and B, based on sieboldigenin and laxogenin [3] (ii) Phytosterols including beta-sitosterol, stigmasterol, pollinostanol and their glucosides (iii) Flavonoids based on kaempferol and quercetin [4] (iv) Miscellaneous; polyphenolic acids, traces of volatile oil etc. R7]. *S. glabra* rhizomes contain a heterodimeric haemagglutinin [5].

MEDICINAL USE: Alterative, anti-inflammatory, anti-rheumatic, antipruritic, antiseptic [R1]. Sarsaparilla was first introduced by the Spanish conquerors in 1563 as a 'sure cure' for syphilis. It has been used for many years as a general 'blood purifier' and treatment for skin diseases, including psoriasis. In a study many years ago patients with psoriasis were treated over a two-year period with 'sarsaponin' tablets prepared from Sarsaparilla; and improvement was noted in 62% of cases [6]. The therapeutic actions of Sarsaparilla are not well-known, although more work has been carried out recently. For example the ethanol extract of *S. regelii* was found to be hepatoprotective in rats, and no toxic effects were observed over a period of 90 days [7], and hypoglycaemic effects have been observed in mice, thought to be due to increasing insulin sensitivity [8]. The anti-inflammatory activity was confirmed in rats [9] and a desmuta-genic effect also noted [10]. In China, other species of *Smilax* are used for similar purposes, for rheumatism, skin diseases, dysentery and even syphilis with apparent success. Sarsaparilla is an ingredient of soft drinks.

PREPARATIONS AND DOSE: Powdered Root, dose: 1–4 g, or equivalent extract.

SPECIFIC REFERENCES: 1. Bernardo R *et al* (1996) *Phytochem.* 43:465. 2. Hobbs C (1988) *HerbalGram* 17(1):10. 3. Mi H-W *et al* (1992) *J. Nat. Prod.* 55(8):1129. 4. Chen G *et al* (1996) *Chung Kuo Chung Yao Tsa Chih* 21:355. 5. Ng T *et al* (2001) *Int. J. Biochem. Cell Biol.* 33(3):269. 6. Thermon F (1942) *N. Eng. J. Med.* 227:128. 7. Rafatullah S *et al* (1991) *Int. J. Pharmacog.* 29(4):296. 8. Fukunaga T *et al* (1997) *Biol. Pharm. Bull.* 20(1):44. 9. Ageel A *et al* (1989) *Drugs Exp. Clin. Res.* 15:369. 10. Ueno S *et al* (2000) *J. Health Sci.* 46(1):29.

SASSAFRAS
SASSAFRAS ALBIDUM (NUTT.) NEES.
Fam. Lauraceae

SYNONYMS: S. varifolium (Salisb.) Kuntze, *S. officinale* Nees and Eberm.

HABITAT: Eastern North America and Canada.

DESCRIPTION: The root bark is a bright, rust-brown colour, in irregular pieces, soft and brittle. The fracture is short and corky, in definite layers, showing numerous oil glands. The root itself is sometimes found as chips; it is brownish-white, showing distinctive concentric rings traversed by narrow medullary rays. Taste: sweetish and slightly astringent; odour: pleasant, aromatic.

PART USED: Root bark, root.

CONSTITUENTS: (i) Volatile oil, containing safrole 80–90%, with 5-methoxyeugenol, asarone, eugenol, alpha- and beta-phellandrene, alpha-pinene, myristicin, thujone, caryophyllene, anethole and others (ii) Alkaloids, boldine, norboldine, isoboldine, norcinnamolaurine, reticuline and others (iii) Lignans; sesamin, desmethoxyaschantin (iv) Miscellaneous; tannins, phlobaphene, resins [R7;1,2,3,4,5,6].

MEDICINAL USE: Carminative, diaphoretic, diuretic, antiseptic, anti-rheumatic [R1]. Safrole is carcinogenic in animals and should not be taken internally [6,7]. Sassafras extract is insecticidal [8]. It is possible to prepare safrole-free extracts but since safrole is responsible for most of the properties of Sassafras, including its odour and flavour, this is rarely used.

REGULATORY STATUS: Root Bark GSL. Oil: for external use only.

SPECIFIC REFERENCES: 1. Sethi M et al (1976) *Phytochem.* 15:1773. 2. Segelman A et al (1976) *JAMA* 236:477. 3. Chowdhary B et al (1976) *Phytochem.* 15:1803. 4. Kamdem D et al (1995) *Planta Med.* 61: 574. 5. Brophy J et al (1993) *J. Ess. Oil Res.* 5:117. 6. Albert K (1997) *Pharm. Ztg.* 142:878. 7. Borchet P et al (1973) *Cancer Res.* 33:375. 8. Jacobson M et al (1975) *Lloydia* 38(6):455.

SASSY BARK
ERYTHROPHLOEUM GUINEENSE G DON
Fam. Caesalpiniaceae

SYNONYMS: Mancona Bark.

HABITAT: Parts of Africa.

DESCRIPTION: In flat or curved pieces, about 5 mm thick, externally warty, greyish, furrowed longitudinally, with a red-brown inner surface, smooth, sometimes with black stains. Fracture: coarsely granular, very hard; taste: astringent, bitter and acrid; odourless.

PART USED: Bark.

CONSTITUENTS: (i) Alkaloids; erythrophleine, erythrophlamine, cassaine, cassaidine, cassamine, cassamidine, norcassamine, norcassamidine, norerythrosuamine and others (ii) Miscellaneous; triterpenes, saponins and catechins [R2;1].

MEDICINAL USE: Narcotic, astringent, laxative [R1]. Used in African traditional medicine for cardiac complaints and migraine, often by intranasal inhalation. The alkaloids are extremely poisonous, they are rapidly cardiotoxic and produce paralysis of the respiratory centre. It has been applied externally as an anti-parasitic, used as a fish poison, and formerly had a role as an ordeal poison or a form of 'divine judgement'.

SPECIFIC REFERENCES: 1. Neuwinger H (2000) African Traditional Medicine, *MedPharm*, Stuttgart.

SAVIN
JUNIPERUS SABINA L.
Fam. Cupressaceae

SYNONYMS: Savin Tops.

HABITAT: Mountainous regions of Switzerland, Italy and Spain.

DESCRIPTION: The shoots bear imbricated, sessile, opposite leaves, the younger of which are oval or hexagonal, becoming rhomboidal or lanceolate with age and less appressed to the stem. An oil gland is visible on the dorsal surface of each leaf. Taste: bitter and resinous; odour: terebinthinate, characteristic.

PART USED: Young shoots.

CONSTITUENTS: (i) Volatile-oil, containing sabinol and sabinyl acetate [1,2] (ii) Lignans including savinin and podophyllotoxin have been reported [3].

MEDICINAL USE: Emmenagogue, diuretic, anthelmintic [R1]. Savin oil is teratogenic and causes abortion, and sabinyl acetate has an anti-implantation effect in animals [1,2]. Savin is toxic and should not be used internally. For actions of podophyllotoxin see Mandrake, American.

SPECIFIC REFERENCES: 1. Pages N *et al* (1996) *Phytother. Res.* 10(6):438. 2. Pages N *et al* (1989) *Planta Med.* 55:144. 3. Hartwell J *et al* (1953) *J. Chem. Soc.* 75:235.

SAVORY, SUMMER
SAVORY, WINTER
SATUREJA HORTENSIS L.
S. MONTANA L.
Fam. Lamiaceae

SYNONYMS: Garden Savory, *Calamintha hortensis* Hort, (= Summer Savory); *S. obovata* Lag., *C. montana* Lam. (= Winter Savory).

HABITAT: Both species are native to southern Europe and North Africa and cultivated elsewhere.

391

DESCRIPTION: Summer Savory is a herbaceous annual; Winter Savory a perennial, woody shrub; both have oblong or linear leaves and blue flowers.

PART USED: Herb.

CONSTITUENTS: (i) Volatile oil; in *S. hortensis* consisting mainly of carvacrol with *p*-cymene, beta-pinene, beta-phellandrene, limonene, borneol and others; in *S. montana* consisting of carvacrol, *p*-cymene and thymol, with alpha- and beta-pinenes, cineole, borneol and others [R2,R19;1,2,3].

MEDICINAL USE: Rarely used medicinally, reputed to be carminative, expectorant and astringent [R1]. Both are used as culinary herbs, Summer Savory particularly. *S. hortensis* oil is antimicrobial, anti-diarrhoeal and spasmolytic [4]. *S. montana* has antiviral activity against HIV-1 *in vitro* [5].

SPECIFIC REFERENCES: 1. Herisset A *et al* (1974) *Plantes Med. Phytother.* 8:287 and 304. 2. Zani F *et al* (1991) *Planta Med.* 57:237. 3. Slavkovska V *et al* (2001) *Phytochem.* 57(1):71. 4. Hajhashemi V *et al* (2000) *J. Ethnopharmacol.* 71(1–2):187. 5. Yamasaki K *et al* (1998) *Biol. Pharm. Bull.* 21(8):829.

SAW PALMETTO
SERENOA REPENS (BARTRAM) J K SMALL
Fam. Arecaceae

SYNONYMS: Sabal, *Sabal serrulata* (Michx.) Benth. and Hook, *Sabal serrulatum* Schult f.

HABITAT: Eastern North America.

DESCRIPTION: The plant is a low, shrubby palm, with a creeping horizontal or ascending stem with vertical stiff palmate leaves divided into segments with sharp teeth. The flowers are small and white, in long panicles, and the fruit is an ovoid drupe, from 2–2.5 cm long and up to 3 cm broad, externally black, with a thin, hard, but fragile pericarp covering a pale brown, spongy pulp and a thin papery endocarp. The seed is pale brown, oval or globular, with a hilum near the base. Taste: soapy; odour: nutty, reminiscent of vanilla.

PART USED: Fruit.

CONSTITUENTS: (i) Fixed oil, consisting of about 25% fatty acids: capric, caprylic, lauric, palmitic, oleic, linoleic and linolenic acids, and neutral fats (ii) Sterols including campesterol, stigmasterol, beta-sitosterol, lupeol and cycloartenol (iii) Long chain alcohols including farnesol, phytol, and polyprenolic alcohols (iv) Flavonoids such as rutin, isoquercitrin and others (v) Miscellaneous; immunostimulant polysaccharides containing galactose, arabinose, mannose, rhamnose, glucuronic acid and others; carotenoids [R2,R7,R8;1].

MEDICINAL USE: Tonic, diuretic, sedative, endocrine agent, anabolic agent [R1]. It was formerly used for debility and wasting diseases, cystitis, prostatitis and similar conditions; however, now it is most widely used to treat urological symptoms associated with prostate enlargement. Although the actual constituents responsible for the activity have not been identified, it has been demonstrated that a mixture known as the liposteroidal fraction has numerous relevant pharmacological effects, and clinical studies support the use of the herb in benign prostatic hyperplasia (BPH). Saw Palmetto extracts inhibit the activity of 5-alpha reductase which, like finasteride (a standard drug for treating BPH), prevents the conversion of testosterone to dehydrotestosterone, a more androgenic derivative [2,3,4]. Extracts also inhibit basic fibroblast-growth-factor-induced proliferation of cultures of human prostate biopsies and affect the distribution of androgens and epidermal growth factor in BPH [5,6,7]. Clinical trials have shown efficacy for Saw Palmetto [8,9,10,11] although long-term treatment is required (as with other therapies) for this condition, and it appears to be safe [7,12]. Review references [R7,R8;1,2,9] should be consulted for further information.

PREPARATIONS AND DOSE: Powdered Berries, dose: 0.5–1 g, or equivalent extract, three times daily.

SPECIFIC REFERENCES: 1. Bombardelli E *et al* (1997) *Fitoterapia* 68(2):99. 2. Brown D (2001) *HerbalGram* 53:22. 3. Weisser H *et al* (1996) *Prostate* 28:300. 4. Bayne C *et al* (1998) *Prostate* 40:232. 5. Paubert-Braquet M *et al* (1998) *Eur. Urol.* 33:340. 6. Bayne C *et al* (2000) *J. Urol.* 164:876. 7. Di Silverio F *et al* (1998) *Prostate* 37:77. 8. Marks L *et al* (2000) *J. Urol.* 163:1451. 9. Wilt T *et al* (1998) *JAMA* 280:1604. 10. Gerber G *et al* (1998) *Urology* 51:1003. 11. Marks L *et al* (2001) *Urology* 57:999. 12. Braekman J *et al* (1997) *Phytother. Res.* 11:558.

SCAMMONY ROOT, MEXICAN
IPOMOEA ORIZABENSIS (PELL.) LED.
Fam. Convolvulaceae

SYNONYMS: Ipomoea, Orizaba jalap.

HABITAT: Mexico.

DESCRIPTION: The root occurs in large transverse or oblique slices, up to 10 cm in diameter and 4 cm thick. It is greyish-brown and wrinkled externally, internally the section shows irregular concentric rings and scattered resin glands, resembling Jalap (q.v.). Taste: acrid and resinous; odour: slight.

PART USED: Root, and resin extracted from it.

CONSTITUENTS: (i) Resins, known as scammonin and alpha-scammonin, which hydrolyse to jalapinolic acid and convolvulenic acids, and the orizabins, which are methyl pentosides of jalapinolic acid (ii) Phytosterols including beta-sitosterol [R3;1].

MEDICINAL USE: Drastic purgative [R1]. Used in a similar way to Jalap (q.v.).

PREPARATIONS AND DOSE: Scammony Resin BPC 1963, dose: 30–200 mg.   393

SPECIFIC REFERENCES: 1. Hernadez-Carlos B *et al* (1999) *J. Nat. Prod.* 62:1096.

SCHISANDRA

SCHISANDRA CHINENSIS (TURCZ.) BAILL.
Fam. Schisandraceae

SYNONYMS: Magnolia vine, Gomishi (Japanese), Wu-Wei-Zi (Chinese), Limonnik Kitajskij (Russian). *Schizandra chinensis*.

HABITAT: Northern China, Korea, Japan, and eastern parts of Russia.

DESCRIPTION: Schisandra is a monoecious vine or liana with a twisting stem, up to 15 m long, usually found climbing round tree trunks. The leaves are elliptical, alternate, cuspidate with a wedge-shaped base, and the flowers white or cream, with a pleasant odour. The berries are small, ovoid, and bright red, occurring in clusters. When dried they are wrinkled, dark reddish brown, with a sticky pulp and a yellow or brown kidney-shaped seed.

PART USED: Berries

CONSTITUENTS: (i) Lignans including schizandrol A (= schizandrin), schizandrol B (= gomisin A), schizandrin A (= deoxyschisandrin or wuweizu A), schizandrin B (= wuweizu B or gamma-schizandrin B), schizanhenol, schisandrin C, schisantherin A (= gomisin C), schisantherin B (= gomisin B), gomisins H, K, L, M etc, gomisin N (= pseudo-gamma-schizandrin), deoxyschisandrin, wuweizu C, schisantherin C and others (ii) Volatile oil containing borneol, 1,8-cineole, citral, sesquicarene, ylangene, beta-bisabolene, chamigranal and chamigrene (iii) Miscellaneous; citric and malic acids, fixed oil (in the seed) [R5;1,2].

MEDICINAL USE: Schisandra has been used in China since antiquity; to prolong life and increase energy (q.v.), to act as a general and sexual tonic in men, and to treat fatigue. It is also used for disorders of the lungs and kidneys, to reduce sweating, detoxify the liver, treat incontinence and suppress cough. There is a lot of pharmacological evidence to support the use of Schisandra although not many clinical studies have been performed. The liver-protectant effects have been well-documented in animal and cell culture studies [2,3] and attributed to the lignan components, particularly schizandrin B, schisandrin C, and gomisin A. These compounds were shown to reduce elevated levels of liver enzymes, and prevent histological damage, in models of liver injury induced by various toxins or immunological agents. These included carbon tetrachloride, cadmium, viruses and aflatoxin, and several mechanisms of action have been proposed [2,3,4,5,6]. The lignans also stimulated glycogen synthesis in the liver, with gomisin A being the most potent [2]. Antioxidant and free-radical-scavenging effects have been described *in vivo* and *in vitro* [7] and the lignans shown to inhibit lipid peroxidation induced by various means [8]. Deoxyschisandrin, gomisin A, B and C increased liver cytochrome P450 enzymes, which supports the detoxifying and anti-cancer properties

proposed for the plant [9] which have been demonstrated in liver [10].
Anti-tumour-promoting and anti-inflammatory properties have also
been shown in skin [11] and the lignans are known to be platelet-
activating-factor antagonists [12]. The adaptogenic and anti-fatigue
properties have been tested in several animal studies; for example
the effect on the physical recovery of race horses was found to be
beneficial, as well as producing an improvement in performance
[13,14]. Schizanhenol and schizandrin B protect against peroxidative
damage associated with ageing and ischemia in the rat brain [15] and
a human study has suggested that intellectual activity can be enhanced,
especially by schizandrin [1,2]. Toxicity studies show that Schisandra
is relatively safe but more clinical trials are needed to assess efficacy
and evaluate any side effects. For further information see reviews
cited [R5, R20;1,2 and refs therein].

PREPARATIONS AND DOSE: Dried berries, dose: 1.5–6 g daily, or
equivalent extract.

SPECIFIC REFERENCES: 1. *Schisandra.* American Herbal
Pharmacopoiea and Therapeutic Compendium (1999). Ed. R Upton.
Pub: AHP, Santa Cruz, USA. 2. Hancke J *et al* (1999) *Fitoterapia*
670:451. 3. Ko K *et al* (1995) *Planta Med.* 61:134. 4. Kubo S *et al*
(1992) *Planta Med.* 58:498. 5. Ip S *et al* (1996) *Biochem. Pharmacol.*
52(11):1687. 6. Ip S *et al* (1996) *Pharmacol. Toxicol.* 78:413. 7. Ko K
et al (1995) *Phytother. Res.* 9(3):203. 8. Lu H *et al* (1992) *Planta Med.*
58:311. 9. Liu K *et al* (1982) *Chem. Biol. Interact.* 39:301 and 315;
and 41:39. 10. Miyamoto K *et al* (1995) *Biol. Pharm. Bull.* 18:1443.
11. Yasukawa K *et al* (1992) *Oncology* 49:68. 12. Jung K *et al* (1997)
Phytomedicine 4:229. 13. Ahumada F *et al* (1989) *Phytother. Res.*
3:175. 14. Hancke J *et al* (1994) *Fitoterapia* 65:113. 15. Xue J *et al*
(1992) *Free Rad. Biol. Med.* 12:127.

SCOPOLIA

SCOPOLIA CARNIOLICA JACQ.
AND OTHER SPP.
Fam. Solanaceae

HABITAT: Central and eastern Europe.

DESCRIPTION: Rhizome knotty, about 1–2 cm in diameter, nearly
black in colour, with numerous depressed stem scars. Fracture: short.

PART USED: Rhizome.

CONSTITUENTS: Tropane alkaloids, including hyoscine and
hyoscyamine, with cuscohygrine, tropine and pseudotropine [R3].

MEDICINAL USE: Narcotic, mydriatic. Used in a similar way to
Belladonna and Henbane (q.v.), which it resembles in action. It has
been suggested as a source of hyoscine [R3].

REGULATORY STATUS: P.

SCULLCAP
SCUTELLARIA LATERIFLORA L.
Fam. Lamiaceae

SYNONYMS: Skullcap, Hoodwort, Quaker Bonnet, Helmet Flower. European or Greater Skullcap is *S. galericulata* L.

HABITAT: North America.

DESCRIPTION: Leaves opposite, cordate-lanceolate, shortly stalked with a tapering apex. Flowers blue, with a helmet-shaped upper lip, in axillary racemes. Hybridization with other species readily occurs and substitution may occur in commerce. Taste: bitter; odour: slight.

PART USED: Herb.

CONSTITUENTS: (i) Flavonoid glycosides including scutellarin, hispidulin, apigenin, luteolin and scutellarein (ii) Iridoids; catalpol is present in both *S. lateriflora* and *S. galericulata* (iii) Volatile oil and waxes, mainly C_{31}, C_{33} and C_{35} hydrocarbons (iv) Tannins [R7;1,2,3,4].

MEDICINAL USE: Sedative, nervine, antispasmodic, anticonvulsant [R1]. Scullcap is highly regarded for hysteria, nervous tension and as an antispasmodic; however experimental work is not yet available to support this, in contrast to the extensive research carried out on *S. baicalensis* (q.v.). Scutellarin has been tested clinically in China for stroke, cerebral thrombosis and cerebral paralysis, with good results [5].

PREPARATIONS AND DOSE: Powdered herb, dose: 1–2 g, or equivalent extract, three times daily.

SPECIFIC REFERENCES: 1. Barberan F (1986) *Fitoterapia* 57(2):67. 2. Popova T *et al* (1972) *Farm. Zh. (Kiev)* 27:58. 3. Kooiman P (1972) *Acta Bot. Neerl.* 21(4):417. 4. Yagmai M *et al* (1979) *J. Nat. Prod.* 42(2):229. 5. Peigen X *et al* (1987) *Phytother. Res.* 1:53.

SCULLCAP, BAICAL
SCUTELLARIA BAICALENSIS GEORGI.
Fam. Lamiaceae

SYNONYMS: Huan qin, Baical Skullcap.

HABITAT: Northern China, Siberia, Manchuria.

DESCRIPTION: Leaves opposite, lanceolate, sessile with an acute apex. Flowers blue, with a helmet-shaped upper lip, in axillary racemes. Taste: bitter; odourless.

PART USED: Root.

CONSTITUENTS: Flavonoids; baicalin, baicalein, wogonin, chrysin, oroxylin A, tenaxin I, ganhuagenin, skullcapflavones I and II, and many other hydroxylated methoxyflavones [R5 and refs therein;1,2,3,4,5].

MEDICINAL USE: Antipyretic, antidote, sedative; used for jaundice, thirst and nosebleeds. Effects of baicalin include anti-inflammatory and anti-allergic properties; it inhibits calcium ionophore-induced leukotriene synthesis in human lymphocytes, the formation of lipoxygenase products and, to a lesser extent, cyclooxygenase products in leukocytes. *S. baicalensis* also inhibits lipid peroxidation in rat liver and has been clinically tested in China on patients with chronic hepatitis, where it improved symptoms in over 70% of patients, increasing appetite, relieving abdominal distension and improving the results of liver function tests. Antioxidant and anti-fungal activity have also been reported for extracts [R5,R7,R20,1,2,3,4,5,6]. Recent work has focused on individual constituents; for example the flavones have been shown to interact with the benzodiazepine binding site of the GABA-A receptor, with wogonin and baicalein being the most potent [7]. Baicalein is anti-genotoxic *in vitro* [8] and inhibits alpha glucosidase [9]. It also inhibits adhesion molecule expression induced by thrombin [10] and cell proliferation of several types of cells, including rat heart endothelial cells [11]; and like baicalin inhibits intracellular calcium ion elevation in rat glioma cells by reducing phospholipase C activity [12]. Baicalin inhibits superantigen-induced inflammatory cytokines and chemokines [13] and is synergistic with beta-lactam antibiotics against methicillin-resistant *Staphylococcus aureus* (MRSA) *in vitro* [14]. Wogonin inhibits nitric oxide production in activated C6 rat glial cells, acting via NF-KappaB inhibition and thus suppressing cell death [15]. It also reduces skin inflammation in mice induced by phorbol ester (TPA) expression of cyclo-oxygenase-2 [16], and inhibits monocyte chemotactic protein-1 gene expression in human endothelial cells [17]. These activities all support the anti-inflammatory use of Skullcap. Wogonin also suppresses production of hepatitis B virus surface antigen [18].

SPECIFIC REFERENCES: 1. Kimura Y *et al* (1981) *Chem. Pharm. Bull.* 29:2308 and 2610; and (1982) 30:219. 2. Kimura Y *et al* (1984) *Planta Med.* 50:290 and (1985)51:132. 3. Kubo M *et al* (1984) *Chem. Pharm. Bull.* 32(7):5051. 4. Kubo M *et al* (1981) *Planta Med.* 43:194. 5. Lim B *et al* (1999) *Phytother. Res.* 13(6):479. 6. Blaszczyk T *et al* (2000) *Phytother. Res.* 14(3):210. 7. Hui K *et al* (2000) *Planta Med.* 66(1):91. 8. Lee B *et al* (2000) *Planta Med.* 66(1):70. 9. Nishioka T *et al* (1998) *J. Nat. Prod.* 61(11):1413. 10. Kimura Y *et al* (2001) *Planta Med.* 67(4):331. 11. Hsu S *et al* (2001) *Eur. J. Pharmacol.* 425(3):165. 12. Kyo R *et al* (1998) *J. Pharm. Pharmacol.* 50(10):1179. 13. Krakauer T *et al* (2001) *FEBS Lett.* 500(1–2):52. 14. Liu I *et al* (2000) *J. Pharm. Pharmacol.* 52(3):361. 15. Kim H *et al* (2001) *Neurosci. Lett.* 309(1):67. 16. Park B *et al* (2001) *Eur. J. Pharmacol.* 425(2):153. 17. Chang Y *et al* (2001) *Mol. Pharmacol.* 60(3):507. 18. Huang R *et al* (2000) *Planta Med.* 66(8):694.

SCURVY-GRASS
COCHLEARIA OFFICINALIS L.
Fam. Brassicaceae

SYNONYMS: Spoonwort.

HABITAT: Grows wild on dry banks, particularly near the coast, throughout Europe.

DESCRIPTION: The basal leaves are long-stalked, kidney-shaped, nearly entire; the stem leaves ovate, becoming sessile upwards, with a few angular teeth. Flowers white and cruciform, in terminal racemes. Taste: pungent and cress-like, less so after drying.

PART USED: Herb.

CONSTITUENTS: (i) Glucosinolates, for example glucoputranjivin, glucocochlearin, glucotropeolin, sinigrin and others, which decompose into mustard oils (ii) Tropane alkaloids; tropine and cochlearine (hydroxybenzyltropine) have been reported (iii) Miscellaneous; flavonoids, ascorbic acid [R2;1].

MEDICINAL USE: Formerly used as an antiscorbutic and diuretic, as a gargle or mouthwash for ulcers and sores in the mouth, and topically for spots and blemishes [R1].

SPECIFIC REFERENCES: 1. Cole R *et al* (1976) *Phytochem.* 15:759.

SELF-HEAL
PRUNELLA VULGARIS L.
Fam. Lamiaceae

SYNONYMS: Siclewort, Heal-all.

HABITAT: A common European and British wild plant.

DESCRIPTION: A low, creeping herb, branched, with quadrangular stems, oblong-ovate leaves, about 2–3 cm long and 1 cm broad, with entire margins. Flowers purplish-blue, in a dense terminal spike, with two kidney-shaped bracts under each whorl. Taste: saline, faintly bitter; odourless.

PART USED: Herb.

CONSTITUENTS: (i) Pentacyclic triterpenes based on ursolic, betulinic and oleanolic acids (ii) Tannins, including prunellin (iii) Flavonoids including rutin (iv) Polysaccharide(s) [R2;1,2,3,4].

MEDICINAL USE: Astringent, vulnerary. Has been taken internally as a haemostatic and for sore throats, and applied externally to wounds [R1]. Anti-inflammatory and anti-allergic activity has been observed for the extract and betulinic and ursolic acid derivatives identified as some of the active ingredients [3] (see also Birch). The extract has antiviral effects [4,5,6,7] due at least in part to prunellin [2] and the polysaccharide [4]. The extract is thought to work by inhibiting reverse transcriptase and also by preventing viral attachment to the CD4 receptor [5]. The polysaccharide has been shown to inhibit replication of herpes simplex viruses 1 and 2 using a plaque reduction assay [4] and the extract reduced HIV-1 induced cytopathogenicity [7]. Self-heal is used as an anti-cancer drug in China, and desmutagenic activity has been observed for the extract [8] as well as antioxidant and free-radical-scavenging effects [9].

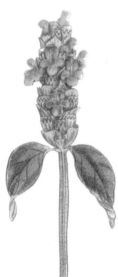

SELF-HEAL

SPECIFIC REFERENCES: 1. Kojema H *et al* (1987) *Phytochem.* 26(4):1107. 2. Tabba H *et al* (1989) *Antiviral Res.* 11:263. 3. Ryu S *et al* (2000) *Planta Med.* 66(4):358. 4. Xu H *et al* (1999) *Antiviral Res.* 44(1):43. 5. Kageyama S *et al* (2000) *Antiviral Chem. Chemother.* 11(2):157. 6. Yao X-J *et al* (1992) *Virology* 187(1):56. 7. Yamasaki K *et al* (1998) *Biol. Pharm. Bull.* 21(8):829. 8. Lee H *et al* (1988) *Mutat. Res.* 204(2):229. 9. Liu F *et al* (2000) *Life Sci.* 66(8):725.

SENEGA
POLYGALA SENEGA L.
Fam. Polygalaceae

SYNONYMS: Snake Root, Rattlesnake Root. In Chinese medicine Senega may also refer to *P. tenuifolia* Willd.

HABITAT: North America.

DESCRIPTION: The root has a knotty crown, from which slender stems arise, with the remains of rudimentary leaves and buds at the base. The root is light yellowish-grey in colour, up to about 1 cm thick, often with a keel-shaped ridge running along the main root on the concave side. Fracture: short and brittle, showing a cleft central column; taste: acrid, odour: rather wintergreen-like. The powder is sternutatory.

PART USED: Root.

CONSTITUENTS: (i) Triterpenoid saponins, the mixture known as 'senegin', based on the aglycones presenegenin, senegenin, hydroxy-senegin, polygalacic acid and senegenic acid. These include the E- and Z-senegins II, III and IV, the E- and Z-senegasaponins a, b and c, and derivatives such as desmethoxysenegin II, and others (ii) Phenolic acids; caffeic, *p*-coumaric, ferulic, sinapic, *p*-methoxycinnamic and others (iii) Oligosaccharide esters, named senegoses A-O, which are mainly glucose and fructose di- and tetrasaccharides esterified with acetic, benzoic and ferulic acids (iv) Miscellaneous; methyl salicylate, sterols, fats etc. *P. tenuifolia* contains similar or related compounds [R7,R3,R9;1,2,3,4,5,6,7,8].

MEDICINAL USE: Expectorant, diaphoretic, emetic. Senega is used especially for chronic bronchitis, catarrh, asthma and croup [R1]. The saponins are considered to be the active constituents; they are anti-inflammatory, molluscicidal and anti-fungal [R7]. Senega extracts, the senegasaponins and the senegins have been shown to be hypogly-caemic in rodents, and the senegasaponins are potent inhibitors of alcohol absorption [8,9,10]. The saponins are irritant and haemolytic but taken orally do not appear to pose many problems. They have immunopotentiating activity to protein and viral antigens and exhibit less toxicity than Quillaia (q.v.) saponins, indicating a potential use as vaccine adjuvant antigens to increase specific immune responses [11]. Senega is usually taken orally as an infusion.

PREPARATIONS AND DOSE: Powdered root, dose: 0.5–1 g; Senega Liquid Extract BPC 1980: dose: 0.3–1 ml, three times daily.

SPECIFIC REFERENCES: 1. Tsukitani Y et al (1973) Chem. Pharm. Bull. 21:791 and 1564. 2. Takiura K et al (1974) Yakugaku Zasshi 94:998 and (1975)95:166. 3. Hamburger M et al (1985) Planta Med. 51: 215. 4. Hamburger M et al (1985) Phytochem. 24:1793. 5. Hamburger M et al (1984) Helv. Chim. Acta 67:1729. 6. Hamburger M et al (1984) J. Nat. Prod. 49:557. 7. Saitoh H et al (1993) Chem. Pharm. Bull. 41:1127, 2125 and (1994)42:641. 8. Yohikawa M et al (1995) Chem. Pharm. Bull. 43(2):350, (12):2115 and (1996) 44(7):1305. 9. Kako M et al (1996) Planta Med. 62(5):440 Kako M et al (1997) J. Nat. Prod. 60(6):604. 11. Estrada A et al (2000) Comparative Immunol. Microbiol. Infect. Dis. 23(1):27.

SENNA

CASSIA SENNA L.
C. ANGUSTIFOLIA VAHL.
Fam. Caesalpiniaceae

SYNONYMS: *C. senna:* Alexandrian Senna, *C. acutifolia* Del.; *C. angustifolia:* Tinnevelly Senna.

HABITAT: *C. senna* is native to tropical Africa and cultivated in Egypt and the Sudan and elsewhere; *C. angustifolia* is native to India and cultivated mainly in India and Pakistan.

DESCRIPTION: Leaves: the leaflets are greyish- to yellowish-green, lanceolate, unequal at the base (*C. senna* being more so), petiolate, varying from 1 to 5 cm long and 0.5 to 1 cm broad. Those of *C. senna* are in general smaller. Pods: kidney-shaped, flat, showing the imprint of the seeds through the pod. *C. senna* pods are shorter and broader and green in colour, without the remains of the style visible; those of *C. angustifolia* are longer and narrower, brown, with stylar remains. Taste: sweetish then rather unpleasant; odour: tea-like, characteristic.

PART USED: Leaves, pods.

CONSTITUENTS: (i) Anthraquinone glycosides; in the leaf; sennosides A and B based on the aglycones sennidin A and sennidin B, sennosides C and D which are glycosides of heterodianthrones of aloe-emodin and rhein. Others include palmidin A, rhein anthrone and aloe-emodin glycosides, some free anthraquinones and some potent, novel compounds of as yet undetermined structure. *C. senna* usually contains greater amounts of the sennosides. In the fruit: sennosides A and B and a closely related glycoside sennoside A1 (ii) Naphthalene glycosides; tinnevellin glycoside and 6-hydroxymusizin glycoside, in both leaves and pods (iii) Mucilage; polysaccharides composed of arabinose, galactose, galacturonic acid and others (iv) Miscellaneous; flavonoids, volatile oil, sugars, resins etc [R2,R3,R7,R9;1,2,3].

MEDICINAL USE: Stimulant laxative [R1]. The glycosides are absorbed from the intestinal tract and the active anthraquinones excreted into the colon where they exert their stimulant effect. At least two mechanisms of action have been identified: a modification of gastrointestinal motility and an accumulation of intra-luminal fluid, inducing peristaltic movement [1]. Senna releases histamine from the colon [4] and prostaglandins and other autacoids are implicated in the effect [5]; however, it is now known that platelet-activating factor is not involved [6]. Senna also increases constitutive calcium-dependent nitric oxide synthase in the colon of the rat [7]. Although genotoxicity of anthraquinones has been postulated from *in vitro* testing [8], these methods are often considered artificial, and antimutagenic effects *in vivo* have also been described with Senna intake [9]. A battery of genotoxicity tests has recently indicated that genotoxicity is not a problem [10] although a discolouration of the colonic mucosa can be observed with Senna intake [11]. Generally Senna is considered to be a safe and effective laxative, which does not normally produce habituation over a long period of use [12]. It is used widely throughout the world. The fruits (pods) may be taken as an infusion.

PREPARATIONS AND DOSE: Powdered leaves, dose: 0.5–2 g. Senna Liquid Extract BP, dose: 0.5–2 ml; Senna Tablets BP, each containing 7.5 mg standardised sennosides, calculated as sennoside B.

SPECIFIC REFERENCES: 1. Mascolo N *et al* (1998) *Phytother. Res.* 12:S143. 2. Lemli J *et al* (1981) *Planta Med.* 43:11. 3. Muller B *et al* (1989) *Planta Med.* 55:99. 4. Autore G *et al* (1990) *Eur. J. Pharmacol.* 191:97. 5. Capasso F *et al* (1986) *J. Pharm. Pharmacol.* 38:629. 6. Capasso F *et al* (1993) *Pharmacol.* 47(Suppl.1):58. 7. Izzo A *et al* (1997) *Eur. J. Pharmacol.* 323:93. 8. Westendorf J *et al* (1990) *Mutat. Res.* 240:1. 9. Al-Dhakan A *et al* (1995) *Pharmacol. Toxicol.* 77:288. 10. Brusick D *et al* (1997) *Environ. Mol. Mutagen.* 29:1. 11. Wittoesch J *et al* (1985) *Dis. Colon Rectum* 1:172. 12. Muller-Lissner S (1993) *Pharmacology* 47:138.

SHATTER STONE
PHYLLANTHUS NIRURI L.
Fam. Euphorbiaceae

SYNONYMS: Stone Breaker, *P. amarus, P. sellowianus, P fraternus,* Bhumyaamlaki.

HABITAT: Indigenous to southern Asia but now common throughout the tropics on waste ground.

DESCRIPTION: An erect annual herb, reaching about 60 cm. The leaves are small, closely arranged, with a short petiole and obtuse apex. The flowers are numerous, unisexual, monoecious and yellowish-green, borne in the axils of the leaves.

PART USED: Leaf, root.

CONSTITUENTS: (i) Lignans including phyllanthin, phyllanthinol, phyllanthinone, phyllnirurin, nirurin, niranthin, hikokinin, corylagin, hydroxysesamin and others (ii) Flavonoids such as astragalin, fisetin, quercetin, phyllochrysin, rutin and others (iii) Phenols and tannins; catechin, ellagic acid, geraniin, epigallocatechin gallate, epigallocatechin, brevifolin and others (iv) Triterpenes; Lupeol, beta-sitosterol

401

and others (v) Alkaloids; norsecurinine and phyllanthine are present in the leaves [R12,R16].

MEDICINAL USE: Diuretic, liver protectant and tonic, choleretic, anti-inflammatory. The plant is used frequently for kidney and gallstones, hence the common name. There is abundant information on the phytochemistry and pharmacology of the herb, but most of the clinical studies are either too small to give significant results, or are of poor quality. Diuretic activity has been confirmed in a small clinical study, and hypotension also observed. Geraniin is an inhibitor of angiotensin converting enzyme [1]. Other documented effects include: hypoglycaemic effects of the ethanolic and flavonoid extracts [2], anti-hepatotoxicity in various animal models of liver injury [3], antiviral properties against several viruses [4], antimalarial effects both *in vitro* and *in vivo* [6,7] and nematocidal properties against the larva of *Toxocara canis* [8]. Inhibition of aldose reductase [9], anti-nociception [10] and protection against cytotoxicity and clastogenicity induced by lead, aluminium and nickel [11,12] have also been reported. For further detail, see [R12,R16 and refs therein].

SPECIFIC REFERENCES: 1. Ueno H *et al* (1988) *J. Nat. Prod.* 51(2):357. 2. Hukeri V *et al* (1988) *Fitoterapia* 59(1):68. 3. Kodakandla, V *et al* (1985) *J. Ethnopharmacol.* 14:41. 4. Ogata T *et al* (1992) *AIDS Res. Hum. Retroviruses* 8(11):1937. 5.Venkateswaran P *et al* (1987) *Proc. Natl. Acad. Sci.* USA 84:274. 6. Tona L *et al* (1999) *J. Ethnopharmacol.* 68(1–3):193. 7. Tona L *et al* (2001) *Ann. Trop. Med. Parasitol.* 95(1):47. 8. Kiuchi F *et al* (1989) *Shoyakugaku Zasshi* 43(4):288. 9. Shimizu M *et al* (1989) *Chem. Pharm. Bull.* 37(9):2531. 10. Santos A *et al* (1995) *Gen. Pharmacol.* 26(7):1499. 11. Dhir H *et al* (1990) *Phytother. Res.* 4(5):172. 12. Agarwal K *et al* (1992) *Fitoterapia* 63(1):49.

SHEEP'S SORREL
RUMEX ACETOSELLA L.
Fam. Polygonaceae

HABITAT: Common on dry places throughout Europe and North America.

DESCRIPTION: A slender, short perennial. Leaves arrow-shaped, narrow, often with a reddish tint. Flowers small, green, often turning red, in spikes, typically dock-like. Taste: acid and astringent; odourless.

PART USED: Herb.

CONSTITUENTS: (i) Anthraquinones, including chrysophanol, emodin and physcion (ii) Flavonoids; rutin, hyperoside, hyperin and others (iii) Miscellaneous; tannins, phytoestrogens (unspecified), minerals and vitamins [1,2,3].

MEDICINAL USE: Diuretic, anti-inflammatory [R1]. In Canada and the North America native people have used the plant as a food and an anti-cancer remedy. The fresh plant juice has been used for urinary conditions. In large amounts it is a laxative, due to the anthraquinones.

SPECIFIC REFERENCES: 1. Tamatayo C *et al* (2000) *Phytother. Res.* 14(1):1. 2. Fairbairn J *et al* (1972) *Phytochem.* 11:263. 3. Zava D *et al* (1998) *Soc. Exp. Biol. Med.* 217:369.

SHEPHERD'S PURSE
CAPSELLA BURSA-PASTORIS (L.) MEDIC.
Fam. Brassicaceae

HABITAT: A common plant growing in many parts of the world.

DESCRIPTION: A very variable annual or biennial. Leaves lanceolate, pinnately lobed, sometimes toothed, sometimes hairy, mainly in a basal rosette with a few on the peduncle. Flowers white, 2–3 mm, cruciferous; pod, an inverted, notched triangle, containing the small seeds, the appearance giving rise to the common name. Taste: pungent; odourless.

PART USED: Herb.

CONSTITUENTS: (i) Flavonoids; diosmetin, hesperetin, luteolin, quercetin and their glycosides (ii) Glucosinolates such as sinigrin (iii) Alkaloids (unidentified) and bases; choline, acetylcholine, histamine, tyramine (iv) Volatile oil containing camphor as the major ingredient (v) Polypeptide (unidentified) (vi) Miscellaneous; carotenoids, fumaric and bursic acids, vitamins [R7;1,2,3,4,5].

MEDICINAL USE: Anti-haemorrhagic, urinary antiseptic, antipyretic [R1]. The polypeptide described above was shown to have contractile activity on rat uterus similar to that of oxytocin [4]. Other experiments showed that extracts produced a transient decrease in blood pressure and haemostatic activity in animals; however, whether this was due to the acetylcholine, choline and tyramine was not clear [1]. Other properties demonstrated included anti-inflammatory, diuretic and anti-ulcer activity [6]. An inhibitory effect of extracts of Shepherd's Purse on Ehrlich solid tumour in mice was found to be due to the fumaric acid content [5]; however, fumaric acid is a ubiquitous compound. Weak antimicrobial activity has been reported, mainly against Gram positive organisms [7]. Despite the pharmacological effects described, the active constituents of Shepherd's Purse have still not been satisfactorily ascertained and little research appears to be continuing.

PREPARATIONS AND DOSE: Powdered herb, dose: 1–4 g or equivalent extract, three times daily.

SHEPHERD'S
PURSE

SPECIFIC REFERENCES: 1. Kuroda K *et al* (1969) *Life Sci.* 8:151. 2. Miyazawa M *et al* (1979) *Yakugaku Zasshi* 99:1041. 3. Park R (1967) *Austr. J. Chem.* 20:2799. 4. Kuroda K *et al* (1968) *Nature* 220:707. 5. Kuroda K *et al* (1976) *Cancer Res.* 36:1900. 6. Kuroda K *et al* (1969) *Arch. Int. Pharmacodyn. Ther.* 178:382 and 392. 7. Moskalenko S (1986) *J. Ethnopharmacol.* 15:231.

SILVERWEED
POTENTILLA ANSERINA L.
Fam. Rosaceae

HABITAT: A common European wild plant.

DESCRIPTION: Leaves often silvery, especially below, pinnate, with 12–15 toothed leaflets. Flowers bright yellow, buttercup-like, solitary, with the petals twice as long as the sepals. Taste: astringent; odourless.

PART USED: Herb.

CONSTITUENTS: (i) Ellagitannins, including catechin (ii) Flavonoids, such as astragalin, kaempferol, myricetin, quercetin and isorhamnetic glycosides (iii) Coumarins; umbelliferone and scopoletin [R2;1,2].

MEDICINAL USE: Astringent, tonic [R1]. The tannins have antimutagenic activity against 2-nitrofluorine induced mutagenicity [2].

SPECIFIC REFERENCES: 1. Kombal R *et al* (1995) *Planta Med.* 61(5):484. 2. Schwimmer O *et al* (1995) *Planta Med.* 61(2):141.

SIMARUBA
SIMARUBA AMARA AUBL.
Fam. Simaroubaceae

HABITAT: South America, Florida, West Indies.

DESCRIPTION: The bark occurs in thin, flat, yellowish or greyish-yellow tough, fibrous, pieces, almost impossible to break, usually folded. Taste: very bitter; odourless.

PART USED: Bark.

CONSTITUENTS: (i) Quassinoids, including simarubolide, simarolide, 2'acetylglaucarubine, 13,18-dehydroglaucarubine and 2'acetylglaucarubinone (ii) Alkaloids; 5-hydroxycanthin-6-one (iii) Limonoids, e.g. melianone and derivatives [R2;1,2].

MEDICINAL USE: Tonic, febrifuge [R1]. Simaruba was formerly taken as an infusion for fevers and dysentery and then fell out of use; however recent research has shown that the quassinoids are in fact amoebicidal and antimalarial *in vivo* in animals and *in vitro* (see Quassia).

SPECIFIC REFERENCES: 1. Ghosh P *et al* (1977) *Lloydia* 40(4):636. 2. Polonsky J *et al* (1978) *Experientia* 34(9):1122.

SKUNK CABBAGE
SYMPLOCARPUS FOETIDUS NUTT.
Fam. Araceae

SYNONYMS: Skunkweed, *Dracontium foetidum* L.

HABITAT: North America.

DESCRIPTION: Rhizome obconical, up to 8 cm long, dark brown, knotted and woody. It is transversely wrinkled and bears numerous roots and root scars. Taste and odour: acrid and unpleasant.

PART USED: Rhizome and root.

CONSTITUENTS: Active constituents largely unknown. (i) Alkaloids (unspecified) (ii) Essential oil and resin (iii) 5-hydroxytryptamine (iii) Anthocyanins; cyanidin and petunidin glycosides [R7;1,2].

MEDICINAL USE: Antispasmodic, diaphoretic, expectorant, sedative [R1]. Used mainly for bronchitis and asthma. It is known to have irritant properties and the fresh plant may cause blistering [R7].

SPECIFIC REFERENCES: 1. Plowman T (1969) *Econ. Bot.* 23:2. 2. Chang N *et al* (1970) *Bot. J. Linn. Soc.* 63:95.

SLIPPERY ELM

ULMUS RUBRA MUHL.
Fam. Ulmaceae

SYNONYMS: Red Elm, *U. fulva* Mich.

HABITAT: Central and northern North America.

DESCRIPTION: The inner bark occurs in flat oblong pieces, about 2–4 mm thick, sometimes folded. The outer surface is light yellowish- to reddish-brown, longitudinally wrinkled or striated, with occasional pieces of dark brown rhizome. The inner surface is paler and finely ridged. Fracture: fibrous. Taste: mucilaginous; odour: slight but characteristic.

PART USED: Inner bark.

CONSTITUENTS: (i) Sterols, including campesterol, beta-sitosterol and cholesterol (ii) Mucilages; a complex mixture of pentoses, methylpentoses and hexoses (iii) Tannins and proanthocyanins (iv) Oleic and palmtic acids [R2;1,2].

MEDICINAL USE: Demulcent, emollient, nutrient [R1]. It is used to make gruel for convalescents and for patients with gastric or duodenal ulcers, by adding boiling water to a small quantity of the powder and flavouring with sugar and cinnamon etc. The mucilage is made by digesting the powder in water, heating gently for an hour and straining. The mucilage swells to form a demulcent and emollient gel, which acts as a form of soluble fibre. The coarsely powdered bark is also made into poultices for wounds, burns, boils and other skin disorders, where it soothes and draws out infection. Slippery Elm has antioxidant properties [2].

SPECIFIC REFERENCES: 1. Beveridge R *et al* (1971) *Carbohydrate Res.* 19:107. 2. Tamayo C *et al* (2000) *Phytother. Res.* 14(1):1.

SMARTWEED

PERSICARIA HYDROPIPER (L.) OPIZ
Fam. Polygonaceae

SYNONYMS: Arsesmart, Water Pepper, *Polygonum hydropiper* L.

HABITAT: Found in damp places throughout Europe, including Britain.

DESCRIPTION: Leaves narrow, lanceolate, sheathed at the base. Flowers white, tinged with pink or green, on a narrow, drooping spike. Taste: pungent and biting; odourless.

PART USED: Herb.

CONSTITUENTS: (i) Sesquiterpenes; polygodial (= tadeonal) and warburganal are present in the leaves, and polygonal, isodrimeninol, isopolygodial, and confertifolin in the seeds (ii) Flavonoids; quercetin, kaempferol, persicarin, hyperoside, isorhamnetin, roseoside, rhamnazin and various sulphated derivatives (iii) Coumarins such as polygonolide and hydropiperoside [1,2,3,4,5].

MEDICINAL USE: Stimulant, diuretic, emmenagogue [R1]. It is taken mainly for amenorrhoea as an infusion. Culpeper states that "the juice destroys worms in the ears, being dropped into them". Presumably worms in the ears were more common in those days. The extract has antimutagenic activity [6]. The sulphated flavonoids, particularly isorhamnetin disulphate, inhibit lens aldose reductase and related enzymes [7]. Polygodial is pungent and irritant. It is also well known as an insect anti-feedant and fish poison [8].

SPECIFIC REFERENCES: 1. Barnes C *et al* (1962) *Aust. J. Chem.* 15:322. 2. Asakawa Y *et al* (1979) *Experientia* 35:1429. 3. Fukujama Y *et al* (1983) *Phytochem.* 22:549. 4. Furutu T *et al* (1986) *Phytochem.* 25:517. 5. Murai Y *et al* (2001) *Planta Med.* 67(5):480. 6. Sato T *et al* (1990) *Mutat. Res.* 241(3):283. 7. Haraguchi H *et al* (1996) *J. Nat. Prod.* 59(4):443. 8. Tripathi A *et al* (1999) *Phytother. Res.* 13(3)239.

SNAKEROOT
ARISTOLOCHIA RETICULATA NUTT.
Fam. Aristolochiaceae

SYNONYMS: Texan Snake Root, Serpentary.

HABITAT: North America.

DESCRIPTION:' Rhizome small, about 2–3 cm long and 3 mm thick, with numerous filiform, branching, longitudinally furrowed roots below and the remains of stem bases on the upper side. Taste: bitter; odour: camphoraceous, aromatic.

PART USED: Rhizome.

CONSTITUENTS: Aristolochic acid and aristored [1].

MEDICINAL USE: Formerly used as a stimulant, diaphoretic, anodyne, antispasmodic, nervine [R1]. These properties are due mainly to the aristolochic acid, for details, see Birthwort. Aristolochic acid is carcinogenic and nephrotoxic.

REGULATORY STATUS: Banned from sale in many countries.

SPECIFIC REFERENCES: 1. Mix D *et al* (1982) *J. Nat. Prod.* 45(6):657.

SOAP BARK

QUILLAJA SAPONARIA MOL.
Fam. Rosaceae

SYNONYMS: Quillaia saponaria, Quillaia, Soap Tree, Panama Bark.

HABITAT: Native to Chile and Peru, cultivated in California and India.

DESCRIPTION: The bark occurs in flat strips up to about 1 cm thick, externally pale yellowish-white with occasional reddish- or brownish-black patches of imperfectly removed rhytidome. The inner surface is pale and smooth. Fracture: splintery and laminate. Large crystals of calcium oxalate may be seen glistening with the naked eye. Taste: acrid and astringent; odourless, but the powder is strongly sternutatory.

PART USED: Inner bark.

CONSTITUENTS: (i) Saponins, the mixture is known as quillaja-saponin, and consists of about 100 individual quillajasaponins (or quillaiasaponins, known as QS 1-100 etc.). They are glycosides of quillaic acid and gypsogenin, with highly complex arrangements of sugar moieties [R3;1,2,3,4,5]. Recently a new saponin based on phytolaccic acid has been isolated [6] (ii) Calcium oxalate (iii) Tannins [R2,R3].

MEDICINAL USE: Expectorant, anti-inflammatory, detergent [R1]. Formerly used to loosen cough in chronic bronchitis and pulmonary complaints. The saponins have been shown to have anti-inflammatory and anti-hypercholesterolaemic activity in animals but also to cause irritation, inflammation of the intestines, cytotoxicity and other untoward effects. In smaller doses they stimulate the immune system [7], and quillajasaponins are used as vaccine adjuncts, due to their property of enhancing the activity of vaccines, in the form of ISCOM (= ImmunoStimulant COMplex) vaccines [8,9]. The saponins induce the production of Interleukin-6 and other cytokines *in vitro* and *in vivo* [10,11]. Quillaia also used externally for dandruff shampoos and as a cleansing and sloughing agent.

PREPARATIONS AND DOSE: Quillaia Tincture BP (2002), dose: 2.5–5 ml.

SPECIFIC REFERENCES: 1. Van Setten D *et al* (1998) *Anal. Chem.* 70:4401. 2. Guo S *et al* (2000) *Phytochem.* 53:861 and 54:615. 3. Higuchi R *et al* (1987) *Phytochem.* 26:229 and 2357; and (1988)27:1165. 4. Nyberg N *et al* (1999) *Carbohyd. Res.* 323(1–4):87. 5. Wolters B (1994) *Deutsche Apot. Ztg.* 134:3693. 6. Nord L *et al* (2000) *Carbohyd. Res.* 329(4):817. 7. Maharaj I *et al* (1986) *Can. J. Microbiol.* 32:414. 8. Bomford R (1987) *Phytother. Res.* 2(4):159. 9. Johansson M *et al* (1999) *Vaccine* 17(22):2894. 10. Behboudi S *et al* (1997) *Cytokine* 9(9):682. 11. Boyaka P *et al* (2001) *J. Immunol.* 166(4):2283.

SOAPWORT

SAPONARIA OFFICINALIS L.
Fam. Caryophyllaceae

HABITAT: Grows wild throughout Europe and cultivated as a garden plant.

DESCRIPTION: A rather straggling, hairless perennial. Leaves opposite, entire, lanceolate. Flowers soft pink, five-petalled, with a long calyx tube. Taste: bitter, acrid; odourless.

PART USED: Herb, root.

CONSTITUENTS: (i) Saponins, about 5%, based on quillaic acid (ii) Flavonoids; saponarine [R2,R3].

MEDICINAL USE: Alterative, detergent [R1]. Used medicinally for skin diseases, and domestically in the past, as a soap substitute and to produce a head on beers. A preparation also containing elderflower and St John's wort (q.v.) has shown antiviral effects and inhibited the replication of various strains of the influenza virus both *in vitro* and *in vivo* (in mice) [1].

SPECIFIC REFERENCES: 1. Serkedjieva J *et al* (1990) *Phytother. Res.* 4(3):97.

SOLOMON'S SEAL

POLYGONATUM MULTIFLORUM (L.) ALL.
Fam. Liliaceae

HABITAT: Largely found as a cultivated plant and garden escape.

DESCRIPTION: A well-known plant, reaching about 0.5 m; the arched stalks bearing alternate elliptical leaves, underneath which hang the bell-shaped white flowers in small clusters. The rhizome is cylindrical, flattened, about 1 cm in diameter, with circular stem scars at intervals and transverse ridges. Fracture: short, waxy, yellowish; taste: mucilaginous, sweet, then acrid and bitter; odourless.

PART USED: Rhizome.

CONSTITUENTS: (i) Saponins, based on diosgenin, known as saponosides A and B [1] (ii) Lectins and ribosome inactivating proteins, in the leaf [2].

MEDICINAL USE: Astringent, demulcent, tonic [R1]. Formerly used as an infusion for pulmonary complaints and as a poultice for bruises and piles. A preparation containing Solomon's Seal, as well as other plant extracts, has shown promise as an anti-obesity agent in a human clinical study [3].

SPECIFIC REFERENCES: 1. Janeczko Z *et al* (1980) *Acta Polon. Pharm.* 37:559. 2. Van Damme E *et al* (2000) *Eur. J. Biochem.* 267(9):2746. 3. Ignjatovic V *et al* (2000) *Pharm. Biol.* 38(1):30.

SORREL
RUMEX ACETOSA L.
Fam. Polygonaceae

HABITAT: Common in moist meadows in Europe, including Britain.

DESCRIPTION: Leaves oblong, arrow-shaped, often with a reddish tinge, with a broad-toothed, membranous, stipular sheath round the stem at the base. Taste: acid and astringent; odourless.

PART USED: Leaves.

CONSTITUENTS: (i) Flavonoids, including hyperoside, orientin and isoorientin (ii) Potassium oxalate, oxalic acid and vitamins and minerals [R4,1,2]. (ii) Anthraquinones; in the roots at least, including chrysophanol, physcion and emodin anthrones [3].

MEDICINAL USE: Refrigerant, diuretic [R1]. Antimutagenic, cytotoxic and anti-tumour properties have been documented for Sorrel [4,5]. The leaves are sometimes eaten in salads and in place of spinach and used to make soup.

SPECIFIC REFERENCES: 1. Kato T *et al* (1990) *Chem. Pharm. Bull.* 38(8):2277. 2. Ladeji O *et al* (1993) *Food Chem.* 48(2):205 and (1997)59(1):15. 3. Tamano M *et al* (1980) *Agric. Biol. Chem.* 46:1913. 4. Ito H *et al* (1980) *Jpn. J. Pharmacol.* 30(Suppl.):111P. 5. Lee N *et al* (2000) *Korean J. Pharmacog.* 32(4):338.

SOUTHERNWOOD
ARTEMISIA ABROTANUM L.
Fam. Asteraceae

SYNONYMS: Lad's Love.

HABITAT: Indigenous to southern Europe, and widely cultivated elsewhere.

DESCRIPTION: An aromatic, perennial shrubby herb with silvery green filiform leaves, up to three times pinnate, on woody stems, and small, whitish green flowers. Taste: bitter; odour: aromatic, pleasant and characteristic.

PART USED: Herb.

CONSTITUENTS: (i) Phenolic acids, including caffeic, ferulic, sinapic, vanillic and salicylic acids (ii) Flavonols (iii) Volatile oil [1,2].

MEDICINAL USE: Anthelmintic, emmenagogue, cholagogue [R1]. It has been used for threadworm infestation in children, and to induce menstruation associated with neuroses. The extract is spasmolytic and shows a dose-dependent inhibition on carbachol-induced contraction of guinea pig trachea. The smooth muscle relaxing effects were attributed to the flavonols [2].

PREPARATIONS AND DOSE: Dried herb, dose: 2–4 g or equivalent extract, three times daily.

SPECIFIC REFERENCES: 1. Swaitek L *et al* (1998) *Pharm. Pharmacol. Lett.* 8(4):158. 2. Bergendorff O *et al* (1995) *Planta Med.* 61(4):370.

SOYA
GLYCINE MAX (L.) MERR.
Fam. Fabaceae

SYNONYMS: Soy, *G. soja* Siebold and Zucc.

HABITAT: Probably indigenous to north-east China but cultivated worldwide.

DESCRIPTION: A low growing, typically leguminous crop plant. The beans are white or yellow.

PART USED: Seeds (beans).

CONSTITUENTS: (i) Isoflavones; genistein, daidzein and their derivatives; ononin, isoformononetin, glycitein, desmethyltexasin and others (ii) Coumestans such as coumestrol, especially in the sprouts (iii) Fixed oil composed mainly of linoleic and linolenic acids (iv) Phytosterols including beta-sitosterol and stigmasterol (v) Protein [1,2].

MEDICINAL USE: Soya is a very important food crop, as well as being used medicinally [R1]. The isoflavones and coumestans are phytoestrogens [1] and are used as a natural form of hormone-replacement therapy. The extract known as 'soya milk' is sometimes used a substitute for animal milks (cow's or goat's) in allergenic individuals, especially babies, and can be made into yoghurt; or fermented into condiments such as 'soy sauce'. The protein is used as a meat substitute, for example as tofu or 'TVP' (= Texturised Vegetable Protein) and the flour can be made into bread and cakes. The fixed oil contains sterols, which can be used as the starting materials for the production of hormones for use in the contraceptive pill, and hormone replacement therapy (HRT). Epidemiological evidence suggests that a diet high in soya reduces hormonal effects associated with the menopause and prostate enlargement, but recent clinical trials are equivocal about the nature of the benefits. Dietary inclusion of whole soya foods in one study resulted in a significant reduction in some clinical risk factors for osteoporosis and cardiovascular disease in menopausal women [2,3 and refs therein]. Lipid profiles were improved and blood pressure reduced, although vasodilation was reduced in one study [4,5]. Another study, however, noted little effect on either lipid profiles or coagulation factors [6], and conflicting results regarding the effect on hot flushes has been observed. In women with breast cancer given a beverage containing 90 mg soya isoflavones, no improvement was noted [7]; but in an open study of 190 healthy post-menopausal women given 35 mg of soy isoflavones, a reduction in the number of hot flushes was found [8]. A high soy diet improved measures of short- and long-term memory in healthy young men and women [9]. There is still much work to be done on the chemopreventative and hormonal effects of the isoflavones in soya, but at present it appears that they are beneficial with few adverse effects. For further information, see [9,10 and refs therein].

SPECIFIC REFERENCES: 1. Price K *et al* (1985) *Food Add. Contam.* 2:73. 2. Scheiber M *et al* (2001) *Menopause* 8(5):384. 3. Vitolins M *et* al (2001) *Curr. Opin. Lipidol.* 12:433. 4. Helena J *et al* (2001) *J. Clin. Endocrinol. Metab.* 86(7):3053. 5. Uesugi T *et al* (2002) *J. Am. Coll. Nutr.* 21(2):97. 6. Dent S *et al* (2001) *J. Nutr.* 131(9):2280. 7. Van Patten C *et al* (2002) *J. Clin. Oncol.* 20(6):1449. 8. Albert A *et al* (2002) *Phytomed.* 9(2):85. 9. File S *et al* (2001) *Psychopharmacol.* 157(4):430. 10. Mason P (2001) *Pharm. J.* 266:16.

SPEARMINT
MENTHA SPICATA L.
Fam. Lamiaceae

SYNONYMS: Garden Mint, *M. viridis* L., *Mentha x cardiaca.*

HABITAT: Europe, Asia, North Africa, North America and elsewhere.

DESCRIPTION: Leaves bright green, almost sessile, opposite, ovate-lanceolate, up to about 7 cm long, with an acute apex and a serrate margin. The lamina has a more or less crumpled appearance. Taste and odour: pleasant, characteristic.

PART USED: Herb, essential oil.

CONSTITUENTS: (i) Essential oil, of variable composition, containing carvone, about 50–70%, with dihydrocarvone, limonene, and phellandrene, and to a lesser extent; menthone, menthol, pulegone, menthofuran and many others (ii) Flavonoids; diosmin and diosmetin (ii) Rosmarinic acid [R2,R19;1,2,3].

MEDICINAL USE: Stimulant, antispasmodic, carminative [R1]. The extract is anti-fungal against the plant pathogen *Fusarium oxysporum* [4] and attenuates benzoyl peroxide-mediated cutaneous oxidative stress and hyperproliferation in mice [5]. Spearmint is widely used as a flavouring.

PREPARATIONS AND DOSE: Spearmint Oil BPC, dose: 0.5–2 ml.

BIBLICAL REFERENCES: Matthew 23:23; Luke 11:42 (Mint).

SPECIFIC REFERENCES: 1. Subramanian S *et al* (1972) *Phytochem.* 11:452. 2. Murray M *et al* (1972) *Crop Sci.* 12:723. 3. Lamaison C *et al* (1991) *Fitoterapia* 62(2):166. 4. Singh J *et al* (1994) *Int. J. Pharmacog.* 32(4):314. 5. Saleem M *et al* (2000) *Food Chem. Toxicol.* 38(10):939.

SPEEDWELL
VERONICA OFFICINALIS L.
Fam. Scrophulariaceae

HABITAT: A common wild plant in Europe, including Britain.

DESCRIPTION: A low, creeping, hairy perennial. Leaves oval, short-stalked, serrated. Flowers lilac-blue, with darker veins, four joined petals and four sepals, in axillary spikes. Taste: bitter and astringent; odour: slightly tea-like when dry.

PART USED: Herb.

CONSTITUENTS: (i) Iridoid glycosides; aucubin, esters of catalpol such as veronicoside, minecoside and verproside, mussaenoside, ladroside and others (ii) Acetophenone glucosides; pungenin, isopungenin and its 6'-caffeate (iii) Flavonoids; apigenin, scutellarin, luteolin and their glycosides (iv) Triterpene saponins [R2;1,2,3,4,5].

MEDICINAL USE: Alterative, expectorant, diuretic [R1]. An extract protected against experimentally induced ulcers in the rat [6].

SPECIFIC REFERENCES: 1. Sticher O *et al* (1982) *Planta Med.* 45:159. 2. Afifi-Yazar F *et al* (1980) *Helv. Chim. Acta* 63:1905. 3. Wojcik E (1981) *Acta Pol. Pharm.* 38:621. 4. Afifi-Yazar F *et al* (1981) *Helv. Chim. Acta* 64:16. 5. Tamas M (1985) *Clujul Med.* 57:169. 6. Scarlat M *et al* (1985) *J. Ethnopharmacol.* 13(2):157.

SPIKENARD, AMERICAN
ARALIA RACEMOSA L.
Fam. Araliaceae

HABITAT: North America.

DESCRIPTION: Rhizome up to 15 cm long, about 2.5 cm in diameter, with prominent concave scars. Roots about 2 cm thick at the base, pale brown, wrinkled. Fracture: short and whitish. Taste and odour: aromatic.

PART USED: Rhizome and root.

CONSTITUENTS: (i) Essential oil, containing the polyacetylenes falcarinone and falcarinolene (ii) Araloside, a glycoside of undetermined structure [R4;1].

MEDICINAL USE: Alterative, diaphoretic [R1]. Little information available, but formerly used for rheumatic and cutaneous disorders.

SPECIFIC REFERENCES: 1. Hansen L *et al* (1986) *Phytochem.* 25(2):285.

SQUAW VINE
MITCHELLA REPENS L.
Fam. Rubiaceae

SYNONYMS: Partridge Berry.

HABITAT: North America.

DESCRIPTION: Stem slender with a deep furrow on one side; leaves opposite, dark green, coriaceous, round to ovate, about 2 cm long, shortly petiolate, with veins prominent on the upper surface. Flowers in pairs, pinkish, bearded inside. Taste: astringent; odourless.

PART USED: Herb.

CONSTITUENTS: Largely unknown. Unspecified alkaloids, glycosides, tannins and mucilages have been reported. No recent or reliable research has been carried out.

MEDICINAL USE: Parturient, astringent [R1]. Used for amenorrhoea, dysmenorrhoea and in preparation for childbirth.

SQUILL
INDIAN SQUILL

DRIMIA MARITIMA (L.) STEARN
D. INDICA (ROXB.) JESSOP
Fam. Hyacinthaceae

SYNONYMS: Scilla. Red and White Squill are derived from different varieties of *D. maritima* (= *Urginea maritima* (L.) Baker). Indian Squill (*D. indica*) = *U. indica* (Roxb.) Kunth.

HABITAT: D. maritima is native to the Mediterranean region; *D. indica* to India.

DESCRIPTION: The bulbs are pear-shaped, about 15–30 cm in diameter, but rarely seen whole in commerce as they tend to start growing; they are sliced transversely (longitudinally in the case of Indian Squill) and dried. White Squill is cream-coloured, and Red Squill as the name suggests has a reddish tinge: Indian Squill is usually darker in colour and several pieces may be joined together unlike the other types. Fracture: short, tough, and flexible. Taste: bitter and acrid.

PART USED: Bulb.

CONSTITUENTS: (i) Cardiac glycosides, bufadienolides based mainly on the aglycone scillarenin (= scillaridin A). The most important glycosides are scillaren A, a rhamnoglucoside of scillarenin, and proscillaridin A, a glucoside of the same. The so-called scillaridin B is a mixture of glycosides. Minor glycosides include scillicyanogenin glucoside, scillipheoside and scilliglaucosidin glucoside. Both Red and White Squills contain similar compounds; however Red Squill contains scilliroside and scillirubroside in addition. Indian Squill contains scilliglaucosidin in addition to the other glycosides (ii) Flavonoids and anthocyanidins; vitexin, isovitexin, dihydroquercetin and in Red Squill, a red pigment [R2,R3;1,2,3,4,5,6].

MEDICINAL USE: Expectorant, emetic, diuretic, cardiac tonic [R1]. Squill is used mainly for its expectorant activity; it is a common ingredient of cough mixtures such as Gee's linctus. In large doses it is emetic. Although cardioactive, the effect is not cumulative and the emetic properties tend to prevent cardiotoxic problems of overdose. Both Squill and Indian Squill have similar potencies and cardiotoxic activities in animals. Red Squill was formerly used as a rat poison and has been used topically as a hair tonic for dandruff and seborrhoea; the active constituent is thought to be scilliroside. The diuretic effects, in common with other cardiac glycosides, are considerable, and Squill had been used for dropsy. It is an ancient medicine; Pliny was conversant with it and knew the two varieties and Dioscorides described a method of making Squill Vinegar which is similar to that used today, involving macerating the bulb in dilute acetic acid (vinegar).

PREPARATIONS AND DOSE: Squill Liquid Extract BP, dose: 0.06–2 ml; Squill Oxymel BP 1998.

413

REGULATORY STATUS: GSL.

SPECIFIC REFERENCES: 1. Court W (1985) *Pharm. J.* 4235:194 5:159. 2. Karawya M *et al* (1973) *Planta Med.* 23:213. 3. Garcia-Casado P *et al* (1977) *Helv. Chim. Acta* 52:218. 4. Kopp B *et al* (1996) *Phytochem.* 42:513. 5. Kopp B *et al* (1996) *J. Nat. Prod.* 59:612.

ST JOHN'S WORT

HYPERICUM PERFORATUM L.
Fam. Hypericaceae

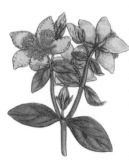

ST. JOHN'S WORT

HABITAT: A native European, including British, plant.

DESCRIPTION: Leaves opposite, sessile, oval to linear, with translucent oil glands on the surface and black dots on the lower surface in some cases. Flowers bright yellow, with numerous stamens, five petals, often black dotted along the margins. The stem has two raised lines along the stem. Taste: bitter and astringent; odour: aromatic, distinctive.

PART USED: Herb.

CONSTITUENTS: (i) Essential oil, containing methyl-2-octane, caryophyllene, alpha-terpineol, geraniol, *n*-nonane, *n*-octanal, *n*-decanal, alpha- and beta-pinene, and traces of limonene and myrcene (ii) Hypericins (naphthodianthrones); hypericin, isohypericin, pseudohypericin, protohypericin and protopseudohypericin (iii) Hyperforin and adhyperforin (prenylated phloroglucinols) and their oxygenated derivatives (iv) Flavonoids, including hyperoside, quercitrin, rutin, amentoflavone, biapigenin and others (v) Caffeic acid derivatives; chlorogenic, caffeic and others (vi) Tannins; mainly (+)- and (−)-epicatechin (vii) Miscellaneous; plant acids, carotenoids, amides and hydrocarbons [R7,R8,R11,R17;1,2,3].

MEDICINAL USE: Anxiolytic, sedative, anti-inflammatory, astringent. St John's wort was formerly used to treat menopausal problems, rheumatism, coughs and colds and used topically as a vulnerary [R1]. Now it is a very important remedy for mild to moderate depression, and numerous clinical trials have confirmed its efficacy. It appears to be as effective as conventional antidepressants with a slightly better short-term safety profile [1,2]. The use in children has also been confirmed [4] and for psychological problems associated with the menopause [5]. The hypericins and hyperforins are known to be pharmacologically active, but no single compound has been identified as the active constituent, and it is likely that a range is necessary for maximum activity [6]. Effects on various neurotransmitters including dopamine, noradrenaline and serotonin have been documented [7,8] and these show that hyperforin is required for antidepressant activity [9,10]. Drug interactions have been observed for St John's wort in conjunction with conventional drugs such as the oral contraceptive pill, protease inhibitors and cyclosporins, but these drugs are already notorious for their interactions [11]. Anti-inflammatory activity has been described and is thought to be due to inhibition of the inflammatory mediator NFkappaB [12], as well as inhibition of interleukin production, by hypericin [13]. Antiviral effects have also been noted and the herb is now under clinical investigation for this indication [14]. St John's wort is still the subject of intense research and there is already a wealth of literature on this plant, although it remains controversial, with a another recent study suggesting that it is ineffective [15]. However; this study was considered to be flawed in several respects (see www.herbalgram.org, the web site for the American Botanical Council). For more detail on uses, adverse events and possible mechanisms of action see [R7,R17;1,2,3 and refs therein].

REGULATORY STATUS: GSL.

PREPARATIONS AND DOSE: Dried herb, dose: 2–4 g or equivalent extract, three times daily. Tablets containing 300 mg of dried extract, standardized to hypericin and hyperforin content, are now available.

SPECIFIC REFERENCES: 1. Barnes J *et al* (2001) *J. Pharm. Pharmacol.* 53:583. 2. Upton R (ed.) *American Herbal Pharmacopoeia* (1997) St John's Wort. Pub: AHP, USA. 3. Bombardelli E *et al* (1995) *Fitoterapia* 66:43. 4. Hubner W *et al* (2001) *Phytother. Res.* 15(4):367. 5. Grube B *et al* (1999) *Adv. Ther.* 16(4):177. 6. Vandenbogaerde A *et al* (2000) *Pharmacol. Biochem. Behav.* 65:627. 7. Wonnemann M *et al* (2000) *Neuropsychopharmacol.* 23:188. 8. Yu P (2000) *Pharmacopsychiatry* 33:60. 9. Chatterjee S *et al* (1998) *Life Sci.* 63:499. 10. Laakman G *et al* (1998) *Pharmacopsychiatry* 31:S54. 11. Schultz V (2001) *Phytomedicine* 8(2):152. 12. Bork P *et al* (1999) *Planta Med.* 65:297. 13. Kang B *et al* (2001) *Planta Med.* 67(4):364. 14. Gulick R *et al* (1999) *Ann. Int. Med.* 130:510. 15. Davison J *et al* (2002) *JAMA* 287:1807.

STAR ANISE
ILLICIUM VERUM HOOK, F.
Fam. Illiciaceae

SYNONYMS: Chinese Anise.

HABITAT: Indigenous to Southeast Asia, cultivated extensively in China.

DESCRIPTION: Fruits about 2 cm in diameter, star-like, formed from eight boat-shaped carpels, open when ripe, each containing one smooth, polished brown seed. Pericarp brown and wrinkled below. Taste and odour: aniseed-like. It should not be confused with the smaller, more irregular Japanese star anise (shikimi fruit, bastard anise, *I. anisatum* = *I. religiosum*), which is highly poisonous.

PART USED: Fruit.

CONSTITUENTS: (i) Volatile oil, containing trans-anethole, 80–90%, with chavicol methyl ether, (= estragole), anisaldehyde, foeniculin, beta-bisabolene, beta-farnesene, caryophyllene, nerolidol and others (ii) Flavonoids; rutin and kaempferol glycosides (iii) Sesquiterpenes; veranisatins A, B and C [R2,R3,R19;1,2,3]. *I. anisatum* contains a volatile oil, together with sesquiterpenes such as the anisatins;

415

shikimic acid, and the toxins sikimotoxin and sikimin [4,5].

MEDICINAL USE: Stimulant, carminative. Uses similar to those of Aniseed (q.v.). The oil has antimicrobial properties related to the anethole content [6]. The veranisatins are neurotoxic at high doses, and analgesics at lower doses [3]. Star Anise is an important spice in Chinese cookery.

SPECIFIC REFERENCES: 1. Kubeczka K *et al* (1982) *Deutsche Apot. Ztg.* 122:2309. 2. Zanglein A (1989) *Z. Phytother.* 10:191. 3. Nakamura T *et al* (1996) *Chem. Pharm. Bull.* 44(10):1908 and (12):2344. 4. Jiang Z-H (1999) *Chem. Pharm. Bull.* 47:421. 5. Huang J-M *et al* (2000) *Chem. Pharm. Bull.* 48:657. 6. De M *et al* (2002) *Phytother. Res.*16(1):94.

STAVESACRE
DELPHINIUM STAPHISAGRIA L.
Fam. Ranunculaceae

HABITAT: Native to the Mediterranean region.

DESCRIPTION: Seeds greyish-black, wrinkled and pitted, more or less triangular or four sided, convex at the back, about 2 cm long and rather less in width. Taste: bitter and tingling; odourless.

PART USED: Seeds.

CONSTITUENTS: (i) Diterpene alkaloids; delphidine, delphinine, delphirine, delphisine, neoline, chellespontine, delstaphisagrine and others (ii) Fatty oil, composed of palmitic and stearic acids, campesterol, avenasterol and beta-sitosterol [1,2,3,4].

MEDICINAL USE: Parasiticide, used for destroying lice and fleas [R1]. The alkaloids are also insect repellents [5]. They are highly poisonous, and care should be taken that they are not ingested or absorbed through the skin.

SPECIFIC REFERENCES: 1. Pelletier S *et al* (1987) *J. Nat. Prod.* 50(3):381. 2. Liang X *et al* (1990) *J. Nat. Prod.* 53(5):1307. 3. Ulubelen A *et al* (1999) *Sci. Pharm.* 67(3):181. 4. Costa de Pasquale R *et al* (1985) *Int. J. Crude Drug Res.* 23(1):5. 5. Ulubelen A *et al* (2001) *Phytother. Res.* 15(2):170.

STOCKHOLM TAR
PINUS SYLVESTRIS L.
AND OTHER SPP.
Fam. Pinaceae

SYNONYMS: Tar, Pine Tar, Pix Liquida.

DESCRIPTION: A viscous, dark brown or black liquid, obtained by the destructive distillation of the stems and roots of various species of *Pinus*. It has a characteristic odour and acid taste.

CONSTITUENTS: A complex mixture of hydrocarbons and phenols, including phenol, cresols, methyl cresols, catechols, guaiacol, with styrene, naphthalene, mesitylene and other hydrocarbons [R3].

MEDICINAL USE: Antiseptic, antipsoriatic, antipruritic, expectorant [R1]. It is an ingredient of some cough mixtures and ointments used for the treatment of eczema and psoriasis. Most tar preparations are now considered to be toxic and are rarely used unless purified to some extent.

STONE ROOT
COLLINSONIA CANADENSIS L.
Fam. Lamiaceae

SYNONYMS: Knob Root, Heal-All.

HABITAT: Canada.

DESCRIPTION: Rhizome greyish-brown, very hard, up to 8 cm long, with knotty, short, irregular branches and numerous shallow stem scars. Bark very thin. Numerous brittle rootlets may be attached. Taste: bitter and unpleasant; odourless.

PART USED: Rhizome.

CONSTITUENTS: (i) Saponins including akeboside-1, and collinsonin and collisonidin, based on collinsonigenin and hederagenin [1] (ii) Flavonoids including baicalein-6,7-dimethyl ether and norwogonin-7,8-dimethyl ether, tectochrysin and other [2].

MEDICINAL USE: Stomachic, diuretic, tonic [R1]. Its main use is in urinary complaints such as kidney and bladder calculi (stones), and as a diuretic, and is a herbalist's favourite for shrinking piles. Little work has been carried out on Stone Root, but for effects of baicalein and wogonin derivatives see Skullcap, Baical.

SPECIFIC REFERENCES: 1. Joshi B et al (1992) J. Nat. Prod. 55(10):1468. 2. Stevens J et al (1999) J. Nat. Prod. 62(2):392.

STORAX
LIQUIDAMBAR ORIENTALIS MILL.
Fam. Hamamelidaceae

SYNONYMS: Styrax, Sweet Gum, Levant Storax. American Storax is from L. styraciflua L.

HABITAT: Native to Asia Minor.

DESCRIPTION: A viscid, treacly liquid, greyish-brown, opaque, heavier than water. It is prepared by beating the tree, causing a flow of balsam, which is then soaked up by the bark; this is boiled in water and pressed, and further purified by warming and straining or by dissolving in alcohol. American storax is collected from natural pockets in the trunk into which it exudes. Taste: sharply pungent and burning; odour: recalling that of the hyacinth.

PART USED: Balsam.

CONSTITUENTS: Cinnamic acid, cinnamyl cinnamate (styracin), phenylpropyl cinnamate, triterpene acids such as oleanolic and their

417

cinnamic esters, volatile oil. American storax is reported to have a similar composition with perhaps a greater proportion of volatile oil [R3;1].

MEDICINAL USE: Antiseptic, expectorant, stimulant [R1]. Its main use is as an ingredient for Friar's Balsam, a useful preparation which is used as an inhalation for coughs and colds and a soothing application for wounds and ulcers.

PREPARATIONS: Compound Benzoin Tincture BPC (Friar's Balsam).

BIBLICAL REFERENCES: See Exodus 30:34. (Could also be Balm of Gilead.)

SPECIFIC REFERENCES: 1. Huneck S (1968) *Tetrahedron* 19:479.

STRAMONIUM
DATURA STRAMONIUM L.
Fam. Solanaceae

SYNONYMS: Thornapple, Jimson Weed, Jamestown Weed.

HABITAT: Common in many parts of the world.

DESCRIPTION: Leaves petiolate, up to about 25 cm long, 15 cm broad, greyish-green when dried and usually found broken in commercial samples. Margins sinuous-dentate, with large irregular teeth, unequal at the base. Flowers white, tubular, with five teeth, funnel-shaped when open; calyx green, tubular. Capsule, when present, spiny, containing black, flat, reticulated, kidney-shaped seeds. Taste: bitter and saline; odour: disagreeable when fresh, tea-like when dried.

PART USED: Leaves, flowering tops, seeds.

CONSTITUENTS: Tropane alkaloids, about 0.2–0.45%; mainly hyoscyamine, hyoscine and to a lesser extent, atropine. The seeds contain about 0.2% alkaloids. Other species, such as *D. metel* and *D. innoxia*, from India, are used as a source of the alkaloids [R3;1 and refs therein].

MEDICINAL USE: Spasmolytic, anti-asthmatic, anticholinergic [R1]. Stramonium has been used to control spasms of the bronchioles in asthma. Its anticholinergic effects are similar to those of atropine, as are the effects of overdosage (see Belladonna). It causes dryness of the mouth; this property can be used to control excessive salivation, for example in Parkinson's disease.

PREPARATIONS AND DOSE: Stramonium Liquid Extract BP 1968, dose: up to 0.6 ml daily; Stramonium Tincture BP, dose: up to 6 ml daily; Compound Lobelia Powder BPC 1949; Compound Stramonium Powder BPC 1934.

REGULATORY STATUS: P.

SPECIFIC REFERENCES: 1. Evans W (1990) *Pharm. J.* 244:651.

STRAWBERRY
FRAGARIA VESCA L.
and varieties
Fam. Rosaceae

HABITAT: Widely cultivated in temperate countries.

DESCRIPTION: The strawberry plant is too well-known to require description.

PART USED: Leaves. The fruit is eaten.

CONSTITUENTS: (i) Flavonoids; glycosides of kaempferol and quercetin [1] (ii) Polyphenols and tannins, including ellagic acid and polyphenols [2,3] (iii) Essential oil, and aromatic components which may be bound as glycosides [4].

MEDICINAL USE: Mild astringent and diuretic [R1]. The procyanidins are free-radical scavengers [3].

SPECIFIC REFERENCES: 1. Henning W (1981) *Lebens. Unters. Forsch.* 173:180. 2.Vennat B *et al* (1988) *Chem. Pharm. Bull.* 36(2):828. 3. Vennat B *et al* (1996) *Boll. Chim. Farm.* 135(6):355. 4. Wintoch H *et al* (1991) *Flav. Frag. J.* 6(3):209.

STROPHANTHUS
STROPHANTHUS KOMBE OLIVER
S. GRATUS.
Fam. Apocynaceae

HABITAT: Tropical East Africa.

DESCRIPTION: A climbing plant producing greenish-brown seeds, about 1 cm long and 3 mm broad, elliptical, with appressed hairs and a long awn.

PART USED: Seeds.

CONSTITUENTS: (i) Cardiac glycosides, based on the aglycone strophanthidin, including K-strophanthoside, K-strophanthin-beta, cymarin and many minor glycosides; the mixture is known as Strophanthin-K. *S. gratus* contains ouabain (= strophanthin-G) [R3;1] (ii) Lignans, in *S. gratus*: pinoresinol, 8-hydroxypinoresinol and olivil have been isolated from the leaf [2].

MEDICINAL USE: Cardiac tonic [R1]. The glycosides have a digitalis-like action [1,3] (see Foxglove) but are poorly absorbed from the digestive tract and are not used orally. Ouabain has been used in the treatment of cardiac arrest since it acts very rapidly when given by injection. It is a sodium pump inhibitor. Recently it has been claimed that ouabain may occur naturally in the human body [4] although this has been disputed [5]. Extracts of the bark of *S. gratus* increase clotting time for blood treated with the venom of the snake *Echis carinatus* [6]. The seeds were formerly used in Africa as an arrow poison.

REGULATORY STATUS: POM.

SPECIFIC REFERENCES: 1. Dzimiri N *et al* (1987) *Br. J. Pharmacol.* 91(1):31. 2. Cowan S *et al* (2001) *Fitoterapia* 72(1):80. 3. Davies M *et al* (1998) *Heart* 80(1):4. 4. Nicholls M *et al* (1995) *Lancet* 346:1381. 5. Hilton P *et al* (1996) *Lancet* 348:303. 6. Houghton P *et al* (1994) *J. Ethnopharmacol.* 44(2):99.

SUMACH, SMOOTH
SUMACH, SWEET

RHUS GLABRA L.
R. AROMATICA AIT.

Fam. Anacardiaceae

SYNONYMS: Sweet Sumach: Fragrant Sumach.

HABITAT: Canada and North America.

DESCRIPTION: The root bark of both species occurs in quilled pieces, with scattered lenticels on the surface. The fracture shows transverse rows of minute, blackish oil glands. The surface of *R. glabra* is dull reddish-brown; that of *R. aromatica* is dull brown with exfoliating patches showing a reddish-brown to whitish cortex. Taste: mucilaginous, with *R. glabra* more astringent; odourless.

PART USED: Root bark. The berries of *R. glabra* are also used.

CONSTITUENTS: Largely unknown (i) Polyphenols including gallic acid, methyl gallate, and 4-methoxy-3,5-dihydroxybenzoic acid [1]. *R. aromatica* contains gallic acid, tannins, essential oil and resin [R4;2]. The genus *Rhus* does not contain the poisonous urushiols present in the closely related genus *Toxicodendron* (formerly *Rhus*), for example Poison Oak and Poison Ivy (q.v.).

MEDICINAL USE: Smooth Sumach: Astringent, tonic [R1]. The bark has been used by North American native peoples as an antimicrobial and for diarrhoea, in the form of a decoction, and externally as a lotion. Antimicrobial activity has been confirmed for the compounds noted above, against Gram positive and Gram negative bacteria [1]. The berries are refrigerant and diuretic and have been used for bowel complaints as an infusion. Sweet Sumach: Astringent, diuretic [R1]. It is mainly used for urinary incontinence and has a reputed anti-diabetic activity. The alcoholic extract demonstrated antimicrobial, antioxidant and free-radical-scavenging abilities [2].

SPECIFIC REFERENCES: 1. Saxena G *et al* (1994) *J. Ethnopharmacol.* 42(2):95. 2. Chakraborty A *et al* (2000) *Pharm. Pharmacol. Lett.* 10(2):76.

SUMBUL

FERULA SUMBUL HOOK
Fam. Apiaceae

SYNONYMS: Musk Root.

HABITAT: Far East, Eastern Europe.

DESCRIPTION: The root occurs in commerce cut into transverse slices about 2 cm thick and 2–5 cm in diameter, more rarely 12 cm. Pieces of the bristly crown and tapering lower part also occur. The external bark is thin, dark brown and papery, the transverse section brownish, resinous, marbled with white. Taste: bitter; odour: aromatic, musky.

PART USED: Root.

CONSTITUENTS: (i) Coumarins including umbelliferone, fesumtuorins A-H, a bicoumarin and many others (ii) Volatile oil, 0.2–0.4% (ii) Resin 5–15% (iii) Sumbulic and angelic acids [R4;1].

MEDICINAL USE: Antispasmodic, tonic. Formerly used for asthma, bronchitis, amenorrhoea etc. [R1]. Some of the coumarins showed anti-HIV activity and very weak inhibition of cytokine release [1].

SPECIFIC REFERENCES: 1. Zhou P *et al* (2000) *Phytochem.* 53:689.

SUNDEW

DROSERA ROTUNDIFOLIA L.
Fam. Droseraceae

HABITAT: Grows throughout Europe on wet heaths and moors and in sphagnum bogs.

DESCRIPTION: Sundew is an insectivorous plant. Leaves radical, six to 10 in number, reddish, orbicular, fleshy, covered with stalked, sticky glands like tentacles. Flowering stem leafless, bearing small, white, five-petalled flowers in a spike.

PART USED: Herb.

CONSTITUENTS: (i) Naphthaquinones: droserone, plumbagin, 7-methyljuglone, and others (ii) Flavonoids including astragalin, quercetin, isoquercitrin, gossypitrin and gossypin [1,2,3,4].

MEDICINAL USE: Antitussive, anti-asthmatic, demulcent, antispasmodic. Used for whooping cough and asthma and for gastric complaints [R1]. The naphthoquinones, particularly plumbagin, have a number of interesting actions; they are antimicrobial *in vitro* against some Gram-positive and Gram-negative bacteria, the influenza virus, pathogenic fungi and parasitic protozoa including some species of *Leishmania* [4,5]. Plumbagin is also antimicrobial against oral bacteria [6].

PREPARATIONS AND DOSE: Dried herb, dose: 1–2 g or equivalent extract, three times daily.

SPECIFIC REFERENCES: 1. Michelitsch A *et al* (1999) *Phytochem. Anal.* 10(2):64. 2. Krenn L *et al* (1995) *Deutsche Apot. Ztg.* 135(10):37. 3. Scholly T *et al* (1993) *Sci. Pharm.* 61(4):277. 4. Schilcher R *et al* (1993) *Z. Phytother.* 14(1):50. 5. Croft S *et al* (1985) *Ann. Trop. Med. Parasitol.* 79(6):651. 6. Didry N *et al* (1998) *J. Ethnopharmacol.* 60(1):91.

SUNFLOWER

HELIANTHUS ANNUUS L.
Fam. Asteraceae

SYNONYMS: Helianthus.

HABITAT: Widely grown throughout the world.

DESCRIPTION: The plant and its seeds are too well-known to require description.

PART USED: Seeds (fruits) and oil expressed from them, flowers.

CONSTITUENTS: Seeds (i) Fixed oil, high in polyunsaturated fatty acids, including alpha- and beta-linoleic acids (ii) Cystatins, known as Sca and Scb, which are proteinaceous cysteine proteinase inhibitors [R3;1]. Flowers: (i) Triterpene saponins; the helianthosides 1,2,3 etc., which are glycosides of oleanolic acid derivatives, and triterpene alcohols such as helianol [2,3,4,5] (ii) Diterpenes; kaur-16-en-19-oic acid, trachyloban-19-oic acid, trachyloban-19-al, kaur-16-en-19-al, loliolide and others [6,7,8] (iii) Sesquiterpenes; the heliannuols A-J, and heliespirone A [9,10,11], and sesquiterpene lactones including 1-O-methyl-4,5-dihydroniveusin A [12] (iv) Aromatic compounds including vanillin, ayapin and others [13] (v) Thiophenes, including alpha-terthienyl and several bithienyls [14] (vi) Polysaccharides [15].

MEDICINAL USE: The seeds have been used medicinally to prepare a decoction used as a demulcent in coughs and colds [R1], and recent research has also shown biological activity for many of the constituents of the flower. For example the saponins are cytotoxic and immunomodulatory in systems such as the YAC-1 and P-815 tumour models, [16,17] and the sesquiterpenes are antimicrobial, insecticidal and phytotoxic in some cases [6,7,8,9]. Sesquiterpene lactones are known to cause allergies and are likely to be mainly responsible for the dermatitis and rhinitis induced by sunflower [12]. The thiophenes are also toxic and can cause photosensitization [14]; however, extracts of the flowers inhibit inflammation induced by the phorbol ester TPA [18]. The seeds are used worldwide as a source of oil for cooking, in salads, and for the manufacture of margarine.

SPECIFIC REFERENCES: 1. Kouzuma Y *et al* (1996) *J. Biochem.* 119(6):1106. 2. Bader G *et al* (1990) *Planta Med.* 56(6):553. 3. Bader G *et al* (1991) *Planta Med.* 57(5):471. 4. Bader *et al* (1997) *Pharmazie* 52(11):836. 5. Akihisa T *et al* (1996) *Chem. Pharm. Bull.* 44(6):1255. 6. Mitscher L *et al* (1983) J. Nat. Prod. 46(5):745. 7. Nakano M *et al* (1995) *J. Food Hygiene Soc. Japan* 36(1):22. 8. St Pyrek J (1984) *J. Nat. Prod.* 47(5):822. 9. Macias F *et al* (1998) *Tet. Lett.* 39(5–6):427. 10. Macias F *et al* (1999) *J. Nat. Prod.* 62(12):1636. 11. Macias F *et al* (1999) *Tet. Lett.* 40(25):4725. 12. Hausen B *et al* (1989) *Contact Dermatitis* 20(5):326. 13. Varga E *et al* (1984) *Fitoterapia* 55(5):307. 14. Tosi B *et al* (1991) *Phytother. Res.* 5(1):59. 15. Fu D *et al* (1990) *Eur. J. Pharmacol.* 183(3):900. 16. Bader *et al* (1996) *Pharmazie* 51(6):414. 17. Plohmann B *et al* (1997) *Pharmazie* 52(12):953. 18. Yasukawa K *et al* (1998) *Phytother. Res.* 12(7):484.

SWAMP MILKWEED

ASCLEPIAS INCARNATA L.
Fam. Asclepiadaceae

HABITAT: North America.

DESCRIPTION: Rhizome about 2–3 cm diameter, yellowish-brown, irregularly globular or elongated, hard, knotty, with a thin bark and tough, whitish wood. Rootlets about 10 cm long, light brown. Taste: sweetish, acrid and bitter; odourless.

PART USED: Root and Rhizome.

CONSTITUENTS: Steroidal pregnane glycosides, at least 29 of which have been isolated from the root, including the cardenolides frugoside and gofruside, together with many tri- and penta-glycosides of isolineolon, ikemagenin, and others [1]. The aerial parts contain a similar number of related glycosides based on metaplexigenin, lineolon and isolineolon derivatives [2].

MEDICINAL USE: Emetic, cathartic [R1]. The cardenolides are cardioactive.

SPECIFIC REFERENCES: 1. Warashina T *et al* (2000) *Chem. Pharm. Bull* 48(4):516. 2.Warashina T *et al* (2000) *Chem. Pharm. Bull* 48(1):99.

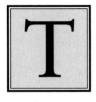

TAMARAC
LARIX LARICINA KOCH.
Fam. Pinaceae

SYNONYMS: American Larch, *L. americana* Michx.

HABITAT: North America.

DESCRIPTION: Dull purplish fragments, with irregular depressions on the outer surface, smooth, finely striated on the inner. Fracture shortly fibrous and laminate. Taste: mucilaginous, astringent; odour: slight.

PART USED: Bark.

CONSTITUENTS: (i) Tannins, 12–15% (ii) Polysaccharides, mainly arabinogalactans [R4;1].

MEDICINAL USE: Formerly used by the indigenous people of North America as an alterative, diuretic and laxative, for gout, jaundice, rheumatism and cutaneous disorders [R1]. The extract has anti-xanthine oxidase activity [1], which supports the traditional use for gout. The gum is used as a gum arabic substitute, and the arabinogalactan as a humectant and additive for skin formulations and as a form of soluble fibre.

SPECIFIC REFERENCES: 1. Owen P *et al* (1999) *J. Ethnopharmacol.* 64(2):149.

TAMARIND
TAMARINDUS INDICUS L.
Fam. Caesalpiniaceae

HABITAT: Native to tropical Asia and Africa, cultivated elsewhere, including China, India, West Indies, Indonesia, Florida etc.

DESCRIPTION: The pods are about 6–15 cm long, with a thin brittle shell containing a pulp, with up to 12 seeds. The pulp is a dark reddish-brown, moist, stringy, sugary mass. The brittle shell may be removed and the fruit preserved in syrup, or the whole fruit salted and pressed into cakes. Taste: sweet, pleasant, acid; odour: aromatic, characteristic.

PART USED: Fruit, pulp, leaf, bark.

CONSTITUENTS: Fruit pulp: (i) Volatile oil, containing 2-acetyl furan, dibutyl phthalate, benzaldehyde geranial, geraniol, limonene, alpha-terpineol, methyl salicylate, safrole, cinnamaldehyde, ethyl cinnamate, piperitone, tamarindineal, alkylthiazoles and pyrazines (ii) Plant acids; nicotinic, tartaric, malic etc., (iii) Polysaccharides particularly xyloglucans, pectin, fats, vitamins, carotenoids etc. Leaf: (i) Flavonols uncluding apigenin, vitexin, isovitexin and orientin (ii) Plant acids such as oxaloacetic, glyoxalic, alpha-oxoglutaric and others. Seed: (i) Cardenolides and bufadienolides based on uzarigenin and scilliphaeoside (ii) Phytosterols and fatty acids, including campesterol and stigmasterol, oleic and linolenic acids etc. [R12;R16;1,2,3,4,5,6,7].

MEDICINAL USE: The fruit is used as a nutritive, laxative and food.

The fruit pulp and leaves are used as an anti-inflammatory in the form of a poultice [R1]. Tamarind fruit is reported to have mild laxative effects, which are destroyed on cooking. In China and India it is also used to treat nausea in pregnancy. Hypoglycaemic and hypolipidaemic effects have been described for the polysaccharides from the fruit, as well as immunomodulatory effects [R12,R16;4]. The fruit extract is antibacterial against various pathogens [8], and molluscicidal, and anti-fungal effects have been noted. See [R12,R16] for further information. Tamarinds are used in Indian and Far Eastern cooking, and to make Worcestershire sauce and various pickles.

SPECIFIC REFERENCES: 1. Ishola M *et al* (1990) *J. Sci. Food Agric.* 51:141. 2. Zhang Y *et al* (1990) *J. Ess. Oil. Res.* 2(4):197. 3. Imbabi E *et al* (1992) *Fitoterapia* 63(6):537. 4. Sreelekha T *et al* (1992) *Anticancer Drugs* 4(2):209. 5. Shankaracharya N *et al* (1998) *J. Food Sci. Technol.* 35(3):193. 6. Bhatia V *et al* (1966) *Phytochem.* 5(1):177. 7. Yadava R *et al* (1999) *Res. J. Chem. Environ.* 3(2):55. 8. Laurens A *et al* (1985) *Pharmazie* 40(7):482.

TANSY

TANACETUM VULGARE L.
Fam. Asteraceae

HABITAT: A common European wild plant.

DESCRIPTION: Leaves dark green, pinnate, up to 12-pointed, toothed segments on each side. Flowers yellow, rayless, button-like, in umbel-like clusters. Taste: bitter; odour: strong, aromatic, characteristic.

PART USED: Herb.

CONSTITUENTS: (i) Volatile oil, of variable composition depending on chemotype: sabinene, camphor, 1,8-cineole, umbellulone, alpha-pinene, bornyl acetate and germacrene D, and some samples contain thujone (ii) Sesquiterpene lactones; parthenolide, partholide, artemorin, tatridin A and B, tanachin, tamirin, 11,13-dehydrodesacetylmatricarin, *l*-epiludovicin-C, crispoloide, and others (iii) Sesquiterpene alcohols such as the tanacetols A and B (iv) Flavonoids; apigenin, diosmetin, quercetin, jaceidin, eupatorin, chrysoeriol, jaceosidin and others [R7;1,2,3,4,5,6,7].

MEDICINAL USE: Anthelmintic, emmenagogue, bitter tonic [R1]. It has been used for expelling worms in children, for amenorrhoea and nausea, and as a lotion for scabies. The oil is anti-microbial [1]. The chloroform extract is anti-inflammatory in the rat paw oedema test [8]. Parthenolide has been shown to be mainly responsible for this activity, with the flavonoids contributing to a lesser extent [9]. It also has anti-ulcerogenic effects, which were attributed to partholide content [10]. Thujone is toxic, although not present in all types, and Tansy should be avoided during pregnancy.

SPECIFIC REFERENCES: 1. Holopainen M *et al* (1989) *Acta Pharm. Fenn.* 98(3):213. 2. Schearer W (1984) *J. Nat. Prod.* 47(6):964. 3. Nano G *et al* (1983) *Fitoterapia* 59(4):135. 4. Ivancheva S *et al* (1995)

425

Fitoterapia 66(4):373. 5. Sanz J *et al* (1991) *J. Nat. Prod.* 54(2):591. 6. Chandra A *et al* (1987) *Phytochem.* 26:1463. 7. Appendino G (1983) *Phytochem.* 22:509. 8. Mordujovich-Buschiazzo P *et al* (1996) *Fitoterapia* 67(4):319. 9. Schinella G *et al* (1998) *J. Pharm. Pharmacol.* 50(9):1069. 10. Tournier H *et al* (1999) *J. Pharm. Pharmacol.* 51(2):215.

TEA

CAMELLIA SINENSIS (L.) KUNTZE
Fam. Theaceae

SYNONYMS: *C. thea* Link, *Thea sinensis* L.

HABITAT: Cultivated China, India, Sri Lanka, Kenya, Indonesia and elsewhere.

DESCRIPTION: Tea is well known. Green Tea is the type produced in China and Japan, it is unprocessed; whereas Black (or Red) Tea is produced in India, Sri Lanka and Kenya, by fermentation and heating. This process inactivates the enzymes and gives rise to different flavour compounds. Oolong Tea is partially fermented [1].

PART USED: Leaf buds and very young leaves.

CONSTITUENTS: (i) Caffeine, 1–5%, with much smaller amounts of other xanthines such as theophylline and theobromine (ii) Polyphenols; in Green Tea these are mainly (–)-epigallocatechin; with theogallin, trigalloyl glucose. Those in Black Tea are oxidized to tea pigments, the theaflavins, thearubigens theaflavic acids, and others (ii) Flavonoids; quercetin, kaempferol and others (iii) Vitamin C, minerals etc; volatile oil. The flavour compounds are very complex. Oolong tea contains similar compounds to both, with the addition of some unique flavones known as oolonghomobisflavins. For detail see [1] and references therein.

MEDICINAL USE: Stimulant, diuretic, astringent, antioxidant [R1]. The fermentation process affects the polyphenol content and flavour; for review, see [1]. The stimulant and diuretic properties are due to the caffeine content, the astringency to the polyphenols. Tea is useful in diarrhoea, and is used in China for many types of dysentery, although in excess it can cause gastrointestinal upsets and nervous irritability due to the caffeine. The polyphenols in Green Tea have recently been shown to have anti-tumour-promoting ability, and many health benefits have been described for Tea, mainly due to the antioxidant properties [2]. Recently even weight loss due to Green Tea extract treatment has been observed [3]. Habitual consumption of Green Tea is generally associated with a lower incidence of cancer, as measured using epidemiological studies, and Black Tea is now known to have similar properties, due to the tea pigments [4]. For example anti-inflammatory and anti-tumourigenic effects have been described, and attributed to inhibition of the transcription factor NF-Kappa-B activation [5,6]. The risk of breast and stomach cancers appears to be lower for Green Tea drinkers [7,8]. Black Tea consumption is associated with a lower risk of death from ischaemic heart disease and also reverses endothelial dysfunction in patients with coronary heart disease [9]. Habitual Tea consumption is associated with a lower incidence of myocardial infarction [10] and higher bone mineral density in adults [11]. Tea is also antimicrobial and anti-cariogenic [12] and a high consumption of Green Tea is associated with a reduced risk of *Helicobacter pylori* infection [13]. For further detail, see [1,14] and references therein. Tea is drunk in nearly every country in the world for its refreshing, stimulating and mildly analgesic effects.

SPECIFIC REFERENCES: 1. Gutman R *et al* (1996) *HerbalGram* 37:33. 2. Benzie I *et al* (1999) *Nutr. Cancer* 34(1):83. 3. Chantre P *et al* (2002) *Phytomed.* 9(1):3. 4. Tomita M *et al* (2002) *Phytother. Res.* 16(1):36. 5. Ahmad N *et al* (2000) *Arch. Biochem. Biophys.* 376(2):338. 6. Das M *et al* (2002) *Phytother. Res.* 16(S1):S40. 7. Inoue M *et al* (2001) *Cancer Lett.* 167(2):175. 8. Setiawan V *et al* (2001) *Int. J. Cancer* 92(4):600. 9. Duffy S (2001) *Circulation* 104(2):151. 10. Geleijse J *et al* (2002) *Am. J. Clin. Nutr.* 75(5):880. 11. Wu C *et al* (2002) *Arch. Int. Med.* 162(9):1001. 12. Hamilton-Miller J (2001) *J. Med. Microbiol.* 50:299. 13. Yee Y *et al* (2002) *J. Gastroenterol. Hepatol.* 17(5):552. 14. Tea. Yong-Su (Ed.) (2002) *Medicinal and Aromatic Plants – Industrial Profiles.* Taylor and Francis, London, UK.

TEA TREE OIL

MELALEUCA ALTERNIFOLIA (MAIDEN ET BETCHE.) CHEEL
Fam. Myrtaceae

SYNONYMS: Ti-Tree.

HABITAT: Indigenous to the northwest coast of Australia.

DESCRIPTION: The oil is the main product found in commerce; distilled from the fresh leaves and twigs; it is colourless or pale yellow with a distinctive odour.

PART USED: Oil.

CONSTITUENTS: Several chemotypes have been described, the most highly regarded are those yielding an oil rich in terpenin-4-ol; with the other varieties mainly being rich in cineole (i) Monoterpenes; terpenin-4-ol, 1,8-cineole, gamma and alpha-terpineol, alpha- and beta-pinene, alpha-terpineol, limonene and cymene (ii) Sesquiterpenes; cubebol, epicubebol, cubenol, epicubanol and delta-cadinene [1,2,3,4]. The composition of the oil may depend also on the method of distillation [1,2].

MEDICINAL USE: The leaves and oil are traditional Aboriginal remedies for bruises, insect bites and skin infections. It is now used worldwide for its antiseptic qualities, in the form of skin creams for acne, pessaries for vaginal thrush, as an inhalation for respiratory disorders and in pastilles for sore throats. It is also popular as a lotion for the treatment of lice and scabies infestations. The oil has broad-spectrum antimicrobial activity against *Staphylococcus aureus,*

427

Escherichia coli and various pathogenic fungi and yeasts, including *Candida albicans* [5,6,7], and also protozoa such as *Leishmania major* and *Trypanosoma brucei* [8]. Many of these properties are due to the terpinen-4-ol content [9,10]. The oil is also anti-inflammatory [11], and terpinen-4-ol suppresses the production of inflammatory mediators by activated human monocytes [12]. Clinical studies have supported many of these uses, including for *Herpes labialis* [13], although many of the studies are small and of variable quality. For details, see [1,4,12 and refs therein].

SPECIFIC REFERENCES: 1. Tea Tree. Southwell I and Lowe, R (Eds). (1999) *Medicinal and Aromatic Plants – Industrial Profiles.* Taylor and Francis, London, UK. 2. Cornwell C *et al* (1995) *J. Ess. Oil. Res.* 7:613. 3. Cornwell C *et al* (2000) *Flav. Frag. J.* 15(5):352. 4. Carson C *et al* (2001) *Contact Dermatitis* 45(2):65. 5. Cox S *et al* (2000) *J. Appl. Microbiol.* 88(1):170. 6. Hammer K *et al* (1998) *J. Antimicrob. Chemother.* 42(5):591. 7. D'Auria F *et al* (2001) *J. Chemother.* 13(4):377. 8. Mikus J *et al* (2000) *Planta Med.* 66(4):366. 9. Buhiraja S *et al* (1999) *J. Manipul. Physiol. Ther.* 22(7):447. 10. Brand C *et al* (2001) *Inflamm. Res.* 50(4):213. 11. Hart P *et al* (2000) *Inflamm. Res.* 49(11):619. 12. Carson C *et al* (2001) *J. Antimicrob. Chemother.* 48(3):450. 13. Syed T *et al* (1999) *Trop. Med. Int. Health* 4(4):284.

TELLICHERRY

HOLARRHENA ANTIDYSENTERICA R. BR.
Fam. Apocynaceae

SYNONYMS: Conessi, Kurchi (Hindi).

HABITAT: Indigenous to India and other Asian countries.

DESCRIPTION: A small deciduous tree or shrub, reaching 13 m in height, with a milky latex. The leaves are opposite, elliptical, shiny on the upper surface and dull and hairy on the lower surface. Flowers are white, borne in terminal cymes. Fruits are cylindrical, found in pairs, dark grey with white flecks, containing light brown seeds with long tufts of hair. The bark is greyish-brown and peels of in flakes.

PART USED: Bark, seeds.

CONSTITUENTS: Alkaloids, including conessimine, conessidine, conimine, conamine, conarrhimine, kurchine, kurchicine, holarrhine, holarrhimine, and the regholarrhenines A-F [R16;1,2,3,4].

MEDICINAL USE: Traditionally used in Ayurvedic medicine for dysentery, and for bleeding disorders such as menorrhagia and haemorrhoids. The stem bark extract has antimicrobial activity against *Staphylococcus aureus, Staph. epidermidis, Escherichia coli, Bacillus subtilis* and others [3]. Amoebicidal and anti-diarrhoeal effects have been described, and conessine considered to be the main active component [4]. The ethanol extract was immunomodulatory, and stimulated phagocyte function in mice [5], and the seeds exhibited hypoglycaemic properties in diabetic rats [6].

PREPARATIONS AND DOSE: Powdered seed or bark, dose: 2–4 g.

SPECIFIC REFERENCES: 1. Bhutani K *et al* (1988) *Phytochem.* 27(3):925 and (1990):29(3):969. 2. Kumar A *et al* (2000) *Fitoterapia* 71(2):101. 3. Chakraborty *et al* (1999) *J. Ethnopharmacol.* 68(1–3):339. 4. Basu N *et al* (1968) *Indian J. Pharmacy* 30:289. 5. Atal C *et al* (1986) *J. Ethnopharmacol.* 18(2):133. 6. Gopal V *et al* (1993) *Indian J. Pharm. Sci.* 56(4):156.

THUJA
THUJA OCCIDENTALIS L.
Fam. Cupressaceae

SYNONYMS: Arbor Vitae, White Cedar.

HABITAT: Native to north-eastern North America and cultivated elsewhere.

DESCRIPTION: Flattened, green twigs, bearing paired, decussate scale-like leaves about 3 mm long, closely imbricated and appressed. Taste: bitter and odour, juniper-like, camphoraceous, characteristic.

PART USED: Leaves and tops.

CONSTITUENTS: (i) Volatile oil, containing thujone as the major component, with isothujone, borneol, bornyl acetate, *l*-fenchone, limonene, sabinene, camphor, 1-alpha-thujene and others (ii) Lignans including deoxypodophyllotoxin, isopicrodeoxypodophyllotoxin, deoxypodorhizone, isopimaric acid and derivatives (iii) Polysaccharides and mucilage (iv) Flavonoids, tannins etc. [1,2,3,4].

MEDICINAL USE: Expectorant, stimulant, emmenagogue, anthelmintic [R1]. The main use of the infusion is as an expectorant in bronchial catarrh and for the treatment of cystitis and amenorrhoea, but as it is a uterine stimulant it should be avoided during pregnancy. Thujone is toxic in large doses and should be taken internally only occasionally. Externally, tincture of Thuja has anti-fungal and antiviral activity and is used as a treatment for warts. Antiviral activity has been demonstrated *in vitro*; however the active principles was not identified [5]. An extract has also been found to stimulate phagocytosis by erythrocytes of Kupfer cells in isolated rat liver [6]. The polysaccharide inhibited expression of HIV-1-specific antigens and HIV-1-specific reverse transcriptase [4]. External application enhanced antibody response to sheep red blood cells [7] and other immunomodulatory effects have been noted [8]. The lignans are cytotoxic [3].

PREPARATIONS AND DOSE: Powdered bark, dose: 1–2 g, or equivalent extract, three times daily.

SPECIFIC REFERENCES: 1. Banthorpe D *et al* (1973) *Planta Med.* 23:64. 2. Tegtmeier M *et al* (1994) *Pharmazie* 49(1):56. 3. Chang L *et al* (2000) *J. Nat. Prod.* 63(9):1235. 4. Offergeld R *et al* (1992) *Leukaemia* 6(Suppl.3):198S. 5. Beuscher N *et al* (1986) *Planta Med.* 52(6):111P. 6. Vomel T (1985) *Arzneim. Forsch.* 35II(9):1437. 7. Bodinet C *et al* (1999) *Planta Med.* 65(8):695. 8. Wustenberg P *et al* (2000) *Deutsche Apoth. Ztg.* 140(19):101.

THYME
THYMUS VULGARIS L.
Fam. Lamiaceae

SYNONYMS: Common Thyme, Garden Thyme.

HABITAT: Thyme is indigenous to the Mediterranean region, and cultivated widely.

DESCRIPTION: A small, bushy herb; leaves opposite, elliptical, greenish-grey, shortly stalked, those of thyme are up to about 6 mm long and 0.5–2 mm broad. Margins entire and recurved. Taste and odour: characteristic.

PART USED: Herb.

CONSTITUENTS: (i) Volatile oil, of highly variable composition; the major constituent is thymol, with lesser amounts of carvacrol, with 1,8-cineole, borneol, geraniol, linalool, bornyl and linalyl acetate, thymol methyl ether and alpha-pinene. (ii) Flavonoids; apigenin, luteolin, thymonin, naringenin and others (iii) Polyphenolic acids; labiatic, rosmarinic and caffeic acids (iv) Polysaccharides composed of arabinogalactans (v) Miscellaneous; tannins etc [R7,R8,R17;1,2,3,4].

MEDICINAL USE: Carminative, antiseptic, antitussive, expectorant, spasmolytic [R1]. Used for coughs, bronchitis, whooping cough and similar complaints. Most of the activity is thought to be due to the thymol, which is expectorant and antiseptic. Thymol and carvacrol are spasmolytic; the flavonoid fraction has also been shown to have a potent effect on the smooth muscle of guinea pig trachea and ileum [1,5]. Thymol is a urinary tract antiseptic, anthelmintic; it is larvicidal, a counter irritant for use in topical anti-rheumatic preparations, and has many other useful actions including inhibition of platelet aggregation [6,7]. The phenolic acids are antioxidants [2] and the polysaccharide has anti-complement activity [4]. It is a popular ingredient of mouthwashes and toothpastes because of its antiseptic and deodorant properties [8]. For review, see [9]. Thymol, however, is toxic in overdose and should be used with care. Thyme is a very useful culinary herb.

PREPARATIONS AND DOSE: Powdered herb, dose: 1–4 g or equivalent extract.

SPECIFIC REFERENCES: 1. Van den Broucke C *et al* (1983) *Pharm. Weekblad* 5(1):9. 2. Nakatani N (2000) *Biofactors* 13(1–4):141. 3. Barberan F (1986) *Fitoterapia* 57(2):67. 4. Chun H *et al* (2001) *Chem. Pharm. Bull.* 49(6)762. 5. Meister A *et al* (1999) *Planta Med.* 65:512. 6. Okazaki K *et al* (1998) *Phytother. Res.* 12:603. 7. Okazaki K *et al* (2002) *Phytother. Res.* 16(4):398. 8. Miura K *et al* (1989) *Chem. Pharm. Bull.* 37:1816. 9. Thyme. Stahl-Biskup E (Ed.) (2002) *Medicinal and Aromatic Plants – Industrial Profiles.* Taylor and Francis, London, UK.

THYME, WILD

THYMUS SERPYLLUM L.
Fam. Lamiacaeae

SYNONYMS: Mother of Thyme, Serpyllum.

HABITAT: Native to Britain and Europe.

DESCRIPTION: A small, bushy herb similar to Thyme (q.v.); with leaves opposite, elliptical, greenish-grey, shortly stalked, broader (about 2 mm), and a little longer longer than thyme. Margins entire, not recurved. Taste and odour: characteristic of Thyme.

PART USED: Herb.

CONSTITUENTS: (i) Volatile oil, with significant amounts of thymol, 1,8-cineole, gamma-terpinene, linalool, cymene, and germacrene D, and also carvacrol, borneol, geraniol, linalool, bornyl and linalyl acetate, thymol methyl ether, thymol acetate, camphor, alpha-pinene and others [1,2,3].

MEDICINAL USE: Carminative, antiseptic, antitussive, expectorant spasmolytic [R1], similar to Thyme (q.v.). The oil is antimicrobial against *Bacillus subtilis*, *Staphylococcus aureus*, and others [1]; it protects against mutagenesis [4] and is insecticidal [5]. For further information, see Thyme.

PREPARATIONS AND DOSE: Powdered herb, dose: 0.6–4 g or equivalent extract, three times daily.

SPECIFIC REFERENCES: 1. Rasooli I *et al* (2002) *Fitoterapia* 73(3):244. 2. Loziene K *et al* (1998) *Planta Med.* 64(8):772. 3. Wolf J (1998) *Pharm. Ztg.* 143(4):42. 4. Milic B *et al* (1998) *Phytother. Res.* 12(Suppl 1)S3. 5. Isman M *et al* (2001) *Fitoterapia* 72(1):65.

TOADFLAX, YELLOW

LINARIA VULGARIS MILL.
Fam. Scrophulariaceae

HABITAT: A common European and British wild flower.

DESCRIPTION: Flowers pale yellow, two-lipped, the mouth closed, with an orange spot on the lower lip and a long straight spur. Leaves grass-like, bluish green.

PART USED: Herb.

CONSTITUENTS: In general, Toadflax is not well-investigated. Related species of *Linaria* such as *L. flava* contain iridoids such as antirrhinoside, 5-deoxyantirrhinoside, 5-glucosylantirrhinoside, antirrhide, linarioside, linaride, arcusangeloside and others [1,2,3] (ii) Diterpenes, including isolinaridial, from *L. saxatilis* [4] (iii) Flavonoids; linarin and pectolinarin [R4].

MEDICINAL USE: Astringent, hepatic [R1]. Isolinaridial is anti-inflammatory, and inhibits 5-lipoxygenase and phospholipase A2 [4]. Toadflax has been used with some success in treating eczemas [5].

431

SPECIFIC REFERENCES: 1. Handjieva N et al (1993) Tetrahedron 49(41):9261. 2. Nikolova-Damyanova B et al (1994) Phytochem Anal. 5(1):38. 3. Bianco A et al (1996) Fitoterapia 67(4):364. 4. Benrezzouk R et al (1999) Life Sci. 64(19)PL205. 5. Dobrescu D et al (1985) Farmacia 33(4):215.

TOBACCO
NICOTIANA TABACUM L
and other species
Fam. Solanaceae

HABITAT: Cultivated worldwide.

DESCRIPTION: Needs no description.

PART USED: Leaf, cured.

CONSTITUENTS: (i) Alkaloids; nicotine, cotinine, anabasine, nornicotine, corcotinine and others [R3] (ii) Volatile oils, flavour ingredients etc.

MEDICINAL USE: None, apart from as nicotine replacement therapy for patients trying to give up smoking cigarettes. Nicotine has interesting pharmacological actions, including stimulation, followed by paralysis, of autonomic ganglia and effects on skeletal muscle but these can hardly be referred to as medicinal. It is very toxic and easily absorbed through the skin, and this is the cause of most cases of poisoning. The addictive effects of tobacco are well-known.

TOLU BALSAM
MYROXYLON BALSAMUM (L.) HARMS
Fam. Fabaceae

SYNONYMS: Balsam Tolu, *M. toluiferum* H.B.K., *Toluiferum balsamum* L.

HABITAT: South America, cultivated in the West Indies.

DESCRIPTION: The resin is collected from incisions in the bark and sapwood of the tree. It is a light brown, fragrant, balsamic resin, softening when warm and becoming brittle when cold. Taste: sweetish, acid; odour: aromatic, vanilla-like.

PART USED: Balsam.

CONSTITUENTS: (i) Cinnamic acid, benzoic acid and their esters such as benzyl benzoate, cinnamyl cinnamate and esters with resin alcohols, coniferyl benzoate, hydroconiferyl benzoate and many others (ii) Miscellaneous; vanillin, ferulic acid, triterpenoids such as oleanolic acid, sumaresinolic acid, and others [R3;1].

MEDICINAL USE: Expectorant, stimulant, antiseptic [R1]. It is used as a mild expectorant and flavouring agent for cough mixture, as a lozenge base and as an ingredient in Friar's Balsam (see also Storax). Tolu Balsam, like many others, can cause allergic reactions.

SPECIFIC REFERENCES: 1. Lund K *et al* (1985) *Deutsche Apot. Ztg.* 125(3):105.

TONKA BEANS

DIPTERYX ODORATA (AUBL.) WILLD.
D. OPPOSITIFOLIA (AUBL.) WILLD.
Fam. Fabaceae

SYNONYMS: Tonco Seed, Tonquin Beans, *Coumarouna odorata* Aubl.

HABITAT: South America.

DESCRIPTION: The beans vary widely in appearance, they are usually 2–5 cm long, about 1 cm in diameter, greyish or black. Odour: like new-mown hay.

PART USED: Seeds.

CONSTITUENTS: (i) Coumarin, about 1–3%, with 7-hydroxycoumarin (= umbelliferone) and coumarin glycosides (ii) Fixed oil, sugars, phytosterols including stigmasterol etc. [R3;1].

MEDICINAL USE: Formerly used as a tonic and aromatic [R1]. Rarely used medicinally now, as coumarin has cardiotoxic and anticoagulant effects, but may be used for flavouring, especially in tobacco, and in perfumery.

SPECIFIC REFERENCES: 1. Sullivan G (1968) *Deutsche Apot. Ztg.* 125(3):105.

TORMENTIL

POTENTILLA ERECTA (L.) RAEUSCHEL
Fam. Rosaceae

SYNONYMS: Tormentilla, *P. tormentilla* Neck et Schranke, *P. officinalis* Curt., *Tormentilla erecta* Wahlenb., *T. officinalis* Curt.

HABITAT: Grows throughout Europe as far as northern Scandinavia and as far south as North Africa, on moors and in grassy places.

DESCRIPTION: A creeping perennial; trefoil root-leaves, stem leaves with about five leaflets, serrate. Flowers: bright yellow, with four petals and sepals and numerous stamens. Root: hard, brown, cylindrical with a rough surface, pitted, showing stem and rootlet scars. Taste: astringent; odourless.

PART USED: Herb, rhizome.

CONSTITUENTS: (i) Tannins, catechins, ellagitannins and gallotannins, including pedunculagin, agrimonine, laevigatives B and F, epigallocate-chin gallate, and others. The catechin tannins may convert during storage to phlobaphenes (= tormentil red) (ii) Procyanidins and flavonoids including kaempferol (iii) Saponins including tormentoside, epipomolic acid and others based on oleanolic and ursolic acids [R2,R8,R9;1,2,3,4,5,6].

MEDICINAL USE: Astringent, antimicrobial, anti-allergic, molluscicidal,

433

tonic [R1]. It has been used internally as an infusion for diarrhoea and gastroenteritis, and externally in the form of a lotion for pressure sores, ulcers, haemorrhoids, wounds and mouth disorders such as gingivitis, laryngitis and pharyngitis. The procyanidins are free-radical scavengers, and inhibit lipoperoxidation and elastase enzymes [4,5].

PREPARATIONS AND DOSE: Powdered herb, dose: 2–4 g or equivalent extract; three times daily.

SPECIFIC REFERENCES: 1. Geiger C et al (1994) *Planta Med.* 60(4):384. 2. Stachurski L et al (1995) *Planta Med.* 61(1):94. 3. Bilia A et al (1994) *J. Nat. Prod.* 57(3):333 (1995). 4. Vennat B et al (1994) *Biol. Pharm. Bull.* 17(2):1613. 5. Bos M-A et al (1996) *Biol. Pharm. Bull.* 19(1):146. 6. Lund K et al (1985) *Deutsche Apot. Ztg.* 125:105.

TRAGACANTH
ASTRAGALUS GUMMIFER LABILL.
AND MANY OTHER SPECIES
Fam. Fabacaeae

SYNONYMS: Gum Tragacanth.

HABITAT: Middle East, especially Turkey and Syria.

DESCRIPTION: It is the dried, gummy exudation from the incised stem. In commerce it occurs as ribbon-like, translucent, horny, white or pale yellow flakes. Taste: mucilaginous; odourless.

PART USED: Gum.

CONSTITUENTS: (i) Polysaccharides and proteinaceous polysaccharides. Tragacanthin is water-soluble, consisting of an arabinogalactan and tragacanthic acid; bassorin is an insoluble methylated fraction. Tragacanth yields on hydrolysis D-galactose, D-galacturonic acid, L-fucose, D-xylose, L-arabinose and others. Both contain residues of hydroxyproline, histidine, aspartic acid and arginine in variable amounts depending upon source (ii) Starch, cellulose, invert sugar, acetic acid [R2,R3,1].

MEDICINAL USE: The main use of Tragacanth is as a suspending or thickening agent for emulsions, mixtures, gels, low calorie syrups and various other pharmaceutical formulations [R2,R3]. It is also used in the food industry and has been shown to be non-carcinogenic [2] at normal dietary levels. Although squamous cell hyperplasia was observed in the forestomach of mice fed with Tragacanth, no other signs of toxicity were apparent, and the oral toxicity was concluded to be negligible [3]. Hypersensitivity reactions have occurred rarely after oral ingestion, and contact dermatitis after external application [R3,R14].

SPECIFIC REFERENCES: 1. Wolf J (1994) *Pharm. Ztg.* 139(49):35. 2. Hagiwara A et al (1992) *Food Chem. Toxicol.* 30(8):673. 3. Hagiwara A et al (1991) *J. Toxicol. Environ. Health* 34(2):207.

TREE OF HEAVEN
AILANTHUS ALTISSIMA (MILL) SW.
Fam. Simaroubaceae

SYNONYMS: Ailanto, Chinese Sumach, *A. glandulosa* Desf.

HABITAT: Asia, northern Australia, China.

DESCRIPTION: Bark brownish grey, with numerous warts, and on some pieces triangular scars. The inner surface is longitudinally striated. Fracture: short, buff coloured; fibrous and porous in the inner part. Taste: bitter; odourless.

PART USED: Bark.

CONSTITUENTS: (i) Quassinoids; ailanthone, ailanthinone, amarolide, acetylamarolide, shinjulactone B and others (ii) Alkaloids; canthin-6-one, 1-methoxycanthin-6-one, methyl 6-methoxy 3-carboline-l-carboxylate etc. (iii) Miscellaneous; flavonols, 2,6-dimethoxy-p-benzoquinone, tannins [1,2,3,4].

MEDICINAL USE: Febrifuge, astringent, antispasmodic, cardiac depressant [R1]. It has also been used for tapeworms, asthma and numerous other complaints, and for the treatment of dysentery. Many quassinoids are amoebicidal, and the constituents of the bark and stem, particularly ailanthone, have antimalarial activity *in vitro* against *Plasmodium falciparum* and in mice against *P. berghei*. The alkaloids do not appear to have these properties [5]. Some of the quassinoids are anti-neoplastic [6].

SPECIFIC REFERENCES: 1. Ohmoto T *et al* (1981) *Chem. Pharm. Bull.* 29(2):390. 2. Varga E *et al* (1980) *Planta Med.* 40:33. 3. Polonsky J (1985) *Prog. Chem. Org. Nat. Prod.* 47:221. 4. Varga E *et al* (1981) *Fitoterapia* 52(4):183. 5. Bray D *et al* (1987) *Phytother. Res.* 1(1):22. 6. Ghosh P *et al* (1977) *Lloydia* 40(4):636.

TURKEY CORN
DICENTRA CUCULLARIA (L.) BERNH
Fam. Papaveraceae

SYNONYMS: Turkey Pea, *Corydalis cucullaria*. Squirrel Corn is *D. canadensis* Walp.

HABITAT: Canada and the North America.

DESCRIPTION: Tubers tawny yellow, about 0.5 cm diameter, subglobular, with a scar on both depressed sides. Taste: bitter; odourless.

PART USED: Root.

CONSTITUENTS: Alkaloids; cularine, cularidine, cryptopine, bicuculline and others. Squirrel corn contains protopine, corydaline, bulbocapnine, cancentrine, dehydrocancentrines A and B [R4;1].

MEDICINAL USE: Tonic, diuretic, alterative [R1].

SPECIFIC REFERENCES: 1. Manske R (Ed.) *The Alkaloids Vol.* 17. Academic press, 1979.

TURMERIC
CURCUMA LONGA L.
Fam. Zingiberaceae

SYNONYMS: **C.** *domestica* Val. or Loir.

HABITAT: Southern Asia, cultivated in other tropical countries.

DESCRIPTION: The rhizomes are sold in both round and long pieces. The round pieces are pyriform, with transverse ridges or leaf scars, the longer pieces are the lateral rhizomes. Both are yellowish-brown internally. In this country turmeric is imported ready prepared and ground into a bright, dark yellow powder. Taste and odour: spicy, characteristic.

PART USED: Rhizome.

CONSTITUENTS: (i) Curcuminoids; the mixture known as curcumin consisting of a mixture of phenolic diarylheptanoids, including curcumin I, II and III, curcumenone, curlone, cyclocumene, curcumenol, turmerin, curzerenone (ii) Volatile oil, containing about 60% of turmerones which are sesquiterpene ketones, including arturmerone, alpha-atlantone, zingiberene; with borneol, alpha-phellandrene, eugenol and others (iii) Polysaccharides such as glycans, the ukonans A-D (iv) Miscellaneous; sugars, ascorbic acid, coumaric acid, phytosterols etc. [R12,R16,1,2,3].

MEDICINAL USE: Turmeric is becoming increasingly used medicinally in the West, as an anti-inflammatory and anti-hepatotoxic agent. It has been widely used in Ayurvedic and other Oriental forms of medicine for many years for these properties and also as a digestive, blood purifier, antiseptic and general tonic. It is given internally and also applied externally to wounds and insect bites. The anti-inflammatory properties are well-documented in a number of models, and some clinical studies. Most of the actions are attributable to the curcuminoids, although some of the essential oil components are also anti-inflammatory. The mechanism of action appears to be by cyclooxygenase inhibition and free-radical-scavenging ability. Curcumins I, II and III are antioxidant and anti-inflammatory and exhibit cytotoxicity against various experimental tumour cell lines. An antioxidant, heat-stable peptide has also been isolated. Turmeric and the curcuminoids are hepatoprotective against liver damage induced by various toxins including paracetamol, aflatoxin and cyclophosphamide. Although the mode of action is not fully understood it is known that they do not act by cleavage to caffeic acid (which is also hepatoprotective). Turmeric protects against stomach ulcers in rats, and has an antispasmodic effect. Turmeric is also hypoglycaemic in animals, and hypocholesterolaemic effects have been observed both in animals and human clinical studies. Immunostimulant activity due to the polysaccharide fraction has been shown, and anti-asthmatic effects have been noted, together with antimutagenic and anti-carcinogenic effects. In addition, turmeric is antibacterial and anti-protozoal *in vitro*. It is the subject of much current research. For further information see references

436

[R7,R12,R16;3,4,5,6,]. Turmeric is used in religious ceremonies for Hindus and Buddhists. It is important in the preparation of curry powders and is increasingly being used as a colouring agent as a result of the increased use of natural ingredients in foods.

PREPARATIONS AND DOSE: Powdered rhizome, dose: 1–4 g daily.

SPECIFIC REFERENCES: 1. Roth G *et al* (1998) *J. Nat. Prod.* 61:542. 2. Krishnamurthy N *et al* 1976) *Trop. Sci.*18:37. 3. Srimal R (1997) *Fitoterapia* 63(6):483. 4. Anton R *et al* (1998) *Pharm. Pharmacol. Comm.* 4:103. 5. Rafatullah S *et al* (1990) *J. Ethnopharmacol.* 29(1):25. 6. Ramsewak R *et al* (2000) *Phytomed.* 7(4):303. 7. Kawamori T *et al* (1999) *Cancer Res.* 51:813. 8. Kin D *et al* (2001) *Neurosci. Lett.* 303(10:57.

TURPENTINE
PINUS PALUSTRIS MILL.
P. PINASTER AIT. AND OTHER SPECIES
Fam. Pinaceae

PART USED: Oil distilled or solvent extracted.

CONSTITUENTS: Mainly monoterpene hydrocarbons, the main ones being alpa- and beta-pinenes, with 3-carene, and to a much lesser extent, beta-phellandrene, camphene, dipentene, terpinolene, beta-myrcene and others [R2,R3].

MEDICINAL USE: Rubifacient, counter-irritant [R1]. It is used externally in liniments and embrocations for rheumatism and muscle stiffness. Turpentine has been taken internally for a number of other complaints but is not recommended since it can cause toxic effects. It is used as a solvent and fragrance ingredient.

PREPARATIONS: Turpentine Oil BP, White Liniment BP 1998.

REGULATORY STATUS: GSL. For external use only.

TURPETH
IPOMOEA TURPETHUM R.BR.
Fam. Convolvulaceae

HABITAT: India, Sri Lanka, Malaysia, northern Australia.

DESCRIPTION: Variable. Wrinkled, dull grey-brown with a nauseous taste.

PART USED: Root.

CONSTITUENTS: (i) Resin, about 4–7%, containing turpethin, jalapin and glycosides based on jalapic, ipomoeic and other acids (ii) Sterols and saponins (unspecified) [R2,R4;1].

MEDICINAL USE: Cathartic, purgative [R1]. Used like Jalap (q.v.).

SPECIFIC REFERENCES: 1. Perry L. (1980) In: *Medicinal Plants of East and Southeast Asia.* MIT Press, Cambridge Mass. USA.

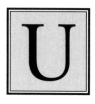

UNICORN ROOT, FALSE
VERATRUM LUTEUM A. GRAY
Fam. Melanthiaceae

SYNONYMS: Starwort, Blazing Star, Helonias Root, *Chamaelirium luteum* (L.) A Gray. *Helonias dioica* Pursh.

HABITAT: North America.

DESCRIPTION: The rhizome is about 2–3 cm long, 0.5–1 cm thick, nearly cylindrical, ringed transversely with a few stem scars on the upper surface and wiry rootlets on the lower. Fracture: horny, greyish-white, showing numerous woody bundles in the centre. Taste: astringent at first, then bitter; odourless.

PART USED: Rhizome.

CONSTITUENTS: Saponins; the glycosides chamaelirin and helonin, based on diosgenin [R4,R7].

MEDICINAL USE: Uterine tonic, diuretic, emetic, anthelmintic [R1]. Used particularly for dysmenorrhoea and amenorrhoea, for threatened miscarriage and also nausea of pregnancy; although modern thought is that all non-essential medication should be avoided during pregnancy. No pharmacological work has been carried out despite the useful indications for this plant.

PREPARATIONS AND DOSE: Powdered rhizome, dose: 1–4 g or equivalent extract; three times daily.

UNICORN ROOT, TRUE
ALETRIS FARINOSA L.
Fam. Melanthiaceae

SYNONYMS: Stargrass, Colic Root, Ague Root.

HABITAT: North America.

DESCRIPTION: Rhizome brownish-grey, flattened, up to 1 cm in diameter but usually less; tufted on the upper surface with leaf bases and marked with circular stem scars; numerous branched wiry rootlets on the lower. Fracture: mealy, white; taste: sweet then bitter and soapy; odour: faint.

PART USED: Rhizome.

CONSTITUENTS: Little recent information available. (i) Saponins, based on diosgenin [1] (ii) Volatile oil, resin etc.

MEDICINAL USE: Tonic and stomachic. It has been used for anorexia and nervous dyspepsia and for debility [R1]. Aletris has been shown to be oestrogenic but the active constituents not identified [2], but are most likely to be the steroidal, saponins.

PREPARATIONS AND DOSE: Powdered rhizome, dose: 0.3–0.6 g or equivalent extract; three times daily.

SPECIFIC REFERENCES: 1. Marker R *et al* (1940) *J. Chem. Soc.* 60:2620. 2. Costello C *et al* (1950) *J. Am. Pharm. Ass.* 39:117.

UVA-URSI
ARCTOSTAPHYLOS UVA-URSI (L.) SPRENG.
Fam. Ericaceae

SYNONYMS: Bearberry.

HABITAT: Britain, central and northern Europe, North America.

DESCRIPTION: A small, evergreen shrub. Leaves dark green on the upper surface, paler beneath, leathery, obovate, spatulate, about 2 cm long and 0.5–1 cm broad, margins entire, slightly revolute. Taste: astringent; odour: slight.

PART USED: Leaves.

CONSTITUENTS: (i) Hydroquinones; mainly arbutin (= hydroquinone beta-glucoside), methylarbutin, 4-hydroxyacetophenone glucoside, galloyl arbutin and others (ii) Iridoids, monotropein, and in the roots, unedoside (iii) Flavonoids, quercitrin, isoquercitrin, myricacitrin and others (iv) Polyphenolic acids and tannins, including gallic acid, methyl gallate and their glycosides (v) Triterpenes; alpha- and beta-amyrin, ursolic acid, and others (vi) Miscellaneous; volatile oil [R2,R7;1,2,3,4].

MEDICINAL USE: Urinary antiseptic, diuretic, astringent. It is used particularly for cystitis, urethritis and pyelitis [R1]. Uva-ursi extracts and arbutin have been shown to have antibacterial effects *in vitro* [5]. A double-blind prospective study using a product (UVA-E) containing Uva-ursi in combination with Dandelion (q.v.), for the prevention of a recurrent cystitis, showed a significant prophylactic effect, although the study was fairly small. No side effects were reported [6]. Diuretic effects have been reported in rats [7] and a reduction in risk factors associated with urolithiasis [8]. The extract also enhances the anti-allergic and anti-inflammatory effect of dexamethasone [9] and inhibits the production of melanin [10], and several of the constituents have anti-tyrosinase activities [4]. It has been suggested that for this reason Uva-ursi may be used as a skin-whitening agent [10]. Arbutin hydrolyses to hydroquinone, which is an effective urinary antiseptic [1]; however, it is also cytotoxic [11] and mutagenic [12], and so excessive doses should be avoided.

PREPARATIONS AND DOSE: Powdered leaf, dose: 1.5–4 g or equivalent extract; three times daily.

REGULATORY STATUS: GSL.

SPECIFIC REFERENCES: 1. Frohne D (1986) *Z. Phytother.* 7(2):45. 2. Jahodar L *et al* (1990) *Pharmazie* 45(6):446. 3. Veit M *et al* (1992) *Planta Med.* 58(Suppl.7):A687. 4. Matsuo K *et al* (1997) *Yakugaku Zasshi* 117(12):1028. 5. Moskalento (1986) *J. Ethnopharmacol.* 15:231. 6. Larsson B *et al* (1993) *Curr. Ther. Res.* 53(4):441. 7. Beaux D *et al* (1998) *Phytother. Res.* 12(7):498. 8. Grases F *et al* (1994) *Int. J. Urol. Nephrol.* 26(5):507. 9. Matsuda H *et al* (1992) *Yakugaku Zasshi* 112(9):673. 10. Matsuda H *et al* (1996) *Biol. Pharm. Bull.* 19(1):153. 11. Assaf M *et al* (1987) *Planta Med.* 53:343. 12. Mueller L *et al* (1996) *Mutat. Res.* 360(3):291.

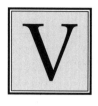

VALERIAN
VALERIANA OFFICINALIS L. *S.L.*
AND OTHER SPECIES OF *VALERIANA*
Fam. Valerianaceae

HABITAT: Native to Europe and Asia, naturalized in North America.

DESCRIPTION: The root consists of a short rootstock, about 2 cm long and 1 cm in diameter, with numerous short, lateral branches, and rootlets up to about 20 cm long, the crown often showing scales from the stem base. The transverse section is horny with a narrow, woody ring and is pale grey-brown. Valerian is unmistakable due to its unpleasant, characteristic, nauseous odour. Tasting is unnecessary.

PART USED: Root.

CONSTITUENTS: (i) Volatile oil, containing valerenic acid, valerenone, valerenal, hydroxyvalerenic acid, alpha-kessyl alcohol, isovaleric acid, citronellyl isovalerate, eugenyl and isoeugenyl isovalerate, bornyl acetate, bornyl isovalerate, faurinone and faurinols (ii) Iridoids known as valepotriates; mainly valtrate and didrovaltrate, with isovaltrate, deacetylisovaltrate, homovaltrate, acevaltrate, homodivaltrate, valechlorine, valeridine, valerosidate and possibly others (iii) Alkaloids; actinidine, valerine, valerianine and chatinine (iv) GABA (gamma-amino benzoic acid) (v) Miscellaneous; choline, flavonoids, sterols, tannins etc. [R2,R7;1,2,3,4]. Indian valerian, *V. wallichii* DC contains valtrate and isovaltrate; *V. thalictroides* Graebn, *V. edulis* (H.B.K.) F G Mey and *V. kilimandschatica* Engl. also have high concentrations of valepotriates [5]; however, they do not appear to contain valerenic acid [1,2]. A great deal of research has been conducted into the chemistry of Valerian; see recent review refs [R2,R7;1,2,3].

MEDICINAL USE: Sedative, hypnotic, nervine, hypotensive [R1]. Valerian is used widely, particularly in Europe, for insomnia, excitability and exhaustion. The sedative activity is thought to be due partly to the valepotriates and some of their degradation products, and partly to valerenic acid, valerenone and other components of the volatile oil, all of which have *in vivo* activity. It has also been suggested that there is an interaction between these constituents; however they both have primary CNS depressant activity. The degradation products of the valepotriates had a higher therapeutic index in mice than didrovaltrate, a significant finding since the valepotriates are notoriously unstable. Valerenic acid and derivatives have been shown to potentiate the effects of GABA, and the herb also contains this sedative neurotransmitter. The valepotriates have cytotoxic and anti-tumour activity in a number of *in vitro* systems; they inhibit the synthesis of DNA and proteins by covalent bonding. Tests in mice show that toxicity is low due to restricted distribution of the drug, and no adverse reactions in humans have been noted. Clinical studies of Valerian show that it improves the quality of sleep as measured by subjective assessment by the patients themselves; this is confirmed to some extent by EEG. It reduced the time taken to fall asleep, particularly in older people and in habitually poor sleepers, and did not cause somnolence in the morning nor affect dream recall. Recent studies have confirmed these results and work continues [6,7,8,9,10,11,12,13]. Recently, in a small pilot study, Valerian was shown to have potential benefits in generalized anxiety disorder [14]. Valerian is generally well-tolerated and few side effects have been recorded. It is often used successfully in combination with other herbal sedatives such as Kava [15], Balm [16], Hops and Wild Lettuce (q.v.). Valerian extracts, valerenic acid and the eugenyl and isoeugenyl esters are spasmolytic. Extracts have been used in skin creams for the treatment of eczema. For detail on all aspects of Valerian, including toxicity, see [R7;1,2,3 and refs therein].

PREPARATIONS AND DOSE: Valerian Liquid Extract BPC 1963, dose: 0.3–1 ml.

REGULATORY STATUS: GSL.

SPECIFIC REFERENCES: 1. Valerian. Houghton P (Ed.) (1997) *Medicinal and Aromatic Plants – Industrial Profiles.* Taylor and Francis, London, UK. 2. *American Herbal Pharmacopoiea* (1999). Ed. Upton R. Pub: AHP, Sacramento, USA. 3. Houghton P (1999) *J. Pharm. Pharmacol.* 51:505. 4. Gao X *et al* (2000) *Fitoterapia* 71:19. 5. Becker H *et al* (1983) *Planta Med.* 49(1):64. 6. Stevinson C *et al* (2000) *Sleep Med.* 1:91. 7. Cerny A *et al* (1999) *Fitoterapia* 70:221. 8. Donath F *et al* (2000) *Pharmacopsychiatry* 33:109. 9. Vonderheid-Guth B *et al* (2000) *Eur. J. Med. Res* 5:139. 10. Cropley M *et al* (2002) *Phytother. Res.* 16(1):23. 11. Pittler M *et al* (2000) *J. Clin. Psychopharmacol.* 20:84. 12. Poyares D *et al* (2002) *Neuropsychopharmacol. Biol. Psychiatry* 26(3):539. 13. Francis A *et al* (2002) *Phytomed.* 9(4):273. 14. Andreatini R *et al* (2002) *Phytother. Res.* 16(7):650. 15. Wheatley D *et al* (2001) *Hum. Psychopharmacol. Clin. Exp.* 16:353. 16. Cerny A *et al* (1999) *Fitoterapia* 70:221.

VERNAL GRASS, SWEET
ANTHOXANTHUM ODORATUM L.
Fam. Graminae

HABITAT: Europe, including Britain, and temperate Asia.

DESCRIPTION: Flowers in dense spikes, tapering at both ends, about 3 cm long and 1 cm wide. It is distinguished from related species by having only two stamens in the flower and by its aromatic, hay-like odour.

PART USED: Flowers.

CONSTITUENTS: Coumarin glycosides. These can be broken down to 4-hydroxycoumarin and furthermore to dicoumarol, if stored under damp conditions [1].

MEDICINAL USE: Has been used for hay fever, internally as a tincture, and as a nasal lotion [R1]. Dicoumarol is a potent anticoagulant and has caused toxic haemorrhagic effects in cattle.

SPECIFIC REFERENCES: 1. Bartol J *et al* (2000) *J. Am. Vet. Med. Ass.* 216(10):1605. 2. Pritchard D *et al* (1983) *Vet. Record* 113(4):78.

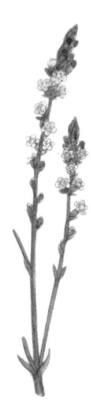

VERVAIN

VERVAIN
VERBENA OFFICINALIS L.
Fam. Verbenaceae

SYNONYMS: Verbena

HABITAT: Grows throughout Europe, particularly in the south.

DESCRIPTION: Leaves pinnately lobed, rough, toothed, opposite, the upper unstalked. Flowers lilac two lipped, petals five lobed, in long, slender, leafless spikes. Taste: very bitter; odour: aromatic when rubbed.

PART USED: Herb.

CONSTITUENTS: (i) Iridoids, verbenin (= aucubin), verbenalin (= verbanaloside), verbascoside (= acetoside), eukovoside and hastatoside (ii) Volatile oil containing verbenone, citral, geraniol and limonene (iii) Triterpenes including ursolic and oleanolic acids, beta-sitosterol (iv) Flavonoids including luteolin-7-glucuronide (v) Miscellaneous; saponin, mucilage [R7;1,2,3,4,5].

MEDICINAL USE: Nervine, tonic, sudorific, emetic [R1]. The medicinal uses of Verbena are varied, including antidepressant and anticonvulsant activity, and for jaundice, coughs and colds and as a digestive aid. Recently immunomodulatory and antiviral effects have been noted [4] and Verbena is reputed to have galactogogue and weak parasympathomimetic activity [R7]. It may be taken as an infusion. Verbenalin is a mild purgative in animals [6], the triterpenes are anti-inflammatory in carrageenan paw oedema models [5], and the flavonoids are antimicrobial [7]. All of these are thought to contribute to the therapeutic efficacy [4]. Verbena appears to be of low toxicity.

REGULATORY STATUS: GSL.

PREPARATIONS AND DOSE: Dried herb, dose: 2–4 g as an infusion, or equivalent extract, three times daily.

SPECIFIC REFERENCES: 1. Lahloub M *et al* (1986) *Planta Med.* 52:47. 2. Carant A *et al* (1995) *Planta Med.* 61(5):490. 3. Mende R *et al* (1998) *Deutsch Apot. Zeit.* 138(31):35. 4. Wichtl. M (1999) *Z. Phytother.* 20(6):353. 5. Deepak M *et al* (2000) *Phytother. Res.* 14(6):463. 6. Inoue H *et al* (1974) *Planta Med.* 25:285. 7. Hernandez N *et al* (2000) *J. Ethnopharmacol.* 73(1–2):317.

VIOLET
VIOLA ODORATA L.
Fam. Violaceae

SYNONYMS: Sweet Violet.

HABITAT: Widely found in Europe, including Britain, and Asia.

DESCRIPTION: A well-known plant. Leaves cordate or ovate, with long stalks. Flowers blue, with a hooked stigma and a short spur inflated at the end and channelled above. Taste: mucilaginous.

PART USED: Flowers, leaves.

CONSTITUENTS: (i) Phenolic glycosides; gaultherin, violutoside (= salicylic acid methyl ester) (ii) Volatile oil, in the flower, containing trans alpha-ionone (= parmone), dihydro-beta-ionone, curcumene, zingiberene, 2,6-nonadien-1-al and undecan-2-one (iii) Saponins; myrosin and violin (iv) Flavonoids; rutin and violarutin (v) Miscellaneous; odoratine, an alkaloid, 2-nitropropionic acid, mucilage [1,2,3].

MEDICINAL USE: Antiseptic, expectorant [R1]. It has been used in syrups for coughs and colds, bronchitis and catarrh; and externally for skin inflammation. Anti-inflammatory and diuretic effects have been reported for a leaf extract [4,5]. It is reputed to be expectorant and antimicrobial due to the saponin content [R2]. The flowers are used in perfumery and to make confectionery.

REGULATORY STATUS: GSL.

PREPARATIONS AND DOSE: Dried herb, dose: 2–4 g as an infusion, or equivalent extract, three times daily.

SPECIFIC REFERENCES: 1. Watt J M *et al* (1962) *In: The Medicinal and Poisonous Plants of Southern and Eastern Africa* 2nd ed. Livingstone, UK. 2. Willaman J *et al* (1970) *Lloydia* 33:1. 3. Uhde G *et al* (1972) *Helv. Chim. Acta* 55:2621. 4. Khattak S *et al* (1985) *J. Ethnopharmacol.* 14(1):45. 5. Rebuelta M *et al* (1984) *Plantes Med. Phytother.* 17(4):215.

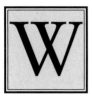

WAFER ASH
PTELEA TRIFOLIATA L.
Fam. Rutaceae

SYNONYMS: Shrubby Trefoil, Swamp Dogwood.

HABITAT: North America and Canada.

DESCRIPTION: The root bark occurs in quilled or curved pieces, 3–20 mm thick, transversely wrinkled with a whitish-brown exfoliating surface of thin, papery layers. The inner surface is nearly smooth, with faintly projecting medullary rays. Transverse fracture short, yellowish-white, the papery layer pale buff. Taste: bitter; odourless.

PART USED: Root bark.

CONSTITUENTS: (i) Alkaloids, including kokusaginine, kokuginine, skimmianine, dictamine, pteleine and maculosidine, and the dimeric derivatives pteledimerine, pteledimeridine and pteledimericine (ii) Coumarins such as isopimpinellin, phellopterin [R2,R4;1,2].

MEDICINAL USE: Tonic, antiperiodic, stomachic [R1]. It has been used in the form of an infusion for fevers, as a tonic and to stimulate the appetite. The bitter substances are reported to have antibacterial activity [R2,R4].

SPECIFIC REFERENCES: 1. Mester I *et al* (1979) *Leibigs Ann. Chem.* 1(11):1785. 2. Petit-Paly G *et al* (1990) *Pharmazie* 45(9):698. 3. Lohar D *et al* (1995) *Indian Drugs* 32(10):506.

WAHOO
EUONYMUS ATROPURPUREUS JACQ.
E. EUROPEA L.
Fam. Celastraceae

SYNONYMS: Spindle Tree

HABITAT: Eastern and central North America and Canada.

DESCRIPTION: Usually occurs in transverse curved pieces or occasionally quills, 2–4 mm thick, very light in weight. The outer surface is light brown, wrinkled, with patches of soft grey rhytidome and few lenticels. Root bark may have root scars and adhering rootlets; stem bark is smoother with lichens usually present. The inner surface is striated, porous, sometimes with adherent patches of yellow wood. Fracture short but friable, showing a narrow brown cork, a whitish cortex and a darker phloem. Taste: bitter and acrid; odour: faint.

PART USED: Stem and root bark.

CONSTITUENTS: This plant has not been well-investigated. (i) Cardenolides, including euatroside and euatrominoside, based on digitoxigenin (ii) Alkaloids such as asparagine and atropurpurine (unconfirmed) (iii) Flavonoids; mainly quercetin and kaempferol glycosides (iv) Sterols; euonysterol, atropurpurol, homo-euonysterol (v) Miscellaneous; lectins, dulcitol, citrullol, fatty acids, tannins etc. [R2,R4;1]. *E. fortunei* contains the triterpenes friedelin, isoarborinol, and their derivatives [2]; *E. phellomana* Loes seed oil and *E. sieboldianus* Blume contain dihydroagarofuran sesquiterpenes [3,4].

MEDICINAL USE: Cholagogue, laxative, diuretic, mild cardiac tonic and circulatory stimulant [R1]. It is reported to be a mild purgative and choleretic and is used mainly in combination with other remedies for liver and gall bladder trouble and dyspepsia, and occasionally for skin problems where these conditions are thought to be a cause. The dihydroagarofuran sesquiterpenes inhibit tumour promotion induced by the phorbol ester TPA [4].

PREPARATIONS AND DOSE: Dried root bark, dose: 0.3–1 g as a decoction, or equivalent extract, three times daily.

SPECIFIC REFERENCES: 1. Grasza B *et al* (1993) *Fitoterapia* 64(4):379. 2. Katakawa J *et al* (2000) *Natural Med.* 54(1):18. 3. Wang H *et al* (2001) *Pharmazie* 56(11):889.

WALNUT
JUGLANS REGIA L.
Fam. Juglandaceae

HABITAT: Native to the Middle East, cultivated widely for the walnuts, which ripen towards the end of September.

DESCRIPTION: Leaves composed of seven to nine leaflets of varying size, averaging 5–10 cm in length and 3–4 cm wide, greenish, parchment-like, turning brown with keeping. The bark is dull, blackish-brown, with traces of a thin, whitish external layer, tough and fibrous and somewhat mealy. Taste: bitter and astringent; leaves: odour characteristic and aromatic; bark: odourless.

PART USED: Leaves, bark. The fruit (walnuts) are eaten in many parts of the world.

CONSTITUENTS: Leaves: (i) Naphthaquinones, mainly juglone (formerly known as nucin or regianin), often as the 4-beta-D-glucoside of alpha lpha-hydrojuglone, and lawsone (ii) Volatile oil, containing beta-eudesmol, eugenol, fatty acids including geranic acid, sesquiterpenes, diterpenes and others (iii) Miscellaneous; tannins, ellagic acid and gallic acids, flavonoids, inositol [R2;1,2].

MEDICINAL USE: Alterative, laxative, antiseptic [R1]. An infusion has been used for herpes, eczema and other conditions, and externally to skin eruptions and ulcers etc. The leaf extract produced vaso-relaxant effects on isolated rat thoracic aorta [3], and both extract and isolated juglone were found to be sedative in mice [4]. The unripe fruits have been used to treat goitre and an extract enhances thyroid-hormone-activity in mice [5]. The volatile oil is anti-fungal *in vitro* and juglone has antimicrobial and anti-neoplastic activity. Walnuts are a food, and have also been used medicinally, for many years: because of its visual resemblance to the brain it was thought, according to the Doctrine of Signatures, to be good for headaches and epilepsy. A dye made from the shells has been used to darken the skin and hair, but it can cause

445

dermatitis and hyper-pigmentation of the skin [6].

PREPARATIONS AND DOSE: Dried herb, dose: 2–6 g as a decoction, or equivalent extract, three times daily.

BIBLICAL REFERENCES: Song of Solomon 6: 11; Genesis 43:11 (nuts).

SPECIFIC REFERENCES: 1. Nahrstedt A *et al* (1981) *Planta Med.* 42(4):313. 2. Lemberkovics E *et al* (1987) *Acta Pharm. Hungarica* 57(3–4):133. 3. Perusquia M *et al* (1995) *J. Ethnopharmacol.* 46(1):63. 4. Girzu M *et al* (1998) *Pharm. Biol.* 36(4):280. 5. Ozturk Y *et al* (1994) *Phytother. Res.* 8:308. 6. Bonamonte D *et al* (2001) *Contact Dermatitis* 44(2):101.

WATER BETONY
SCROPHULARIA AQUATICA L.
Fam. Scrophulariaceae

SYNONYMS: Water Figwort, *Betonica aquatica.*

HABITAT: Common by streams or ponds and in wet places in Britain and parts of Europe.

DESCRIPTION: Stem four-angled, winged, bearing leaves in opposite pairs with winged petioles. The leaves are oval, with serrated margins, pointed at the apex, and sometimes with one or two small lobes at the base. The flowers are up to 1 cm across, brownish-purple with greenish undersides, with a tubular base opening into five small petal lobes, the upper two of which are joined. Taste: bitter; odourless.

PART USED: Herb.

CONSTITUENTS: Unknown. Other species of *Scrophularia* contain iridoids (see Figwort).

MEDICINAL USE: Vulnerary [R1]. Used as a poultice or ointment for ulcers, sores and wounds.

WATER DOCK
RUMEX AQUATICA L.
Fam. Polygonaceae

HABITAT: Northern Europe and Great Britain, mainly by rivers and ditches.

DESCRIPTION: The leaves are triangular, up to three times as long as wide, alternate, with a sheath round the stem at the base of the leaves. The root has a blackish or dark brown outer surface, the remains of a few branches, and transverse rings of rootlet scars. Taste: astringent and sweetish; odourless.

PART USED: Root.

CONSTITUENTS: Anthraquinones, about 0.6%; tannins, about 20%, (unspecified) [R2,R4].

MEDICINAL USE: Alterative, deobstruent, detergent [R1]. An infusion has been used internally and the powdered root has been used as a dentifrice.

WATER DROPWORT

OENANTHE CROCATA L.
Fam. Apiaceae

SYNONYMS: Hemlock Water Dropwort, Dead Men's Fingers.

HABITAT: Found in damp grassy places in Britain, France and other parts of Europe.

DESCRIPTION: A tall, hairless, perennial; flowers typical white umbels, leaves 3–4 pinnate, with broad, wedge-shaped toothed leaflets; stem, grooved. The root bears pale fleshy tubers, hence the synonym. Odour: reminiscent of parsley.

PART USED: Root.

CONSTITUENTS: Oenanthetoxin, a polyunsaturated higher alcohol, and oenanthetol, oeanthetone, and dihydroenanthetoxin [1].

MEDICINAL USE: None. Formerly used for epilepsy but cannot be recommended. The plant has been responsible for numerous cases of poisoning, in mistake for parsley, celery etc. [2].

SPECIFIC REFERENCES: 1. King L *et al* (1985) *Hum. Toxicol.* 4(4):355. 2. Filippini R *et al* (1993) *Pharmacol. Res.* 27(Suppl.1):7.

WATER FENNEL

OENANTHE AQUATICA (L.) POIR.
Fam. Apiaceae

SYNONYMS: Fine-leaved Water Dropwort, *Oenanthe phellandrium* Lamk.

HABITAT: In damp places throughout Europe.

DESCRIPTION: A much branched, hairless perennial. Leaves 3–4 pinnate, upper with pointed lobes, lower lobes linear to threadlike. Flowers white, umbels opposite to leaves as well as terminal. Fruits about 5 mm long and 2 mm in diameter, tapering towards the apex, and crowned with four teeth. Taste: acrid; odour: strong, aromatic, characteristic.

PART USED: Fruit.

CONSTITUENTS: (i) Essential oil, about 1.5–2% [2] (ii) Flavonoids; tricetin, myricetin and rhamnetin (iii) Fixed oil, about 20% (iii) Polyacetylenes [1,2]. The herb contains the poisonous oenanthetoxin (see Water Dropwort) [R4].

MEDICINAL USE: Expectorant, alterative, diuretic [R1]. Rarely used and not recommended.

SPECIFIC REFERENCES: 1. Vincieri F *et al* (1985) *Planta Med.* 51(2):107. 2. Ram A *et al* (1983) *Indian J. Bot.* 6(1):21.

WATER GERMANDER
TEUCRIUM SCORDIUM L.
Fam. Lamiaceae

HABITAT: Europe, rarely in Britain.

DESCRIPTION: Leaves opposite and sessile, oval-oblong, about 2 cm long and 0.5 cm broad, narrowed at the base, coarsely serrate at the margin, softly hairy on both sides. Taste: bitter; odour: when the fresh leaves are rubbed, rather alliaceous.

PART USED: Herb.

CONSTITUENTS: (i) Iridoids, including harpagide and acetyl harpagide (ii) Diterpenes, of the clerodane type, teucrin F, teucrin G and 6-hydroxyteuscordin [1] (iii) Miscellaneous; tannins, essential oil etc. [2].

MEDICINAL USE: Antiseptic, diaphoretic, stimulant [R1]. It was recommended in ancient times as a sudorific and antiseptic, and taken as an infusion. Gerard even declares that "after battle, the bodies found lying on these plants were much slower in decaying than those not".

SPECIFIC REFERENCES: 1. Fikenscher L *et al* (1969) *Plantes Med. Phytother.* 3(3):181. 2. Kalodera Z *et al* (1996) *Farm. Glasnik* 52(11):273.

WHITE POND LILY, AMERICAN
NYMPHAEA ODORATA SOLAND.
Fam. Nymphaceae

SYNONYMS: Water Nymph, Water Cabbage. *N. alba* and *N. tuberosa* are also used.

HABITAT: North America.

DESCRIPTION: The rhizome occurs in irregular pieces up to about 5 cm in diameter. The outer surface is dark greyish-brown to black, with the remains of leaf bases up to about 1 cm in diameter and root scars. Buds may also be present; these have a dense covering of fine grey hairs. The transverse surface is yellowish-brown, with a ring of porous depressions immediately inside the cork. Fracture: short; taste: mucilaginous; slightly pungent; odour: faint.

PART USED: Rhizome.

CONSTITUENTS: Unidentified. *N. tuberosa* contains tannic acid and gallic acid; and alkaloids, sterols and flavonoids [1]; and *N. alba* is reputed to contain the alkaloids nymphaeine and nupharine, glycosides and tannins [R2,R4]. Little recent work has been carried out on this genus.

MEDICINAL USE: Antiseptic, astringent, demulcent [R1]. It may be taken in the form of an infusion internally for chronic diarrhoea, as a douche for leucorrhoea and vaginitis, as a gargle for sore throat and as a poultice with Slippery Elm and Linseed for boils. *N. tuberosa* has some anti-tumour effects in hamsters. The tannic acid and gallic acid are antimicrobial [1] and astringent. *N. alba* is hypotensive in animals and is reported to have low toxicity [2].

PREPARATIONS AND DOSE: Dried rhizome, dose: 1–2 g as an infusion, or equivalent extract, three times daily.

REGULATORY STATUS: 1. Su K *et al* (1983) *Lloydia* 36:72 and 80.
2. Odinstova N *et al* (1960) *Farmakol. i Toxicol.* 23:132.

WILD INDIGO
BAPTISIA TINCTORIA R. BR.
Fam. Fabaceae

SYNONYMS: Indigo Weed, False or Yellow indigo.

HABITAT: Indigenous to Canada and North America.

DESCRIPTION: Crown of root with knotty branches; the roots vary in diameter from 0.2–1.5 cm, external surface brownish, longitudinally wrinkled and grooved, somewhat warty due to detached rootlets. Fracture tough and fibrous, showing a thick bark and whitish wood with concentric rings. Taste: bitter, acrid, disagreeable; odour: faint.

PART USED: Root, leaves.

CONSTITUENTS: (i) Isoflavones; genistein, biochanin A, baptigenin, pseudobaptigenin, maackiain, formononetin, baptisin and trifolirhizin (ii) Alkaloids including cytisine, N-methylcytisine, anagyrine and sparteine (iii) Coumarins such as scopoletin (iv) Polysaccharides, mainly arabinogalactans [R2;1,2,3,4].

MEDICINAL USE: Antimicrobial, antiseptic, antipyretic, laxative, mild cardiotonic [R1]. Wild Indigo is used for infections of the respiratory tract, in the form of an infusion for tonsillitis, pharyngitis and other conditions, particularly with associated catarrh, and as a mouthwash for aphthous ulcers and sore gums. It may be applied topically to boils, and in the form of an ointment for sore nipples and indolent ulcers. It is used as a douche in vaginitis and leucorrhoea. The isoflavones are oestrogenic (for further information see Red Clover). The polysaccharide fraction has been shown to enhance antibody production in sheep red blood cells and stimulate phagocytosis of erythrocytes in isolated perfused rat liver. It demonstrates numerous other immunomodulatory activities, which supports the anti-infective use [1,3,5].

PREPARATIONS AND DOSE: Dried root, dose: 0.5–1 g by decoction, or equivalent extract, three times daily.

REGULATORY STATUS: 1. Beuscher N *et al* (1985) *Planta Med.* 51:381 and (1989)55:358. 2. Markham K *et al* (1970) *Phytochem.* 9:2359.
3. Wagner H *et al* (1985) *Arzneim. Forsch.* 35:1069. 4. Gocan S *et al* (1996) *J. Pharm. Biomed. Anal.* 14(8–10):1221. 5. Egert D *et al* (1992) *Planta Med.* 58(2):163.

WILD MINT

MENTHA AQUATICA L.
Fam. Lamiaceae

SYNONYMS: Water Mint, Marsh Mint, Hairy Mint, *M. sativa* L.

HABITAT: Europe and the British Isles.

DESCRIPTION: Similar to Peppermint (q.v.), which is a hybrid of this species. The leaves are wider, less sharply toothed and the flowers more hairy. Odour and taste: characteristic.

PART USED: Herb.

CONSTITUENTS: (i) Volatile oil, composed of mainly methofuran, with menthol, menthyl acetate, beta-caryophyllene, 1,8-cineole, germacrene-D, viridoflorol, linalool, pulegone and others (ii) Polyphenols, including rosmarinic acid. [R2;1,2].

MEDICINAL USE: Stimulant, emetic, astringent; it has been used for difficult menstruation and diarrhoea [R1].

SPECIFIC REFERENCES: 1. Avao P *et al* (1995) *Sci. Pharm.* 63(3):223. 2. Lamaison C *et al* (1991) *Fitoterapia* 62(2):166.

WILD YAM

DIOSCOREA VILLOSA L.
Fam. Dioscoriaceae

SYNONYMS: Colic Root, Rheumatism Root.

HABITAT: Common in eastern and central North America and in some tropical countries.

DESCRIPTION: Tubers cylindrical, pale brown, compressed, about 10–15 cm long and 1–2 cm thick, curved, branched at intervals, showing stem scars on the upper surface and rootlets on the other. Occurs in commerce as hard, pale yellowish-brown chips of rhizome and narrow, fibrous roots. Fracture: short, hard; taste: insipid at first, then acrid; odourless.

PART USED: Root and rhizome.

CONSTITUENTS: (i) Steroidal saponins, based on diosgenin: dioscin, dioscorin, and others (ii) Alkaloids; dioscorine (unconfirmed) [R2,R4]. Many other species of *Dioscorea* are used as sources of saponins for the preparation of steroids for the pharmaceutical industry.

MEDICINAL USE: Anti-inflammatory, cholagogue, spasmolytic, mild diaphoretic [R1]. The main use is in various types of rheumatism and for bilious and intestinal colic. It is also used for dysmenorrhoea and cramps. Recently Wild Yam has been promoted as a natural form of hormone replacement therapy, used as a cream. The rationale behind such use is that increasing the level of steroid precursors in the body will lead to an increase in natural hormone levels. Clinical studies have not supported this theory and in a recent double-blind, placebo-controlled crossover study in 23 healthy peri-menopausal women, no significant effects were observed. No toxicity was observed either [1].

PREPARATIONS AND DOSE: Dried root and rhizome, dose: 2–4 g as an infusion or decoction, or equivalent extract, three times daily.

SPECIFIC REFERENCES: 1. Komesaroff P *et al* (2001) *Climacteric* 4(2):144.

WILLOW
SALIX ALBA L.
S. FRAGILIS L.
S. CINEREA L.
AND OTHER SPECIES
Fam. Salicaceae

SYNONYMS: White Willow, European Willow.

HABITAT: Indigenous to Britain, central and southern Europe.

DESCRIPTION: The bark occurs in thin channelled pieces up to about 2 cm wide and 2 mm thick. Outer surface glossy in young bark, wrinkled and duller in older bark, greenish- or greyish-brown; inner surface striated, fibrous, yellowish or reddish-brown. Taste: astringent and bitter; odour: faint.

PART USED: Bark.

CONSTITUENTS: (i) Phenolic glycosides; salicin, picein and triandrin, with esters of salicylic acid and salicyl alcohol, acetylated salicin, salicortin and salireposide; concentrations etc. depending on species (ii) Miscellaneous; tannins, catechin, *p*-coumaric acid and flavonoids [R2,R3,R7,R9;1,2,3].

MEDICINAL USE: Analgesic, anti-inflammatory, febrifuge, tonic [R1]. Willow is an ancient remedy, which has been used in various forms for rheumatism and gout, fevers and aches and pains of all kinds. It is usually considered to be the natural form and origin of the modern aspirin. Several clinical trials have confirmed the therapeutic effects in the treatment of rheumatism, osteoarthritis and other painful inflammatory conditions [4,5,6,7]. In the body, the glycosides are hydrolyzed to salicylic acid and this was until recently considered to be the active principle. However, it is now known that effective dose levels of Willow bark produce lower blood levels of salicylic acid than would be expected to be active, and the side effects on the gastrointestinal system experienced were much less than those with aspirin [6]. This suggests an enhanced effect for the extract, rather than it being merely a source of salicylic acid, and confirms that the total extract is more efficaceous than a single isolated substance [6,7].

REGULATORY STATUS: GSL.

PREPARATIONS AND DOSE: Dried bark, dose: 2–4 g as a decoction, or equivalent extract, three times daily.

BIBLICAL REFERENCES: Leviticus 23:40; Job 40:22; Psalm 137:2; Isaiah 15:7 and 44:4; Ezekiel 17:5.

SPECIFIC REFERENCES: 1. Willow Bark. *American Herbal Pharmacopoiea* (1999), Ed. Upton R Pub: AHP, Sacramento, USA. 2. Meier B *et al* (1985) *Pharm. Acta Helv.* 60:269. 3. Julkunen-Tiitto R (1986) *Phytochem.* 25:663. 4. Mills S *et al* (1996) *Br. J. Rheumatol.* 35:874. 5. Chubrasik S *et al* (2000) *Am. J. Med.* 109:9. 6. Schmid B *et al* (2001) *Phytother. Res.* 15(4):344. 7. Schmid B *et al* (2001) *Eur. J. Clin. Pharmacol.* 57(5):387.

WINTER'S BARK

DRIMYS WINTERI FORST.
Fam. Winteraceae

SYNONYMS: True Winter's Bark, Pepper Bark. *D. granadensis* is often substituted. False Winter's Bark is *Cinnamodendron corticosum.*

HABITAT: Central and South America.

DESCRIPTION: Rare in commerce. In short pieces, 5–8 mm thick, dark brown throughout. Fracture short and granular, showing pale medullary rays which project on the inner surface, giving it a striated appearance. Taste: pungent; odour: faint.

PART USED: Bark.

CONSTITUENTS: (i) Sesquiterpene derivatives; mainly polygodial, 1-beta-(*p*-methoxycinnamyl)-polygodial, astilbin and taxifolin [1,2].

MEDICINAL USE: Used mainly for indigestion, flatulence and colic; and various types of pain [R1], usually as an infusion. The methanol extract, and polygodial and its derivatives, have anti-allergic, anti-inflammatory [1] and anti-nociceptive activity in mice [1,2], and support the use of this plant for the treatment of pain. False Winter's Bark is used for similar purposes.

SPECIFIC REFERENCES: 1. Cechinel Filho V *et al* (1998) *J. Ethnopharmacol.* 62(3):223. 2. Malheiros A *et al* (2001) *Phytochem.* 57(1):103.

WINTER CHERRY

PHYSALIS ALKEKENGI L.
Fam. Solanaceae

HABITAT: Indigenous to Asia and parts of Europe, cultivated in gardens in Britain and America.

DESCRIPTION: The dried berries are dull red, about 0.5 cm in diameter, globular, bilocular, containing numerous whitish, ovoid flattened seeds. Taste: first sweet and then bitter; odourless. The plant sold in florists and garden centres as 'Winter Cherry' is usually *Solanum pseudocapsicum.*

PART USED: Berries.

CONSTITUENTS: (i) Steroidal triterpenes; known as physalins A, B, C, D etc.; up to physalin R at present, and various hydro- and dehydro-derivatives (ii) Tropane alkaloids; calystegins A5, B1, B3,

C1 and others, cuscohygrine, tropine and tigloidine (iii) Flavonoids, including luteolin-7-glucoside [1,2,3,4,5].

MEDICINAL USE: Diuretic, febrifuge [R1]. Has been employed in intermittent fevers, in urinary disorders and gout. Extracts of *Physalis* have oestrogen antagonistic activity in female rats measured by various methods, and significantly reduce the numbers of pups born per litter [6,7]. The calystegins inhibit glycosidase enzymes, such as almond beta-glucosidase and bovine liver beta-galactosidase [5]. Physalins B and F were shown to inhibit the growth of several human leukaemia cell lines *in vitro* [8].

SPECIFIC REFERENCES: 1. Makino B *et al* (1995) *Bull. Chem. Soc. Japan* 68(1):219. 2. Makino B *et al* (1995) *Tetrahedron* 51(46):12529. 3. Kawai M *et al* (2001) *J. Asian Nat. Prod. Res.* 3(3):199. 4. McGaw B *et al* (1982) *J. Pharm. Pharmacol.* 34(Suppl.1):18P. 5. Asano N *et al* (1995) *Eur. J. Biochem.* 229(2):369. 6. Vessal M *et al* (1991) *J. Ethnopharmacol.* 34(1):69. 7. Vessal M *et al* (1995) *Comp. Biochem. Physiol.* (B) 111(4):675, and (1996)5(2):267; and (C) (1995) 112(2):229. 8. Chiang H-C *et al* (1992) *Anticancer Res.* 12(4):1155.

WINTERGREEN

GAULTHERIA PROCUMBENS L.
Fam. Ericaceae
BETULA LENTA L.
Betulaceae

SYNONYMS: Teaberry, Checkerberry (*G. procumbens*). Wintergreen oil is now more frequently obtained from *B. lenta* than *G. procumbens* although it is has a similar composition [R3].

HABITAT: Native to North America and Canada.

DESCRIPTION: Leaves obovate or broadly ellipitical, short-stalked, faintly serrate at the margin, leathery, glossy green above, paler beneath. Taste: astringent and aromatic; odour: characteristic.

PART USED: Leaves.

CONSTITUENTS: (i) Phenolic compounds; gaultherin, salicylic acid, pyrocatechuic, gentisic, vanillic, caffeic and other acids (ii) Volatile oil, 0.5–1%, containing methyl salicylate, about 98%, which is produced by enzymatic hydrolysis of gaultherin during maceration and steam distillation [R2,R3,R14;1].

MEDICINAL USE: Anti-inflammatory, anti-rheumatic, diuretic [R1]. An infusion of the leaves is occasionally taken internally but oil of Wintergreen is used mainly in the form of an ointment or liniment for rheumatism, sprains, sciatica, neuralgia and all kinds of muscular pain.

PREPARATIONS: Methyl Salicylate Liniment BPC; Compound Methyl Salicylate Ointment BPC; Methyl Salicylate Ointment BPC.

REGULATORY STATUS: GSL.

453

SPECIFIC REFERENCES: 1. Freidrich H et al (1974) Planta Med.
26:327 8(1):219.

WITCH HAZEL

HAMAMELIS VIRGINIANA L.
Fam. Hamamelidaceae

HABITAT: Indigenous to North America and Canada.

DESCRIPTION: Leaves broadly oval, up to 15 cm long, 7 cm
broad, the margin dentate or crenate, the apex acute and the base
asymmetrically cordate. When dried the lamina is papery, dark
greenish-brown. Venation pinnate, very conspicuous on the lower
surface. Bark quilled or channelled, usually in pieces up to 10 cm
long and 2 cm broad, 1–2 mm thick, with a silvery grey external
surface with numerous lenticels and a pinkish-brown striated inner
surface. Fracture: fibrous and laminated; taste: very astringent;
odour: slight.

PART USED: Leaves, twigs, bark.

CONSTITUENTS: Leaves: (i) Tannins; 8–10%, composed mainly of
gallotannins with some condensed catechins and proanthocyanins.
These include 'hamamelitannin' which is a mixture of related tannins,
including galloylhamameloses (ii) Flavonoids; quercetin, kaempferol,
astragalin, myricitrin and others (iii) Volatile oil, containing hexenol,
n-hexen-2-al, alpha- and beta-ionones and others [R2,R3,R7,R17;
1,2,3,4]. Bark: (i) Tannins; 1–7%, mainly the alpha-, beta- and
gamma-hamamelitannins, with some condensed tannins such as
d-gallocatechin, *l*-epigallocatechin and *l*-epicatechin (ii) Miscellaneous;
saponins, resin etc. [3,4].

MEDICINAL USE: Astringent, haemostatic. Witch Hazel extract is very
highly regarded for the treatment of haemorrhage, piles and varicose
veins [R1]. The tannins and other polyphenols are anti-inflammatory
in croton oil-induced oedema, and carrageen and adjuvant-induced
rat paw oedema [5,6] and inhibit 5-lipoxygenase enzyme [7]. They
have potent free-radical-scavenging and antioxidant properties [8,9]
and protect against cytotoxicity induced by the superoxide anion
radical [10]. The proanthocyanins, particularly the catechin and
gallocatechin oligomers, exhibit antimutagenic effects against
nitroaromatic compounds [11]. Antiviral activity has been described
against *Herpes simplex* type 1 [6] and a cream containing a special
extract was beneficial in treating *Herpes labialis* [12]. Hamamelitannin
inhibits tumour necrosis factor (TNF)-induced endothelial cell death
in vitro [13]. Several clinical studies have demonstrated efficacy of
topically applied Witch Hazel in inflammatory conditions, including
UV irradiated burning [14,15,16] and atopic dermatitis [17]. A
randomized trial comparing hamamelis water with ice and a
proprietary formula found no difference between the three forms
of treatment in women suffering episiotomy pain following childbirth
[18]. The distilled extract is widely and successfully used as a

treatment for sprains and bruises, spots and blemishes, in eye drops [19], haemorrhoids [20], after shave lotions and in cosmetic preparations; for example as a skin tonic and anti-wrinkle cream.

PREPARATIONS: Leaves: Hamamelis Dry Extract BPC; Hamamelis Liquid Extract BPC; Hamamelis Ointment BPC. Twigs: Distilled Extract of Witch Hazel BP (= Hamamelis water).

REGULATORY STATUS: GSL.

SPECIFIC REFERENCES: 1. Kaul P (2001) *Deutsch Apot. Ztg.* 141(5):115. 2. Vennat B *et al* (1992) *Pharm. Acta Helv.* 67(1):11. 3. Engel R *et al* (1998) *Planta Med.* 64(3):251. 4. Haberland C *et al* (1994) *Planta Med.* 60(5):464. 5. Duwiejua M *et al* (1994) *J. Pharm. Pharmacol.* 46(4):286. 6. Erdelmeier C *et al* (1996) *Planta Med.* 62(3):241. 7. Hartisch C *et al* (1997) *Planta Med.* 63(2):106. 8. Da Silva A *et al* (2000) *Phytother. Res.* 14(8):612. 9. Masaki H *et al* (1995) *Biol. Pharm. Bull.* 18(1):162. 10. Masaki H *et al* (1993) *Free Rad. Res. Comm.* 19(5):333. 11. Dauer A *et al* (1998) *Planta Med.* 64(4):324. 12. Baumgartner M *et al* (1998) *Z. fur Allgemeinmed.* 74(3):158. 13. Habtermariam S (2002) *Toxicon* 40(1):83. 14. Korting H *et al* (1993) *Eur. J. Clin. Pharm.* 44(4):315. 15. Hughes-Formella B *et al* (1998) *Dermatology* 196(3):316. 16. Hughes-Formella B *et al* (2002) *Skin Pharmacol. Appl. Skin Physiol.* 15(2):125. 17. Swoboda M *et al* (1991) *Z. Phytother.* 12(4):114. 18. Moore W *et al* (1989) *J. Obstet. Gynaecol.* 10(1):35. 19. Titcomb L (2000) *Pharm. J.* 264(7082):212. 20. Knoch H *et al* (1992) *Forschr. Med.* 110(8):69.

WOOD BETONY

STACHYS OFFICINALIS (L.) TREV.
Fam. Lamiaceae

SYNONYMS: Bishopswort, *Betonica officinalis* L.

HABITAT: Europe, including Britain, in open woods, hedge banks, grasslands and heaths.

DESCRIPTION: Basal leaves up to 7 cm long, ovate or oblong, obtuse, cordate at base, coarsely crenate. Stems upright and hairy, bearing smaller leaves, 2–3 pairs. Flowers bright reddish-purple, in tight oblong spikes, the tube longer than the calyx. Taste: slightly bitter; odour: faint.

PART USED: Herb.

CONSTITUENTS: (i) Alkaloids; stachydrine and betonicine
(ii) Diterpenes such as the betonicosides A-D and betaconolide
(iii) Miscellaneous; betaine, choline, tannins etc. [R4;1].

MEDICINAL USE: Sedative, bitter, aromatic, astringent [R1]. Used, often in combination with other remedies, for nervous headache, neuralgia and anxiety. Some herbalists use it to advantage in tackling withdrawal from benzodiazepines. Parkinson states. "...it is said also to hinder drunkenness being taken beforehand and quickly to expel it

455

afterwards." This use has not been tested in modern times and cannot be relied upon.

SPECIFIC REFERENCES: 1. Miyase T *et al* (1996) *Chem. Pharm. Bull.* 44(8):1610.

WOODRUFF

GALIUM ODORATUM (L.) SCOP.
Fam. Rubiaceae

SYNONYMS: Asperula odorata L.

HABITAT: Grows in woods in Britain and Europe.

DESCRIPTION: A short perennial, unbranched, with slender, quadrangular, brittle stems and whorls of 6–9 elliptical, pointed leaves edged with tiny, forward-pointing bristles. Flowers small, with four petal lobes, white, in loose clusters. Odour: when dry, of new-mown hay.

PART USED: Herb.

CONSTITUENTS: (i) Iridoids; asperuloside (about 0.05%) and monotropein (ii) Miscellaneous; coumarins, tannins, anthraquinones, flavonoids, nicotinic acid [R2;1,2].

MEDICINAL USE: Diuretic, tonic, antispasmodic, sedative, hepatic [R1]. Asperuloside and monotropein are mildly purgative in animals [3]. Woodruff extract has anti-inflammatory activity in animals [4] and shows hepatoprotective effects in a pentobarbital-induced hypnosis model in mice [5]. It is sometimes used as a fragrance ingredient.

SPECIFIC REFERENCES: 1. Markham K *et al* (1970) *Phytochem.* 9:2359. 2. Wolf G (1998) *Pharm. Zeit.* 143(7):48. 3. Inoue H *et al* (1974) *Planta Med.* 25:285. 4. Mascolo N *et al* (1987) *Phytother. Res.* 1(1):28. 5. Deliorman D *et al* (1999) *Gazi Univ. Eczacilik. Fakultesi Dergisi* 16(2):77.

WOOD SAGE

TEUCRIUM SCORODONIA L.
Fam. Lamiaceae

SYNONYMS: Garlic Sage.

HABITAT: Grows in open woods and on heaths and scrubs throughout western Europe.

DESCRIPTION: A short, downy perennial. Leaves cordate, bluntly toothed, wrinkled, sage-like. Flowers greenish-yellow, two-lipped, with prominent maroon stamens. Taste: bitter; odour: slightly aromatic.

PART USED: Herb.

CONSTITUENTS: (i) Iridoids; harpagide, reptoside and acetyl harpagide (ii) Diterpenes of the clerodane type; teupolin, teuscorolide, teuscorodol, teuscorodal, teuscorodin, teuflin, teuplin-1 (iii) Flavonoids; luteolin, cirsiliol, cirsimarin [R2;1,2,3,4].

MEDICINAL USE: Anti-rheumatic, astringent, carminative,

antimicrobial, diaphoretic, vulnerary [R1]. It is used for feverish colds, rheumatic conditions and flatulent dyspepsia, normally as an infusion. As a poultice it has been applied to boils and abscesses.

PREPARATIONS AND DOSE: Dried herb, dose: 2–4 g as an infusion, or equivalent extract, three times daily.

REGULATORY STATUS: GSL.

SPECIFIC REFERENCES: 1. Marco J *et al* (1982) *Phytochem.* 21:2567 and (1983)22:727. 2. Bruno M *et al* (1985) *Phytochem.* 24(11):2597. 3. Fikenscher L *et al* (1969) *Plantes Med. Phytother.* 3(3):181. 4. Velasco-Negueruela A *et al* (1990) *Phytochem.* 29:1165.

WOOD SORREL
OXALIS ACETOSELLA L.
Fam. Oxalidaceae

HABITAT: Common in woods throughout Europe.

DESCRIPTION: Leaves, bright green, trifoliate, stalked, the leaflets broadly obcordate. Flowers white, bell-shaped, with purplish veins. Taste: acidic; odourless.

PART USED: Herb.

CONSTITUENTS: (i) Flavonoid glycosides; orientin, vitexin and isovitexin (ii) Oxalic acid [R2;1].

MEDICINAL USE: Diuretic, refrigerant [R1]. Has been used for fevers and urinary disorders, in both in the form of an infusion and boiled in milk.

SPECIFIC REFERENCES: 1. Tschesche R *et al* (1976) *Chem. Berlin* 109:2901.

WORMSEED
CHENOPODIUM AMBROSIOIDES L.
C. AMBROSIOIDES L. VAR *ANTHELMINTICUM* (L.) A GRAY
Fam. Chenopodiaceae

SYNONYMS: American Wormseed.

HABITAT: Tropical America; also cultivated in India and China.

DESCRIPTION: Fruit sub-globular, about 2 mm in diameter, greenish or brown. The single seed is glossy, black, lenticular, with an obtuse edge. Taste: acrid, astringent; odour: camphoraceous and terebinthinate (turpentine-like).

PART USED: Seeds.

CONSTITUENTS: (i) Oil, containing ascaridole, an unsaturated terpene peroxide, in highly variable amounts up to 90%, with geraniol, cymene, terpinene, methyl salicylate, and butyric acid (ii) Flavonoids; mainly kaempferitrin (iii) Triterpenes, triacontyl alcohol, alpha-spinasterol [R2;1,2,3].

MEDICINAL USE: Anthelmintic [R1]. The active constituent is

457

ascaridol; it is highly active against roundworms, hookworms and small, but not large, tapeworms. Positive results have recently been shown to some extent in lambs infected with *Trichostrongyle* nematodes; however total eradication was not achieved as the lambs continued to shed eggs in the faeces [4]. The leaf extract is antipyretic and anti-inflammatory in the rat paw oedema test, and no toxic effects were observed [5]. Ascaridole is also anti-inflammatory [1]. Wormseed increases gastrointestinal propulsion in mice [5] but clinically it was usually used in conjunction with a purgative. It must be used with great care if at all, as it is highly toxic and can cause unpleasant side effects such as headache, dizziness, vomiting, convulsions and even death in overdose. The oil is explosive [R2].

PREPARATIONS AND DOSE: Powdered seed, dose: 1–4 g.

REGULATORY STATUS: P.

SPECIFIC REFERENCES: 1. Okuyama E *et al* (1993) *Chem. Pharm. Bull.* 41(7):1309 2901. 2. Gohar A *et al* (1997) *Phytother. Res.* 11(8):564. 3. Mata R *et al* (1987) *Phytochem.* 26(1):191. 4. Kato S *et al* (2000) *J. Herbs Spices Med. Plants* 7(2):11. 5. Olajide O *et al* (1997) *Fitoterapia* 68(6):529.

WORMSEED, LEVANT
ARTEMISIA CINA BERG.
Fam. Asteraceae

SYNONYMS: Santonica.

HABITAT: Native to eastern Europe and Russia, cultivated elsewhere.

DESCRIPTION: Dried, unexpanded flower-heads containing three to five minute, tubular flowers without pappus. The flower-heads are about 3 mm long and 1.5 mm in diameter, greenish-yellow when fresh, brown when kept for some time; each has numerous oblong-obtuse scales closely overlapping each other. Taste: bitter; odour: aromatic, characteristic.

PART USED: Unexpanded flower-heads.

CONSTITUENTS: (i) Volatile oil, containing 1,8-cineole as the major component, up to about 80%, with alpha-terpineol and carvacrol (ii) Sesquiterpene lactones; about 2–6% L-alpha-santonin and alpha-hydroxysantonin (= artemisin) [R2,R3;1].

MEDICINAL USE: Vermifuge [R1]. Santonin is particularly active against roundworms, and to some extent against threadworms, but is ineffective against tapeworm. Wormseed has been taken combined with honey or treacle or as a decoction or infusion; however high doses are toxic.

REGULATORY STATUS: Pharmacy only.

SPECIFIC REFERENCES: 1. Wagner H *et al* (1984) *In: Plant Drug Analysis* Springer-Verlag Germany.

WORMWOOD
ARTEMISIA ABSINTHIUM L.
Fam. Asteraceae

SYNONYMS: Absinthium.

HABITAT: Native to Europe, North Africa and western
Asia, cultivated in North America and elsewhere.

DESCRIPTION: A shrubby perennial reaching about 1 m;
leaves pinnately divided, up to 12 cm long, the lobes obovate
or lanceolate, entire or toothed. Both surfaces are covered with
fine, whitish, silky hairs. The flowers are small, nearly globular,
with no pappus, greenish-yellow, arranged in an erect leafy
panicle. Taste: very bitter; odour: characteristic, aromatic.

PART USED: Herb.

CONSTITUENTS: (i) Volatile oil, of variable composition,
usually containing alpha- and beta-thujone as the major
components, with thujyl alcohol, azulenes including
chamazulene, 3,6- and 5,6-dihydrochamazulene; bisabolene,
cadinene, camphene, sabinene, *trans*-sabinylacetate, pinene, phellandrene and others (ii) Sesquiterpene lactones; artabsin, absinthin,
anabsinthin, artemetin, arabsin, artabin, artabsinolides A, B, C and
D, matricin, isoabsinthin, artemolin and others (iii) Acetylenes, in the
root; *trans*-dehydromatricaria ester, C13 and C14-trans-spiroketalenol
ethers and others (iv) Flavonoids; quercetin 3-glucoside and
3-rhamnoglucoside, spinacetin 3-glucoside and 3-rhamnoglucoside
and others (v) Phenolic acids; *p*-hydroxyphenylacetic, chlorogenic,
p-coumaric, protocatechuic, syringic, vanillic and other acids (vi)
Lignans; diayangambin and epiyangambin [R2,R3,R9;1,2,3,4,5,6].

WORMWOOD

MEDICINAL USE: Choleretic, anthelmintic, stomachic, anti-
inflammatory [R1]. Wormwood has been used for hundreds of years
for many types of disorders; for colds, rheumatism, as a cardiac
stimulant, carminative, antispasmodic, emmenagogue, pain reliever
during childbirth, tonic and antiseptic. The azulenes are anti-inflammatory (see Chamomile), and the water soluble extract of Wormwood
was shown to be antipyretic in rabbits [6]. Choleretic effects have been
demonstrated in man [7]. The extract has anticholinesterase activity *in
vitro* [8] and is hepatoprotective against paracetamol-induced toxicity
in rats [9]. Thujone, however, is highly toxic; it has hallucinogenic and
addictive properties, which have led to the suggestion that it interacts
with a common receptor in the central nervous system to that of
tetrahydrocannabinol, the active constituent in Indian Hemp (q.v.)
[10]. Wormwood was the basis for the alcoholic drink 'absinthe',
which was popular in the 19th century but subsequently banned
because of its dangerous properties. In large doses it causes insomnia,
nightmares, vomiting and convulsions, and was reputed to cause
insanity: for example the artist Van Gough is thought to have cut off
his ear whilst under the influence of absinthe. It is, however, possible
to make a thujone-free extract of the herb [11]. The anthelmintic

459

properties are probably due to the sesquiterpene lactones present (see Wormseed, Levant). Wormwood is widely used as a flavouring agent in liqueurs. For review see [12].

PREPARATIONS AND DOSE: Dried herb, dose: 1–2 g, or equivalent extract, three times daily.

REGULATORY STATUS: GSL.

BIBLICAL REFERENCES: Deuteronomy 29:18; Proverbs 5:4; Jeremiah 9:15 and 23:15; Lamentations 3:15, 19; Amos 5:7; Revelation 8:11. May refer to similar species.

SPECIFIC REFERENCES: 1. Vostrowski O *et al* (1981) *Z. Naturforsch. C.* 36(5–6):369. 2. Beauhaire J *et al* (1982) *J. Chem. Soc. Perk. Trans.* 861. 3. Beauhaire J *et al* (1981) *Tet. Lett.* 22(24):2269. 4. Greger H (1978) *Phytochem.* 17:208. 5. Swiatek L *et al* (1998) *Pharm. Pharmacol. Lett.* 8(4):158. 6. Khattak S *et al* (1985) *J. Ethnopharmacol.* 14(1):45. 7. Baumann I *et al* (1975) *Z. Allgemein Med.* 51(17):784. 8. Wake G *et al* (2000) *J. Ethnopharmacol.* 69(2):105. 9. Gilani A *et al* (1995) *Gen. Pharmacol.* 26(2):309. 10. Del Castillo J *et al* (1975) *Nature* 253:365. 11. Stahl E *et al* (1983) *Z. Lebens. Unters. Forsch.* 176(1):1. 12. Artemisia. Wright C (Ed.) (2001) *Medicinal and Aromatic Plants – Industrial Profiles.* Pub: Taylor and Francis, London, UK.

WORMWOOD, SWEET
ARTEMISIA ANNUA L.
Fam. Asteraceae

SYNONYMS: Qinghaou, Annual Wormwood, Annual Wormweed.

HABITAT: Native to temperate parts of Asia, particularly China; introduced elsewhere.

DESCRIPTION: A prostrate or erect annual with woody stems; leaves pinnately divided, the lobes filiform or lanceolate, with an entire or toothed margin. The flowers are small, yellowish, arranged in panicles. Taste: very bitter; odour: characteristic, sweet, aromatic.

PART USED: Herb.

CONSTITUENTS: (i) Sesquiterpenes including artemisinin, arteannuins A-O, artemisitine, artemisinic acid, hydroarteannuin, and others (ii) Volatile oil, containing artemisia ketone, cadinene, camphene, camphor, beta-caryophyllene, cuminal, beta-farnesene, 1,8-cineole and others (iii) Flavonoids; artemetin, bonazin, eupalitin and chrysosplenetin (v) Coumarins such as scopoletin, (iv) Sterols including oleanolic acid, stigmasterol, beta-sitosterol [1,2,3,4,5,6,7].

MEDICINAL USE: Sweet Wormwood has been used for thousands of years in China for fevers, chills, and disorders of the liver and gall-bladder. More recently the herb was found to be highly effective for the treatment of malaria, especially resistant strains of *Plasmodium berghei* and *P. falciparum,* and this is now the major use of the plant. The active principle is artemisinin (also known as qinghaosu) which is one of the most rapidly acting anti-plasmodial compounds known. Several more stable and effective derivatives, such as artemether, arteether and artesunate have now been developed and are being used clinically for both the prophylaxis and treatment of malaria [4,8,9 and refs therein]. The herb is being introduced into other parts of the world, particularly Central Africa, with some success [10]. Arteannuin B is anti-fungal [3]. Other properties of Sweet Wormwood include anti-ulcer effects, attributed to the sesquiterpene content [11], and immunomodulatory properties, shown by inhibition of the classical pathway of complement and T-cell proliferation. These were not due to artemisinin [12]. The herb appears to be fairly non-toxic although some of the terpenes and flavonoids are cytotoxic *in vitro* [13] and teratogenic effects have been observed in mice [1]. For review, see [14].

SPECIFIC REFERENCES: 1. Bharel S *et al* (1996) *Fitoterapia* 67(5):387. 2. Gulati A *et al* (1996) *Fitoterapia* 67(5):403. 3. Hai Q-T *et al* (2000) *Planta Med.* 66(4):391. 4. Woerdenbag H *et al* (1993) *Flav. Frag. J.* 8(3):131. 5. Yang S *et al* (1990) *J. Pharm. Pharmacol.* 42(Suppl.1):96P. 6. Wei Z *et al* (1992) *Planta Med.* 58(3):300. 7. Sy L-K *et al* (2001) *Phytochem* 58(8):1159. 8. Balint G (2001) *Pharmacol. Ther.* 90(2–3):261. 9. Van Agtmael *et al* (1999) *Trends Pharm. Sci.* 20(2):199. 10. Mueller M *et al* (2000) *J. Ethnopharmacol.* 73(3):487. 11. Dias P *et al* (2001) *Phytother. Res.* 15(8):670. 12. Kroes B *et al* (1995) *Phytother. Res.* 9(8):551. 13. Zeng G-Q (1994) *Planta Med.* 60:54. 14. Artemisia. Wright C (ed) (2001) *Medicinal and Aromatic Plants – Industrial Profiles.* Pub: Taylor and Francis, London, UK.

WOUNDWORT

STACHYS PALUSTRIS L.
Fam. Lamiaceae

SYNONYMS: All Heal, Marsh Woundwort. Hedge Woundwort is *S. sylvatica* L.

HABITAT: Grows in damp places throughout Europe, including Britain.

DESCRIPTION: Leaves narrowly lanceolate, nearly sessile, hairy. Flowers purple. *S. sylvatica* has ovate and cordate leaves, long stalked, hairy; and reddish-purple flowers. Both taste astringent; odour unpleasant.

PART USED: Herb.

CONSTITUENTS: *S. palustris*: (i) Iridoids, harpagide and acetyl harpagide (ii) Flavonoids; based on isoscutellarein and oroxylin-A. *S. sylvatica:* (i) Alkaloids; betonicine, stachydrine and trigonelline (ii) Allantoin (iii) Betaine and choline [R2;1,2].

MEDICINAL USE: Antiseptic, antispasmodic, vulnerary [R1]. Both are used for gout, cramp, vertigo, and haemorrhage, and as a poultice applied to wounds. Betonicine (= achilleine) is haemostatic [3].

SPECIFIC REFERENCES: 1. Kooiman P (1972) *Acta Bot. Nederland* 21:417. 2. Barbera F (1986) *Fitoterapia* 57:67. 3. Miller F *et al* (1954) *J. Am. Chem. Soc.* 76:1353.

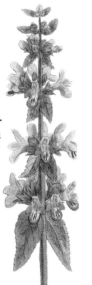

WOUNDWORT

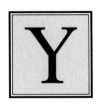

YARROW
ACHILLEA MILLEFOLIUM L.
Fam. Asteraceae

SYNONYMS: Milfoil, Nosebleed.

HABITAT: Native to Eurasia and naturalized in North America, also found in most temperate zones of the world.

DESCRIPTION: A widely varied aggregate species. Stem angular, tough. Leaves opposite, dark green, bipinnatifid, about 6–10 cm long, clasping the stem at the base, the segments very narrow, downy, and feathery in appearance. Flowers in terminal, flattened, corymbose cymes, ray florets usually white or pinkish, disc florets cream. Taste: insipid; odour: faintly aromatic.

PART USED: Herb.

CONSTITUENTS: (i) Volatile oil, of highly variable composition, containing azulenes, including chamazulene (achillea azulene) and guaiazulene, alpha- and beta-pinene, borneol, bornyl acetate, camphor, caryophyllene, eugenol, farnesene, myrcene, sabinene, isoartemisia ketone, terpineol, thujone, alpha-bisabolol, nerolidol, spathulenol and others (ii) Sesquiterpenes and sesquiterpene lactones (also found in the oil); achillin, achillicin, hydroxyachillin, balchanolide, leucodin, millifin, millifolide, longipinene and achillifolin and their derivatives, achimillic acids A, B and C, alpha- and beta-peroxyachifolide, epi-artabsin derivatives and many others (iii) Flavonoids; apigenin, luteolin, quercetin and their glycosides, artemetin, casticin, rutin, orientin, isovitexin and others (iv) Alkaloids and bases; betonicine (= achilleine), stachydrine, achiceine, moschatine, trigonelline and others (v) Miscellaneous; polyynes, cyclitols, salicylic acid etc [R2,R7;1, and refs therein, 2,3,4,5,6,7].

MEDICINAL USE: Antipyretic, anti-inflammatory, haemostatic, spasmolytic, diuretic, diaphoretic, hypotensive [R1]. Yarrow is used for very many complaints, throughout the world, with justification; and particularly for rheumatism, colds, catarrh, fevers, amenorrhoea and hypertension. The sesquiterpenes are anti-oedematous [4] and anti-inflammatory. They inhibit mouse ear oedema produced by croton oil, and although the mechanism of action was not established it did not involve interference with the transcription factor NF-KappaB [8]. Achimillic acids A, B and C have anti-tumour activity against mouse P-388 leukaemia cells *in vivo* [6]. Extracts of the herb possess anti-spermatogenic effects in mice [9] and may be hepatoprotective [10]. Apigenin is anti-inflammatory, anti-platelet and spasmolytic [11]; the azulenes (where present) are also anti-inflammatory, as is salicylic acid. Eugenol has local anaesthetic activity (see Clove). The alkaloid betonicine (achilleine) has been shown to be haemostatic [12]. It has also been used as an eye lotion, and for diarrhoea, dyspepsia, ulcers and rashes. Yarrow is generally regarded as

462

non-toxic although the peroxyachifolides are known to be allergenic [3].

PREPARATIONS AND DOSES: Dried herb, dose: 2–4 g as an infusion, or equivalent extract, three times daily.

REGULATORY STATUS: GSL.

SPECIFIC REFERENCES: 1. Chandler R *et al* (1982) *Econ. Bot.* 36:203. 2. Orth M (1999) *Z. Phytother.* 20(6):345. 3. Rucker G *et al* (1991) *Arch. Pharm.* 324(12):979. 4. Kastner U *et al* (1993) *Planta Med.* 59(Suppl.7):A669. 5. Valant-Vetschera K (1984) *Sci. Pharm.* 52(4):307. 6. Tozyo T *et al* (1994) *Chem. Pharm. Bull.* 42(5):1096. 7. Kastner U *et al* (1996) *Pharmazie* 51(7):503. 8. Lyss G *et al* (2000) *Pharm. Pharmacol. Lett.* 10(1):13. 9. Montanari T *et al* (1998) *Contraception* 58(5):309. 10. Gadgoli C *et al* (1995) *Fitoterapia* 66(4):319. 11. Middleton E *et al* (1984) *Biochem. Pharmacol.* 33:3333. 12. Miller F *et al* (1954) *J. Am. Chem. Soc.* 76:1353.

YELLOW DOCK
RUMEX CRISPUS L.
Fam. Polygonaceae

SYNONYMS: Curled Dock.

HABITAT: A common European weed.

DESCRIPTION: Leaves large, typically dock-like, lanceolate, with strongly wavy margins. The root is found in commerce cut and split; with a thick grey-brown cork, yellowish cortex and pale wood, showing concentric rings and a radiate structure.
Taste: mucilaginous, bitter; odourless.

PART USED: Root.

CONSTITUENTS: (i) Anthraquinone glycosides, based on chrysophanol, physcion, nepodin and emodin (ii) Miscellaneous; volatile oil, tannins, rumicin, proanthocyanidins and oxalates [R7;1,2,3,4] [183].

MEDICINAL USE: Laxative, cholagogue, alterative, tonic [R1]. It is used for chronic skin disease, jaundice and constipation. Fatalities have been recorded after ingestion of the leaves [5], and large doses should be avoided due to the oxalate content.

PREPARATIONS AND DOSES: Dried root, dose: 2–4 g as a decoction, or equivalent extract, three times daily.

SPECIFIC REFERENCES: 1. Fairbairn J *et al* (1972) *Phytochem.* 11:263. 2. Midiwo J *et al* (1985) *Phytochem.* 24:1390. 3. Demirez L (1994) *Pharmazie* 49(5):378. 4. Dabi-Lengyel E *et al* (1991) *Herba Hung.* 30(1–2):91. 5. Reig R *et al* (1990) *Vet. Hum. Toxicol.* 32(5):468.

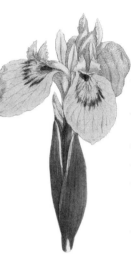

YELLOW FLAG

IRIS PSEUDOACORUS L.
Fam. Iridaceae

SYNONYMS: Yellow Iris, *I. lutea*, Fleur-de-Lys.

HABITAT: Native to Europe and Africa and a worldwide garden plant.

DESCRIPTION: The flowers and leaves are well-known. Rhizome brownish externally, cylindrical, compressed, with transverse leaf scars above and root scars beneath. Taste: very acrid; odourless.

PART USED: Rhizome.

CONSTITUENTS: Not well investigated. A glycoside, irisin, iridin or irisine, is reportedly present, with myristic acid [R4].

MEDICINAL USE: Astringent [R1]. Used formerly in dysmenorrhoea, and for leucorrhoea in the form of a lotion.

YELLOW FLAG

YERBA SANTA

ERIODICTYON CALIFORNICUM (HOOK. ET ARN.) TORR.
Fam. Hydrophyllaceae

SYNONYMS: Eriodictyon, Mountain Balm, Bearsweed,
E. glutinosum Benth.

HABITAT: California, Oregon and parts of Mexico.

DESCRIPTION: A low, evergreen shrub, with woody rhizomes from which arise lanceolate leaves, up to 15 cm long and about 2 cm broad, irregularly dentate at the margins. The upper surface is green and appears to be varnished with resin, the lower surface is reticulated and white with hairs. Taste: balsamic; odour: pleasant and aromatic.

PART USED: Leaves.

CONSTITUENTS: (i) Flavonoids; homoeriodictyol (= eriodictyone), eriodictyol, chrysoeriodictyol, xanthoeriodictyol, 3,-methyl-4, -isobutyleriodictyol, pinocembrin, sakuranetin, naringenin 4,-methyl ether, cirsimaritin, hispidulin, chrysin and others (ii) Resin, containing triacontane, cerotic acid, eriodonol, and pentatriacontane, [R19;1].

MEDICINAL USE: Aromatic, tonic, expectorant; it is used mainly for bronchitis and asthma [R1]. Eriodictyol is vasodilatory in isolated rat thoracic aorta [2] and many of the flavonoids have chemopreventant activity by inhibiting the metabolism of the carcinogen benzo(a)pyrene in hamster embryo cells in tissue culture [1].

SPECIFIC REFERENCES: 1. Liu Y-L *et al* (1992) *J. Nat. Prod.* 55(3):357.
2. Ramon Sanchez de Rojas V *et al* (1999) *Planta Med.* 65(3):234.

YEW
TAXUS BACCATA L.
Fam. Taxaceae

HABITAT: Grown as an ornamental in Britain, America and other parts of the world.

DESCRIPTION: A large evergreen tree, with male and female flowers on separate plants. The leaves are 1–2 cm long, lanceolate, dark green; the flowers small and green, followed by pink, waxy, cup-like berries. All parts of the plant, excepting the pulp of the fruit, are poisonous.

PART USED: Bark, leaves (= needles).

CONSTITUENTS: (i) Diterpene (taxine) alkaloids, or 'taxoids', including taxol (= paclitaxel), derivatives such as 10-deacetylpaclitaxel, taxicine I and II, baccatin III and 10-deacetylbaccatin III, 2-deacetoxy-taxinine J, 13-decinnamoyltaxchinin B, 2-deacetoxyaustospicatine and others (ii) Miscellaneous; lignans such as isotaxiresinol, rhododendrol, hibalactone, berevifoliol; phenolics, and others [1,2,3,4,5].

MEDICINAL USE: Yew is mainly used as a source of taxanes, including paclitaxel, and its derivatives such as docetaxel, which are anti-mitotics with a unique mode of action now being clinically used for ovarian and breast cancer [R14,6 and refs therein]. Other properties of the plant include antimicrobial activity [7,8]; however the plant is still highly toxic, due principally to the content of alkaloids, and should not be used as an extract [9].

SPECIFIC REFERENCES: 1. Jenniskens L *et al* (1996) *J. Nat. Prod.* 59(2):117. 2. Das B *et al* (1998) *Nat. Prod. Sci.* 4(2):78, 4(4):185. 3. Das B *et al* (1999) *Nat. Prod. Lett.* 13(1):71. 4. Breeden S *et al* (1996) *Planta Med.* 62(1):94. 5. Mroczek T *et al* (2000) *Biomed. Chrom.* 14(8):516. 6. Fumoleau P *et al* (2995) *Breast Cancer Res. Treatment* 33(1):39. 7. Erdemoglu N *et al* (2001) *Fitoterapia* 72(1):59. 8. Srinivasa Reddy P *et al* (2001) *Pharm. Biol.* 39(3):236. 9. Shankar K *et al* (2002) *J. Ethnopharmacol.* 79(1):69.

YOHIMBE BARK
PAUSINYSTALIA YOHIMBE (K. SCHUM) PIERRE
Fam. Rubiaceae

HABITAT: Cameroon.

DESCRIPTION: The bark occurs in flat or slightly quilled pieces up to 75 cm long and 2 cm thick; the outer surface is grey-brown, cracked and fissured, often covered with lichen; the inner surface is reddish-brown and striated. Taste: bitter; odourless.

PART USED: Bark.

CONSTITUENTS: Indole alkaloids; the major one is yohimbine, minor ones include alpha- and beta-yohimbane, pseudoyohimbine and coryantheine [1].

465

MEDICINAL USE: Aphrodisiac [R1]. Yohimbine is an alpha-adrenergic blocker and has a long-standing reputation as a sexual stimulant [2,3]. It should be used only under the advice of a medical herbalist or physician, although the use is rarely justifiable since better and less toxic drugs are now available to treat erectile dysfunction. The dose of yohimbine is very important since too high a dose leads to general depression.

REGULATORY STATUS: POM.

SPECIFIC REFERENCES: 1.Wagner H *et al* (1984) *In: Plant Drug Analysis* Pub: Springer-Verlag, Stuttgart, Germany. 2. Riley A (1994) *Br. J. Clin. Practice* 48(3):133. 3. Meletis C (2000) *Alt. Comp. Ther.* 6(4):207.

YUCCA
YUCCA SCHIDIGERA ROEZL EX ORTIGES
Y. BREVIFOLIA ENGELM.
Y. FILAMENTOSA L.
Y. GLAUCA NUTT EX J FRASER
Y. SCHOTTI.
AND OTHERS
Fam. Agavaceae

SYNONYMS: Mohave Yucca, *Y. mohavensis* Sarg. (= *Y. schidigera*); Joshua Tree, *Y. arborescens* Trel., (= *Y. brevifolia*); Bear Grass (= *Y. filamentosa* L.)

HABITAT: South-western North America.

DESCRIPTION: Yuccas are medium-sized trees, with simple or branched trunks, and lanceolate leaves. The Mohave yucca is smaller, reaching about 4.5 m, with leaves up to 1.5 m long; whereas the Joshua tree reaches 20 m and has leaves up to 35 cm, usually in dense clusters at the end of the branches. Bear Grass is, as the name suggests, smaller and grass-like.

PART USED: Leaves.

CONSTITUENTS: (i) Saponins based on the aglycones sarsapogenin, yuccagenin, tigogenin, markergenin, kammogenin, higogenin, hecogenin, gloriogenin, smilagenin and others [R3,R7,R19;1,2,3]. *Y. filamentosa* L. leaves contain spirostane derivatives [4] (ii) Stilbene derivatives including resveratrol, and the yuccaols A, B and C [5].

MEDICINAL USE: Anti-inflammatory, anti-arthritic and anti-diabetic. The leaf extract of *Y. schotti* is anti-inflammatory against carrageenan-induced oedema in the rat [2] and a saponin extract showed beneficial effects in a small clinical study [R7]. It also reduced blood pressure and high cholesterol blood levels in another study of arthritic and hypertensive patients [6]. The saponin fraction is cytotoxic to B16 melanoma cells *in vitro* [R7]. An aqueous extract of *Y. schidigera* increased gastrointestinal transit time in mice, but did not induce diarrhoea, and an effect on gastrointestinal propulsion was suggested, rather than cathartic activity [7]. It also reduced serum urea levels in treated rats [8]. An extract of this species also inhibited the growth of some micro-organisms, mainly *Clostridium* and *Fusarium* species [9], and that of *Y. filamentosa* had leishmanicidal activity [4]. Anti-giardial effects were noted in gerbils and lambs, in that cyst shedding was reduced, but infection persisted and it was suggested that further concentration of the extracts was needed [10]. Yucca species are used as a source of steroidal sapogenins for the production of steroid hormones, for use in the contraceptive pill and for hormone replacement therapy. Young plants (with a lower concentration of saponins) were an item of food for Native Americans.

SPECIFIC REFERENCES: 1. Dewidar A *et al* (1970) *Planta Med.* 19:87. 2. Backer R *et al* (1972) *J. Pharm. Sci.* 61:1665. 3. Oleszek W *et al* (2001) *J. Agric. Food Chem.* 49(9):4392. 4. Plock A *et al* (2001) *Phytochem.* 57(3):489. 5. Oleszek W *et al* (2001) *J. Agric. Food Chem.* 49(2):747. 6. Bingham R *et al* (1978) *J. Appl. Nutr.* 30:127. 7. Yamazaki T *et al* (1999) *Pharm. Pharmacol. Comm.* 5(6):415. 8. Duffy C *et al* (2001) *J. Agric. Food Chem.* 49(7):3408. 9. Katsunuma Y *et al* (2000) *Animal Sci. J.* 71(2):164. 10. McAllister T *et al* (2001) *Vet. Parasitol.* 97(2):85.

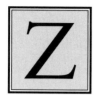

ZEDOARY
CURCUMA ZEDOARIA (CHRISTMANN) ROSCOE.
Fam. Zingiberaceae

HABITAT: Indigenous to India, cultivated elsewhere in the Far East.

DESCRIPTION: The rhizome usually occurs in transverse slices, about 2–4 cm in diameter and 0.5–1 cm thick; outer surface greyish, with a few circular striae and small, spiny points of root bases. The transverse section is greyish-white, hard and horny. Taste: bitter; odour: camphoraceous, and recalling that of cardamoms and ginger.

PART USED: Rhizome.

CONSTITUENTS: (i) Sesquiterpenes, known as curcuminoids; curcumenone, curcumanolide A and B, desmethoxycurcumin, bisdemethoxycurcumin, procurcuminol, epi-procurcuminol and others (ii) Volatile oil, containing zingiberene, 1,8-cineole, camphor, camphene, borneol, curcumol, curcuminol, cedarone, (+)germacrone-4,5-epoxide, isofuranogermacrene and others [R2;1,2,3].

MEDICINAL USE: Aromatic, stimulant [R1]. Used in a similar manner to Ginger (q.v.). The rhizome is used to treat certain types of tumour in China and has shown cytotoxicity in some systems [4]. Anti-inflammatory activity has been demonstrated and attributed to the sesquiterpenes and curcuminoids, which inhibit release of tumour necrosis factor (TNF)-alpha from macrophages [3]. The extract shows hepatoprotective properties [5]. Mitogenic effects were demonstrated *in vitro*, although the substances responsible were denatured by proteases, and may therefore either not normally be bioavailable, or only present in certain extracts [6].

SPECIFIC REFERENCES: 1. Shiobara Y *et al* (1985) *Phytochem.* 24(11):2629. 2. Hikino H *et al* (1970) *Chem. Pharm. Bull.* 18:752. 3. Mi K-J *et al* (2001) *Planta Med.* 67(6):550. 4. Matthes H *et al* (1980) *Phytochem.* 19:2643. 5. Rana A *et al* (1992) *Fitoterapia* 63(1):60. 6. Tachibana Y *et al* (1992) *Planta Med.* 58(3):250.

Glossary of Medical Terms

T his glossary has been only slightly changed from the original. It is included to explain some of the terms used in herbal medicine as these are often of a more vague or general nature than those used in conventional medicine and are in accordance with the more holistic methods of treatment used. They are not intended as a recommendation to particular remedies where used in the text but are an indication of the current and historical usage of the plant, whether or not validated.

Abortifacient Causing abortion

Adaptogen Aiding adaptation of the body, particularly to stress

Alterative A vague term indicating a substance hastening renewal of the tissues to improve function

Amenorrhoea Absence of menstruation

Analgesic Pain-relieving

Androgenic Having qualities similar to the male hormone testosterone

Anodyne Pain-easing

Anthelmintic Causing death or removal of worms in the body

Anti-bilious Against biliousness or excess bile

Antihypertensive Reducing blood pressure

Anti-lithic Against stones, e.g. kidney or bladder

Antioxidant Preventing the production of harmful oxygen radicals

Antiperiodic Preventing the return of recurrent fevers, e.g. malaria

Anti-platelet Inhibiting the aggregation of blood platelets, to reduce thrombosis

Antiscorbutic Preventing scurvy, i.e. a source of vitamin C

Antiphlogistic Relieving pain and inflammation

Anti-scrophulous Preventing or curing scrophula, an old-fashioned term for diseases causing swelling of the lymph glands, especially in the neck, also known as king's evil

Antiseptic Preventing putrefaction or infection

Antispasmodic Preventing spasm

Antitussive Preventing cough

Aperient Promoting a mild or natural movement of the bowels

Aphrodisiac Exciting the sexual organs

Aromatic Having an aroma

Astringent Causing contraction of the tissues, binding

Atherosclerosis Deposition of fatty tissue, cholesterol etc. on the lining of blood vessels

Ayurveda The ancient medical system of India

Bitter Applied to bitter-tasting substances used to stimulate the appetite

469

Cardiac Having an effect on the heart

Carminative Easing griping pains and expelling flatulence

Cathartic Producing evacuation of the bowels

Cholagogue Producing a flow of bile

Choleretic Stimulating bile production

Cognition Memory and the processing of information

Corrective Restoring to a healthy state

Cytochrome P450 A family of liver enzymes responsible for metabolizing many drugs

Demulcent Applied to drugs that soothe and protect the alimentary canal

Deobstruent Clearing away obstructions by opening the natural passages of the body

Depurative A purifying agent

Dermatic Applied to drugs with an action upon the skin

Detergent Cleansing

Diaphoretic Promoting perspiration

Diuretic Increasing the flow of urine

Digestive Aiding digestion

Dysmenorrhoea Painful menstruation

Emetic Causing vomiting

Emmenagogue Promoting menstrual flow

Emollient Softening and soothing, usually the skin

Erythema Reddening and inflammation of skin

Expectorant Aiding expectoration, loosening phlegm

Febrifuge Reducing fever

Flatulence Having gases in the intestine, distension; windiness

Free-Radical Scavenger A substance which complexes with and removes harmful free radicals

Galactagogue Milk-inducing

Haematoma Bleeding under the skin, bruising

Haemolysis Breakdown or opening of red blood cells

Haemostatic Controlling or stopping bleeding

Hallucinogen Producing visions or hallucinations

Hepatic Affecting the liver

Hepatoprotective Protecting the liver from toxins

Hypnotic Producing sleep

Hyperglycaemia Elevated blood sugar

Hypercholesterolaemia Elevated blood levels of cholesterol

Hyperlipidaemia Elevated blood levels of fats

Hyperplasia Thickening of layers on cells (usually the skin)

Hypertension High blood pressure

Hypocholesterolaemia Low blood levels of cholesterol

Hypolipidaemia Low blood levels of fats

Hypoglycaemia Low blood sugar

Hypotension Low blood pressure

Ischaemia The absence or reduction of blood flow

Immunomodulator Having an effect on the immune system (usually enhancement)

Insecticide A substance that kills insects

Irritant Causing irritation

Counter Irritant, against irritation, often by having a warming or rubifacient effect (q.v.)

Laxative Bowel stimulant

Lipolysis Breakdown of fat

Lymphocyte White blood cells of several types involved with the immune system

Mastalgia Painful or swollen breasts

Menorrhagia Heavy menstrual bleeding from the uterus

Metrorrhagia Bleeding from the uterus

Mydriatic Causing dilation of the pupil of the eye

Myotic Causing contraction of the pupil of the eye

Narcotic Applied to drugs producing stupor or insensibility

Nematocide A substance that kills nematode worms

Nervine Restoring the nerves, mildly tranquillizing

Nutritive Nourishing

Oestrogenic Having qualities similar to the female hormone oestrogen

Orexigenic Stimulating the appetite

Oxytocic Stimulating contractions of the womb

Parasiticide A substance that kills parasites

Parturient Applied to substances used to facilitate childbirth

Pectoral Having an effect upon the lungs

Phagocytosis Ingestion and removal of pathological organisms or tissue by white blood cells

Protozoicidal A substance that kills protozoa, e.g. amoebae

Purgative A substance that evacuates the bowels, more drastic than an aperient or laxative

Rasayana A general tonic and rejuvenator in Ayurveda (q.v.)

Refrigerant Relieving thirst and giving a feeling of coolness

Rubefacient Causing reddening of the skin, applied to substances producing inflammation or sometimes used as a rub for muscular pain

Sedative Causing sedation, reducing nervous excitement

Spasmolytic Relieving spasm, usually of smooth muscle (e.g. digestive system)

Spermatogenesis Production of spermatozoa

Sternutatory Producing sneezing by irritation of the mucous membranes

Stimulant Energy producing

Stomachic Applied to drugs that ease stomach pain

Styptic A substance that stops bleeding by clotting the blood, applied externally

Sudorific Producing copious perspiration

Taenicide A substance that expels tapeworms

Teratogen A substance causing damage to the foetus

Thrombosis Blood-clotting, whilst in the body

Tonic A substance that gives a feeling of well-being to the body

Uterotonic Having a tonic effect on the uterus; causing rhythmic contractions

Vermifuge A substance that expels worms from the body

Vesicant Causing blistering

Vulnerary Used in healing wounds

Forms of Medicinal Preparations

Infusions

Infusions are often known as herbal teas, and are aqueous preparations made by pouring boiling water over finely chopped botanical drugs. The usual quantities used for infusion are 500 ml (or 1 pint) of water to 30 g (or 1oz) of drug. The infusion is then allowed to stand for up to 30 minutes with occasional stirring, and the clear liquid then decanted or strained. Being extemporaneous preparations, infusions should be taken in divided doses throughout the day of preparation. The amount of infusion to be taken would be proportionate to the amount of the drug dosage required. They are used when the drug to be extracted has a light structure, as with leafy herbs.

Decoctions

These are made by pouring cold water on to the finely divided botanical drug and then allowing the mixture to simmer. This method is used for hard materials such as roots and barks. Decoctions are generally made in strengths of 30 g (or 1 oz) to 500 ml (or 1 pint) but, as the water boils away, it is often preferable to use excess and allow it to simmer down to the required volume. When cool the decoction is strained and taken in divided doses proportionate to the required dosage of the drug. As with infusions, decoctions are usually not preserved and should be prepared fresh daily.

Liquid Extracts

Liquid extracts provide a more permanent and convenient form of preserving the constituents of vegetable drugs in a concentrated form. They are prepared by percolation, or maceration of the comminuted drug, with water or a mixture of water and alcohol. When extraction is complete it is evaporated under vacuum to a suitable volume. This produces a liquid extract where a unit of volume represents a unit weight of drug; for example a 1:1 extract means that the medicinal value of 1 g of drug is contained in 1 ml extract.

SOLID EXTRACTS

i. Soft Extracts

These are prepared by evaporating down either the freshly expressed juices of the herb, or the liquors produced as explained above. If alcohol and water mixtures are used as solvents the alcohol is distilled off and recovered before evaporating the residual extract to the required consistency, rather like treacle.

ii. Dry Extracts

These are prepared by removing the remaining water in the solid (soft) extract by drying under vacuum. Solid extracts and dry extracts represent a much larger quantity of the drug from which they are prepared than do liquid extracts, tinctures or infusions.

Tinctures

These are liquid preparations using differing strengths of alcohol as their solvent. Tinctures, like liquid extracts, are more permanent

473

preparations. They are particularly suitable for extracting drugs containing resinous and volatile principles. Tinctures are prepared at room temperature, and the solvent acts selectively. For example alcohol precipitates unwanted gums and proteins so that the tinctures may be filtered to yield a clear, more elegant preparation, which is better preserved from deterioration. Tinctures are usually made in strengths of 1 in 5, where 5 ml tincture represents the medicinal value of 1 g drug, or 1 in 10, where 10 ml represents 1 g.

Pills

Pills were formerly widely used, but have been superseded by tablets, as a convenient and tasteless method of taking unpleasant substances. They are small spherical bodies usually containing concentrated herbal extracts, often combined with powdered crude herbs, and an excipient to form a firm plastic mass, soluble in the stomach. Pills may be sugar-coated or even silver-coated.

Tablets

These are made by compressing vegetable drug extracts and herbal powders using suitable excipients for binding the ingredients, compressing them and aiding disintegration after administration.

Capsules

These may be hard or soft gelatin single dose units in a convenient size for swallowing. They are used for taking nauseous substances, such as Cod Liver Oil, Garlic Oil, Saw Palmetto oily extract, and other drugs difficult to administer in their naturally occurring form.

Suppositories

These are small cones, or torpedo-shaped solid dosage forms, usually made of a cocoa butter, a synthetic or glycero-gelatin base, carrying the medicament, which is to be introduced into the rectum. The base is easily soluble at body temperature. They provide a valuable treatment for haemorrhoids and other disorders of the rectum but can also carry medicines for systemic absorption.

Pessaries

These are similar to suppositories but are used to introduce medicaments into the vagina, and usually for local rather than systemic application.

Glossary of Botanical Terms

Achene A one-seeded fruit, or part of a compound fruit, dry, not opening when ripe, distinguished from a seed by the remains of a stigma or style

Acrid Leaving a burning sensation in the mouth

Acuminate Tapering to a fine point

Acute Pointed

Alliaceous Garlic or onion-like

Alternate Arranged in two rows, not opposite, often including a spiral arrangement

Amplexicaul Clasping the stem

Anastomosing Joining up to form loops

Annular, Annulated Ring-like, ringed

Anther Part of the stamen containing the pollen grains

Apetalous Without petals. When only one layer of floral leaves is present, even if coloured, this is considered to be the calyx

Apiculate With a small, broad point at the apex

Apocarpous Having the carpels free from one another

Appressed Pressed close to but not united with another organ, e.g. hairs against the stem

Arillus A fleshy growth from the point of attachment of a seed, e.g. mace around a nutmeg

Ascending Sloping or curving upwards

Awn A stiff, bristle-like projection, e.g. terminating the flower scales in grasses

Axillary Arising from the axil or angle of a leaf or bract

Balsamic Balsam-like, e.g. odour, sweet, like benzoin

Barbed Furnished with sharp points, curved backwards

Berry A fleshy fruit, usually containing many seeds, without a stony layer surrounding them

Biennial Completing the life-cycle within two years, without flowering in the first year

Bifid Deeply split into two divisions

Bipinnatifid Twice divided, in a pinnate or feather-like way, in a leaf about halfway to the stalk or midrib

Bract A leaf-like structure under a flower

Bracteole The bracts under the flower, when there are other bracts present under the inflorescence

Bristles Stiff or rigid hairs

Bulb An underground organ composed of fleshy modified leaves, often with thin or membranous outer scales, containing the next year's plant

Bulbil A small bulb rising in an axil in the aerial parts

Calyx The sepals or outer layer of floral leaves

Campanulate Bell-shaped

Capsule A dry fruit, opening when ripe, composed of more than one carpel

Carpel A unit of the ovary which may be separate and distinct, or joined or fused

Catkin A spike of male or female flowers, usually from a tree and without petals or calyx

Cauline Of leaves, borne on the aerial part of the stem, not subtending a flower or inflorescence

Chlorophyll The green pigment of plants

Clavate Club-shaped

Compound Of an inflorescence, with the axis branched; of flower-heads, made up of many small florets; of leaves, composed of several distinct leaflets

Conchoidal Shell-like, e.g. of a fracture, concave with curved lines

Cordate Heart-shaped

Coriaceous Leathery in texture

Corm A short, swollen, underground stem, often with membranous scales, from which the next year's plant arises, e.g. crocus

Corolla The petals, or inner row of floral leaves, either distinct or united, e.g. into a tube

Cortex The outer, separable portion of the stem or fruit

Corymb A raceme of flowers where the pedicels are of different lengths, so that all the flowers are at the same level at the top, the outer flowers opening first. Adj. corymbose

Cotyledons The first leaves of a plant, present in the seed, containing nourishment for the seedling and usually different from subsequent leaves

Crenate With rounded teeth

Crenulate Diminutive form of crenate

Cruciform Cross-shaped, e.g. wallflower

Cuneate Wedge-shaped

Cuneiform Wedge-shaped with the thin end at the base

Cuticle The waxy layer outside the epidermis, e.g. in leaves

Cyme An inflorescence where the growing points terminate in a flower, hence the central flower opens first and the oldest branches or flowers are normally at the apex. Adj. cymose

Deciduous Dropping off, losing the leaves in autumn

Decumbent Lying on the ground, usually rising at the end

Decurrent Having the base prolonged down the axis, e.g. in leaves where the base continues down the petiole to form a winged stem

Decussate Of leaves, opposite but with pairs oriented at right angles to each other

Dehiscence Opening to shed seeds or spores

Dentate Sharply toothed

Denticulate Diminutive of dentate

Digitate Finger-like, having five or more narrow segments, e.g. like the leaves of the lupin

Dioecious Having the sexes on different plants

Disc, disk The fleshy part of the receptacle, e.g. in the compositae

Divaricate Diverging at a wide angle

Drupe A more or less fleshy fruit, with one or more seeds, each surrounded with a stony layer, e.g. sloe

Elliptic Shaped like an ellipse

Emarginate Notched or indentated at the apex

Embryo The young plant in the seed

Endocarp The inner layer of the fruit, corresponding to the inner layer of the carpel, e.g. in the plum, the endocarp is the stone, the mesocarp forms the flesh and the epicarp the skin

Endosperm The nutritive tissue in the seed

Entire Not toothed nor cut at the margin

Epicalyx A calyx-like structure outside the true calyx

Epicarp See Endocarp

Epidermis The outer skin, e.g. of the leaf

Epigeal Above ground, e.g. germination where the cotyledons are raised above ground

Epigynous Where the stamens etc. are inserted on a level with or above the top of the ovary, e.g. into the pistil

Epipetalous Inserted upon the corolla

Exfoliating Splitting off in layers, e.g. some barks

Falcate Scythe-shaped

Filament The stalk of the anther

Filiform Thread-like

Fimbriate Fringed

Florets The small individual flowers in the flower-heads of the compositae; the central ones being the tubular or disc florets, the outer, long ones being the ray or ligulate florets

Fracture The way in which an organ breaks, e.g. tough, layered, fibrous, short (= brittle or not fibrous) and its appearance

Fusiform Spindle-shaped

Gamopetalous Having the petals joined into a tube or at the base

Gamosepalous Having the sepals joined

Gibbous Having a rounded, solid projection

Glabrous Without hairs

Gland A small, globular or oblong vesicle containing oil, resin etc.

Glandular Furnished with glands

Glaucous Bluish

Gynoecium The female part of the plant, made up of the ovary or ovaries, stigma and style

Hastate Shaped like a halberd or arrow-tip

Heartwood The central portion of a tree-trunk, sometimes filled with resin or colouring matter

Hermaphrodite Having both stamens and ovary

Hilum The scar on a seed where it has been attached by a stalk to the ovary; also applied to the more or less central spot or marking on a starch grain

Hirsute Clothed with long, not stiff, hairs

Hispid Clothed with coarse, stiff hairs

Hybrid A plant originating by fertilization of one species or subspecies by another

Hypogeal Below ground, e.g. in germination where the cotyledons remain below ground

Hypogynous Calyx or corolla situated below the ovary

Imbricate Having the edges overlapping, like roof tiles

Imparipinnate A pinnate leaf having an odd leaf at the apex

Indehiscent Not opening to release seeds or spores

Inferior When the ovary is inserted into or fused with the receptacle

Inflorescence Flowering branch, above the last stem leaves, including bracts and flowers

Internodes The interval between branches or leaves on a root or stem

Involucre A ring of bracts forming a calyx-like structure around or below an inflorescence or flower-head, e.g. in the compositae

Involute With the margins rolled upwards

Keeled Having a projecting line resembling the keel of a boat

Lamina Layer, the flat part or blade of a leaf etc.

Lanceolate Oval and pointed at both ends

Latex Milky juice, e.g. of poppies

Leaflet Each individual part of a compound leaf

Legume A fruit consisting of one carpel, opening on one side, e.g. pea

Lenticel Breathing pores in the bark

Lenticular Lens-shaped, e.g. lentil

Lichen Cryptogamic plants, usually greyish or yellowish, growing on rocks and tree-trunks.

Ligulate Strap-shaped

Linear Of leaves, narrow and short with parallel margins

Lobed Of leaves, divided, but not into separate leaflets

Loculus Cavity, often applied to fruits containing seeds

Membranous Thin, dry and flexible, not green

Medullary Ray Slender lines of parenchyma tissue connecting the pith with the bark, seen as radiating lines in the wood

Mericarp A one-seeded portion split off from a syncarpous ovary at maturity, e.g. caraway, fennel

Micropyle The pore of a seed through which the embryo emerges

Monoecious Having unisexual flowers, but both sexes on the same plant

Mucronate Having a short, narrow point

Mycelium The thread-like mass of fungi from which the fruiting body emerges; in mushrooms it is cottony and known as mushroom spawn; in ergot it is compacted into a hard mass and known as a sclerotium

Node The point on a stem from which leaves arise

Nodule A small, more or less globular, swelling

Nut A fruit composed of three fused carpels, containing one seed

Ob- *prefix:* Inverted, e.g. an ovate leaf is broader above the middle, an obovate leaf below the middle

Obtuse Blunt

Ochrea A sheath, formed from fused stipules, e.g. polygonaceae

Opposite Applied to leaves where two arise from opposite sides of the same stem node

Ovary The part of the gynoecium containing the ovules and young seeds, composed of one or more carpels

Ovate Egg-shaped

Ovoid Nearly egg-shaped

Paleae Delicate, membranous bracts; in the compositae forming the bracts of the disc florets and in grass flowers enclosing the pistils and stamens

Palmate Consisting of more than three leaflets arising from the same point

Panicle A branched, racemose inflorescence

Papillae Small, raised points or elongated projections

Pappus The calyx in a composite flower developed in the form of simple or feathery hairs, membranous scales, teeth or bristles. May or may not be present

Pedicel The stalk of a single flower

Peduncle The stalk of an inflorescence

Peltate Of a leaf, when the stalk is inserted on the under surface, not at the edge

Perennial Living for more than two years, normally flowering every year

Perianth The floral leaves as a whole, including petals and sepals

Perianth segment The separate leaves of the perianth, especially when petals and sepal cannot be distinguished

Perigynous Arising from a ring between the ovary and the floral parts

Petals The corolla or inner, usually coloured, layer of floral leaves

Petiole The stalk of a leaf

Pilose Hairy, with long, soft hairs

Pinnate A leaf composed of more than three leaflets arranged in two rows along a common stalk

Pinnatifid Pinnately cut, but not completely, the lobes still being joined at the lamina

Pinnatisect As pinnatifid but cut more deeply, some leaflets may be free

Placenta The part of the ovary to which the ovules are attached

Pollen The male gamete, produced by the anthers

Polypetalous Having many petals

Polysepalous Having many sepals

Procumbent Lying loosely along the ground, rising at the ends

Prostrate Lying flat on the ground

Pubescent Shortly and softly hairy

Punctate Dotted or shallowly pitted, usually with glands

Pungent Biting or piercing

Pyriform Pear-shaped

Quill Applied to a bark which is inrolled into a tube, e.g. cinnamon

Raceme An inflorescence, usually conical in outline, in which the pedicels are of approximately equal length, and the lowest flowers open first. Adj. racemose

Rachis or rhachis The central rib or axis of a pinnate leaf

Radical Of leaves, arising from the base of the stem or rhizome

Receptacle The upper part of the stem from which the floral parts arise

Recurved Bent backwards in a curve

Reniform Kidney-shaped

Reticulate Marked with a network, usually of lines or veins

Revolute Rolled back at the edges

Rhizome An underground stem lasting more than one growing season

Rhomboid More or less diamond-shaped

Rosette Of leaves, closely and spirally arranged

Rotate Of a corolla, wheel-like

Rugose Wrinkled

Ruminate Usually of seeds, looking as though chewed, infolded

Scarious Thin, rather stiff and dry, not green

Schizocarp A dry fruit which splits into separate one-seeded parts when mature, e.g. caraway, dill

Scyphi The wineglass-shaped reproductive organ bearing fruit in some lichens

Sepals The leaves of the calyx

Serrate Having oblique teeth like a saw

Sessile Without a stalk

Sinuate Having a wavy outline

Spathulate or **spatulate** Paddle-shaped

Spike An inflorescence in which sessile flowers are arranged in a raceme

Spine The hardened, projecting vein of a leaf, e.g. holly or thistle

Spore A small, asexual reproductive body

Spur A tubular projection at the base of the corolla, e.g. toadflax

Stamen The male reproductive organ, consisting of the two anthers containing pollen, and the filament

Staminode An infertile, often reduced stamen, e.g. scrophulariaceae

Stellate Star-shaped

Stigma The sticky apex of the style to which the pollen grains adhere

Stipule A small, leaf-like structure usually at the base of the petiole

Stipulet or Stipel A stipule-like structure at the base of a leaflet in a compound leaf

Stolon A creeping stem of short duration produced from a central rosette or erect stem, usually above ground

Stoma, Stomata Pore(s) in the leaf through which exchange of gases takes place.

Striations More or less parallel line markings

Style The thread connecting the stigma and ovary

Sucker Underground shoots which arise some distance away from the plant

Superior Of ovary, with the perianth inserted below the base

Syncarpous Of ovary, having the carpels united to one another

Tendril A climbing organ derived from the stem, leaf or petiole, e.g. pea

Terebinthinate Turpentine-like

Terminal At the end of a shoot or branch

Ternate Divided into three distinct segments

Thallus A flat, branching, undifferentiated plant body, e.g. seaweed

Tomentose Covered with dense, short, cottony hairs

Tortuous Twisted and undulating

Trued Split into three

Trifoliate Having three distinct leaflets, e.g. clover

Truncate Appearing as if cut off at the end

Tuber A swollen part of an underground stem, of one year's duration, bearing leaf buds and capable of new growth, e.g. potato

Tubercle A more or less spherical or ovoid swelling

Umbel An inflorescence where the petioles all arise from the top of the stem, umbrella-like

Unisexual Flowers having either stamens or pistils, but not both

Vascular Consisting of the conductive tissue, vessels or tubes

Villous Shaggy

Viscid Sticky

Vitta The oil gland of an umbelliferous fruit, seen as a dark line between the ridges

Whorl A circle of leaves around a node

Index

483

485

491

"THE ESSENCE OF POTTER'S"

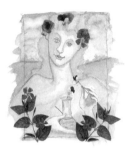

'Spring'
(Product Code: PS 01)

Potter's products are well recognised for their natural content, but over the years 'science' has played its part in ensuring purity, quality and efficacy for every Potter's product manufactured.

Potter's wanted an image that could be used to bring science and nature together and also look good in their promotional material.

Potter's decided to commission a competition with students at Liverpool Art College, asking them for their personal visual interpretations. The brief was 'to provide images, in whatever medium, to illustrate Potter's traditional herbalist roots alongside the science in development of herbal medicines'.

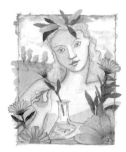

'Summer'
(Product Code PS 02)

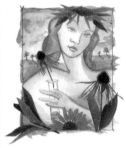

'Autumn'
(Product Code: PA 01)

Kate Weymouth, a third year student at the Art College, captured exactly what Potter's were looking for in her four separate illustrations - Spring, Summer, Autumn and Winter. Each was carefully researched by Kate and illustrated in water colours as a collage. The effort that had had gone into the project impressed Potter's as much as the beautiful illustrations themselves.

Potter's are so delighted with the illustrations that they have decided to make them available as limited editions, either as a set of four or as individual prints.

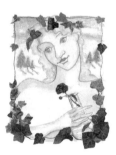

'Winter'
(Product Code: PW 01)

If you would like further details about these prints please contact George Woodward at Potter's, 01942 405100.

EST. 1812

Herbal Medicine consumers are seeing more of Potter's products through various advertising, marketing and PR campaigns, all aimed at increasing product awareness.

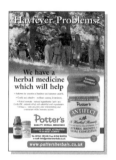
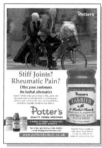
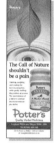
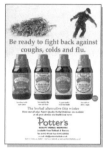

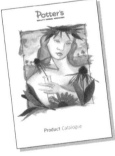
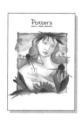
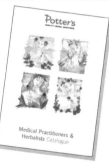

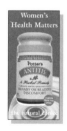
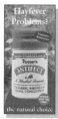
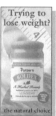
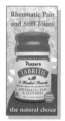
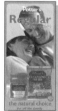
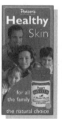
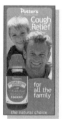

To get to know more about our herbal medicines, visit either of these websites.

www.pottersdirect.com
www.pottersherbals.co.uk

EST. 1812

505